PHARMACOLOGY AND APPLICATIONS OF CHINESE MATERIA MEDICA

VOL. II

PHARMACOLOGY AND APPLICATIONS OF CHINESE MATERIA MEDICA

VOL. II

Edited by

Hson-Mou CHANG (Ph.D.)
Paul Pui-Hay BUT (Ph.D.)

Translated by

Sih-Cheng YAO (M.D.)
Lai-Ling WANG (B.A.)
Shem Chang-Shing YEUNG (M.Sc.)

Chinese Medicinal Material Research Centre
The Chinese University of Hong Kong

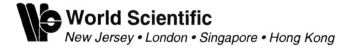
World Scientific
New Jersey • London • Singapore • Hong Kong

Published by

World Scientific Publishing Co. Pte. Ltd.
P O Box 128, Farrer Road, Singapore 912805
USA office: Suite 1B, 1060 Main Street, River Edge, NJ 07661
UK office: 57 Shelton Street, Covent Garden, London WC2H 9HE

British Library Cataloguing-in-Publication Data
A catalogue record for this book is available from the British Library.

First published 1987
Reprinted 1996, 1998, 2001

PHARMACOLOGY AND APPLICATIONS OF CHINESE MATERIA MEDICA (Vol. II)

ISBN 981-02-3694-8 (pbk)

Printed in Singapore by Mainland Press

PHARMACOLOGY AND APPLICATIONS OF CHINESE MATERIA MEDICA

(Chinese Edition)

Editor-in-Chief   WANG Yusheng

Assistant Editors   BI Chunsheng   Deng Wenlong

Consulting Editor   ZHANG Yi

Editorial Committee

LIAO Nengge	DAI Guangjun	YE Songbai	YUAN Wei
CHEN Quansheng	GONG Xuling	BAO Dingyuan	YIN Caiyuan

Consultants (arranged by the number of character-strokes)

BIAN Rulian	WANG Jianhua	WANG Xiankai	WANG Zhenwang
LIU Tianpei	JIANG Mingxing	XU Zhiqi	WU Baojie
ZHANG Jiaquan	ZHANG Qiguang	ZHANG Tanmu	SU Chengye
LI Zhangwen	ZHOU Chaofan	YUE Songjian	JIN Guozhang
XU Shuyun	SUN Jiajun	SUN Ruiyuan	TU Guorui
XIA Chengke	JIANG Junming	PENG Xiang'e	ZHAO Yi

WAMG Liwen	WANG Junmo
CHEN Xianyu	CHEN Xiu
LI Wenhan	LI Tingqian
RAO Manren	LING Yikui
HUANG Wenxing	HUANG Qingzhang
ZHAO Gengsheng	PAN Qichao

People's Medical Publishing House, Beijing (*First published in 1983)

CONTENTS

KUXINGREN 苦杏仁

<Kuxingren>, also known as <Xingren>, is the seed obtained from *Prunus armeniaca* L. var. *ansu* Maxim., *P. sibirica* L., *P. mandshurica* (Maxim.) Koehne, or *P. armeniaca* L. (Rosaceae). It tastes bitter, has a "warm" property and is slightly toxic. It has antitussive, antiasthmatic, and laxative actions and is indicated for the treatment of cough and asthma of various origins, and constipation.

CHEMICAL COMPOSITION

<Kuxingren> contains about 3% of amygdalin and several free amino acids. It also contains emulsin, amygdalase, and prunase. Decomposition of amygdalin by amygdalase and prunase yields hydrocyanic acid and benzaldehyde. Comparison of the various methods of processing the seeds revealed that the hydrocyanic acid content was better retained and the enzymes better destroyed by rapid introduction of 100°C steam, maintained for 10 minutes and followed by drying at a low temperature. For this reason, <Kuxingren>should be added later when preparing decoctions (1).

PHARMACOLOGY

1. Antitussive and Antiasthmatic Effects

It is believed that when a small amount of <Kuxingren> is ingested, amygdalin disintegrates in the body, gradually producing traces of hydrocyanic acid; this slightly depresses the respiratory center, thus producing antitussive and antiasthmatic effects (2).

2. Effect on the digestive System

Either *in vitro* or in the body of healthy individuals or ulcer patients, benzaldehyde has been proved to inhibit the digestive function of pepsin (3).

3. Antineoplastic Effect

In vitro studies showed that the crude infusion of <Kuxingren> inhibited human carcinoma of the cervix JTC-26 strain by 50–70% (4). A weak antineoplastic action was exhibited *in vitro* by hydrocyanic acid, benzaldehyde, and amygdalin. The antineoplastic effect could be enhanced by the combined use of hydrocyanic acid and benzaldehyde, or by amygdalin and β-glucosidase. Treatment of rats with amygdalin etc. starting on the fifth day after transplantation of Walker carcinoma 256 produced the following results: the average survival period of the amygdalin group was 33 days, and that of amygdalin plus β-glucosidase group 41 days, whereas that of the control group was 23 days (5). Long-term aspiration of hydrocyanic acid vapour in young rats arrested body weight increase, delayed the growth of transplanted Jensen sarcoma and caused tumor degeneration; however, the effective dose was very close to the lethal dose (6). The growth of transplanted Ehrlich ascites carcinoma in mice fed freely with the herb was inhibited, and the survival period of the animals was prolonged (7).

The antineoplastic effect is made even greater by the preponderance of glycolysis in cancer cells which produces the final product lactic acid — an acidic environment enhances the activity of β-glucosidase in hydrolysing amygdalin into hydrocyanic acid and benzaldehyde. Moreover, as cancer cells contain less rhodanase than normal cells, they are therefore less capable of detoxifying hydrocyanic acid. Hence <Kuxingren> has a definite selective action on neoplastic cells (8).

4. Toxicity

Poisoning is easily produced by oral ingestion of large amounts of <Kuxingren>. The first symptom is stimulation of the vomiting, respiratory, vagus, and vasomotor centers of the medulla, followed by coma, convulsion, and paralysis of the whole CNS, and lastly, death from paralysis of the respiratory center (6). Poisoning is attributed to hydrocyanic acid contained in the herb, which readily interacts with the trivalent iron of cytochrome oxidase in the mitochondria to form a cytochrome oxidase-cyanide complex that inhibits cellular respiration resulting in tissue asphyxia and death (9).

The LD_{50} of amygdalin in mice by intravenous injection was 25 g/kg. Its LD_{50} in rats by intravenous injection was 25 g/kg and by intraperitoneal injection was 8 g/kg. Its LD_{80} in rats by mouth was 0.6 g/kg. The MTD in mice, rabbits, and dogs by intravenous or intramuscular injection was 3 g/kg, and by mouth 0.075 g/kg; the MTD in man by intravenous injection was 5 g (about 0.07 g/kg). Oral ingestion of 55 pieces of this herb containing about 1.8 g (about 0.024 g/kg) of amygdalin is lethal to man. The toxicity of the orally administered amygdalin is about 40 times greater than that of the intravenous injection, because it readily decomposes in the gastrointestinal tract to release hydrocyanic acid (5).

CLINICAL STUDIES

1. Respiratory Diseases

<Kuxingren> is often used with the stem of *Ephedra* plant in the treatment of respiratory diseases; for example, the Ephedra-Prunus-Gypsum-Glycyrrhiza Decoction (modified to suit individual cases). Refer to the monograph on <Mahuang>.

2. Cancer

<Kuxingren> is useful in the treatment of Hodgkin's disease, bronchial carcinoma, spindle cell sarcoma, seminoma, chronic myelocytic leukemia, carcinoma of the pleura, malignant lymphoma, multiple rectal carcinoma, and carcinoma of the breast complicated with bone metastasis. Amygdalin can be given by mouth at doses of 0.5–1.0 g on the first day followed by 0.1 g daily for 10 days, and for detoxication, sodium thiosulfate may be given intravenously (5), thus achieving the desired therapeutic effect and also preventing the occurrence of toxic reactions.

3. Aplastic Anemia

The addition of the oral doses of <Kuxingren> by mouth in the therapeutic regimen of two cases of chloramphenicol-induced aplastic anemia markedly enhanced the therapeutic effect (10). It is deduced that hydrocyanic acid contributes to tissue anoxia, thereby stimulating the kidney to produce erythropoietin which promotes hematopoiesis (11).

ADVERSE EFFECTS AND EMERGENCY TREATMENT OF INTOXICATION

The inadvertent oral ingestion of <Kuxingren> in large quantities leads to poisoning due to the formation of hydrocyanic acid in the body. The toxic manifestations include vertigo, headache, shortness of breath, vomiting, palpitation, cyanosis, coma, and convulsion (12–16). Without appropriate emergency treatment the intoxicated patient may die. The chief antidotes are nitrites and sodium thiosulfate. The nitrites should be given first to change the hemoglobin into methemoglobin which will compete with cytochrome oxidase for the cyanide radical to form cyanomethemoglobin, thus reactivating cytochrome oxidase. Then sodium thiosulfate is given. Under the influence of rhodanase, the drug reacts with cyanide to form the relatively nontoxic thiocyanate which is rapidly excreted in the urine.

REFERENCE

1. Lu BS. Shanghai Zhongyiyao Zazhi (Shanghai Journal of Traditional Chinese Medicine) 1980 (6):38.
2. Zhu Y. Pharmacology and Applications of Chinese Medicinal Materials. People's Medical Publishing House. 1958. p. 139.
3. Kleeberg J. Archives Internationales de Pharmacodynamie et de Therapie 1959 120:152.
4. Sato A. Kampo Kenkyu 1979 (2):51.
5. Reitnauer PG. Arzeimettel Forschung 1972 22(8):1347.
6. Sollmann T. A Manual of Pharmacology. 8th edition. 1957. p. 982.

7. Editorial Group, Institute of Medical Information of the Chinese Academy of Medical Sciences (abstract translator). Medical References 1975 (6):270.

8. Liu YG. Zhejiang Zhongyiyao (Zhejiang Journal of Traditional Chinese Medicine) 1978 (1):5.

9. Goodman LS et al. The Pharmacological Basis of Therapeutics. 5th edition. 1975. p. 904.

10. Li JH et al. Acta Academiae Medicinae Changwei 1980 (3):38.

11. Shanghai First Medical College et al. Medical Biochemistry. People's Medical Publishing House. 1979. p. 168.

12. Luo QX et al. Chinese Journal of Paediatrics 1956 7(6):451.

13. Ma PR et al. Chinese Journal of Paediatrics 1956 7(6):455.

14. Yu ZJ. Chinese Journal of Paediatrics 1956 7(6):456.

15. Jiang ZZ. Chinese Journal of Paediatrics 1956 7(6):457.

16. Wu YZ. Chinese Journal of Paediatrics 1956 7(6):457.

(Gong Xuling)

KULIANPI 苦楝皮

<Kulianpi> refers to the bark and root bark of *Melia azedarach* L. or *M. toosendan* Sieb. et Zucc. (Meliaceae). It is bitter, "cold" and slightly toxic. As an anthelmintic, it is indicated in ascariasis and oxyuriasis. It is also a remedy for erysipelas, rubella, scabies, and tinea favosa.

CHEMICAL COMPOSITION

<Kulianpi> mainly contains toosendanin $C_{30}H_{38}O_{11}$ and a soluble component $C_{30}H_{40}O_{12}$. It also contains margoside, kaempferol, resin, tannin, n-triacontane, β-sitosterol, and the triterpene kulinone.

PHARMACOLOGY

1. Anthelmintic Effect

The active antiascaris constituent is toosendanin which is more potent than the ethanol extract of <Kulianpi> (1). Compared with santonin, toosendanin had a slower onset but a more lasting effect (2). *Mode of action*: Toosendanin at low concentrations (1:5000–9000) exerted a marked excitatory action on the whole swine ascaris as well as on the worm segments (head and middle part). This was manifested in the increased spontaneous movement, abnormally strong intermittent contractions, loss of rhythmic movement (i.e., strong movements alternated with weak ones) of the worms; these effects lasted 10–24 hours, and ultimately, spastic contraction developed. At these concentrations, its neuromuscular excitatory effect on the ascaris could not be blocked by atropine (1.25×10^{-4} and 3.07×10^{-5}), indicating that toosendanin is not a cholinergic agent, and that it acted directly on the muscle of the worm (3). At higher concentrations (over 1:1000), toosendanin exerted a paralyzing effect on the swine ascaris, especially on the worm head (4–5). This effect might be due to the intermittent spastic contraction resulting from the drug's prolonged influence on the worm.

Experiments on whole worms with ligated mouth and anus, and sealed genital pores showed that toosendanin penetrated the skin and acted on the muscle of the worm. The drug did not influence cholinesterase activity in worm homogenates as proved by Ammon's method nor respiratory enzymolysis in the worm muscle homogenates as proved with Warburg's apparatus. These results suggest that toosendanin does not act on glycolysis. From the studies on 32P uptake by the worm, and the incorporation of 32P into ATP of the worm muscle and inorganic phosphate, toosendanin was shown to accelerate the catabolism of ATP in the worm body resulting in the shortage of energy, spastic contraction, fatigue, detachment of the worm from the intestinal wall, and finally, to its expulsion. This explains the rather slow excretion of worms (24–48 hours) and the retained motility of the excreted worms observed clinically (3). The ethanol extract of the herb had a paralyzing effect on swine ascaris, particularly on the head of the worm (6). The extract of this herb at high concentrations (25–50%) also exhibited a paralyzing effect on mouse pinworms (7).

2. Miscellaneous Actions

Intravenous or intramuscular injection of toosendanin 8 mg/kg, or injection of 0.4 mg/kg directly into the respiratory center in the medulla of rats caused respiratory failure, indicating depression of the respiratory center. Respiratory stimulation elicited by nikethamide was slightly antagonized by toosendanin. The drug did not exhibit a significant influence on the spontaneous cortical electrical activity of conscious rabbits (8). Experiments with rat diaphragms showed that at the concentration of $1.7-2.5 \times 10^{-4}$ toosendanin is a specific presynaptic neuromuscular blocker (9). Electron microscopy of the phrenic neuromuscular junctions of mice poisoned by toosendanin revealed marked changes in the subcellular structures, mainly widening of synaptic cleft of the nerve endings and marked reduction of synaptic vesicles (10). Enhanced muscle tone and contractility of *in situ* or isolated rabbit intestines were observed after intragastric administration of 200 mg/kg or upon contact with toosendanin at 2.0×10^{-5}. At a higher concentration (2.0×10^{-4}), toosendanin caused spastic contraction. Therefore, purgatives are not needed with this drug clinically. The stimulant action of toosendanin could be antagonized by diphenhydramine but could not be blocked by atropine (11).

3. Toxicity

The LD_{50} of toosendanin was determined to be 2194 mg/kg PO in mice, whereas that of santonin was 671.9 mg/kg PO; the toxicity of toosendanin was 3.26 times lower than that of santonin (2). The toxicity varies widely with the purity and content of the product. The LD_{50} reported in Sichuan, Yunnan, and Guangxi provinces ranged from 277 to 1146 mg/kg. The LD_{50} in rats by intragastric administration was 120.67±38.5 mg/kg and the MLD in cats 3–4 mg/kg, suggesting that the toxicity of toosendanin widely varies with animal species. The following animals showed sensitivity to toosendanin in decending order: pig, cat, monkey, dog, rabbit, rat, and mouse (12). Intragastric administration of 20–40 mg/kg of toosendanin to rats produced gastric mucosal edema, inflammation and ulcer. Hence, this agent should be used with caution in ulcer patients. Vomiting was observed in some dogs after intragastric administration of 8–10 mg/kg. Intragastric administration of 5 doses of toosendanin to dogs at 10 mg/kg and to rabbits at 40 mg/kg per dose on alternate days, or a single intragastric dose to monkeys at 20 mg/kg resulted in swelling degeneration of hepatocytes, extreme narrowing of the hepatic sinusoides, and increases in GPT and GOT. Swelling degeneration of hepatocytes was reversible. When 5 doses of 8 mg/kg were given intragastrically to dogs, or a single intragastric dose of 15 mg/kg was administered, no elevation of transaminase was observed.

High dosages given intragastrically could cause acute poisoning; the chief cause of death was increase in vascular permeability which led to internal bleeding, hypotension, and acute circulatory failure (12).

The action of toosendanin is slow but prolonged; the drug is completely excreted in a period of more than a week and it has a cumulative effect. It is, therefore, not recommended for continuous administration. In short, toosendanin is less toxic than santonin; it has a lower therapeutic dosage and is safer to use. The epiderm of the bark is more toxic and should be discarded.

CLINICAL STUDIES

1. Worm Expulsion

The decoction of fresh <Kulianpi> 90–120 g was given to 116 children with ascariasis, of whom 98% expelled worms. In 1348 adult patients with ascariasis, M. azedarach Cortex Syrup (2.5 g fresh herb/ml) at 35–40 ml by mouth achieved an expulsion rate of 100%. Toosendanin Tablet (25 mg each) can be given to adults at 8–10 tablets/dose without using purgatives. The dose should be reduced for patients under 16. A mean of 79.4% of 3793 cases with relatively complete case history expelled worms; the percentage in children was higher than in adults; it was 84.8% in 2326 children under 16 against 74.8% in 687 adults. Of 2765 cases with the stool examined, 75.6% was negative for the ova. Worm expulsion began 1–6 hours after medication, peaked in 24–48 hours, and usually continued for 3–4 days, or for a maximum of 8 days. The therapeutic effect of toosendanin resembled that of santonin, but was better than bephenium hydroxynaphthoate (13–15). <Kulianpi> is also effective in treating oxyuriasis, taeniasis, and trichuriasis.

2. Scabies

The powdered <Kulianpi> mixed with vinegar is used locally for scabies in folk medicine.

ADVERSE EFFECTS

The therapeutic dose of toosendanin is usually devoid of severe side effects. Occasionally, it may cause dizziness, abdominal pain, vomiting, diarrhea, flushing, and drowsiness, and in individual patients, blurred vision and pruritus. Most symptoms disappear within 2–3 hours, though in a few patients they may last for longer than one day, and disappear spontaneously without special treatment. Toosendanin has fewer side effects than piperazine citrate and santonin (11). However, severe reactions may appear when the dose is over 0.8 mg in adults; the chief manifestations are peripheral neuritis, arrhythmia, hypotension, and dyspnea. Thus, it is to be used with caution, or avoided in patients with severe heart disease, gastric ulcer, anemia and in those with weak constitutions. It is contraindicated in patients with lever diseases.

REFERENCE

1. Liu GD. Acta Physiologica Sinica 1958 22(1):18.

2. Zhang MY et al. Journal of Traditional Chinese Medicine 1959 (4):42.

3. Wu TJ et al. Collections of Research Information. 4th edition. Sichuan Institute of Chinese Materia Medica. 1966. p. 59.

4. Shi LD et al. Yunnan Medical Journal 1963 5(2):32.

5. Guangxi Institute of Medical and Pharmaceutical Sciences. Collected Information on Mersosin. Guangxi Institute of Medical and Pharmaceutical Sciences. 1970. pp. 27, 37.

6. Hu CJ. The National Medical Journal of China 1948 34(10):437.

7. Feng YS et al. Acta Scientiarum Naturalium Universitatis Shandong 1956 2(3):102.

8. Tian WH et al. Acta Physiologica Sinica 1980 32(4):338.

9. Shi YL et al. Acta Physiologica Sinica 1980 32(3):293.

10. Huang SK et al. Acta Physiologica Sinica 1980 32(4):385.

11. Zhang MY et al. Collections of Research Information. 4th edition. Sichuan Institute of Chinese Materia Medica. 1966. p. 67.

12. Mersosin Research Group, Scientific Research Committee of Guangxi Medical College. Health Journal of Guangxi 1979 (5):46.

13. Sichuan Institute of Chinese Materia Medica. Production Techniques of Toosendanin. 1971. p. 15.

14. Wang YB. Journal of Traditional Chinese Medicine 1959 (4):46.

15. Sichuan Institute of Chinese Materia Medica. Journal of Traditional Chinese Medicine 1959 (4):43.

(Zang Qizhong)

HUZHANG 虎杖

<Huzhang> comes from the root and rhizome of *Polygonom cuspidatum* Sieb. et Zucc. (Polygonaceae). It is also called <Yinyanglian>, <Dayeshezongguan>, and <Huabanzhu>. The leaves may also be used as medicine.

<Huzhang> is bitter and slightly "cold". It is credited with latent-heat-clearing, antipyretic, detoxicant, anti-inflammatory, antirheumatic, diuretic, expectorant, antitussive, stasis-eliminating and channel-deobstruent actions. It is mainly used in the treatment of jaundice, rheumatic pain, strangury with turbid urine and leukorrhea, dysmenorrhea, retained lochia, abdominal mass, bleeding hemorrhoids, and anal fissure, wounds and injuries, scalds and burns, swelling and pains of unknown etiology, and snake bites.

CHEMICAL COMPOSITION

The root and rhizome of *P. cuspidatum* contain anthraquinones emodin, chrysophanol, rheic acid, emodin monomethyl ether (physcion), polygonin, and physcion-8-β-D-glucoside. The root contains 0.1–0.5% of hydroxyanthraquinone. The root and rhizome also contain stilbene derivatives polydatin (piceid) and resveratrol, polysaccharides, and large amounts of condensed tannins. The stem and leaf contain anthraquinone glycosides. The leaf also contains quercetin, isoquercitrin, reynoutrin, and vitamin C (1,2).

PHARMACOLOGY

Refer to the monograph on <Dahuang> for the pharmacological actions of anthraquinones emodin, chrysophanol and rheic acid contained in this herb.

1. Antibacterial Effect

In vitro studies showed that the <Huzhang> decoction (25–200%), polygonin, and polydatin (10 mg/ml) were inhibitory to *Staphylococcus aureus*, *Staphylococcus albus*, *Neisseria catarrhalis*, alpha and beta streptococci, *Escherichia coli*, *Proteus vulgaris*, *Pseudomonas aeruginosa*, *Salmonella typhi*, and *Shigella flexneri*. It also had a lethal effect on leptospira *in vitro* (3,4).

2. Antiviral Effect

The 10% <Huzhang> decoction inhibited Asian influenza virus type A Jingke 68–1 strain, ECHO$_{11}$, and herpes simplex virus. A stronger inhibitory action was exhibited by the 2% decoction against adenovirus type III, poliomyelitis virus type II, Coxsackie virus groups A and B, $ECHO_{11}$ group, encephalitis B virus Jingweiyan I, and herpes simplex I strain; the MIC against these viruses were 1:1600, 1:400, 1:400, 1:2560, 1:10,240, >1:3200 and 1:51,200, respectively. The 20% <Huzhang> solution had a significant inhibitory action against hepatitis B antigen (HBAg) (5). The active principles I and II of the herb were able to decrease the HBAg titer by 8 times (6).

3. Antitussive and Antiasthmatic Effects

Intraperitoneal injection of polydatin or its crude preparation at a dose of 1.5 or 3.0 mg/animal produced an antitussive effect in mice with cough induced by ammonia spray. The antitussive effect could also be achieved by: intragastric administration of the <Huzhang> decoction 12 g/kg; intravenous injection of Compound Yinyanglian Decoction (Rhizome Polygoni Cuspidati, *Mahonia bealei*, Folium Eriobotryae) 6 g/kg; intravenous injection of 50 mg/kg or intragastric administration of 75 mg/kg of polydatin to anesthetized cats following electrical stimulation of the superior laryngeal nerve. The herb decoction and Compound Yinyanglian Decoction (7.5×10^{-2}) could also significantly antagonize contraction of isolated guinea pig bronchi induced by histamine (6.25×10^{-6}) (3).

4. Effect on the Cardiovascular System

Intravenous injection of polydatin 50–60 mg/kg to anesthetized cats lowered the blood pressure. It did not affect the pressor effect of norepinephrine or epinephrine, but inhibited the pressor response to blockade of the common carotid artery and electrical stimulation of the afferent sciatic nerve. While the blood pressure in cats was lowered by polydatin, the rate and contraction amplitude of the heart *in vitro* were unchanged (7). Polydatin at a dose of 300 µg markedly increased the contraction amplitude of isolated guinea pig hearts. Cumulative dosing produced an initial stimulation followed by inhibition (8). The 10% solution of the <Huzhang> decoction markedly increased the contraction of isolated toad hearts (9). In dogs with catheterized coronary arteries, intravenous injection of polydatin 1.12–1.9 mg/kg increased the coronary flow and significantly decreased the coronary resistance; its action was much slower and more prolonged than that of aminophylline (10).

Polydatin dilated the constricted blood vessels of burned rabbit ears thereby increasing the number of activated capillaries and reducing thrombosis (11). It also dilated the bronchial and mesenteric capillaries of rats (12,13).

5. Anticholesterolemic Effect

Whereas daily intragastric administration of polydatin 200 mg/kg to normal rats for 7 days significantly lowered the serum cholesterol level, the <Huzhang> decoction was not significantly active; this could be due to the small amount of polydatin contained in the herb (14).

6. Miscellaneous Actions

Intraperitoneal injection of polydatin 500 mg/kg to mice markedly prolonged sleep induced by pentobarbital sodium and urethane (3). The stilbene derivatives exerted hemostatic and astringent actions when applied locally (15).

7. Toxicity

The LD_{50} of polygonin in mice by intrapertoneal injection was 1363.9±199.4 mg/kg, and that of polydatin was 1000.0±57.3 mg/kg. Polydatin at dosage levels of 50, 150, and 700 mg/kg injected intraperitoneally to separate groups of rats for 42 days caused different degrees of hepatic necrosis, peritonitis, and accumulation of fat in the bone marrow of some rats. The high-dosage group also developed leukopenia (3). Intragastric administration of the anthraquinone derivatives of the herb (containing mainly emodin and also some anthraquinones and a small amount of polydatin) to mice at 9 g/kg caused no deaths during one week of observation (2).

CLINICAL STUDIES

1. Acute Inflammatory Diseases

<Huzhang> and compound formulae containing this herb had good therapeutic effects in acute lung infections, appendicitis, appendiceal abscess, and tonsillitis (4,16–21). Good results were achieved in 45 cases of pneumonia treated with the herb decoction or Compound P. cuspidatum Decoction (Rhizome Polygoni Cuspidati, Herba Houttuyniae, Herbs Commelinae, Herba Scutellariae Barbatae, Rhizoma Fagopyri Cymosi). Body temperature dropped back to normal in 1–1.5 days in most cases (16,17). Twenty-six cases of acute appendicitis, 14 cases of appendiceal abscess and 4 cases of perforated appendix complicated with peritonitis were all cured by the herb decoction (20). Appendicitis Syrup (Rhizoma Polygoni Cuspidati, Herba Hedyotis Diffusae, Herba Taraxaci, Radix et Rhizoma Rhei) was used in the treatment of 107 cases of appendicitis complicated with diffuse peritonitis; 100 cases obtained marked effects and cure in the short-term; there were no deaths (21).

2. Scalds and Burns

Various preparations of <Huzhang>, its tannins, and its compound formulae promoted eschar formation and possessed antiseptic action. They reduced exudation, prevented loss of water and electrolytes, and hastened the healing of wounds. Clinical observations indicate that the herb preparations had a good therapeutic effect on burns (4,22–28). There was a report on 60 cases of second- and third-degree burns involving 10–71% of body area treated with the ointment, powder and dressing prepared from the concentrated herb decoction; 15 of these cases were already infected. Fifty-nine patients were cured; 1 died. Second-degree burns healed in 4–6 days, whereas third-degree burns required 20–42 days (22). In 153 cases of burns treated with the tannins of the herb, 86 cases obtained marked effects, 55 cases moderate effects, and 12 cases unsatisfactory results. The agent was more effective in second-degree scalds and burns (1), but less satisfactory in wounds with severe infection (24).

3. Hepatitis

The treatment of acute viral hepatitis with the anthraquinone glycosides of the herb was studied. For control, Compound Polygonum-Artemisia Decoction (Rhizome Polygoni Cuspidati, Herba Artemisiae, Fructus Ziziphi Jujubae) and Western drugs for liver protection were used. The results in the three treatment groups were the same, i.e., gradual recovery after the acute stage, satisfactory short-term effect, and clinical cure. However, based on the remission time of subjective symptoms and of positive physical signs, and the recovery time of liver functions, the anthraquinone glycosides were better than Compound Polygonum-Artemisia Decoction and were much superior to the Western drugs (29). There are many reports concerning the good therapeutic effects of the decoction, extract tablets, powder, and syrup of the herb and of its compound formula (Rhizoma Polygoni Cuspidati, Herba Hyperici Japonici, Herba Artemisiae, etc.) in the treatment of hepatitis. Generally speaking, these drugs were more effective in acute icteric viral hepatitis, and effective to some extent in chronic persistent hepatitis, but they appeared to be ineffective in chronic hepatitis (30–77).

4. Chronic Bronchitis

Compound Yinyanglian Crude Extract Tablet, which chiefly contains the herb <Huzhang>, is reported to have good antitussive and expectorant effects but poor antiasthmatic effect in chronic bronchitis. The tablet is also effective in reducing dry and moist rales (38). It is likewise effective in relapse cases (39). The therapeutic effect of the tablet was consistent irrespective of the locality and climate (40–42). There is also a report on the treatment of chronic bronchitis with the herb plus the leaf of *Elaeagnus pungens* and the whole plant of *Houttuynia cordata* (43,44).

5. Neonatal Jaundice

The 50% <Huzhang> syrup was used to treat 175 cases of neonatal jaundice 8 of which had severe jaundice (including hemolytic jaundice); 151 cases were cured, 7 improved, and 17 unchanged. Jaundice subsided more quickly when the herb was used with steroids than when Western medicines were used alone (45).

6. Leukopenia

<Huzhang> and its anthraquinones have a significant incremental effect on white blood cells (WBC) in leukopenia due to radiation and chemicals (benzene, naphthalene). The herb tablet or granule preparation was employed to treat 67 cases of leukopenia (in tumor patients) due to radiotherapy. After the fourth week of medication, the WBC count in 40 of 59 patients who continued with the ratiotherapy was increased by more then $1000/mm^3$; out of 8 patients who temporarily discontinued the radiotherapy, 7 had an increase of $1000/mm^3$. As the medicines had prolonged effects, patients who were sensitive to radiation were able to complete the radiotherapeutic course as scheduled (46,47).

7. Arthritis

A satisfactory therapeutic effect was achieved in more than 100 cases of rheumatic arthritis, rheumatoid arthritis, lumbar hypertrophy, and osteoarthritis treated with the ethanol preparation of this herb (48,49). There is also a report on the treatment of rheumatic arthritis with the decoction of the roots of *P. cuspidatum, Fagopyrum cymosum*, and *Ficus pandurata* (50).

8. Miscellaneous

<Huzhang>, polygonin, or <Huzhang> plus <Qiyelian>, or the compound formulae was used to treat hyperlipidemia (51), psoriasis (52,53), herpes zoster (54), cervix erosion (55), chronic osteomyelitis, vaginal candidiasis, hepatolithiasis, and snake bites (16).

ADVERSE EFFECTS

The side effects of <Huzhang> and its preparations are rather mild. Oral administration might cause digestive symptoms such as xerostomia (dry mouth), bitter aftertaste, nausea, vomiting, abdominal pain, and diarrhea. No irritation from local application, except occasional euphoria and sensitivity to low temperatures, has been reported (25,33,38,46).

REFERENCE

1. Shanghai Institute of Pharmaceutical Industry et al. Xinyiyaoxue Zazhi (Journal of Traditional Chinese Medicine) 1977 (7):45.

2. Chinese Materia Medica Analytical Laboratory, Shanghai Institute of Pharmaceutical Industry. Pharmaceutical Industry 1976 (10):34.

3. Chemistry Department, 173 Guangzhou Unit of the Chinese PLA. Xinyiyaoxue Zazhi (Journal of Traditional Chinese Medicine) 1973 (12):31.

4. New Medical Information (Teaching Hospital of Zunyi Medical College) 1971 (11):10.

5. Infectious Diseases Section, Tianjin Sanitation and Anti-epidemic Station. Tianjin Medical Journal 1975 (7):343.

6. Infectious Diseases Section of the Internal Medicine Department, Second Teaching Hospital of Chongqing Medical College. Chinese Journal of Internal Medicine 1976 (3):192.

7. Lei QJ. Selected Information of Scientific Research (Military Medical College of the Chinese PLA) 1974 (6):64.

8. Yang JC. Selected Information on Scientific Research (Military Medical College of the Chinese PLA) 1974 (6):36.

9. Class 1974 et al. Selected Information on Scientific Research (Military Medical College of the Chinese PLA) 1975 (Supplement):51.

10. Zhen HJ et al. Selected Information on Scientific Research (Military Medical College of the Chinese PLA) 1974 (6):74.

11. Zhao KS et al. Medical Journal of Chinese PLA 1980 5(2):75.

12. Pharmacology Department, First Military Medical College. Selected Information on Scientific Research (First Military Medical College of the Chinese PLA) 1976 (8):74.

13. Zhou XH et al. Selected Information on Scientific Research (First Military Medical College of the Chinese PLA) 1977 (10):56.

14. Pharmacology and Biochemistry Sections, Shanghai First Medical College. Internal information.

15. Editorial Group (Nanjing College of Pharmacy). Chinese Traditional Pharmacy. Vol. 2. Jiangsu People's Publishing House. 1976. p. 156.

16. Wang Q et al. (reviewer). Journal of Barefoot Doctor 1977 (8):29.

17. Internal Medicine Department. New Medical Information (Teaching Hospital of Zunyi Medical College) 1970 (4):7.

18. Liu GP. Xinzhongyi (Journal of New Chinese Medicine) 1977 (5):23.

19. Fuyang District First People's Hospital. Study of New Chinese Medicine (Fuyang District First People's Hospital, Anhui) 1972 (1):41.

20. Yingshan County People's Hospital. Hubei Science and Technology — Medicine 1975 (6):20.

21. Surgery Department, Guangji County (Hubei) First People's Hospital. Tianjin Medical Journal 1978 (1):13.

22. Surgery Department, Baise District Hospital. Health Bulletin (Baise District Health Bureau, Guangxi) 1972 (4):19.

23. Burns Group, Teaching Hospital of Sichuan Medical College. Sichuan Communications on Chinese Traditional and Herbal Drugs 1974 (1):38.

24. Surgery Department, Jinjiang District Second Hospital. Xinyiyaoxue Tongxun (Bulletin of New Chinese Medicine) (Jinjiang District Second Hospital) 1972 (2):15.

25. 171st Hospital of the Chinese PLA. New Medical Information (Jiangxi School of Pharmacy) 1970 (3):11.

26. Teaching Hospital of Zunyi Medical College et al. Chinese Medical Journal 1973 (4):246.

27. Health Department of Changde Submilitary Region. Chinese Traditional and Herbal Drugs Communications 1974 (6):51.

28. Burns Therapy Group. New Medical Information (Teaching Hospital of Zunyi Medical College) 1970 (2):8.

29. Third Internal Medicine Department, 88th Hospital of the Chinese PLA. Medical Information (Health Division of the Logistics Department of Fuzhou Military Region of the Chinese PLA) 1976 (2):83.

30. Infectious Diseases Department, 181st Hospital of the Chinese PLA. Health Journal of Guangxi 1975 (5):27.

31. Infectious Diseases Department, 47th Army Hospital of the Chinese PLA. Chinese Traditional and Herbal Drugs Communications 1973 (1):43.

32. Wuhan Ninth Hospital. Xinyiyaoxue Zazhi (Journal of Traditional Chinese Medicine) 1973 (2):22.

33. Infectious Diseases Ward, 3rd Branch of the 176th Hospital of the Chinese PLA. Medical Information (Health Division of the Logistics Department of Fuzhou Military Region of the Chinese PLA) 1972 (2):23.

34. Traditional Chinese Medicine Department, Xiangfan People' s Hospital. Xiangfan Science and Technology — Medicine and Health 1977 (3):23.

35. Bazhong County Sanitation and Anti-epidemic Station. Sichuan Communications on Chinese Traditional and Herbal Drugs 1973 (2):12.

36. Scientific Research Group, Pingnan County Health Bureau. Revolution in Health (Yulin District Health Bureau, Guangxi) 1975 (3):26.

37. 175th Hospital of the Chinese PLA. Medical Information (Health Division of the Logistics Department of Fuzhou Military Region) 1972 (2):26.

38. Guangxi PLA Units Coordinating Research Group on Chronic Bronchitis. Clinical Trials of Compound Polygonum cuspidatum Therapy of Chronic Bronchitis (1971–73). Health Division of the Logistics Department of Guangzhou Military Region. p. 60.

39. Bronchitis Group, 303rd Hospital of the Chinese PLA. Clinical Trials of Compound Polygonum cuspidatum Therapy of Chronic Bronchitis (1971–73). Health Division of the Logistics Department of Guangzhou Military Region. p. 45.

40. Bronchitis Group, 303rd Hospital of the Chinese PLA. Clinical Trials of Compound Polygonum cuspidatum Therapy of Chronic Bronchitis (1971–73). Health Division of the Logistics Department of Guangzhou Military Region. p. 5.

41. 220th Hospital of the Chinese PLA. Clinical Trials of Compound Polygonum cuspidatum Therapy of Chronic Bronchitis (1971–73). Health Division of the Logistics Department of Guangzhou Military Region. p. 11.

42. 145th Hospital of the Chinese PLA. Clinical Trials of Compound Polygonum cuspidatum Therapy of Chronic Bronchitis (1971–73). Health Division of the Logistics Department of Guangzhou Military Region. p. 18.

43. Mobile Medical Team, 502nd Hospital of the Chinese PLA et al. Health Bulletin (Baise District Health Bureau, Guangxi) 1972 (2):1.

44. Debao County Chronic Bronchitis Group. Health Bulletin (Baise District Health Bureau, Guangxi) 1972 (2):6.

45. Surgery Department, Guangdong People's Hospital. Medical Trends (Guangdong Institute of Medicine and Health) 1972 (3):11.

46. Pharmaceutical Factory, May 7th Cadre's School of the Ministry of Health of the People's Republic of China. Radiomedicine and Radiation Protection (PO Box 753, Beijing) 1974 (2):37.

47. Shanghai Compilation of New Drugs (confirmed in 1976). Shanghai Institute of Scientific and Technological Information. p. 193.

48. Dou GX. Xinyiyaoxue Zazhi (Journal of Traditional Chinese Medicine) 1974 (7):32.

49. Combined Western and Traditional Chinese Therapy Unit, Zhenhai County People's Hospital. Zhenhai Medicine and Health 1977 (1):20.

50. Dexing County Coordinating Group of Barefoot Doctors for the Identification of Chinese Traditional Drugs. Cultivation, Preparation and Uses of Chinese Medicinal Materials (Dexing County Health Bureau) 1975 (3–4):19.

51. Huainan Pharmaceutical Factory (Shanghai) et al. Medical References — Special Issue on Coronary Disease (Henan College of Traditional Chinese Medicine et al.) 1973 (1):154.

52. Dermatology Department, Huashan Teaching Hospital of Shanghai First Medical College. Xinyiyaoxue (Journal of Traditional Chinese Medicine) 1977 (7):48.

53. Dermatology Department, Yangzhou District People's Hospital. Dermatological Research Communications (Jiangsu Institute of Dermatology) 1976 (2):90.

54. Yang JX. Medical Communications (Information Unit of Xiamen Health Bureau et al.) 1975 (1):29.

55. Health Team for Fentou Commune, Qianyang District (Hunan) People's Hospital. New Chinese Medicine 1977 (1):51.

(Liu Changwu)

HUGU AND GOUGU 虎骨與狗骨

<Hugu> refers to the tiger bone, *Panthera tigris* L. (Felidae). It is pungent and has a "warm" property. It is reputed to be analgesic and fortifying to the bones, tendons and muscles, and is thought to prevent palpitation associated with fear. It is commonly used to treat atrophy of the leg and knee, and rheumatism.

<Gougu> is the tibial bone of the dog, *Canis familiaris* L. (Canidae). It has a sweet and salty taste and a "warm" property. It is antirheumatic, "spleen"-invigorative, channel-harmonizing, blood-stimulant and tissue-generative. Therapeutically, it is used in rheumatism and arthritis. It is now used by some people as a substitute for <Hugu>.

CHEMICAL COMPOSITION

The bones of the dog and tiger contain collagen, fats, calcium phosphate, calcium carbonate and magnesium phosphate. Collagen is the active component. The amino acid compositions of the gelatin of tiger and dog bones are more of less similar; the former contains 17 amino acids, the latter one more amino acid, tyrosine.

PHARMACOLOGY

1. Anti-inflammatory Effect

Both tiger and dog bones possess significant anti-inflammatory action. Experiments showed that the suspension of the bone powder of either animal given intragastrically at 1 g/kg to rats significantly inhibited paw swelling due to injection of formaldehyde or egg white. Both bone powders inhibited the increase in total WBC and lymphocyte and the reduction in the neutrophil in the peripheral blood of rats with formaldehyde-induced paw swelling. Bilateral adrenalectomy or anesthesia with pentobarbital sodium abolished the anti-inflammatory action of the bone powders. Thus, the anti-inflammatory action of the bone powders is thought to be realized through central control of the pituitary-adrenocortical function. Intragastric administration of either bone powder to rabbits at 2 g/kg could also inhibit the increase in cutaneous capillary permeability induced by xylene (1).

The gelatins from dog and tiger bones have similar anti-inflammatory effects. Experiments showed that oral administration of either gelatin at 0.3 g/kg inhibited formaldehyde-induced paw swelling in rats. There was no significant difference in the potency of the gelatins. The degelatinized dog bone powder still exhibited a very weak anti-inflammatory action at 1.5 g/kg; this is attributed to incomplete extraction of gelatin which is thought to be the bioactive component (2,3). The dog tibia fried with peanut oil also had an anti-inflammatory effect, but the gelatin of the skull, spine, and rib of the animal and the autoclaved tibia had no such effect (4).

As the gelatins from tiger, dog and pig bones shared similar chemical compositions and amino acids, some investigators tried using pig bones in lieu of tiger bones. Experiments on rats showed that the injection prepared from pig bones had significant inhibitory action on paw swelling due to egg white and granulation induced by implanted cotton pledget. The active constituents were considered to be peptides and not amino acide (5).

2. Analgesic Effect

Intragastric administration of the gelatin of tiger or dog bones at 1 g/kg was proved to have an analgesic effect in the experiment of exposing an animal's tail to focused radiant heat; it elevated the pain threshold and delayed the onset of pain reaction (2,3).

3. Sedative Effect

In experiments using the cage-trembling tracing method, spontaneous activity of experimental mice was reduced after intragastric administration of the gelatin of tiger or dog bones at 1 g/kg (3).

4. Healing of Fractures

Roentgenography, determination of the resistance to fracture, and also histology of rabbit models of artificial fracture of the femur showed that Compound Bone Union Pill (Os Tigris, Pyritum, Eupolyphaga seu Steleophaga, Sanguis Draconis, Moschus, etc.) promoted the healing of fractures, resulting in rapid and abundant formation of callus and in strong and mature bone. Component analysis of the compound formula revealed that the healing effect of the tiger bone and pyrite was better than the others, and the bone strength was particularly high when they were used together in equal amounts (6).

5. Toxicity

Intragastric administration of the powder of tiger or dog bones to mice at 1 or 2 g/kg/day for two weeks did not affect the growth of the animals (1).

CLINICAL STUDIES

1. Rheumatic and Rheumatoid Arthritis, etc.

Tiger bones are commonly used in atrophy of bones in the lower extremities, spasm of limbs, low-back pain, chills, and ostalgia. They can be soaked in wine for oral administration, or used in compound prescriptions; for instance, together with the fruit of *Chaenomeles speciosa*, rhizome of *Ligusticum chuanxiong*, root of *Angelica sinensis*, rhizome of *Gastrodia elata*, root of *Achyranthes bidentata*, root bark of *Acanthopanax gracilistylus*, flower of *Carthamus tinctorius*, root of *Dipsacus asper*, rhizome of *Polygonatum odoratum* var. *pluriflorum*, root of *Gentiana macrophylla*, root of *Ledebouriella divaricata*, and tender stem of *Morus alba* as in Tiger Bone-Papaya Wine. Fifty cases of arthritis with severe "cold and damp" syndrome were reported to have been treated with Tiger Bone Myrrh Pill (Os Tigris, Myrrha, Scorpio and Scolopendra) (7).

In view of the scarcity of tiger bones, dog bones which have a similar anti-inflammatory action are being used nowadays in lieu of the former. Various preparations of dog bones achieved good therapeutic effect in rheumatic and rheumatoid arthritis. For instance, there is a report on 38 cases of arthritis (including acute, subacute and chronic rheumatic, rheumatoid arthritis and osteoarthritis) treated orally with the dog bone gelatin at doses of 3–4 g twice daily, 30 days as a therapeutic course; 18 cases were symptom-free or had marked effects, and 17 had moderate effects. Relief of sensitivity of joints to cold was very pronounced, but the onset of the analgesic effect was slow (8,9). In another series of 222 cases of rheumatic and rheumatoid arthritis, Dog Bone Gelatin Medicinal Wine containing dog bone gelatin and the rhizome of *Dioscorea nipponica*, etc., was used at doses of 20–30 ml, 2–3 times a day with an aggregate effective rate of 92.7% and a marked effective rate of 65.7%. It was more effective for rheumatic arthritis, and to a certain extent, for rheumatoid arthritis. It controlled the symptoms, reduced swelling and pain, and also improved the patients' health (10–12). Antirheumatic Injection prepared from dog bones and muskmelon seeds was effective in 84%, and offered temporary relief to 21.2% of 280 cases of rheumatic arthritis (13,14). Another preparation called Antihyperplasia No. 1 Injection, containing dog and sheep bones, the root of *Angelica sinensis*, and the bark of *Eucommia ulmoides*, was proven effective for bone hyperplasia (15).

2. Miscellaneous

Compound Fracture Union Pill, prepared mainly from tiger bones, was effective for fractures; it was able to reduce swelling, stop pain, and enhance the healing or fractures (6). The efficacy of the dog bone powder and alunite in the treatment of infantile diarrhea has also been reported (16).

REFERENCE

1. Cui ZG et al. Collections of Research Information. 5th edition. Sichuan Institute of Chinese Materia Medica. 1965. p. 327.

2. Zhang MY et al. Collections of Research Information. 2nd edition. Sichuan Institute of Chinese Materia Medica. 1959. p. 69.

3. Zhang MY et al. Collections of Research Information. 5th edition. Sichuan Institute of Chinese Materia Medica. 1965. p. 333.

4. Cui ZG et al. Collections of Research Information. 3rd edition. Sichuan Institute of Chinese Materia Medica. 1960. p. 101.

5. Caixi County (Shandong) Health Bureau et al. Chinese Traditional and Herbal Drugs Communications 1977 (12):22.

6. Liu RT et al. Tianjin Medical Journal 1962 4(8):457.

7. Yan DX. Harbin Zhongyi (Harbin Journal of Traditional Chinese Medicine) 1965 8(8):40.

8. Nan' an District (Chongqing) Second People' s Hospital. Collections of Research Information. 5th edition. Sichuan Institute of Chinese Materia Medica. 1965. p. 339.

9. First Workers' Sanatorium of Sichuan Workers' General Union. Research Information on Chinese Traditional Drugs (Sichuan Institute of Chinese Materia Medica) 1973 (10):53.

10. Shandong Coordinating Group on Dog Bone Gelatin Medicinal Wine. Chinese Traditional and Herbal Drugs Communications 1976 (12):12.

11. Shandong Medicinal Materials Company. Chinese Traditional and Herbal Drugs Communications 1976 (8): 45.

12. Shandong Medicinal Materials Company. Chinese Traditional and Herbal Drugs Communications 1977 (5):21.

13. Science and Education Group, Caixi County (Shandong) Health Bureau. Chinese Traditional and Herbal Drugs Communications 1977 (1):15.

14. Scientific Research Group, Caixi County (Shandong) Health Bureau. Chinese Traditional and Herbal Drugs Communications 1977 (12):30.

15. Liu H. Zaozhuang Yiyao (Zaozhuang Medical Journal) 1979 (2):18.

16. Sun TS. Liaoning Zhongji Yikan (Liaoning Journal of Paramedics) 1978 (4):59.

(Deng Wenlong)

BAIJIANG 敗醬

<Baijiang> comes from the whole plant or the rhizome of *Patrinia scabiosaefolia* Fisch. or *P. villosa* Juss. (Valerianaceae). The latter is also called <Kuzhaigong>.

<Baijiang> has a bitter and pungent taste, and a "cool" property. It is latent-heat-clearing, antipyretic, detoxicant, anti-inflammatory, stasis-eliminative and pus-discharging. It is employed in the treatment of intestinal carbuncle including acute appendicitis, abscess of the liver, dysentery in enteritis, postpartum abdominal pain due to blood stasis, carbuncle, and deep-rooted ulcer.

CHEMICAL COMPOSITION

The rhizome and root of *P. scabiosaefolia* contain about 0.1% of volatile oil (called Huanghualongyajing) composed of more than 15 constituents. Patrinene and isopatrinene are the principal constituents. Another constituent is isopentanoic acid which imparts a unique, foul smell (1). The rhizome and root also contain patrinosides which yield the aglycone oleanolic acid after hydrolysis (2). The root and rhizome of *P. villosa* contain villoside, morroniside, and loganin (3).

PHARMACOLOGY

1. Sedative Effect

It has been reported that the *P. scabiosaefolia* grown in northeastern China possesses a sedative action; its active constituent is believed to be saponins (4). Recent studies proved that oral administration of the ethanol extract or the volatile oil of *P. scabiosaefolia* to mice produced a marked sedative effect and potentiated the hypnotic action of pentobarbital sodium. But the ethanol extract of the drug residue which is devoid of the volatile oil and the total saponins was without any sedative action. Patrinene and isopatrinene were reported to be the chief active constituents of the volatile oil, whereas isopentanoic acid was inactive (1,5,6). The sedative action of <Baijiang> was found to be twice as strong as that of a related species, *Valeriana officinalis* (5).

2. Antibacterial Effect

The <Baijiang> extract had a weak inhibitory action *in vitro* on *Staphylococcus aureus*, *Staphylococcus albus*, and *Corynebacterium paradiphtheriae*; it was inactive against *Streptococcus hemolyticus*, *Corynebacterium diphtheriae*, *Diplococcus pneumoniae*, *Bacillus anthracis*, and *Clostridium tetani* (7). On the other hand, the decoction of *P. villosa* was found to have no significant inhibitory action against influenza virus in the chicken embryo (8).

3. Miscellaneous Actions

<Baijiang> promoted the regeneration of liver cells and prevented hepatocellular degeneration (5). Whether its action is causally related to oleanolic acid deserves further studies since the latter has a liver-protective action (9). The infusion of the root at 500 µg/ml had an inhibition rate of 100% against cancer cells of the human cervix; conversely, it promoted multiplication of normal cells (10).

4. Toxicity

No adverse reactions occurred in albino mice following intragastric administration of the *P. scabiosaefolia* extract at 24 g (crude drug)/kg (11). The ethanol extract, 30 g/kg PO, caused mild respiratory depression and diarrhea in mice (5). Huanghualongyajing fed to mice at dose levels corresponding to 400, 700 and 1500 times the human dose did not produce any abnormalities in a week (6). *P. scabiosaefolia* is, therefore, considered to be non-toxic.

CLINICAL STUDIES

1. Neurasthenia

Sixty-two cases of neurasthenia with insomnia as the chief symptom and 284 cases of severe psychosis at the convalescent stage with residual neurasthenic syndrome were treated with the 20% *P. scabiosaefolia* tincture 10 ml per dose, or the dried extract tablet (Mian Er Jing Tablet, 1 g of crude drug each) at 2–4 tablets 2–3 times daily. The aggregate effective rats of these preparations for improving insomnia were 92 and 80%, and the marked effective rates 30.7 and 33.5%, respectively. It was also effective for other symptoms caused by increased excitation of the CNS such as dizziness, heaviness of the head, palpitation, photophobia, phonophobia, emotional instability, anorexia, and decreased mental activity (5,11). The same therapeutic effect was achieved with Huanghualongyajing Capsule (6). It has a characteristic slow onset with marked effects usually appearing after 3 to 6 days of treatment. The drug does not produce dizziness and drowsiness the morning after medication.

2. Mumps

The fresh *P. scabiosaefolia* plus crushed gypsum and mixed with egg white may be used for external dressing. The herb decoction may be used concomitantly in cases with complications at doses of 10–15 g three to four times daily. In over 200 cases treated locally, 90% were symptom-free within 24 hours of treatment. A second application in severe cases also abolished the symptoms (i.e., 48 hours) (12).

3. Acute Bacterial Inflammation

One hundred and thirty-four cases of acute suppurative tonsillitis, pneumonia acute appendicitis, biliary tract infection, and acute pancreatitis were treated with the distillate of *P. villosa* (2 g crude drug/ml) at doses of 2–4 ml two to four times daily by intramuscular injection for a course of 2–15 days; 69% were cured, while the remaining cases achieved different degrees of improvement (13). The treatment of appendiceal abscess with a compound prescription containing the herb plus the kernel of *Coix lachryma-jobi* and the stem of *Sargentodoxa cuneata* has also been reported (14).

4. Infiltrative Pulmonary Tuberculosis

The therapeutic effect achieved by intramuscular injection of the distillate or oral administration of the syrup of *P. villosa* was reported to be similar to that obtained from the combined use of isoniazid and streptomycin (15).

5. Influenza

The granule infusion and injection preparation of *P. villosa* had an antipyretic effect in influenza (16).

6. Chronic Nonspecific Colitis

Retention enema with the decoction of the kernel of *Coix lachryma-jobi*, the lateral root tuber of *Aconitum carmichaeli*, and <Baijiang> (species not given) was effective (17).

ADVERSE EFFECTS

Side effects and toxic reactions from the preparations of *P. scabiosaefolia* are rarely seen. Individual patients may develop xerostomia and gastric discomfort (11). The side effects of Huanghualongyajing are even rarer; the drug does not affect the liver and kidney functions and the WBC count (6). In a clinical trial where 134 cases of acute bacillary dysentery were treated with P. villosa Injection, WBC counts were reduced to 2200–2800 in 3 cases on the 2nd, 5th and 7th day of treatment, respectively, but were restored to normal about one week after discontinuation of the drug (13), suggesting a possible antineoplastic action from *P. villosa*.

REFERENCE

1. Advanced Class for Chemists of Chinese Traditional Drugs, Faculty of Pharmacy of Beijing Medical College. Journal of Beijing Medical College 1976 (1):17.

2. Sidorovich TI. Apt Delo 1966 15(6):38.

3. Taguchi H et al. Journal of the Pharmaceutical Society of Japan (Tokyo) 1973 93(5):607.

4. Gao YQ. Graduate Theses of Shenyang College of Pharmacy. 1966.

5. Psychiatry Department, Third Teaching Hospital of Beijing Medical College. Journal of Beijing Medical College 1974 (1):23.

6. Chinese Traditional Drug Chemistry Group, Faculty of Pharmacy of Beijing Medical College. Journal of Neurological and Psychiatric Diseases 1979 (1):4.

7. Zhang WX. Chinese Medical Journal 1949 67:648.

8. Hu Q et al. Chinese Traditional and Herbal Drugs Communications 1979 (7):30.

9. Xu LZ et al. Chinese Traditional and Herbal Drugs Communications 1979 (8):25.

10. Sato A. Journal of Oriental Medicine 1979 7(1):12.

11. Psychiatry Department, Third Teaching Hospital of Beijing Medical College. Xinyiyaoxue Zazhi (Journal of Traditional Chinese Medicine) 1976 (5):26.

12. Jinshan Health Clinic of Fencheng County. Jiangxi Medical Information 1972 (1):29.

13. Chongqing Clinical Observation Group of Patrinia scabiosaefolia Injection. Chongqing Journal of New Chinese Medicine 1972 (1):17.

14. Sun GW. Jiangsu Zhongyi (Jiangsu Journal of Traditional Chinese Medicine) 1965 (5):20.

15. Chongqing Institute of Tuberculosis. Chongqing Yiyao (Chongqing Medical Journal) 1975 (4):65.

16. Yichun District Coordinating Research Group on Influenza. Internal information. 1977.

17. Internal Medicine Department, Third Teaching Hospital of Zhongshan Medical College. New Chinese Medicine 1974 (6):268.

(Xue Chunsheng)

KUNMINGSHANHAITANG 昆明山海棠

<Kunmingshanhaitang>, also known as <Diaomaocao> or <Liufangteng>, is the root, or peeled root of *Tripterygium hypoglaucum* (L' evl.) Hutch. (Celastraceae). It is bitter, puckery, and "warm". Its actions are believed to be blood-activating, channel-deobstruent, and antirheumatic. Hence, it is chiefly used in rheumatism, rheumatoid arthritis, lupus erythematosus, and lepra reaction.

CHEMICAL COMPOSITION

The chemical composition of <Kunmingshanhaitang> is quite similar to that of *T. wilfordii* (1). <Kunmingshanhaitang> contains alkaloids, saponins, lactones, terpenes, and pigments. It was recently reported that it contains triptolide, 0.0005%, hypolide, and dulcitol (2,3).

PHARMACOLOGY

Refer to the monograph on <Leigongteng> for the pharmacological actions of triptolide — one of the chief active constituents of the herb.

1. Anti-inflammatory Effect

<Kunmingshanhaitang> has a significant anti-inflammatory action. Animal experiments showed that administration of the peeled root decoction markedly inhibited the increase in cutaneous capillary permeability in mice due to xylene, histamine, or chicken egg white, inhibited extravasation of dye into the peritoneal cavity due to intraperitoneal injection of acetic acid, and antagonized egg white- and formaldehyde-induced paw swelling in rats. The potency of 20–40 g/kg of the decoction was equivalent to that of 50–100 mg/kg of cortisone acetate.

In rats with croton oil-induced granulocyst, <Kunmingshanhaitang> significantly inhibited exudation and reduced inflammatory blood-stained exudates. It also markedly inhibited granulation induced by cotton pledget (4). Intraperitoneal injection of the crude extract to rats also significantly inhibited paw swelling induced by turpentine, and the increase in capillary permeability of the auricle due to histamine injection (5). It is inferred that the anti-inflammatory activity of <Kunmingshanhaitang> is not causally related to the pituitary-adrenocortical function since the herb still produced a significant anti-inflammatory activity in bilaterally adrenalectomized rats, though it failed to prolong the survival period of adrenalectomized young rats and to inhibit the compensatory hypertrophy of the remaining adrenal of unilaterally adrenalectomized animals, and since under the usual anti-inflammatory dosage, it did not cause thymic atrophy in young mice, though high dosages could not decrease the vitamin C content of the adrenal glands of rats (4).

2. Effect on the Immunologic Function

<Kunmingshanhaitang> has a signficant immunosuppressive effect. It inhibited reticuloendothelial phagocytosis of carbon particles in mice and suppressed the formation of hemolytic antibodies following immunization with sheep red blood cells. Its effect increased with duration of medication (6,7). The herb produced a strong, dose-dependent inhibitory action on delayed allergic reaction induced by 2,4-dinitrochlorobenzene on the auricle of mice. It had no additive or synergistic action with cortisone, cyclophosphamide, and 6-mercaptopurine. It also significantly inhibited BCG-induced delayed skin hypersensitivity in guinea pigs (6). Likewise, it markedly suppressed rejection of skin allograft in rats (5). In the case of adjuvant arthritis in rats, <Kunmingshanhaitang> markedly suppressed the primary lesions and especially the secondary ones. However, it had no marked inhibitory effect on immediate hypersensitivity in guinea pigs due to egg white or in mice due to the root of *Trichosanthes kirilowii* (6). All these results suggest that <Kunmingshanhaitang> inhibits the function of monocytes, the humoral and cellular immunities, and the types III and IV allergic reactions. Its action was strongest against cellular immunity. On the other hand, the usual effective dosage of the herb did not cause atrophy of the immune organs such as the thymus and spleen but their weights were increased by sufficient dosage (4,6,7).

3. Antineoplastic Effect

The inhibition rate of the ethanol extract of the herb against the cervix cancer U_{14} in mice was 40% (8). In experiments on four groups of mice, the inhibition rates of the crude extract of herb against sarcoma 180 and sarcoma 37 in mice were between 33 and 52% (9). The crude extract was reported to have a significant therapeutic effect on leukemia L_{615}; its active component was reported to be triptolide (10).

4. Miscellaneous Actions

The writhing reaction elicited by intraperitoneal injection of acetic acid in mice was inhibited by intragastric administration of 40 g/kg of the herb decoction, suggesting the presence of analgesic action (11). Daily administration of the aqueous or ethanol extract of the herb at 5 g/kg inhibited malaria in rats; the plasmodium inhibition rate of the alkaloid at 15 mg/kg/day was 77% (12).

5. Toxicity

The toxicity of *T. hypoglaucum* varies with the time of harvest, plant parts used, and methods of preparation. Various animals showed different degrees of tolerance to it. Generally speaking, the root bark was more toxic than the peeled root, and prolonged processing at high temperatures would greatly reduce the toxicity. The LD_{50} of the root was reported to be 35.2 g/kg, the LD_{100} 70 g/kg, and safety dose 10 g/kg (8). The LD_{50} of the 50% ethanol extract was 12–14 g/kg (9). In another paper, the LD_{50} of the decoction of the peeled root in mice by intragastric administration was reported to be 64–68 g/kg, whereas the LD_{50} of the root bark decoction was 40.9 g/kg, and that of the tablet, prepared by film evaporation of the alcohol-precipitated decoction of the peeled root, was 94.8 g/kg. The LD_{50} of the 70% ethanol extract in mice was 7.0–14.9 g/kg and that in rats over 40 g/kg.

Subacute toxicity tests showed that the tablet of the alcohol-precipitated decoction of the peeled root administered intragastrically to rats at 40 g/kg daily for 30 days did not produce any significant toxic effect, but the 70% ethanol extract tablet at 20 g/kg/day for 5 days readily caused hepatic and renal disorders (11).

The LD_{50} of dulcitol in mice was over 7 g/kg (1).

CLINICAL STUDIES

1. Rheumatoid Arthritis, Fibrositis, etc.

<Kunmingshanhaitang> is used as a folk remedy for rheumatoid arthritis and rheumatic pain. It has been reported that the wine preparation of the herb had a good therapeutic effect in rheumatoid arthritis and fibrositis (13,14). Large numbers of clinical trials support this fact (15,16). For instance, a report claims that when 200 g of the dried roots macerated in 1000 ml of white wine for one week was given to 600 cases of rheumatoid arthritis at doses of 10–20 ml thrice daily, 117 cases (19.5%) were basically relieved of symptoms, 191 cases (31.8%) had marked effects and 274 cases (45.7%) were improved. The aggregate effective rate was 97% (16) . The 50% ethanol extract tablet, which could be conveniently administered, was also very effective in rheumatoid arthritis (17–19). Out of 45 cases so treated, 92.3% were relieved of morning stiffness, 97.8% pain, 100% swelling, 100% tenderness, and 62.8% had improved functional state (17). The various components of the herb, the crude alkaloids, pigments, steroids, terpenes, and lipids, were reported to exhibit different degrees of effectiveness, with the ethanol extract giving the most potent effect (20). Others reported later that dulcitol (21) and alkaloid A of the herb (22) were also quite effective. For example, 10 cases treated with alkaloid A obtained complete remission within 5 weeks (22).

The most prominent effect manifested was the improvement of symptoms. In some patients there were improvement or normal recovery of the biochemical parameters of the blood, including erythrocyte sedimentation rate, antistreptolysin "O", rheumatoid factor and mucoprotein, as well as corresponding normalization of the hemoglobin, white blood cell and platelet values. X-Ray examination performed after 3 to 4 months of medication revealed different degrees of improvement in soft tissue swelling, bone decalcification and joint cleft narrowing.

2. Lupus Erythematosus

Good effects were achieved with <Kunmingshanhaitang> in lupus erythematosus (9,23). Out of 25 cases treated with the tablet prepared from the 50% ethanol extract of the root, 11 cases obtained marked effects and 8 moderate effects. Improvement of various symptoms and signs was achieved. In patients with systemic lupus erythematosus, the medication achieved optimal effects on skin lesions and some improvement on lesions of internal organs as well as on laboratory parameters such as normalization of WBC count, lowering of the erythrocyte sedimentation rate, disappearance of proteinuria, rheumatoid factors and antinuclear antibodies, elevation of C_3, and reduction of γ-globulin, IgG and IgA. Hemorheology revealed improvement of microcirculatory disorders in the tongue and nailfold, and improvement or normalization of blood or plasma viscosity, cellular electrophoretic timd, hematocrit, and fibrinogen (9).

3. Chronic Nephritis

A marked decrease in urinary protein, increase of urine output, subsidence of edema, increase of plasma protein, albumin and globulin were observed in 40 cases following a 2-week course with the 50% ethanol extract tablet. Eight cases obtained a short-term cure, 14 cases had marked effects and 3 moderate effects; the therapeutic effect was enhanced by increasing the dosage. The drug might also be effective in cases unresponsive to adrenocorticosteroids or cyclophosphamide. The complementary use of this drug in steroid-treated patients would facilitate the tapering and withdrawal of steroids. The drug was most effective in cases with a short history, in young patients, and in those with minimal pathological changes manifested mainly as proteinuria (24).

4. Psoriasis

The extract tablet along with other drugs was used to treat 123 cases, of which 119 were of the common type. Fifteen cases were cured, 56 had marked effects, 40 were improved, and 12 unchanged; the aggregate effective rate was 90.2% and the marked effective rate, 57.7%. Drug effects usually appeared after 1 to 2 weeks of treatment, and marked effects were apparent after 2 to 4 weeks. It was equally effective in the common, arthritic, and pustular types. Three to 12 months of follow-up revealed that 18 our of 26 responsive cases relapsed within 6 to 12 months, but the new skin lesions were milder than before. Remission was still obtained by repeating the treatment, except in a few patients. PHA skin test, PHA lymphocyte transformation test and serum IgG, IgA and IgM determination performed in some patients showed no typical changes (25).

5. Lepra Reaction

<Kunmingshanhaitang> is reported to be very effective in lepra reaction. The peeled root decoction at doses of 20–30 g daily could promptly control fever, pain, and development of new skin lesions (26).

6. Miscellaneous

It had been reported that <Kunmingshanhaitang> is effective in different degrees in angiitis (26), erythema multiforme (27), primary thrombocytopenic purpura (28), allergic subsepticemia (29), hyperthyroidism (30), malaria (12), and some cancers (31).

ADVERSE EFFECTS

T. hypoglaucum is toxic, especially its branch and leaf which, when eaten by cows, sheep and other domestic animals, cause hair loss. For this reason, it is known as <Diaomaocao> or "the herb that causes hair falling". No poisoning has been reported in man when given the root for treatment. However, *T. hypoglaucum* should be used with caution as it shares a similar chemical composition with *T. wilfordii* Hook. f. a species to which it is very closely related, whose toxicity has repeatedly been reported. The common side effects of the herb are gastrointestinal symptoms gastric pain, nausea, vomiting, diarrhea or constipation, and decrease of appetite. Secondary reactions include WBC reduction, facial pigmentation, and subcutaneous hemorrhage, with oligomenorrhea and amenorrhea being most prominent (8,16,17–20,25).

The herb <Kunmingshanhaitang> has a significant but reversible inhibitory effect on menstruation. Its use was associated with the development of amenorrhea in 60 out of 397 cases, and in 42 out of 177 premenopausal cases below 41 years old. The incidence rate was 23.7%. Amenorrhea mostly occurred in 1–6 months after medication. In some patients, menstruation returned spontaneously during the treatment period, or after treatment with Chinese herbal medicines or hormonal therapy, and in other patients it returned on discontinuation of the herb. Vaginal smears in amenorrheal patients usually revealed low levels of estrogen, but the progesterone tests were mostly positive. In very few patients, there were various degrees of genital atrophy. The results of the studies on the 17-hydroxycorticosteroid, thyroid ^{131}I uptake and X-ray of the sella turcica, in conjunction with other findings, attribute the amenorrheal effect to interference or inhibition of the function of some parts of the anterior pituitary gland (32). This side effect was more marked with the ethanol extract than with the aqueous extract.

REFERENCE

1. Shen JS. Identification of the chemical constituents of the roots of Tripterygium wilfordii and Tripterygium hypoglaucum. In: Proceedings of the Shanghai Regional Symposium on Pharmacy — Botany. Chinese Pharmaceutical Association (Shanghai Branch). 1978. p. 54.

2. Phytochemistry Department, Yunnan Institute of Botany et al. Chinese Traditional and Herbal Drugs Communications 1977 (7):10.

3. Phytochemistry Department, Yunnan Institute of Botany et al. Kexue Tongbao (Science Bulletin) 1977 22(10):458.

4. Deng WL et al. Chinese Traditional and Herbal Drugs 1981 12(8):22.

5. Liu CR. Selected Information (Kunming Medical College) 1979 (4):14.

6. Deng WL et al. Chinese Traditional and Herbal Drugs 1981 12(10):26.

7. Immunology Unit of the Microbiology Section, Kunming Medical College et al. Acta Academiae Medicinae Kunming 1980 1(2):1.

8. Pharmaceutical Bulletin (Beijing Institute of Pharmaceutical Industry) 1975 (12):7.

9. Shanghai No. 2 Pharmaceutical Factory. Clinical observation of Tripterygium hypoglaucum therapy in lupus erythematosus. 1978.

10. Zhang TM et al. Chinese Pharmaceutical Bulletin 1980 5(46).

11. Deng WL et al. General pharmacology and toxicity III. In: Pharmacological Studies of Tripterygium hypoglaucum. 1980.

12. Chinese Traditional Drugs Group, Chemistry Section of Kunming Medical College. Selected Information (Kunming Medical College) 1978 (2):86.

13. Dongshan Health Clinic of Yaoan County. Yunnan Yiyao (Yunnan Medical Journal), 1974 (2):57.

14. Internal Medicine Department, 64th Hospital of the Chinese PLA. Xinyiyaoxue Zazhi (Journal of Traditional Chinese Medicine) 1976 (11):24.

15. Rheumatoid Arthritis Research Group, First Teaching Hospital of Kunming Medical College. Zhonghua Yixue Zazhi (National Medical Journal of China) 1976 (6):384.

16. Shu SY et al. Chinese Traditional and Herbal Drugs Communications 1978 9(12):27.

17. Wound and Fracture Department, OPD of Longhua Teaching Hospital et al. Chinese Traditional and Herbal Drugs Communications 1978 (6):33.

18. Yang BC et al. Shanghai Zhongyiyao Zazhi (Shanghai Journal of Traditional Chinese Medicine) 1979 (1):33.

19. Rheumatoid Arthritis Ward, Guanghua Hospital of Shanghai. Summary of the clinical use of Tripterygium hypoglaucum in rheumatoid arthritis. 1978.

20. Traditional Chinese Medicine Department, First Teaching Hospital of Kunming Medical College et al. Selected Information (Kunming Medical College) 1976 (1):19.

21. Zhu YL et al. Chinese Traditional and Herbal Drugs 1979 10(12):26.

22. Shu SY. Chinese Traditional and Herbal Drugs 1980 11(1):33.

23. Dermatology Department, First Teaching Hospital of Kunming Medical College. Dermatological Research Communications 1978 (1):5.

24. Shen JS. Xinyiyaoxue Zazhi (Journal of Traditional Chinese Medicine) 1979 (3):36.

25. Dermatology Department, First Teaching Hospital of Kunming Medical College. Acta Academiae Medicinae Kunming 1980 (1):60.

26. Sichuan Institute of Dermatology. Sichuan Achievements in Medicine and Health. Sichuan Centre of Medical and Technological Information. 1979. p. 57.

27. Sichuan Institute of Dermatology. Dermatological Research Communications 1978 (1):9.

28. Yang MB et al. Selected Information (Kunming Medical College) 1979 (4):21.

29. Yang MB et al. Selected Information (Kunming Medical College) 1979 (4):78.

30. Endocrinology Section of the Internal Medicine Department, First Teaching Hospital of Kunming Medical College. Selected Information (Kunming Medical College) 1976 (1):25.

31. Tumor Department, First Teaching Hospital of Kunming Medical College. Selected Information 1977 (2):27.

32. Shu SY. Acta Academiae Medicinae Kunming 1980 (3):38.

(Deng Wenlong)

LUOBUMA 羅布麻

<Luobuma>, also called <Zeqima>, is the whole plant of *Apocynum* Linn. (Apocynaceae). While two sources of the herb have been confirmed, viz., *A. lancifolium* Russam and *A. hendersonii* Hook., much of the current research is concentrated on *A. lancifolium* (1–3).

<Luobuma> tastes bitter and pungent and has a slightly "cold" property. It is able to r relieve intense "heat", and is credited with hypotensive, cardiotonic, and diuretic activities. The herb is recommended for hypertension, heart diseases, neurosis, and edema in nephritis.

CHEMICAL COMPOSITION

The root of *A. apocynum* contains four cardiotonic agents: cymarin, strophanthidin, K-strophanthin-β and an unknown acetyl compound with mp 167–169.5°C (4). The root also contains α-amyrin lupeol and p-hydroxyacetophenone (5).

The stem contains cardiac glycosides, lauric acid, isoquercitroside (isoquercitrin), quercetin (6,7), phenolic compounds, sterols, steroid saponins and triterpenoides (6).

PHARMACOLOGY

1. Effect on Cardiac Contractility and Heart Rate

Intravenous injection of the root decoction to anesthetized cats at 0.05–0.2 g/kg did not increase the contractility of the normal heart, but significantly increased the contractility of the heart weakened by pentobarbital sodium poisoning. Its action resembled that of K-strophanthin 0.042–0.084 mg/kg by intravenous injection (8). Two minutes after intravenous injection of the 8% root decoction to dogs and cats at 0.05–0.2 g/kg, decrease of the heart rate was seen on the ECG, became very distinct in 10–20 minutes and gradually recovered after 30 minutes. Intragastric administration of this decoction to dogs or cats at 0.4 g/kg decreased the heart rate on the ECG; a 12.6% reduction was obtained after 1 dose, 30% after 3 doses, and 50% after 5 doses (8). There is also a report that intravenous injection of the leaf decoction 0.25 g/kg, or the flavonoid glycoside from the leaf 10–15 mg/kg to dogs markedly decreased the heart rate on the ECG 1–10 minutes after medication. The heart rate was reverted to normal after 30 minutes. When the dose of the decoction was increased to 1 g/kg, or that of the flavonoid glycosides to 20 mg/kg, arrhythmia, ST depression, and distorted T waves appeared, suggesting that both agents were toxic to the heart (9).

When the concentration of the cardiotonic component of the root reached 1:60,000, the contraction amplitude of the isolated frog heart was doubled, the heart was markedly slowed down, and finally cardiac arrest occurred at the mid-systolic phase. Perfusion of the same agent to isolated frog hearts at the concentration of 1:40,000 promptly triggered arrhythmia, conduction block, and cardiac arrest at the systolic phase (10). When this cardiotonic component was injected intravenously to anesthetized cats at 0.64–0.82 mg/kg, cardiac contractility was enhanced and the heart rate was reduced (from 190 to 168 beats/min) 1.5 minutes later; arrhythmia developed after 15 minutes; and after 30 minutes, the atria stopped at the diastolic phase ahead of the ventricles; and typical ventricular fibrillation developed before ventricular arrest (10,11). In the case of cat hearts weakened by pentobarbital sodium poisoning, intravenous injection of the cardiotonic component at a dose of 0.25 mg/kg increased the contraction amplitude after 3–6 minutes; 20 minutes later 50–70% of the original measurement was recovered. The action of the cardiotonic component was weaker than that of K-strophanthin (11). Two minutes after intravenous injection of the cardiotonic component to cats at 1.55 mg/kg, the ECG showed flat and inverted T waves, and prolonged P-P interval; some animals failed to recover after 24 or even after 72 hours (10). In cats intravenous infusion of the 6% cardiac glycoside solution of the root at 1 ml per minute resulted 10 minutes later in the decrease of heart rate on the ECG, which became more pronounced after 20 minutes. Cove-shaped digitalis effect appeared which was followed by ventricular tachycardia, multifocal premature beats, ventricular flutter, ventricular fibrillation, and death (11).

2. Effect on Coronary Flow and Myocardial Oxygen Consumption

Intravenous injection of the root decoction at 0.05–0.2 g/kg to anesthetized cats, or of the cardiac glycoside of the root at 0.2 mg/kg to anesthetized dogs, resulted 10–20 minutes later in an increase in the coronary flow and a slight increase in myocardial oxygen consumption. However, these changes were statistically insignificant (8,11).

3. Effect on Blood Pressure

Intravenous injection of the leaf decoction to dogs or cats at 0.25 g/kg markedly lowered the blood pressure to 69.4% of the normal level. Intravenous injection of the flavonoid glycosides of the leaf to dogs or cats at 5–15 mg/kg also reduced the blood pressure by 12.6–36.7%. The hypotensive action of a single dose lasted 3–10 minutes. Tachyphylaxis developed with the flavonoid glycosides but not with the decoction (9).

When the leaf decoction was intragastrically administered to dogs with experimental renal hypertension at 1, 5 and 10 g/kg, it was found that the 1-g dose produced a poor hypotensive effect, whereas the 5-g dose lowered the blood pressure form 194/140 to 152/100 mmHg after 2 hours for 3 days (12). Perfusion of the flavonoid glycosides into the blood vessels of isolated rabbit auricles at 5 mg caused marked vasodilation, suggesting that the hypotensive mechanism is related to direct vasodilation (9).

Intravenous injection of the cardiac glycosides of the root to anesthetized dogs at 0.2 mg/kg slightly increased the blood pressure (11).

4. Effect on Smooth Muscles

At the concentration of 1:1000, the leaf decoction did not significantly modify the amplitude and frequency of the contraction of isolated smooth muscles of rat uteri, whereas at 1:2000 it significantly reduced the amplitude and frequency of the contraction of isolated rabbit intestines and rat uteri (9).

5. Miscellaneous Actions

The leaf decoction at 0.25 g/kg SC given to mice did not produce significant sedation; the same dosage intravenously administered to rabbits did not increase the urine output during 30 minutes of observation (9).

6. Toxicity

The LD of the root decoction in cats was 0.46±0.12 g/kg (10). The LD_{50} of the leaf decoction in mice was 10.6 g/kg IP or 66.9 g/kg PO (12). No significant difference from the control group was observed after a single oral administration of the leaf decoction to rats at 15, 30, or 50 g/kg during 2 weeks of observation (12). The LD_{50} of the flavonoid glycosides in mice was 398 mg/kg IP (9). The average LD of the cardiac glycosides of the root in cats was 3.2 mg/kg (10); another paper, however, reported it to be 0.8 mg/kg (11). In cats killed by intravenous injection of the cardiac glycosides at 1.55 mg/kg (about one-half the LD) plus supplementary doses given at 1, 1.5 and 3 days after the injection, drug accumulation was 61.7% in 1 day, 58% in 1.5 days, and 34.3% in 3 days (8). Another report also showed the mean drug accumulation one day after medication to be 67±9.9% (11).

CLINICAL STUDIES

1. Chronic Cardiac Insufficiency

The 8% root decoction 100 ml twice daily, or the fluidextract of the root 5 ml (containing 8 g of the crude drug) twice daily was given. When the heart had slowed down, the patients were given the decoction 50 ml once daily or the fluidextract 3 ml. In 62 cases so treated, 50 cases had marked effects, 10 moderate effects and 2 were unchanged (13,14). Fifty cases of chronic congestive heart failure were treated similarly, achieving marked effects in 31 cases, moderate effects in 16 and no response in 3 (8,15). The fluidextract of the root was reported to be effective in 5 cases of rheumatic heart disease with heart failure and 3 cases of hypertensive heart disease with heart failure, but ineffective in 2 cases of pulmonary heart desease (16).

2. Edema

When the root 12–15 g was given every day as a decoction in two doses to 34 cases of edema of various etiologies (renal edema 10 cases, cardiac edema 10 case, edema of liver cirrhosis 6 cases, edema due to pregnancy 5 cases, and others 3 cases), 10 cases obtained marked effects and 19 cases moderate effects (17). This decoction was tried in 30 cases of acute nephritis with edema. The edema began to subside on the 4th day of medication; in 27 cases edema subsided completely on the 10th day, and in the remaining 3, it disappeared within 12 days after medication (18).

3. Hypertension

The tea, prepared by boiling 3–6 g of the leaves, was administered to 196 hypertensive patients of whom 169 had never taken any other antihypertensive drugs. Abatement or disappearance of symptoms was observed in 81.7%, and various degrees of reduction in the blood pressure were seen in 70.4%. In 427 patients unresponsive to other antihypertensive remedies, the tea produced symptomatic relief or improvement in 76.8%, and different degrees of blood pressure reduction in 68.4%. It was also proved clinically that the effective rate of the tea increased with the duration of the treatment, but that the history of illness had no significant effect (19). Two hundred and eleven hypertensive patients were concurrently treated with the tea and two doses (noon and evening) of the leaf decoction daily for a course of 4–8 weeks. This scheme produced marked effects in 104 cases, moderate effects in 60 cases, and no response in 47 cases; the aggregate effective rate was 77.7% (20). The leaf extract tablet alone, or combined with other antihypertensive drugs such as verticil (chiefly containing reserpine) was also effective for the various stages of hypertension (21).

The syrup prepared from the aerial part of *A. hendersonii* was administered to 100 cases of hypertension at 10 ml thrice daily. It was effective in 71% and ineffective in 29% (22).

4. Chronic Bronchitis

The cigarette prepared from the leaves is reported to be useful in preventing and treating chronic bronchitis. It was effective in cough, asthma, expectoration, symptomatic improvement, and recovery of physical strength (23,24).

5. Common Cold

The prophylactic use of the 20% decoction 50–100 ml twice daily or of the 50% herb injection 2 ml (corresponding to 1 g of the crude drug) intramuscularly 2–3 times daily in 184 persons decreased the incidence of common cold by 52.2%. The cure rate in 120 cases reached 89.2% (25).

ADVERSE EFFECTS

The adverse effects of the decoction or fluidextract by mouth include nausea, vomiting, diarrhea, upper abdominal discomfort, and possibly bradycardia and premature beats (10,13,14,22). The cigarette prepared from the herb may cause headache, dizziness, cough, nausea, and insomnia (23).

REFERENCE

1. Dong ZJ. Luobuma. Science Press. 1958.

2. Editorial Group. General Uses of Luobuma. Science Press. 1978.

3. Wei MJ. Xinyiyaoxue Zazhi (Journal of Traditional Chinese Medicine) 1978 (3):47.

4. Xu C et al. Acta Pharmaceutica Sinica 1966 13(8):589.

5. Cheng DL et al. Journal of Lanzhou University 1979 (4):85.

6. Qian XS et al. The References of Traditional Chinese Medicine 1975 (2):31.

7. Zhang ZJ et al. Chinese Traditional and Herbal Drugs Communications 1974 (1):21.

8. Shaanxi Coordinating Research Group on Coronary Disease. Shaanxi Medical Journal 1974 (5):10.

9. Shaanxi Coordinating Research Group on Coronary Disease. Xinyiyaoxue Zazhi (Journal of Traditional Chinese Medicine) 1975 (2):45.

10. Shao YD et al. Acta Pharmaceutica Sinica 1962 9(7):413.

11. Shaanxi Coordinating Research Group on Coronary Disease. Shaanxi Medical Journal 1974 (6):56.

12. Shanghai Institute of Materia Medica, Chinese Academy of Sciences. Research on the Medicinal Uses of Luobuma. Part I. 1972. p. 11.

13. First Teaching Hospital of Xi' an Medical College. Research on the Medicinal Uses of Luobuma. 1972. p. 13.

14. First Teaching Hospital of Xi' an Medical College. Shaanxi Medical Journal 1973 (4):8.

15. Shaanxi Coordinating Research Group on Coronary Disease. Chinese Medical Journal 1975 55(2):269.

16. Sanyuan County (Shaanxi) Hospital. Research on the Medicinal Uses of Luobuma. Part I. 1972. p. 19.

17. First Teaching Hospital of Xi' an Medical College. Research on the Medicinal Uses of Luobuma. Part I. 1972. p. 27.

18. Sanyuan County (Shaanxi) Hospital. Research on the Medicinal Uses of Luobuma. Part I. 1972. p. 30.

19. <Luobuma> Experimental Farm of Xianyang, Northwest Institute of Botany. Chinese Traditional and Herbal Drugs Communications 1972 (4):12.

20. Cardiovascular Diseases Prevention and Treatment Pilot Area of Yancheng County et al. Henan Scientific and Technological References 1977 (6):18.

21. Cardiovascular Section of the Internal Medicine Department, Teaching Hospital of Xinjiang Medical College. New Medical Communications (Xinjiang) 1975 (15):61.

22. Qinghai College of Traditional Chinese Medicine. Health Journal of Qinghai 1974 (1):41.

23. Health Clinic of Shijingshan Electric Company (Beijing). General Uses of Luobuma. Science Press. 1978. p. 100.

24. Health Clinic of Shijingshan Electric Company (Beijing) et al. General Uses of Luobuma. Science Press. 1978. p. 104.

25. 371st Hospital of Wuhan Military Region of the Chinese PLA. General Uses of Loubuma. Science Press. 1978. p. 73.

(Bao Dingyuan)

ZHIMU 知母

<Zhimu> is the rhizome of *Anemarrhena asphodeloides* Bunge (Liliaceae). Bitter to the taste and "cold", it is reputed to have latent-heat-clearing, antipyretic, and tranquilizing effects as well as "lung-heat"-purgative and "kidney"-nourishing actions. It is used to quench thirst due to fever, in dry cough and hectic fever.

CHEMICAL COMPOSITION

The rhizome of *A. asphodeloides* contains about 6% of saponins, of which timosaponins A-I, A-II, A-III, A-IV, B-I, and B-II were isolated and named. Sarsasapogenin is the major aglycone of the saponins of the rhizome and its amount in the dried root is about 0.5%. Timosaponin A-III is a diglyceride of sarsasapogenin and timobiose (β-glucose-(1→2)-β-galactose). Timosaponin A-I is sarsasaponin-β-0-pyranogalactoside. The rhizome also contains markogenin, neogitogenin, chimonin (mangiferin) and isomangiferin.

PHARMACOLOGY

1. Antipyretic Effect

Injection of the extract of *A. asphodeloides* rhizome 4 g/kg SC to rabbits prevented and treated hyperpyrexia due to *Escherichia coli*; its action was prolonged (1).

2. Effect on Adrenocortical Hormones

Mean plasma corticosterone level was significantly increased in rabbits following intragastric administration of the rhizomes of *Rehmannia glutinosa*, *Anemarrhena asphodeloides* and *Glycyrrhiza uralensis* plus dexamethasone, or after concurrent dosing of one, two or all of these herbs with dexamethasone for 5 days. The most significant effect was produced by the rhizome of *A. asphodeloides*. In the absence of adrenocortical hormones, plasma corticosterone level of rabbits was not significantly modified by these herbs whether used individually or in combination. Thus, the incremental effect on plasma corticosterone is not attributed to the simple promotion of ACTH secretion by the anterior pituitary nor to a direct action in the adrenal cortex (2).

In normal subjects with no liver diseases or endocrine disorders continuous administration of the rhizomes of *R. glutinosa*, *A. asphodeloides* and *G. uralensis* for 1–3 days, followed by concomitant use of these herbs with dexamethasone for 2 nights, antagonized the inhibitory effect of dexamethasone on the early-morning peak plasma cortisol level. Fourteen cases of nephrotic syndrome were given 30 g of the rhizome of *R. glutinosa*, and 9 g each of the rhizomes of *A. asphodeloides* and *G. uralensis* daily for 1–3 days, followed by a regimen of steroids and the herbs for 2 weeks on average. Eight out of these treated cases registered negative for urinary protein after treatment. In most cases the side effects of the steroids — moon face, mental excitation and insomnia — were mitigated (3). *In vitro* studies prove that the rhizome of *A. asphodeloides* weakened the ring-opening reduction at the $C_{4:5}$ double bond in cortisol and reduced the changes in the two hydroxyl groups on $C_{17,20}$ and in the ketone group on C_{20}. As it prevented the reduction of the $C_{4:5}$ double bond and C_3 ketone group in the A ring cortisol and the degradation of the hydroxyl groups on C_{17} and C_{21} and of the ketone group on C_{20} of the side chain, the herb was thus able to retard the catabolism of cortisol by the liver cells (4). These experimental results explain why medicines that are reputed to nourish the "yin" and relieve intense "heat", such as the rhizome of *A. asphodeloides*, are able to prevent the suppression of the adrenal cortex by exogenous cortical hormones. They also indicate that one of the regulatory actions of these medicines is to directly modulate the corticosteroid level in the blood.

3. Antibacterial Effect

The 100% *A. asphodeloides* rhizome decoction was shown to inhibit many kinds of pathogenic organisms *in vitro* (5,6). The inhibitory effect of the ethanol extract, the ether extract, and the crude crystal obtained by treating the ether extract with acetone was strongest against *Mycobacterium tuberculosis* var. *hominis* $H_{37}RV$ in Proskauer-Beck medium. The MIC of the ethanol extract against this bacteria *in vitro* was 1:8000 irrespective of the presence or absence of serum. For the ether extract, the MIC without the serum was 1:64,000 and with serum 1:16,000. The MIC of the crude crystal was 1:16,000 without serum and 1:8000 with serum. the ether extract showed a stronger antitubercular action, whereas the saponins were inactive (7).

Optimal therapeutic effects were achieved in guinea pigs with experimental tuberculosis, given feeds containing the herb (3%) for 3–4 months; the pulmonary lesions were found to be one-third to one-half of those seen in the control (8). However, in mice with experimental tuberculosis, the mortality rate was not reduced although the animals showed milder pulmonary lesions than the control. When the proportion of the herb in the feed was increased to 5%, the mortality rate of the test animals was paradoxically even higher than that of the control, although the pulmonary tuberculosis index approximated that of isoniazid. This effect could be due to the toxicity of the herb itself (9). The 8–20% herb decoction inhibited common pathogenic skin fungi in Sabouraud agar (10). The 100% decoction also inhibited *Candida albicans* (11).

4. Effect on Blood Glucose

The aqueous extract of *A. asphodeloides* rhizome could lower the blood glucose level in normal rabbits. The action was more marked in rabbits with alloxan-induced diabetes mellitus (12,13). This extract injected at 0.15 g/kg IP to mice with alloxan-induced diabetes mellitus lowered blood glucose by 200 mg% in 5 hours and reduced urinary ketone bodies. Intraperitoneal injection of the extract of White Tiger Decoction of Ginseng (Rhizome Anemarrhenae, Radix Ginseng, Radix Glycyrrhizae) to mice with experimental diabetes mellitus at 0.5–1 g/kg also afforded a hypoglycemic effect; the blood glucose level was lowered by 120 mg% 6 hours after medication (14).

The herb did not promote glucose oxidation in normal rats, but it enhanced glucose uptake in the diaphragm and adipose tissues, increasing phrenic glycogen but reducing liver glycogen (15). However, early reports claimed that the dried extract of the herb injected into rabbits at 6 g/kg did not affect the blood glucose level (16), whereas the ethanol extract increased it (17).

5. Miscellaneous Actions

The original neutral herb fluidextract injected intravenously to rabbits at a dose of 0.5 ml had no effect on the blood pressure and respiration, whereas the 1–2 ml doses inhibited respiration and slightly lowered the blood pressure, and the 7-ml dose depressed the respiratory center and lowered the blood pressure, resulting in death. The herb extract at the concentration of 0.01% had no significant effect on the toad heart, whereas the 0.01–0.1% extract weakened cardiac contraction, and the 1% extract induced cardiac arrest. No significant action was exhibited by the herb extract on the isolated uteri of pregnant rabbits (1).

CLINICAL STUDIES

1. Epidemic Hemorrhagic Fever

One hundred and thirty patients, most with mild and moderate symptoms and 10 with shock and renal failure, were treated with the White Tiger Decoction; 115 cases were given the oral dose, 6 cases the intramuscular injection, and 9 cases the intravenous injection for a course of 3–7 days. While fever subsided in 2.9 days on average, which was not much different from the average obtained in the groups treated with other medicines, there was nevertheless a marked reduction in the intensity of fever, and 91.5% of the cases, with a temperature of over 40°C, had a normal body temperature within 2 days of medication. Marked improvement of generalized toxic symptoms was attained in most patients, and none developed profuse bleeding. One patient died, the mortality rate being 0.8%. The average period of hospitalization was 21.1 days (18).

2. Encephalitis B

Therapeutic effects were achieved in 132 cases by intravenous infusion of the Encephalitis Injection (Radix Isatidis, Folium Isatidis, Fructus Forsythiae, Rhizome Phragmitis, Gypsum Fibrosum, Rhizoma Anemarrhenae, Radix Rehmanniae, berberine, Radix Curcumae) (19).

3. Pulmonary Tuberculosis with Hectic Fever

The herb can be given as a decoction at 6–15 g daily (20).

4. Diabetes Mellitus

The decoction of the herb, the root of *Trichosanthes kirilowii*, the root tuber of *Ophiopogon japonicus*, each 12 g, and the rhizome of *Coptis chinensis* 4.5 g may be given by mouth (20).

5. Chronic Bronchitis ("Heat" Type)

The decoction of the herb, the root of *Scutellaria baicalensis*, the root bark of *Morus alba*, the sclerotium of *Poria cocos*, the root tuber of *Ophiopogon japonicus* each 9 g, the root of *Platycodon grandiflorum* and the root and rhizome of *Glyryrrhiza uralensis* each 3 g may be given by mouth (20).

6. Acute Infectious Diseases

In cases of high fever, prolonged sweating, thirst, smooth and solid pulse, White Tiger Decoction (Rhizome Anemarrhenae 15 g, Gypsum Fibrosum 30 g, Radix Glycyrrhizae 6 g) is recommended (20).

REFERENCE

1. Jing LB. Chinese Reports of the Institute of Physiology (National Peiping Research Institute) 1935 (2):39.
2. Chen RQ et al. Acta Academiae Medicinae Primae Shanghai 1979 (6):393.
3. Shen ZY et al. Acta Academiae Medicinae Primae Shanghai 1979 (5):313.
4. Zhang LL et al. Acta Academiae Medicinae Primae Shanghai 1980 7(1):37.
5. Liu GS et al. Chinese Journal of New Medicine 1950 1(2):95.
6. Liao YX. Bulletin of Northwestern Veterinary College 1953 (4):5.
7. Pharmacology Section, Yanbian Medical College. Papers of Yanbian Medical College. 2nd edition. 1963. p. 52.
8. Wang JG et al. Acta Academiae Medicinae Lanzhou 1962 (1):79.
9. Feng YQ. Acta Academiae Medicinae Primae Shanghai 1964 2(2):241.
10. Sun X. Chinese Journal of Dermatology 1958 (3):210.
11. Medical Laboratory, First Teaching Hospital of Wuhan Medical College et al. Xinyiyaoxue Zazhi (Journal of Traditional Chinese Medicine) 1973 (5):28.
12. Pharmacology Section, Shandong Medical College. Pharmacology of Chinese Traditional Drugs. 1976 p. 144.

13. Eda et al. Japan Centra Revuo Medicina 1972 285:572.

14. Kimura M. Japan Centra Revuo Medicina 1966 221:265.

15. Nagata E. Japan Centra Revuo Medicina 1971 276:347.

16. Jing LB. Chinese Reports of the Institute of Physiology (National Peiping Research Institute) 1936 (3):8.

17. Piungki M. Chemical Abstracts 1931 25:1286.

18. Health Team of the 43rd Battalion, 4th Division of the Production and Construction Corps of Heilongjiang Military Region. Heilongjiang Yiyao (Heilongjiang Medical Journal) 1976 (1):31.

19. Combined Western and Traditional Chinese Medicine Unit, Chongqing Hospital of Infectious Diseases. Chongqing Yiyao (Chongqing Medical Journal) 1973 (4):47.

20. Zhu Y. Pharmacology and Applications of Chinese Medicinal Materials. People's Medical Publishing House. 1958. p. 172.

(Yuan Wei)

CHUIPENCAO 垂盆草

<Chuipencao> is the plant *Sedum sarmentosum* Bunge (Crassulaceae). Also known as <Fojiacao> or <Shuyabanzhilian>, this herb has a sweet, bland and slightly sour taste, and a "cool" property. It is attributed with latent-heat-clearing, antipyretic, diuretic, detoxicant and anti-inflammatory actions. Hence, it is a recommended remedy for chronic persisting hepatitis, carbuncle and deep-rooted ulcer.

CHEMICAL COMPOSITION

S. sarmentosum mainly contains carbohydrates, cyanophoric glycosides, amino acids, flavonoids, triterpenes and phytosterols. The amino acids are mainly 1-asparagine, 1-aspartic acid, 1-α-alanine, 1-levcine, 1-tyrosine, and 1-valine.

PHARMACOLOGY

1. Liver-Protective Effect

S. sarmentosum administered to mice at 0.33 g(crude drug)/day PO for 6 days reduced hepatic necrosis due to carbon tetrachloride poisoning (1). The herb also significantly protected rats from subacute liver damage due to carbon tetrachloride; he treatment group showed markedly lower levels of γ-globulin and milder liver fibrosis than the control (1,2). The water-soluble fraction of the dilute ethanol extract markedly decreased SGPT and sodium bromsulphalein retention in rats with subacute liver damage (3). There are data indicating that amino acids were the active principles responsible for reducing SGPT, and that although the alkaloids were also active, they did not protect liver from carbon tetrachloride-induced liver damage as the amino acids did (4,5). In experimental acute icteric hepatitis produced by administration of pentobarbital sodium prior to carbon tetrachloride poisoning, the serum bilirubin level in the control group was 1.6 mg%, whereas in the *S. sarmentosum* treatment group it was 0.5 mg% (3).

Pathological changes in mice resembling the "autoimmune type" of hepatitis were induced using hepatocellular membrane extract of heterogenous animals as antigen. Serum was collected in the 2nd, 5th, and 9th weeks after immunization for counter-immunoelectrophoresis. Examination of the liver slices revealed hyperplasia of Kuppfer' s cells, infiltration of neutrophils and monocytes at the portal area, and punctate necrosis, indicating that *S. sarmentosum* had no significant effect on the pathological changes (3). Determination of the bile flow in rats by catheterizing the common bile duct did not show any choleretic action from this herb. Also, *S. sarmentosum* had no significant effect on the weights of the thymus and spleen of mice (3).

2. Antibacterial Effect

In vitro, S. sarmentosum injection at concentrations over 1:50 strongly inhibited *Staphylococcus albus*, and to a lesser extent, *Staphylococcus aureus* (6). No bacteriostatic action was exhibited by its components — triterpenes, phytosterols, cyanophoric glycosides, and alkaloids. The distillate injection, containing 2 g of the crude drug per ml, was active against *Staphylococcus aureus, Staphylococcus albus, Escherichia coli, Salmonella typhi, Pseudomonas aeruginosa*, alpha streptococcus, beta streptococcus, *Candida albicans*, and *Shigella flexneri* (7).

3. Toxicity

The LD_{50} of the fluidextract of *S. sarmentosum* in mice was 54.2 g/kg IP. Intragastric administration of the fluidextract to dogs at 30 g/kg/day for 8 weeks produced vomiting and diarrhea, but no abnormalities in the blood picture, GPT, bilirubin, urea nitrogen and serum protein, and no distinct pathological changes in the various organs. Based on these findings, and clinical dosages (2), it can be said that *S. sarmentosum* has a low toxicity.

CLINICAL STUDIES

1. Acute and Chronic Hepatitis

One thousand cases of acute and chronic hepatitis were treated with the tablets prepared from the fresh or dried herb (total daily dose of 250 and 30 g, respectively) thrice daily for 2 weeks. Consequently, SGPT was normalized in 73.6%, improved in 14..8% and unchanged in 11.6% (8). The "Jingchui Tablet" (each containing about 8 mg of *S. sarmentosum* glycoside) was used to treat 200 cases of chronic hepatitis at the dosage of 9 tablets daily. It normalized the transaminase level of 167 cases (82%) within 2 weeks but failed to alter significantly other parameters of the liver function (TT, ZNZ, SB, A/C. γ-G), nor did it cause the disappearance of HBAg (2). The "Jingchui Tablet" was also used in 54 cases of intractable chronic persisting hepatitis at a dose of 90 mg glycoside per day for a course of 2 months. Transaminase examination revealed that the medication produced marked effects in 47 cases and moderate effects in 7 cases. Thymol turbidity was normalized in 65.2% and zinc turbidity in 37.3%. No significant changes in the post-treatment γ-globulin and HBAg measurements were observed. However, the lymphocyte transformation rate, the phagocytic rate and the phagocytic index of macrophages in the treated patients were markedly decreased, suggesting that the effectiveness of *S. sarmentosum* is a result of transient suppression of the cellular immunity. Consequently, most patients relapsed 6 months after discontinuation of the medication (2). In anther paper, a transient therapeutic effect was achieved with the syrup prepared from *S. sarmentosum* and <Pingdimu> in the treatment of chronic persisting hepatitis (9), but it was not comparable to that obtained from *S. sarmentosum* used alone.

2. Corneal Ulcer and Prevention of Infection in Eye Operations

For surface anesthesia dicaine was instilled into the diseased eye, then the *S. sarmentosum* injection 0.8 ml in 2% procaine 0.4 ml was injected into the lower bulbar conjunctiva. Treatment was given once daily for 5 days as a therapeutic course; vitamins were given as adjuvant therapy. Out of 92 cases of corneal ulcers of various etiologies so treated, 45 were essentially cured, 39 improved and 8 cases unchanged. And, of 95 cases of intraocular operation in which the lower bulbar conjunctiva was injected with the *S. sarmentosum* injection 1 ml postoperatively, in addition to sulfamethoxypyridazine 0.5 g/day PO for 4 days, none developed postoperative infection (7).

3. Miscellaneous

It was reported that the crushed fresh herb used as a local dressing is an effective treatment for viper bites and insect stings.

REFERENCE

1. Shanghai Institute of Traditional Chinese Medicine. Scientific Papers (1966–75) (Shanghai College of Traditional Chinese Medicine) 1978 (11):90.

2. Shanghai Institute of Scientific and Technological Information. Shanghai Compilation of New Drugs Confirmed in 1976. Shanghai Sci-Tech Literature Publishing House. 1977. p. 127.

3. Li XY. Abstracts of the First National Symposium of the Society of Pharmacology. 1979. p. 59.

4. Scientific Information Unit, Ministry of Petrochemical Industry. Developments in Chinese Traditional Drugs (Hunan Institute of Medical and Pharmaceutical Industry) 1977 (8):4.

5. Pathology Department, 178th Hospital of the Chinese PLA. Compiled Information on Clinical Pathology. Coordinating Research Group on Pathology of Fuzhou Military Region. 1977. p. 80.

6. Wu GJ. New Chinese Medicine 1975 (3):145.

7. Wu GJ. Wuhu Yiyao (Wuhu Medical Journal) 1978 (2):64.

8. Shanghai Institute of Traditional Chinese Medicine et al. Medical Exchanges (Chinese Medical Association, Shanghai Branch) 1973 (7):27.

9. Lin YY. New Chinese Medicine 1974 5(7):324.

(Wen Zhijian)

SHIJUNZI 使君子

<Shijunzi> is the ripe fruit of *Quisqualis indica* L., or *Q. indica* L. var. *villosa* Clarke (Combretaceae). It has a sweet taste and "warm" property. Its actions are considered to be anthelmintic, digestant, and "spleen"-invigorative. It is prescribed in abdominal pain due to ascariasis, malnutrition in children due to improper feeding, infantile dyspepsia, and in abdominal distention of dysentery.

CHEMICAL COMPOSITION

The ripe fruit contains potassium quisqualata, large amounts of fixed oil, 20–27%, trigonelline, and pyridine. The shell and leaf also contain potassium quisqualata.

PHARMACOLOGY

1. Ascaricidal Effect

<Shijunzi> is a commonly used effective traditional Chinese folk remedy for ascariasis. *In vitro* studies showed that it strongly inhibited the earthworm, leech, and swine ascarides. For instance, it was reported that the 10% aqueous extract of this herb comatized or killed earthworms within 2 hours of contact, whereas the 95% ethanol extract was inactive (1). The 50% ethanol extracts of 20 kinds of Chinese herbs were studied for their lethal effect on the swine ascaris, earthworm and leech. <Shijunzi> topped the list of 8 herbs including the fruit of *Carpesium abrotanoides*, the processed fruit of *Ulmus macrocarpa*, the seed of *Areca catechu*, the rhizome of *Dryopteris crassirhizoma*, the fruit of *Melia toosendan*, the sclerotium of *Polyporus mylittae*, and the ripe fruit of *Evodia rutaecarpa* (2). Kymocyclography of swine ascaris head revealed that the extract of the kernel produced a strong paralyzing effect often preceded by excitation. The active principle was water-soluble; the concentrated ethanol, petroleum ether, and chloroform extracts as well as the ash of the kernel were all inactive (3). Most authors considered that the active principle was potassium quisqualata (4–7). This constituent exerted a significant inhibitory effect against the whole swine ascaris *in vitro*, but failed to kill them (6). Clinical studies also showed that the anti-ascaris activity of potassium quisqualata was similar to that of the fresh or baked kernel (7). Quisqualic acid, which was first obtained by Japanese workers from *Q. indica* L. var. *villosa* (8), was also found to be markedly active against the intact swine ascaris by causing dyskinesia; the MIC was 1:1000 (9). Some authors, however, isolated pyridine and its analogues (about 1/1000) from <Shijunzi> which have been shown to have vermicidal and anthelmintic effects. Thus, the anti-ascaris action of <Shijunzi> is probably due to these compounds (10). Another report claims that the mixture of the <Shijunzi> oil and castor oil has a marked anti-ascaris activity (11).

2. Oxyurifugal Effect

The <Shijunzi> powder, or the powder of <Shijunzi> and <Baibu> (*S. japonica*) exhibited an oxyurifugal action in mice naturally infected with pinworms (*Enterobius vermicularis*). The <Shijunzi> powder was ineffective against young worms; the mixed powder was slightly effective (12).

3. Effect on Skin Fungi

In vitro, the aqueous extract of <Shijunzi> inhibited to different extents the following skin fungi: *Trichophyton violaceum*, *Trichophyton concentricum*, Schlemm's *Dermatophyton favosa*, *Microsporum audouini*, *Microsporum ferrugineum*, *Microsporum lanosum*, *Epidermatophyton inguinale*, and *Nocardia asteroides* (13).

4. Toxicity

<Shijunzi> is not very toxic, but significant toxic reactions have been noted with parenteral administration. In an early report, subcutaneous injection of the water-soluble extract of the herb to mice produced marked toxic reactions within a few minutes, and after 1–2 hours, mild generalized spasm and respiratory failure leading to death. The MLD was about 20 g/kg (14). Oral administration of the crude preparation of <Shijunzi> to dogs at 26.6 g/kg caused depression, hiccup, and vomiting; the same reactions were observed with the resin of the herb administered at 0.83 g/kg. However, the oil extracted from <Shijunzi> had no toxic effects except mild diarrhea (15). No toxic manifestations were noted in mice or rabbits after intragastric administration of this oil 5–10 g/kg (11).

CLINICAL STUDIES

1. Ascariasis

Satisfactory therapeutic effects can be achieved with the use of <Shijunzi> in ascariasis. Usually the crude or stir-fried herb, or the herb decoction is given by mouth. The leaf decoction is also effective. Clinical reports of the therapeutic effect of <Shijunzi> on ascariasis are numerous (1,16–26). Summarizing 12 of these papers, an author reported the following data: 30 to 86% of treated cases usually expelled worms, and 30–40% registered negative for the ova in the stool examination (a minimum of 15.4%); the therapeutic effect depended on the freshness of the drug, method of use and dosage; taking the decoction was less effective than chewing the herb; one large dose was better than divided doses, and 2–3 days of medication was less effective than one single dose; the therapeutic effect was directly proportional to the dosage, and the fresh herb was superior to the old; magnesium sulfate or sodium sulfate 3 hours after <Shijunzi> potentiated the therapeutic effect; the recommended dosage was 1 g per year of age with a maximum dosage of 16 g (27). A report claimed that the effect of <Shijunzi> was improved and its side effects reduced when it was combined with the seed of *Areca catechu* (18). Potassium quisqualata 0.125 g PO without purgatives was 82% effective for ascariasis; a slightly higher percentage was achieved with santonin (7).

2. Oxyuriasis

<Shijunzi> is reported to be quite effective in oxyuriasis; it killed all the worms which were then expelled with stool. *Dosage and administration*: patient's age plus one = dosage in grams, twice daily for 3 days; or children 3–15 pills/day, adults 15–30 pills/day divided in 3 doses, for 15 days. A second course of 15 days was given after a one month interval (17,28–30).

3. Intestinal Trichomoniasis

<Shijunzi> stir-fried to yellow color, or in powder form, is taken by mouth. *Dosage and administration*: under 1 year, 3 g/day in 1–2 doses; 1–3 years 4.5 g/day; adults 15 g/day. A course lasts 3 to 5 days. The course can be repeated once or twice when the desired effect has not been achieved 3 to 5 days after the first course. Seven cases so treated were all cured (31).

ADVERSE EFFECTS

The common reactions are hiccup, and dizziness. Also, there may be mild abdominal pain, diarrhea, nausea and vomiting which usually disappear spontaneously. It has been reported that hiccups occur less often with the roasted kernel medication (7). Tea is contraindicated, either before or after treatment with this herb, because it may enhance the side effects.

REFERENCE

1. Zhou TC et al. Kexue (Science) 1947 29(5):143.
2. Wu YR et al. The National Medical Journal of China 1948 34(10):437.
3. Hu CJ. The National Medical Journal of China 1950 36(12):619.
4. Chen SY et al. Kexue (Science) 1948 30(11):329.
5. Chen SY et al. Chinese Medical Journal 1952 38(4):319.
6. Chen SY et al. Journal of Nanjing College of Pharmacy 1959 (4):27.
7. Duan YQ et al. Acta Pharmaceutica Sinica 1957 5(2):287.
8. Takemoto T. Journal of the Pharmaceutical Society of Japan (Tokyo) 1975 95:176, 326.
9. Shi QD et al. Journal of Parasitology 1973 22(4):1.
10. Zhao CG et al. Science Record 1951 4(1):75.

11. Wu YR et al. Abstracts of the First Congress of the Chinese Society of Physiology (Pharmacy). 1956 p. 27.

12. Feng YS et al. Acta Academiae Medicinae Qingdao 1957 (1):20.

13. Cao RL et al. Chinese Journal of Dermatology 1957 (4):286.

14. Tsuruta S. Nagasaki Igakkai Zasshi 1924 2:471.

15. Wu KM. The National Medical Journal of China 1926 12(2):161.

16. Wang YX et al. Chinese Medical Journal 1955 41(5):456.

17. Guo XX. Chinese Medical Journal 1955 41(10):977.

18. Shi PD. Chinese Medical Journal 1956 42(2):167.

19. Liu DQ. Journal of Traditional Chinese Medicine 1956 (1):23.

20. Li JW. Shanghai Zhongyiyao Zazhi (Shanghai Journal of Traditional Chinese Medicine) 1958 (10):26.

21. Wang YX. Acta Academiae Medicinae Shandong 1958 (1):62.

22. Liu QR. Shanxi Medical and Pharmaceutical Journal 1959 3(1):50.

23. Chen ZA. Northeastern Region Medical Journal 1952 (10):929.

24. Tang DJ et al. Shandong Medical Journal 1958 (1):14.

25. Zhong YH et al. Acta Academiae Medicinae Jiangxi 1956 (1):1.

26. Liu JA. Chinese Journal of Paediatrics 1966 15(1):47.

27. Jiangsu College of New Medicine. Encyclopedia of Chinese Materia Medica. Vol. 1. Shanghai People's Publishing House. 1977. p. 1374.

28. Zhao J et al. Zhongji Yikan (Intermediate Medical Journal) 1954 (8):11.

29. Kang SY. Chinese Journal of Paediatrics 1955 4(2):162.

30. Chen SR. Jiangsu Zhongyi (Jiangsu Journal of Traditional Chinese Medicine) 1960 (2):34.

31. Liu JJ. Jiangsu Zhongyi (Jiangsu Journal of Traditional Chinese Medicine) 1964 (10):16.

(Deng Wenlong)

CEBAIYE 側柏葉

<Cebaiye> refers to the leafy twigs of *Biota orientalis* (L.) Endl. (Cupressaceae). It is bitter and puckery to the taste with a slightly "cold" property. It has astringent, hemostatic, latent-heat-clearing, and antipyretic actions and is thought to be able to remove pathogenic "heat" from the blood. Hence, it is used to treat hemoptysis, epistaxis, hematuria, metrorrhagia, cough, and bacillary dysentery.

CHEMICAL COMPOSITION

<Cebaiye> contains 0.6–1.0% of volatile oil which is composed of thujene, thujone, fenchone, and pinene. It also contains flavonoids aromadendrin and quercetin, isopimaric acid, and tannin.

PHARMACOLOGY

1. Antitussive Effect

Intraperitoneal injection of the alcohol-precipitated substance of the <Cebaiye> decoction, or the ethanol extract at 10 g/kg, or the flavone isolated from the herb at 250 mg/kg produced an antitussive effect in mice with SO_2-induced cough (1,2). Likewise, the petroleum ether extract of the herb, the ether dialysate, and the phenolic substances produced a significant antitussive effect in mice with cough induced by ammonia fumes (3). A marked antitussive activity was also exhibited by the herb in cats following electrical stimulation of the superior laryngeal nerve, suggesting a central action (1,2).

2. Expectorant Effect

The phenol red excretion test in mice showed that the ethanol extract, the petroleum ether extract, or the alcohol-precipitated substance of <Cebaiye> had a marked expectorant effect (3,4). An active expectorant principle, isopimaric acid, had been isolated recently (5). However, the alcohol-precipitated fraction of the decoction did not significantly increase bronchial secretion in rats (1).

2.1 *Mechanism of expectorant effect.* The petroleum ether extract of <Cebaiye> was found to increase phenol red excretion in the respiratory tract of rabbits, and the expectorant effect persisted even after bilateral vagotomy. Hence, this effect is probably not mediated by neuroreflex. However, the petroleum ether extract did not significantly influence the speed of chicken bronchial ciliary transport of Indian ink (6). Consequently, it is preliminarily held that the expectorant effect is due to a direct action on the bronchial mucosa.

3. Antiasthmatic Effect

The alcohol-precipitated <Cebaiye> decoction relaxed the isolated bronchial smooth muscle of mice and guinea pigs and also partially blocked the action of acetylcholine. Further experiments showed that the active principle resided in the portion extracted by ethyl acetate (1,2). However, this extract did not significantly protect guinea pigs from asthma induced by histamine (1–4). <Cebaiye> was also reported to reduce the oxygen consumption of the tracheal-pulmonary tissue of rats (7).

4. Hemostatic Effect

The <Cebaiye> decoction significantly shortened the bleeding time in mice and the capillary coagulation time in rabbits, suggesting the presence of hemostatic effect. The hemostatic effect of carbonized <Cebaiye> was, however, slightly poorer than that of the crude herb (8).

5. Sedative Effect

The <Cebaiye> decoction markedly minimized the spontaneous activity in mice and prolonged pentobarbital sodium-induced sleep, but did not antagonize caffeine-induced convulsion (1,2). On the other hand, prolonged use of thujone in rats at 10 mg/kg did not affect the spontaneous activity of the animals or alter their conditioned behavior; on the contrary, it produced more coordinated movements. Even at a high dosage, thujone did not affect the respiration of the cerebral cortex (9).

6. Effect on the Circulatory System

Intravenous or intragastric administration of the alcohol-precipitated substance of the <Cebaiye> decoction to anesthetized cats caused a slight fall of the blood pressure and vasodilation of the isolated rabbit ear (1,2).

7. Antibacterial Effect

In vitro, the <Cebaiye> decoction inhibited *Staphylococcus aureus, Neisseria catarrhalis, Shigella dysenteriae, Salmonella typhi, Corynebacterium diphtheriae*, beta streptococcus and *Bacillus anthracis* (2,4,10). The aqueous extract at 1:100 or the ethanol extract at 1:180,000 inhibited *Mycobacterium tuberculosis* and also synergized with isoniazid (11,12); another report, however, claimed that it was inactive against the same organism (13). The herb decoction (1:40) also had inhibitory action against influenza virus Jingke 68–1 and herpes virus (14).

8. Miscellaneous Actions

The alcohol-precipitated <Cebaiye> decoction, at a single dose of 60 g/kg or a daily dose of 30 g/kg for 3 days, did not alter the vitamin C content of rat adrenals, suggesting no causal relationship with the pituitary-adrenocortical function (1,2). The same preparation showed a significant relaxant effect on the isolated intestines of guinea pigs (1,2).

9. Toxicity

No death was observed within 72 hours of administration of the <Cebaiye> decoction at 60 g/kg PO to mice; the LD_{50} in mice was 15.2 g/kg IP. The LD_{50} of the alcohol-precipitated <Cebaiye> decoction was 30.5 g/kg IP in mice, indicating a significant decrease in toxicity after alcohol precipitation (2). The LD_{50} of the petroleum ether extract was 2964 mg/kg PO (3). Only reduced activity and poor appetite were observed in separate groups of albino rats given the herb decoction intragastrically at doses 20 times (24 g/kg) and 40 times (48 g/kg) the clinical dose, for 6 weeks, and there were no significant effects on the growth, liver function, blood picture and pathological picture (1).

CLINICAL STUDIES

1. Chronic Bronchitis

The effective rate in 2802 cases treated with <Cebaiye> preparations was 70% (15). Various preparations of the extracts of the herb or of its compound prescriptions afforded an aggregate effective rate of 94.5% and a marked effective rate of 63.9% in 819 cases of bronchitis, of which 95 received <Cebaiye> preparations plus other herbs reputed to increase body resistance (the root tuber of *Dioscorea opposita* and the whole plant of *Epimedium sagittatum*, each 15 g). The SIgA level in the respiratory tract was markedly increased after the treatment, indicating recovery of the reduced immunologic function (16,17). Another paper reported an effective rate of 80.9% in 277 cases treated with the decoction of the cone at 60 g/day divided into 2 doses, 15 days as a therapeutic course (18).

2. Pulmonary Tuberculosis

The tablet prepared from <Cebaiye> was used at a dose of 45 g(crude drug)/day for a course of 6 months in the treatment of 224 active cases; 64.1% of the patients who had received this therapy for the first time and 36.3% who had repeated the course registered negative for bacillus tubercle in the post-treatment sputum test. The drug was also effective for the cavities and symptoms (12,19). Other authors used the tablet and the injection of the herb extract in the treatment of 153 cases of infiltrative pulmonary tuberculosis at 120 g(crude drug)/day for a course of 3–5 months. Out of 119 cases treated with <Cebaiye> alone, 73.95% showed absorption of lesions, 23.33% had healing of cavities and 58.14% were pathogen-free in the sputum test. Cough, expectoration, sweating, hemoptysis, and lassitude disappeared or improved in most cases (20). Also, the injection was used in 55 cases of pulmonary tuberculosis, achieving an effective rate of 85.5%. In 46 infiltrative types so treated, 92.8% showed absorption of lesions and 25%, closed cavities (21).

3. Whooping Cough

The fresh leaves and young branches of *B. orientalis* 30 g decocted into 100 ml with 20 ml of honey added can be administered as follows: under 2 years, 15–25 ml thrice daily; the dosage is to be adjusted according to age. Out of 56 cases treated for 4 to 10 days, 11 were cured, 9 markedly improved, and 6 unresponsive (22).

4. Acute and Chronic Bacillary Dysentery

Administration of the dilute alcohol (18% ethanol) extract of <Cebaiye> to 114 cases at a dose of 50 ml trice daily for 7 to 10 days cured 100 cases,s the cure rate being 87.7% (23).

5. Peptic Ulcer with Bleeding

Stool tests for occult blood in 50 patients turned negative in an average of 2.8 days after oral administration of the <Cebaiye> decoction 15 g, in contrast to 4.5 days achieved in the same number of control cases (24).

6. Alopecia

The ethanol extract of the fresh leaves and branches rubbed onto the bald areas was effective in 160 cases of various types of alopecia (25).

7. External Use in Burns

Ointment prepared from the fine powder of carbonized <Cebaiye> and boiled sesame oil or soya bean oil may be used to treat first-degree burns covering small or moderate areas. Application of this agent over the wound after primary management produced anti-inflammatory and antiseptic effects (26).

8. Miscellaneous

Clinically this herb had also been used in neurasthenia, palpitation, insomnia, asthenia, constipation (27) and alopecia (28) etc.

REFERENCE

1. Chronic Bronchitis Research Section, Institute of Materia Medica of Zhejiang People's Academy of Health. Scientific Research Compilation. Zhejiang People's Academy of Health. 1973. p. 175.

2. Chronic Bronchitis Research Section, Institute of Materia Medica of Zhejiang People's Academy of Health. Scientific Research Compilation. Zhejiang People's Academy of Health. 1972. p. 130.

3. Pharmacology Group of Chronic Bronchitis Research Unit, Fourth Military Medical College of the Chinese PLA. Scientific and Technical Information (Fourth Military Medical College) 1973 (5):10.

4. Jiangsu Coordinating Research Group on Biota orientalis. Clinical Trial of Biota orientalis in the Treatment of Chronic Bronchitis. 1973.

5. Medicinal Chemistry Group of Chronic Bronchitis Research Unit, Fourth Military Medical College of the Chinese PLA. Scientific and Technical Information (Fourth Military Medical College) 1975 (6):1.

6. Pharmacology Group of Chronic Bronchitis Research Unit, Fourth Military Medical College of the Chinese PLA. Scientific and Technical Information (Fourth Military Medical College) 1976 (3):21.

7. Pharmacology Section, Hebei College of New Medicine. Research of new Traditional Chinese Medicine (Hebei College of New Medicine) 1972 (3):2.

8. Pharmacology Section, Shandong Institute of Traditional Chinese Medicine. Studies on Traditional Chinese Medicine (Shandong Institute of Traditional Chinese Medicine) 1965 (3):48.

9. Pinto-Scognamiglio W. Chemical Abstracts 1969 70:76275j.

10. Hunan Sanitation and Anti-epidemic Station. Hunan Communications on Sanitation and Epidemic Prevention 1974 (1):112.

11. Beijing Institute of Tuberculosis. Chinese Journal of Prevention of Tuberculosis 1964 5(3):481.

12. Shandong Coordinating Research Group on Biota orientalis. Medical Communications 1975 (1):1.

13. Guiyang Hospital of Tuberculosis. Chinese Journal of Prevention of Tuberculosis 1959 2(6):37.

14. Virus Section, Institute of Chinese Materia Medica of the Academy of Traditional Chinese Medicine. Xinyiyaoxue Zazhi (Journal of Traditional Chinese Medicine) 1973 (1):26.

15. Zhejiang Coordinating Research Group on Biota orientalis. Zhejiang Compiled Information on Chronic Bronchitis 1972 (6):23.

16. Clinical Bronchitis Research Unit, Fourth Military Medical College of the Chinese PLA. Scientific and Technical Information (Fourth Military Medical College) 1976 (3):24.

17. Clinical Bronchitis Research Unit, Fourth Military medical College of the Chinese PLA. Scientific and Technical Information (Fourth Military Medical College) 1976 (3):41.

18. Xuyi County (Jiangsu) Health Bureau. Xinyiyaoxue Zazhi (Journal of Traditional Chinese Medicine) 1974 (2):23.

19. Tuberculosis Department, 116th Hospital of the Chinese PLA. Anqing Science and Technology — Medicine and Health 1974 (1):11.

20. Tuberculosis Department, 309th Hospital of the Chinese PLA. People's Military Medicine 1976 (7):57.

21. Tuberculosis Department. Huolu Airforce Hospital of the Chinese PLA. People's Military Medicine 1976 (7):88.

22. Pediatrics Department, Guilin Workers' Hospital. Chinese Journal of Pediatrics 1960 (2):146.

23. 171st Hospital of the Chinese PLA. New Medical Information (Jiangxi School of Pharmacy) 1971 (6):11.

24. Ni DR. Chinese Journal of Internal Medicine 1960 8(3):249.

25. Medical Clinic of Jieyang (Guangdong) Nitrogenous Fertilizer Plant. Chinese Medical Journal 1973 53(8):459.

26. Editorial Group (Zhongshan Medical College). Clinical Applications of Chinese Traditional Drugs. 1st edition. Guangdong People's Publishing House. 1975. p. 258.

27. Chengdu College of Traditional Chinese Medicine (editor). Chinese Traditional Pharmacy (Trial Teaching Materials for Traditional Chinese Medicine Course). Shanghai People's Publishing House. 1977. p. 196.

28. Ye KZ. New Chinese Medicine (Zhongshan Medical College) 1972 (9):53.

(Chen Quansheng)

JINQIANCAO 金錢草

<Jinqiancao> refers to the plant *Lysimachia christinae* Hance (Primulaceae). This herb, which has a bland taste and slightly "cold" property, is known for its latent-heat-clearing, antipyretic, choleretic, cholagogic, lithagogic, and diuretic effects. Hence, it is used for the treatment of jaundice of the "damp-heat" type, hepatobiliary lithiasis, urolithiasis, and various infections.

Other species also used as <Jinqiancao> are *L. hemsleyana* Maxim., *Dichondra repens* Forst. (Convolvulaceae), *Desmodium styracifolium* (Osb.) Merr. (Leguminosae), *Hydrocotyle sibthorpioides* Lam., *H. sibthorpioides* Lam. var. *batrachium* (Hance) Hand.-Mazz, *H. maritima* Honda (*H. wilfordii* non Maxim.), (Umbelliferae), and *Glechoma hederacea* L. (Labiatae). Though these plants belong to very different genera, and their degrees of efficacy vary, all are effective in the treatment of calculi as well as of diseases of the liver and gallbladder (1–4).

CHEMICAL COMPOSITION

<Jinqiancao> contains flavonoids, glycosides, tannin, volatile oil, amino acids, choline, sterols, potassium chloride, and lactones.

The volatile oil of *G. hederacae* contains 1-pinocamphone, 1-menthone, α-pinene, β-pinene, limonene, 1,8-cineole, p-cymene, stachyose, and ursolic acid.

PHARMACOLOGY

1. Cholagogic, Choleretic and Lithagogic Effects

Bile secretion and excretion were promoted in rats given *L. hemsleyana* 5 ml/day PO for 6 weeks, and 3 ml before anesthesia on the day of biliary drainage (4).

Intravenous infusion of *D. styracifolium* injection into the femoral vein, or intraduodenal administration of the decoction, at 8 g(crude drug)/kg to dogs also markedly increased the bile collected (5).

Drainage of the human duodenum showed that *L. hemsleyana* had a choleretic action. Since rats do not have gallbladders, it is inferred that the choleretic effect of this herb is not a result of the reflex contraction of the gallbladder. Bile excretion is probably promoted by the relaxation of the Oddi's sphincter following the increase in intraductal pressure consequent to the increase of bile secreted by the liver cells. the choleretic action facilitated the excretion of sandy stones, abated biliary obstruction and pain, and caused the subsidence of jaundice (1,5). In both acute and chronic experiments, bile flow from the gallbladder was greatly increased in dogs given "Paishi Tang" (Lithagogue Decoction) in which the herb is the chief ingredient. Furthermore, bile secretion was increased by 3–20 times, and concretion components in the bile were markedly decreased in 6 out of 7 anesthetized dogs 10–20 minutes after administration of this decoction. Simultaneously, the Oddi's sphincter relaxed coinciding with the peak choleretic effect. A 20–60% increase in bile secretion associated with relaxation of the Oddi's sphincter in 4 cases of biliary fistulae was achieved after administration of this decoction (5–10). *In vitro* studies using fresh bile obtained from patients suffering from bile pigment stones also showed that Lithagogue Decoction prevented the precipitation of the stone-forming elements, indicating that this herb has an antilithiasis effect. The action of Lithagogue Decoction was said to relate to the inhibition of β-glucuronidase activity in the bile (11). The decoction appeared to minimize the formation of new stones in rabbits with transplanted cholesterol gallstones (12).

2. Diuretic an Lithagogic Effects

Experiments on rabbits with acute urinary bladder fistulae showed that the decoction of *G. hederacea* 20 g(crude drug)/kg and its ash solution (equivalent to 20 g/kg of the crude drug) had a significant diuretic effect probably caused by the potassium salt content of the herb, whereas the tincture preparation was inactive. This diuretic action did not differ from that obtained with potassium acetate (13). Experiment with rats revealed that *D. styracifolium* and *D. repens* had significant diuretic and natriuretic effects (14). Similar results were obtained in chronic experiments on rats given the herb decoction at 20 g(crude drug)kg/day PO, but the diuretic action was weakened after dosing for 6 days. No diuretic action was obtained with the ethanol extract (13).

The <Jinqiancao> decoction 120 g (equivalent to 10 times the human dosage) injected into the duodenum of anesthetized dogs increased the ureteral peristalsis and concurrently the urine output, similar to the responses elicited by hydrochlorothiazide (16). Intravenous infusion of *D. styracifolium* 8 g(crude drug)/kg into the femoral vein of dogs, or intraduodenal injection of the herb decoction to the same species very markedly increased the urine output (6). Perfusion of the small intestine of dogs with the "Niaolu Paishi Tang" (Urolithagogue Decoction) markedly increased the amplitude of ureteral peristalsis and urine output. Oral administration of this decoction to patients with ureteral calculi resulted in greater urine output than that obtained with the same amount of plain water (16). Prophylactic and therapeutic effects were achieved in rats with experimental oxalate calculi given Lithagogue Decoction No. 3, a proven effective remedy for urolithiasis. Scattered sandy stones were seen in the urinary bladders of treated rats, indicating that the drug had probably reduced the size of the stones by decomposing them so that they could finally be expelled from the body (5,17). Other articles report that the orally administered herb rendered the urine acidic, promoting the dissolution of stones formed under alkaline conditions (18,19).

3. Effect on the Cardiovascular System

Intravenous administration of the *D. styracifolium* decoction at 8 g(crude drug)/kg to anesthetized dogs significantly increased coronary and renal blood flows; the coronary flow was increased by

197.4%. Cerebral and femoral arterial blood flows were also increased and the carotid arterial pressure was lowered. Heart rate was decreased simultaneously with marked decreases in the coronary resistance index and myocardial oxygen consumption. The injection of the *D. styracifolium* decoction protected rabbits and dogs against diminution of the coronary flow and against acute myocardial ischemia induced by pituitrin (6). The ^{86}Rb uptake study showed that the crude flavones extracted from *D. styracifolium* significantly increased the myocardial flow in mice in a dose-dependent manner. The increase in ^{86}Rb uptake achieved by the dose of 1 g(crude drug)/10 g was equivalent to that elicited by 1 mg/10 g of dipyridamole. Intravenous injection of the *D. styracifolium* flavones at 200 mg(20 g crude drug)kg to anesthetized dogs significantly augmented the coronary flow for 5–10 minutes. Concurrently, the arterial blood pressure, heart rate, and coronary resistance were decreased. When 20 mg/kg of the flavones was injected into the carotid artery of these animals, a significant increase in the cerebral blood flow promptly ensued lasting 3–9 minutes; a decrease in cerebrovascular resistance and transient fall of the blood pressure were also observed (20–21). The ethyl acetate extract, and in particular the n-butanol extract (flavones with high polarity) of *D. styracifolium* at 60 mg/kg markedly increased the cerebral blood flow and lowered the arterial pressure as well as the cerebrovascular resistance (22).

Experiments on mice under normobaric hypoxic conditions revealed that the flavones of *D. styracifolium* enhanced the tolerance of the animals to hypoxia, and prolonged the survival of the animals dose-dependently. At 0.5 g(crude drug)/10 g, the survival period was prolonged by 30.23% (P<0.001) which was lower than that achieved with propranolol 0.2 mg/10 g(45.33% P<0.001). The flavones also antagonized potassium chloride-induced spasm of isolated rabbit arterial strips (18).

The phenolic compounds of *D. styracifolium* also increased the myocardial blood flow in mice (20).

<Jinqiancao> precipitated the euglobulin of dog blood and had a anticoagulant effect *in vitro* (21).

In addition, the herb also enhanced bile secretion by the liver, and probably interfered with the enteronepatic circulation of cholesterol in man, thus accelerating the excretion of cholesterol. Consequently, <Jinqiancao> is thought to be an effective drug for coronary disease and cerebral arteriosclerosis (16,21).

4. Antibacterial Effect

In vitro, the decoction and tincture of *D. repens* strongly inhibited *Corynebacterium diphtheriae* and was also active against *Staphylococcus aureus, S. hemolyticus, Bacillus subtilis*, and *Escherichia coli* (23). The decoction of *L. hemsleyana* also inhibited *Staphylococcus aureus* (24), while that of *G. hederacea* inhibited *Staphylococcus aureus, Salmonella typhi, Shigella dysenteriae*, and *Pseudomonas aeruginosa* (25). The ethanol extract of *D. styracifolium* inhibited *Candida albicans*; the decoction was less active (26).

5. *Toxicity*

<Jinqiancao> has a low toxicity. No death occurred in rats given *G. hederacea* 20 g/kg PO daily for 6 days. A single dose of 100 g PO to dogs did not affect the blood picture, although deep and quick respiration developed (5). The LD_{50} of the *D. styracifolium* flavones in mice was 1583 ± 251 mg/kg PO (20). Lithagogue Decoction administered to dogs and mice did not produce any effect on cardiac and hepatic functions at dosage levels 5 and 200 times higher than the clinical dose (27).

CLINICAL STUDIES

1. *Hepatobiliary Diseases*

The effects of <Jinqiancao> and compound prescriptions containing the herb on hepatobiliary stones and biliary infection were reported to be salutary (4–9,29), and even more so in cases with sandy stones. The fresh plant was superior to the dried herb (28). The commonly used prescriptions and methods of treatment are as follows:

1.1 *Cholelithiasis*.

1.1.1   Decoction prepared from 60–250 g of Herba Lysimachiae, once daily by mouth, for 2–3 months.

1.1.2   Decoction using fresh plants of *Hydrocotyle sibthorpioides, Dichondra repens, Lygodium japonicum*, and *Plantago asiatica*, 50 g each, one dose daily.

1.1.3   "General attack lithagogic therapy" (5–8,10,30). This is a new and advanced combined approach in the treatment of cholelithiasis using both Chinese herbs and Western medicines. The advantages of this approach are: high incidence of stone passage, short therapeutic course, and low incidence of operation.

   The therapeutic regimen and principle of "general attack lithagogic therapy".

Time	Therapeutic regimen	Principle
8:30	Lithagogue Decoction 200 ml PO	Use Chinese herbal medicines having liver soothing, choleretic, latent-heat clearing, damp-eliminative and purgative activities to drugs which constrict the Oddi's sphincter such as morphine should be given to induce bile retention and increase the pressure in the gallbladder to a tolerable extent. Lastly, use magnesium sulfate, amyl nitrite or electro-acupuncture to open the Oddi's sphicter and constrict the gallbladder, thereby flushing the stones out all at once or accelerating their expulsion.
9:30	Morphine 5 mg SC	
10:10	Amyl nitrite 1 amp inhalant	
10:15	33% magnesium sulfate 40 ml PO	
10:20	0.5% dilute HC1 30 ml PO	
10:25	Rich meal (2–3 fried eggs)	
10:30	Electroacupuncture: right "Danyu" (Anode), "Reyue" or "Liangmen", "Taichong" (cathode) for 30 min	

Lithagogue Decoction is particularly useful in cases of hepatobiliary lithiasis without severe infection or biliary obstruction (stricture, stone obstruction). It is also effective in inoperable cases with extensive intrahepatic lithiasis. It is, however, less effective in cases of gallbladder stones. The stones were mostly passed after 6–7 days of treatment with the simple decoction. In a report of 59 cases of choledocholithiasis managed by the general attack therapy, 61% of the cases passed stones, usually after 1–2 treatments.

Precautions: Lithagogue Decoction produces few adverse effects. There may be occasional vomiting, headache and abdominal pain. Intermittent medication is advocated whenever appetite is impaired. During the general attack therapy, signs may occur at the time of large stone passage; they include gallbladder colic, fever, fast pulse rate or jaundice, but these reactions often disappear quite suddenly. Close monitoring is mandatory during treatment. Whenever persistent distention and pain or paroxysmal severe pain of the upper abdomen, chills, reappearance of jaundice, and low blood pressure occur, the possibility of acute obstruction requiring operation should be considered. Morphine must be used with care because it causes spasm of the Oddi's sphincter, which in some very sensitive individuals may not be relieved by Chinese herbal medicines, or atropine, and will aggravate the ailment. Therefore, morphine is contraindicated or its use minimized during acute attacks, and overdosage should be avoided during the remission period.

Lithagogue Decoction No. 5 (Herba Lysimachiae 100 g, Radix Aucklandiae 15 g, Fructus Aurantii 15 g, Radix Scutellariae 15 g, Fructus Meliae Toosendan 15 g, Radix et Rhizoma Rhei 10 g) divided into 2 doses daily is useful during the remission period of cholangiolithiasis.

Moreover, Lithagogue Decoction No. 6 (Rhizome Polygoni Cuspidati or Radix Berberidis 100 g, Radix Aucklandiae 25 g, Fructus Aurantii 25 g, Radix et Rhizoma Rhei 25 g, Herba Lysimachiae (or Herba Artemisiae) 100 g, Fructus Gardeniae 20 g, Rhizoma Corydalis 25 g) given as a single dose of 200 ml is useful in the acute stage, or as one of the drugs in the general attack regimen. Patients with strong constitutions and mild adverse responses may be given the general attack therapy on alternate days, 2–3 times a week. Those with weak constitutions and severe responses received only 1 treatment per week. Some patients needed only 1 treatment, the maximum being 16, and the average being 5.

1.2 *Cholecystitis.* A decoction prepared from <Jinqiancao> 30–60 g and Radix Polygoni Cuspidati 15 g is to be taken orally. Radix Curcumae Aromaticae 15 g may be added in case of pain.

1.3 *Icteric hepatitis.*

1.3.1 A decoction prepared from <Jinqiancao>, Herba Artemisiae Capillaris, Rhizoma Polygoni Cuspidati, each 9 g, Herba Ardisiae Japonicae 15 g, Herba Agrimoniae Pilosae 12 g, is to be taken once daily.

1.3.2 A decoction prepared from <Jinqiancao>, Herba Taraxaci, and Radix Isatidis, each 30 g, is to be taken once daily.

2. Urolithiasis

<Jinqiancao> and its compound formulae afforded satisfactory therapeutic results in urolithiasis (2,31–40).

2.1 A decoction of <Jinqiancao> 60–250 g may be administered once daily for 2–3 months.

2.2 *Treatment with Chinese herbs and Western medicines.* The therapeutic principle is similar to that of the general attack lithagogic therapy for cholelithiasis. In 677 cases of urolithiasis treated with Urolithagogue Decoction plus Western medicines, satisfactory results were obtained with respect to dissolution of stones, stone expulsion, and decrease in relapses.

The basic formula of Urolithagogue Decoction consists of Herba Lysimachiae 30 g, Semen Plantaginis 9–30 g, Folium Pyrrosiae 15–30 g, Talcum 15–30 g, Herba et Spora Lygodii 9–30 g, Fructus Malvae Verticillatae 9–15 g, Radix Cyathulae 98 g, Cortex Magnoliae Officinalis 9 g, Fructus Aurantii 9 g, and Semen Vaccariae 9 g.

Another paper reported that an oral decoction of *D. styracifolium* 60 g given in two doses daily caused rapid disappearance of ascites and amelioration of symptoms in one patient with advanced schistosomiasis with ascites (41).

3. Miscellaneous

3.1 Fresh *H. sibthorpioides* 250 g were soaked in 100 ml of 75% ethanol for one week, and the filtrate was mixed with 6 g of realgar powder. Local application of this preparation on erysipelas and herpes zoster 2–3 times daily produced a salutary effect. The preparation is, however, contraindicated in cases with broken skin (42).

3.2 As antidote for *Tripterygium wilfordii* Hook. f. poisoning. Forty such cases achieved good effects chiefly with *D. styracifolium* (43).

ADVERSE EFFECTS

Adverse effects are rare. No side effects were seen in 10 cases of cholelithiasis treated with *L. hemsleyana* at 150–250 g daily by mouth for over six months, and no toxic effects in one case treated for as long as 318 days. No adverse reaction was observed in another case of ureteral calculi given one catty of the herb daily for 7 days (1,4). Occasional leukopenia was seen during the clinical trial of *H. sibthorpioides*; this condition was reversed spontaneously after medication was discontinued (2).

REFERENCE

1. Institute of Chinese Materia Medica, Academy of Traditional Chinese Medicine. Journal of Traditional Chinese Medicine 1960 (1):41.

2. Xie ZW et al. Bulletin of Chinese Materia Medica 1959 (1):26.

3. Xie ZW et al. Chinese Pharmaceutical Bulletin 1960 (2):94.

4. Surgery Department, Teaching Hospital of the Academy of Traditional Chinese Medicine. Journal of Traditional Chinese Medicine 1960 (1):12.

5. Acute Abdomen Research Unit, Zunyi Medical College. Information on Medical Sciences and Technology (Zunyi Medical College) 1974 (5):25.

6. Chen RD et al. Chinese Journal of Surgery 1964 (Supplement):74.

7. He RL et al. Chinese Journal of Surgery 1965 (2):103.

8. He RL et al. Scientia Sinica 1974 (2):206.

9. Second Teaching Hospital, Hunan Medical College. Compiled Medical Information. Second Teaching Hospital of Hunan Medical College. 1974. p. 244.

10. Coordinating Research Unit for Combined Western and Traditional Chinese Medicine Therapy of Cholelithiasis, Second Teaching Hospital of Hunan Medical College. Hunan Information on Science and Technology (Hunan Centre of Scientific and Technological Information) 1979 (2):16.

11. Cholelithiasis Unit of the Surgery Department, Third Teaching Hospital of Beijing Medical College. Journal of Traditional Chinese Medicine 1979 (6):358.

12. Pei DK. New Chinese Medicine 1980 (2):71.

13. Ji ZX. Wuhan Medical Journal 1964 (5):392.

14. Wang LW et al. Chinese Traditional and Herbal Drugs 1980 11(5):222.

15. Lin MZ et al. Communications on Combined Western and Traditional Chinese Therapy of Acute Abdomen 1978 (4):57.

16. Acute Abdomen Research Unit, Zunyi Medical College. Information on Medical Sciences and Technology (Special Issue on Acute Abdomen) (Zunyi Medical College) 1974 (5):15.

17. Yang LX. Journal of Traditional Chinese Medicine 1980 (3):73.

18. Li ZH et al. Chinese Journal of Surgery 1960 (6):564.

19. Xiao YC. Journal of Traditional Chinese Medicine 1955 (5):21.

20. Xu SB. Chinese Traditional and Herbal Drugs 1980 (6):205.

21. Hematology Research Unit, Hunan Medical College et al. Compiled Information on Combined Western and Traditional Chinese Therapy of Acute Abdomen. Hunan Coordinating Research Group on Acute Abdomen. 1977. p. 102.

22. Jian JY et al. Chinese Traditional and Herbal Drugs 1980 11(8):362.

23. Chen GQ et al. Fujian Zhongyiyao (Fujian Journal of Traditional Chinese Medicine) 1964 (2):33.

24. Zhejiang People's Academy of Health. Scientific Research Compilation (1966–1971). Zhejiang People's Academy of Health. 1972. p. 90.

25. Shanghai College of Traditional Chinese Medicine. Chinese Traditional Pharmacy. Shanghai College of Traditional Chinese Medicine. 1974. p. 252.

26. Dermatology Department, Second Teaching Hospital of Zhongshan Medical College. Guangdong Medical Information (Guangdong Institute of Medicine and Health) 1975 (9):15.

27. Lin ZH et al. Jiangsu Yiyao (Jiangsu Medical Journal) — Traditional Chinese Medicine 1979 (3):22.

28. Pharmacognosy Department, Institute of Chinese Materia Medica of the Academy of Traditional Chinese Medicine. Journal of Traditional Chinese Medicine 1958 (11):794.

29. Cholelithiasis Research Section, Institute of Surgery, Academy of Traditional Chinese Medicine. Journal of Traditional Chinese Medicine 1963 (11):1.

30. Acute Abdomen Research Unit, Zunyi Medical College. Information on Medical Sciences and Technology (Zunyi Medical College) 1974 (5):6.

31. New Chinese Medicine Department, Xuwen County (Guangdong) People' s Hospital. New Pharmaceutical Communications (Guangzhou Health Bureau) 1971 (4–5):27.

32. New Chinese Medicine Department, Xuwen County (Guangdong) People' s Hospital. New Pharmaceutical Communications (Guangzhou Health Bureau) 1971 (4–5):27.

33. Xue F et al. Acta Academiae Medicinae Primae Shanghai 1957 (3):35.

34. Lang SZ et al. Chinese Journal of Surgery 1960 (5):503.

35. Liang RF. Guangdong Zhongyi (Guangdong Journal of Traditional Chinese Medicine) 1956 (5):10.

36. Chen GY. Journal of Traditional Chinese Medicine 1965 (11):9.

37. Wang YQ et al. Shanghai Zhongyiyao Zazhi (Shanghai Journal of Traditional Chinese Medicine) 1966 (2):58.

38. Wenzhou College of Traditional Chinese Medicine. Notes on Science and Technology — Medicine and Health (Zhejiang Information Centre of Medical Sciences and Technology) 1971 (5–6):48.

39. Urology Department, Guang' anmen Teaching Hospital of the Academy of Traditional Chinese Medicine. Zhonghua Yixue Zazhi (National Medical Journal of China) 1976 (3):151.

40. Yang WX et al. New Chinese Medicine 1973 (1):33.

41. Li QR. Guangdong Zhongyi (Guangdong Journal of Traditional Chinese Medicine) 1958 (5):25.

42. Health Group, Taojiang County (Hunan) Revolutionary Committee. Chinese Traditional and Herbal Drugs Communications 1973 (4):54.

43. Zhitangjie District Hospital of Herbal Medicine (Taojiang County, Hunan). Hunan Yiyao Zazhi (Junan Medical Journal) 1974 (4):46.

(Liao Nengge)

JINYINHUA 金銀花

<Jinyinhua>, also called <Shuanghua>, refers to the flower buds or newly bloomed flowers of *Lonicera japonica* Thunb., *L. hypoglauca* Miq., *L. confusa* DC, and *L. dasystyla* Rehd. (Caprifolaceae). The vine and leaf, called <Rendongteng>, are also used as medicines.

<Jinyinhua> has a sweet taste and "cold" property. It has latent-heat-clearing, antipyretic, detoxicant and anti-inflammatory actions. It is, therefore, prescribed to treat fever due to common cold, febrile diseases, dysentery, carbuncles, furuncles, and virulent swellings.

CHEMICAL COMPOSITION

<Jinyinhua> contains chlorogenic acid, isochlorogenic acid, neochlorogenic acid, 4-0-caffeoylquinic acid, 4,5-dicaffeoylquinic acid, 3,5-dicaffeoylquinic acid, 3,4-dicaffeoylquinic acid, flavonoids (such as luteolin), lonicerin, inositol, and saponins.

PHARMACOLOGY

1. Antimicrobial Effect

In vitro, both the flower and vine inhibited many kinds of pathogenic organisms such as *Staphylococcus aureus, Streptococcus hemolyticus, Escherichia coli, Shigella dysenteriae, Vibrio cholerae, Salmonella typhi*, and *Salmonella paratyphi*; they were also effective against *Diplococcus pneumoniae, Neisseria meningitidis, Pseudomonas aeruginosa*, and *Mycobacterium tuberculosis* (1–5). The aqueous extract is more potent than the decoction, and the leaf decoction is more active than the flower decoction (1,5). A wider antibacterial spectrum was obtained when the herb was used in combination with the fruit of *Forsythia suspensa* (6). Used with penicillin, it potentiated the action of the latter agent against the drug resistant *Staphylococcus aureus*, probably by inhibiting the synthesis of bacterial proteins (7). Chlorogenic acid and isochlorogenic acid were thought to be the chief active principles of this herb (8,9), but luteolin was also shown to have strong antibacterial action (10). *In vitro*, the aqueous extract exhibited various degrees of inhibitory effect against skin fungi such as *Microsporum ferrugineum* and *Nocardia asteroides* (11).

In the monolayer primary culture of the epithelial cells of human embryonic kidney, <Jinyinhua> decoction inhibited the influenza virus, ECHO virus, and herpes virus. The aqueous extract of the vine was also shown to delay cellular pathological changes due to ECHO virus (12).

In vitro, decoction of <Jinyinhua> and its vine also inhibited leptospirae. Intraperitoneal or subcutaneous injection of a preparation from the vine and the aerial part of *Senecio scandens* was effective in treating leptospirosis in rabbits and preventing this disease in guinea pigs (13).

More than half of the mice given the LD$_{90}$ of *Pseudomonas aeruginosa* or its endotoxin survived after injection of <Jinyinhua> at 7.5 g/kg IP. Injection of the distillate of the herb at 6 g/kg IV was therapeutically effective in mice poisoned by *Pseudomonas aeruginosa* endotoxin. The untreated animals showed markedly low body temperature and total WBC count, with a left shift of the leukocytic nuclei, whereas the treatment group exhibited a slight increase in the body temperature and WBC count, with no significant abnormality in the differential count. Poisoning of rabbits by the same endotoxin was checked by injection of "Jinhuang Injection" (Flos Lonicerae and Radix Scutellariae in equal amounts) at 7.5 g/kg IV; the injection reduced the toxic symptoms and mortality (14).

Another paper reported that an antipyretic and detoxifying formula containing <Jinyinhua>, the fruit of *Forsythia suspensa*, and the plants *Taraxacum mongolicum* and *Viola yedoensis* was effective in mitigating the toxic effects of *Salmonella typhi* (15).

2. Anti-inflammatory and Antipyretic Effects

Intraperitoneal injection of <Jinyinhua> extract at 0.25 g/kg to rats inhibited carrageenin-induced paw swelling (16). Another report claimed that at 30–40 g/kg, the <Jinyinhua> injection abated paw swelling induced by egg white (17). Intraperitoneal injection of the <Jinyinhua> extract to rats at 8 g/kg twice daily for 6 days also achieved antiexudative and antihyperplastic effects on croton oil-induced granuloma (16). Early reports claimed that <Jinyinhua> had a significant antipyretic action (18). However, experiments on rabbits with fever induced by injecting cholera vaccine, or lysate of *Bacillus atterimus* or *B. subtilis* into the animals' vein showed that <Jinyinhua> decoction at 5 g/kg PO produced no antipyretic effect. This could be attributed to the variations in the preparations, doses, and animal's tolerance (19).

3. Enhancement of the Defensive Function

The diluted decoction of <Jinyinhua> (1:1280) was still able to promote leukocytic phagocytosis (20). Intraperitoneal injection of the herb to mice also markedly enhanced the phagocytic activity of the inflammatory cells (17).

4. Central Stimulant Effect

Experiments using electric shock and the revolving cage showed that oral administration of chlorogenic acid to rats and mice resulted in central excitation; the strength of the stimulant effect was equal to one-sixth that of caffeine. No additive or potentiating effect was observed when these two agents were used together (21,22).

5. Antilipemic Effect

<Jinyinhua> at 0.5 g/kg PO decreased the intestinal absorption of cholesterol and the plasma

cholesterol level (23). *In vitro* experiments showed that <Jinyinhua> conjugated with cholesterol. However, in rabbits with experimental atherosclerosis, no observable antilipemic effect and cholesterol reduction on arterial walls were achieved with the "Simiao Yong' an Decoction" (Flos Lonicerae, Radix Scrophulariae Ningpoensis, Radix Angelicae Sinensis, Radix Glycyrrhizae) (24).

6. Miscellaneous Actions

In vitro screening of the aqueous and ethanol extracts of <Jinyinhua> proved that they possessed significant cytotoxic activity against sarcoma 180 and Ehrlich ascites carcinoma (25).

A mild prophylactic effect was achieved against experimental gastric ulcer in rats given the herb extract orally (26).

Large doses of chlorogenic acid by mouth increased gastrointestinal peristalsis, and promoted gastric and bile secretion. Chlorogenic acid and its degradation products had a stimulant effect on the isolated rat uterus (5,27). Chlorogenic acid also slightly enhanced the pressor effect of epinephrine and norepinephrine in cats and rats, but did not influence the nictitating membrane reaction of cats (22).

7. Toxicity

Intragastric administration of the aqueous extract of the herb to rabbits and dogs produced no significant toxic effects, nor any alterations in the respiration, blood picture, and urine output. The LD_{50} of this extract was determined to be 53 g/kg SC in mice (23). Allergic reactions were associated with chlorogenic acid, but these reactions were absent with oral administration, intestinal secretion transforming it into a non-allergenic substance (28).

CLINICAL STUDIES

1. Acute Infections

<Jinyinhua> is therapeutically effective in upper respiratory tract infections, lobar pneumonia, lung abscess, bacillary dysentery, acute mastitis, acute conjunctivitis, furuncle, carbuncle, pustules and erysipelas. Decoction of 6–15 g of the flowers or 15–100 g of the vines is commonly prescribed to be taken by mouth daily, or as a local wash (29,30).

The <Jinyinhua> injection used intramuscularly in 55 cases of acute tonsillitis afforded good therapeutic effects in lowering body temperature and reducing inflammatory reaction and exudation (31). A recent report stated that a preparation containing chlorogenic acid as the chief ingredient was effective in 70% of 85 cases of acute tonsillitis (32). "Yin Qiao San" (Lonicera-Forsythia Powder) was also quite effective for common cold at the early stage. The intramuscular dose of the <Jinyinhua> injection given to 12 cases of pulmonary tuberculosis complicated with bronchitis and

25 cases of pneumonia improved or relieved fever, chest pain, cough, expectoration, and dyspnea within a few days (33,34).

2. Infectious Hepatitis

The vines are useful for the amelioration of the symptoms and signs of infectious hepatitis and for the recovery of the hepatic function. Twenty-two cases were treated with the vine decoction at 60 g twice daily, 15 days as a therapeutic course; 12 were cured and 6 improved (35).

3. Infantile Diarrhea

The fine powder of the dried <Jinyinhua> suspended in water as a retention enema can be used as an adjunctive therapy in dyspepsia in young children. *Dosage and administration*: under 6 months, 1 g in 10 ml of water; 6–12 months, 1.5 g in 15 ml of water; 1–2 years, 2–3 g in 20–30 ml of water. The enema is to be used twice daily (36).

4. Leptospirosis

A 96.3% cure rate was achieved with the injection containing <Jinyinhua> and the aerial part or whole plant of *Senecio scandens* used in 109 cases of leptospirosis; symptoms and signs disappeared mostly within 2–4 days (13).

5. Hyperlipidemia

In 30 cases of hyperlipidemia treated with <Jinyinhua> by intravenous injection, no significant lowering of the serum cholesterol level was achieved. However, serum triglyceride was markedly decreased especially when the herb was also used orally concomitantly. Clinical improvement in the coronary blood supply was also observed concurrent with the reduction in blood lipids. This might be due to dilation of the coronary vessels caused by luteolin (24,37).

6. Miscellaneous

Decoction of fresh <Jinyinhua> given orally was effective for the treatment of urticaria (38). The fluidextract of the herb or the powders of the herb and the root and rhizome of *Glycyrrhiza uralensis* applied intravaginally with cotton balls were reported to be effective in the treatment of cervical erosion (39,40).

REFERENCE

1. Zhang JQ. New Chinese Medicine 1975 6(3):155.

2. Li XX et al. Chinese Medical Journal 1955 41(10):952.

3. Liu GS. Chinese Journal of New Medicine 1950 1(2):95.

4. Traditional Chinese Medicine and Materia Medica Research Unit of the Internal Medicine Department, Teaching Hospital of Chongqing Medical College et al. Collection of Papers on Science and Technology (Chongqing Medical College) 1959 (3):37.

5. Jiangxi Institute of Traditional Chinese Medicine and Materia Medica. Jingxi Zhongyiyao (Jiangxi Journal of Traditional Chinese Medicine) 1960 (1):34.

6. Wenzhou District (Zhejiang) Health Bureau. South Zhejiang Herbal. New edition. 1975. p. 340.

7. Yu YC et al. Acta Microbiologica Sinica 1959 7(3):231.

8. Lin QS. Chemical Studies of Traditional Chinese Drugs. Science Press. 1977. pp. 93, 146.

9. Shanghai No. 1 Chinese Medicine Factory. Summary of the Studies on the Active Constituents of Flos Lonicerae. 1972.

10. Takeda R. Chemical Abstracts 1961 50:5247c.

11. Cao RL et al. Chinese Journal of Dermatology 1957 (5):286.

12. Virus Section, Institute of Materia Medica of the Academy of Traditional Chinese Medicine. Xinyiyaoxue Zazhi (Journal of Traditional Chinese Medicine) 1973 (1):26.

13. Leptospirosis Research Group, Qianyang District (Hunan) Sanitation and Anti-epidemic Station. Studies on Epidemic Prevention 1975 (2):114.

14. Feng YC et al. Journal of Shenyang College of Pharmacy 1979 (11):73.

15. Nankai (Tianjin) Hospital. Chinese Medical Journal 1973 (1):33.

16. Xu JF et al. Compiled Information on Traditional Chinese Medicine (Jilin Medical College) 1973 (1):95.

17. Zhu QN et al. Compiled Information on Combined Western and Traditional Chinese Therapy of Acute Abdomen. Vol. 2. Teaching Hospital of Hubei Medical College. 1979. p. 64.

18. Zhang HQ et al. Shandong Medical Journal 1960 (10):22.

19. Huang YL et al. Studies on Traditional Chinese Medicine 1965 (3):43.

20. Hangzhou Second People's Hospital. Hangzhou Medical Information. 1977. p. 62.

21. Czok G et al. Chemical Abstracts 1961 55:20218i.

22. Valette G. Chemical Abstracts 1971 74:97900g.

23. Li XX. Abstracts of the 1962 Symposium of the Chinese Pharmaceutical Association. 1963. p. 342.

24. Coronary Disease Research Section. Zhejiang Institute of Traditional Chinese Medicine. Communications on Traditional Chinese Medicine and Materia Medica. 1974. p. 70.

25. Laboratory of the Surgery Department, First Teaching Hospital. Bulletin of Science and Technology (245 Unit of the Chinese PLA) 1973 (3):41.

26. Tomizawa S. The Journal of Society for Oriental Medicine in Japan 1962 13(1):5.

27. Czok G. Chemical Abstracts 1966 65:12755g.

28. Freedman SO et al. Chemical Abstracts 1965 63:18775e.

29. Editorial Group. National Collection of Chinese Materia Medica. Vol. 1. People's Medical Publishing House. 1975. p. 540.

30. Zhu Y. Pharmacology and Applications of Chinese Medicinal Materials. People's Medical Publishing House. 1954. p. 18.

31. EENT Department, 222nd Hospital of the Chinese PLA. Chinese Medical Journal 1974 54 (8):492.

32. Pharmaceutical Factory of Guilin Medical School. Clinical Data (Guilin Medical School) 1976 (3):33.

33. Sun QB et al. Fujian Zhongyiyao (Fujian Journal of Traditional Chinese Medicine) 1959 4(6):17.

34. Combined Western and Traditional Chinese medicine Research Group, Pediatrics Department of Chaoyang People's Hospital. Liaoning Yiyao (Liaoning Medical Journal) 1971 (1):32.

35. 26th Hospital of the Chinese PLA. Shaanxi Medical Journal 1972 (3):41.

36. Xu WJ. Zhongji Yikan (Intermediate Medical Journal) 1965 (4):207.

37. Xia SY. Notes on Science and Technology (Information Institute of Zhejiang Bureau of Science and Technology) 1973 (11):12.

38. Xu SS et al. Chinese Journal of Dermatology 1960 8(2):118.

39. Teaching Hospital of Obstetrics and Gynecology, Shanghai First Medical College. Chinese Journal of Obstetrics and Gynecology 1959 7(2):107.

40. Liang MC et al. Chinese Journal of Obstetrics and Gynecology 1960 8(1):38.

(Zhang Zunyi)

YUXINGCAO 魚腥草

<Yuxingcao> is the plant *Houttuynia cordata* Thunb. (Saururaceae). The fresh plant, which is more efficacious than the dried herb, is often used medicinally. It has a pungent taste and "cool" property. It is regarded as latent-heat-clearing, antipyretic, detoxicant, anti-inflammatory, and diuretic. It is, therefore, used in the treatment of virulent carbuncle, lung abscess, cough with thick sputum, leukorrhea, and edema.

CHEMICAL COMPOSITION

The fresh plant contains volatile oil, 0.005% as reported in Japan or 0.1% as usually reported in China. The volatile oil is composed of decanoyl acetaldehyde, methyl-n-nonylketone, myrcene, lauric aldehyde, α-pinene, camphene, d-limonene, linalool, bornyl, acetate, and caryophyllene (1).

The flower, leaf and fruit contain quercitrin and isoquercitrin. The flower bud also contains a large amount of potassium salts and a small amount of cordarine.

PHARMACOLOGY

1. Antimicrobial Effect

The fresh juice of *H. cordata* inhibited *Staphylococcus aureus* as shown in the well diffusion method, but its action was attenuated by heating (2). Various *in vitro* studies proved that the herb decoction was inhibitory to *Staphylococcus aureus, Staphylococcus albus, Streptococcus hemolyticus, Diplococcus pneumoniae, Neisseria catarrhalis, Corynebacterium diphtheriae, Proteus vulgaris, Shigella shigae, S. schmitzii, S. flexneri, S. sonnei, Salmonella enteritidis, Vibrio cholerae suis,* and leptospirae (3–6). A number of reports, however, claimed that the herb decoction had no significant antibacterial action (7–9); this could be due to the evaporation of the active principles — decanoyl acetaldehyde and methyl-n-nonylketone with steam. Thus, differences in the duration and condition of storage and in the heating time during processing could lead to divergent experimental results. The ether extract of the herb had been reported to markedly inhibit *Mycobacterium tuberculosis in vitro*, the MIC being 1:32,000, which was reduced to 1:2000 with the addition of serum. Feeds containing 2.5 and 7.5% of *H. cordata* prolonged the survival and decreased the mortality rate of mice injected with *Mycobacterium tuberculosis* $H_{37}RV$ into the caudal vein, but only slightly reduced pulmonary lesions (10). In the monolayer primary culture of the epithelial cells of human embryonic kidney, the *H. cordata* decoction inhibited Asian influenza virus type A Jingke 68-1 strain and also delayed cellular pathological changes caused by $ECHO_{11}$ virus (11).

The chief antibacterial principle of *H. cordata*, decanoyl acetaldehyde, is a labile compound which promptly polymerizes upon purification (12). But its adduct with sodium acetaldehyde has a significant activity against many bacteria (including acid fast bacilli) and fungi, it and a number of its derivatives were successfully synthesized and screened for antibacterial and antifungal activities (14).

The adduct of decanoyl acetaldehyde and sodium hydrogen sulfite synthesized in China was named "houttuynine" and the adduct of dodecanoyl acetaldehyde and sodium hydrogen sulfite as "neohouttuynine". *In vitro* bacteriostatic tests showed that houttuynine markedly inhibited many gram-positive and gram-negative bacteria. The most sensitive organisms were *Staphylococcus aureus* and its penicillin-resistant strains, *Diplococcus pneumoniae*, alpha streptococcus, and *Hemophilus influenzae*. *Neisseria catarrhalis* and *Salmonella typhi*, ranked second; *Escherichia coli, Pseudomonas aeruginosa* and *Shigella dysenteriae* showed marginal sensitivity. Its MIC against *Staphylococcus aureus* and the penicillin-resistant strains was determined to be 62.5–80 μg/ml, *Hemophilus influenzae* 1.25 mg/ml, and *Mycobacterium tuberculosis* $H_{37}RV$ strain in Proskauer-Beck medium 16 μg/ml (51), and in the modified semi-solid Sauton agar, 25 μg/ml. The MIC of the potassium salt of houttuynine against the same tubercular bacillus in the modified semi-solid Sauton agar was 12.5 μg/ml. Houttuynine markedly prolonged the survival of tuberculous mice (16). Houttuynine also significantly inhibited *Candida albicans, Cryptococcus neoformans, Sporotrichum, Aspergillus, Chromomycosis fungus, Epidermophyton rubrum, Tinea imbricata, Microsporum gypseum, Microsporum ferrugineum*, and sharkskin fungus, MIC was 2 mg/ml (15). On the other hand, neohouttuynine had an inhibitory action against *Diplococcus pneumoniae, Salmonella typhi, Staphylococcus aureus, Escherichia coli* and *Sporotrichum in vitro* (17,18). The synthetic houttuynine isoniazone showed strong inhibitory action against *Mycobacterium tuberculosis* both *in vitro* and in vivo with an MIC of 0.78–3.1 μg/ml. Intraperitoneal injection of this agent to tuberculous mice at 1 mg/mouse prolonged the survival period of the animals by 62 days; the therapeutic effect was enhanced when the drug was mixed with the animal feed (16).

2. Enhancement of Immunologic Function

In vitro studies showed that the *H. cordata* decoction markedly promoted the phagocytic ability of human peripheral leukocytes against *Staphylococcus aureus* (19). During treatment of chronic bronchitis with the houttuynine, leukocytic phagocytosis of *Staphylococcus albus* was greatly increased. Intramuscular injection of this agent to rabbits at 8 mg/day for 3 days markedly increased the serum properdin level determined on 4th and 8th days. The properdin level in patients with chronic bronchitis given houttuynine orally at 90 mg thrice daily for 7 days also tended to increase (20). In patients with chronic bronchitis, the combined therapy of houttuynine and *Aster ageratoides* greatly enhanced lysozyme activity in the blood and sputum, decreased serum lactate dehydrogenase activity, and markedly reduced lactate dehydrogenase in the sputum (21). The role of *H. cordata* and its active principles in strengthening the body resistance is of great importance in the treatment of infectious diseases.

3. Diuretic Effect

The *H. cordata* powder exerts a diuretic effect owing to quercitrin and large amounts of potassium salt it contains. Perfusion of the toad kidney or frog web with the herb extract produced a diuretic effect which might be causally related to its vasodilatory effect and its incremental effect on the renal blood flow (22–25).

4. Miscellaneous Actions

The *H. cordata* decoction had a distinct anti-inflammatory action on formaldehyde-elicited paw swelling in rats (26). It suppressed serous effusion and fostered tissue regeneration. The herb also exerted analgesic and hemostatic effects (27). Intraperitoneal injection of the *H. cordata* decoction produced an antitussive effect in mice with ammonia spray-induced cough (28). The herb was also reported to possess an antineoplastic activity (29). Subcutaneous injection of the water-soluble portion of the herb produced mild sedative and anticonvulsant effects in mice. It inhibited spontaneous activity, prolonged cyclobarbital sodium-induced sleep and antagonized strychnine-induced convulsion. Intravenous injection of this agent to dogs at doses of 20–40 mg/kg lowered the blood pressure by 40–50 mmHg and also depressed the isolated toad heart (30). Decanoyl acetaldehyde inhibited the germination of seeds (31).

5. Pharmacokinetics

The absorption half-life of houttuynine 200 mg/kg in the rat gastrointestinal tract was determined to be 3.5 hours. Twenty minutes after intravenous injection of 20 mg/kg, drug level was found to be highest in the lungs, next in the heart, liver, and kidneys, and minimally in the serum. No drug was detected in various tissues 2 hours after the injection. Two hours after 500 mg/kg PO, the drug was undetectable in the heart, liver, lungs, kidneys and serum. Incubation of houttuynine with various isolated tissues caused rapid transformation of the drug. Biotransformation of the drug was fastest in the renal tissue which within one hour metabolized 77–83% of the administered dose, compared with the metabolic rate of 51–64% in the lungs, liver, heart, and serum. Whether by intravenous or oral administration, drug excretion in the urine was very low and in the stool nil. Experiments also demonstrated that houttuynine could reversibly bind to plasma proteins.

That houttuynine was absorbed slowly from the gastrointestinal tract and distributed abundantly in the lungs after intravenous injection implies that it is of therapeutic value in the management of respiratory diseases; however, its rapid and almost complete biotransformation in the different tissues and organs indicates fast elimination from the blood and tissues (32). On the other hand, another paper reported the slow disappearance of radioactivity from the blood of albino mice injected with ^{14}C-houttuynine at 20 mg/kg IV. The radioactivity detected 30 minutes, 1, 2, 4, 8, 24 and 48 hours after medication accounted for 95, 89, 84.9, 85.8, 56, 24 and 11.1% of the administered dose, respectively. The highest drug level was in the bronchi, especially 1 and 4 hours following medication; descending concentrations were found in the gallbladder, liver, ovary, intestine, spleen, kidneys, and lungs. The highest drug level 24 hours after a single oral dose of 100 mg/kg was also detected in the bronchi. The total radioactivity in the expired air during 4 hours after the intravenous injection was equivalent to 68.1% of the administered dose, whereas urinary excretion accounted for only 4.5% in 48 hours. These results suggest that the main excretion route of houttuynine is the respiratory tract (33).

6. Toxicity

H. cordata has a very low toxicity. The fresh plant is often used as edible vegetable or porcine feed. Oral ingestion of large quantities of the herb is not known to cause intoxication. The LD_{50} of the synthetic houttuynine in mice was 1.6 ± 0.081 g/kg PO. Daily injection at 75–90 mg/kg IV to albino mice was not lethal. Soon after the injection, ataxia and spasm were seen in rodents, but these features were self-limiting and required no discontinuation of the injection. Intravenous infusion of 38 or 47 mg/kg to dogs did not cause any abnormalities or histopathological changes in the heart, lungs, liver, kidneys, spleen, stomach and intestine, but increasing the dosage to 61–64 mg/kg caused severe pulmonary hemorrhage.

Subacute toxicity tests showed that daily oral dosing of 80 or 160 mg/kg of the synthetic houttuynine to dogs for 30 days did influence the appetite, blood picture and liver function but caused vomiting and salivation of different extents (15).

CLINICAL STUDIES

1. Respiratory Tract Infections

The various preparations of *H. cordata* afforded satisfactory therapeutic effects on upper respiratory tract infections and chest infections such as bronchopneumonia, lobar pneumonia, lung abscess, and chronic bronchitis. The available preparations are *H. cordata* decoction, injection of the steam distillate of the herb, and houttuynine injection. The herb can be used alone or in compound formulae (34–55). The *H. cordata* injection had been used in 8 cases of lobar pneumonia, 7 of which had a fever of over 39°C; all cases recovered within 1–3 days and lesions were absorbed in an average period of 12.8 days (34). Others also reported the efficacy of *H. cordata* prescribed together with the root of *Platycodon grandiflorum* in lobar pneumonia (35). The *H. cordata* docoction (36), mixture (37), injection (38) and compound formulae (39,40) were reported to be effective in the treatment of lung abscess. Reports regarding the treatment of pneumonia in children with houttuynine are many; most of them claim that the agent has therapeutic value (42–48). It was reported that out of 91 cases treated with houttuynine, 72 were cured, 12 improved and 7 unresponsive (49). The efficacy the *H. cordata* injection administered into acupoints in the treatment of severe cough due to upper respiratory tract infections has also been reported (55). In addition, optimal effects were also achieved with houttuynine in chronic bronchitis in the elderly (56–59). In 587 elderly patients with chronic bronchitis treated with *H. cordata* and *Gnaphalium affine*, the effective rate was 94.1% and the marked effective rate, 55.1% (59).

2. Prevention and Treatment of Leptospirosis

The *H. cordata* tablet 15–30 g administered daily by mouth upon contact with contaminated water (60), or the *H. cordata* injection 3 ml intramuscularly every 5 days (61) afforded a prophylactic effect against leptospirosis. Other authors reported the efficacy of *H. cordata* alone or together with *Artemisia annua* in the management of leptospirosis (62,63).

3. Surgical Infections

H. cordata has curative and prophylactic values in postoperative infections (64,65) and acute phlebitis following infusion or transfusion (66). It could also be applied locally in skin infections such as boils (67).

4. Chronic Cervicitis and Others

Cotton impregnated with houttuynine solution, or the houttuynine tablet, was used in 243 cases. The medication was applied to the lesions overnight. Five applications comprised one course. The effective rate was reported to be 81–92% (68). Neohouttuynine was also quite effective in cervicitis, adnexitis, and pelvic inflammation (17).

5. Otorhinolaryngological Infections

Out of 100 cases of chronic suppurative otitis media treated with ear drops of the distillate of *H. cordata*, 95 cases were cured (69). Thirty-one of 33 cases of atrophic rhinitis benefitted from the nose drop preparation (70). Perfusion of the *H. cordata* extract was also very efficacious in the treatment of chronic maxillary sinusitis (71).

6. Miscellaneous

Eating the herb raw to increase appetite is a folk practice. Various preparations of *H. cordata* were also reported to be used with different beneficial effects to treat tinea infection of the hands (72), chronic nephritis (73,74), cancer (75), pulmonary tuberculosis, psoriasis (57,76,77) and for disinfection of the (78). A recent paper claimed that neohouttuynine had an excellent effect in the treatment of sporotrichosis (18).

ADVERSE EFFECTS

The side effects associated with houttuynine are generally mild. Oral ingestion of the herb produces a fishy smell on the breath, and pain at sites of intramuscular injection has been reported by a minority of patients. Intravaginal medication has been known to cause congestion of the vagina in individual patients. These untoward effects are self-limiting and disappear upon discontinuation of the medication. However, subsequent reports claimed that anaphylactic shock (79,80) and even death (81), atrophic dermatitis medicamentosa (82), and peripheral neuritis (83) developed following the *H. cordata* injection; thus caution be exercised while using this herb.

REFERENCE

1. Liu YL et al. Pharmaceutical Abstracts. Chinese Pharmaceutical Association (Beijing Branch). Sept 1978. p. 231.

2. Yan GH et al. Chinese Pharmaceutical Bulletin 1960 8(2):57.

3. Antibacterial Section, Institute of Materia Medica of the Chinese Academy of Medical Sciences. Chinese Pharmaceutical Bulletin 1960 8 (2):59.

4. Leptospirosis Research Unit, Chengdu College of Traditional Chinese Medicine. Scientific Research Compilation. 3rd edition. Chengdu College of Traditional Chinese Medicine. 1972. p. 59.

5. Leptospirosis Section, Sichuan Institute of Chinese Materia Medica. Research Information on Chinese Traditional Drugs (Sichuan Institute of Chinese Materia Medica) 1971 (6):34.

6. Yang HC et al. Chemical Abstracts 1953 47:8175d.

7. Zhejiang People's Academy of Health. In Vitro Bacteriostatic Tests of 110 kinds of Chinese Traditional Drugs. 1972.

8. Guiyang Medical College. Preliminary Report on the Bacteriostatic Tests of 516 kinds of Chinese Traditional Drugs. 1972.

9. Wuhan Sanitation and Anti-epidemic Station. Hubei Science and Technology — Medicine (Hubei Institute of Scientific and Technological Information) 1972 (6):37.

10. Feng YQ. Acta Academiae Medicinae Primae Shanghai 1964 (2):241.

11. Virus Section, Institute of Chinese Materia Medica of the Academy of Traditional Chinese Medicine. Xinyiyaoxue Zazhi (Journal of Traditional Chinese Medicine) 1973 (1):26.

12. Kosuge T. Journal of the Pharmaceutical Society of Japan (Tokyo) 1975 72 (10):1227.

13. Isogai Y. Chemical Abstracts 1953 47:2832a.

14. Kosuge T et al. Journal of the Pharmaceutical Society of Japan (Tokyo) 1953 75(5):435; 1956 76(4):386; 1954 74(8):819; 1956 76(4):390; 1954 74(10):1086; 1956 76(4):393.

15. Pharmaceutical Factory of the May 7 Cadre's School, Ministry of Health of the People's Republic of China et al. Jiangxi Medical Information (Jiangxi School of Pharmacy) 1972 (2):12.

16. Materia Medica Section, Bacteriology-Immunology Department, Beijing Institute of Tuberculosis. Pharmaceutical Abstracts. Chinese Pharmaceutical Association (Beijing Branch). 1978. p. 264.

17. Qui CQ et al. New Chinese Medicine 1979 10(12): 601.

18. Li SC et al. Guangdong Medical Journal 1981 (2):22.

19. Hangzhou Second People's Hospital. Hangzhou Medical Information. Centre of Medical and Health Information of Hangzhou Health Bureau. 1977. p. 62.

20. Bronchitis Unit, Third People's Hospital of Shanghai Second Medical College. Xinyiyaoxue Zazhi (Journal of Traditional Chinese Medicine) 1973 (7):25; Pharmaceutical Industry 1972 (8):9.

21. Medical Laboratory, Teaching Hospital of Jiangxi College of Traditional Chinese Medicine. New Medical Information (Jiangxi College of Traditional Chinese Medicine) 1975 (2):46.

22. Nakamura H et al. Chemical Abstracts 1938 32:5833(3).

23. Masuzawa H. Chemical Abstracts 1943 37:1773(1).

24. Ohta T. Chemical Abstracts 1950 44:11030a.

25. Kimura Y et al. Chemical Abstracts 1953 47:4550i.

26. Cui ZG et al. Compiled Research Information (Institute of Traditional Chinese Medicine and Materia Medica, Sichuan Branch of Chinese Academy of Sciences) 1960 (3):101.

27. Japan Centra Revuo Medicine 1954 112:668; Jiangsu College of New Medicine. Encyclopedia of Chinese Materia Medica. Vol. 1. Shanghai People's Publishing House. 1977. p. 1439.

28. Guangzhou Institute for Drug Control. New Medical Communications (Guangzhou Health Bureau) 1971 (6):64.

29. Lee C et al. Chemical Abstracts 1975 83:152250h.

30. Suzuki Y. Folia Pharmacologica Japonica 1980 76(4):146p.

31. Isogai Y. Chemical Abstracts 1954 48:7125f.

32. Materia Medica Unit, Jiangxi Second People's Hospital. Zhonghua Yixue Zazhi (National Medical Journal of China) 1976 56(7):454.

33. Jiangxi College of Traditional Chinese Medicine et al. New Medical Information (Jiangxi College of Traditional Chinese Medicine) 1977 (1):38.

34. Peng PC. Shanghai Zhongyiyao Zazhi (Shanghai Journal of Traditional Chinese Medicine) 1979 (4):28.

35. Li ZC et al. Chinese Medical Journal 1956 42(10):926.

36. Zhu YC et al. Shanghai Journal of Traditional Chinese Medicine 1960 (3):137.

37. Internal Medicine Department, Anbo Branch of Luda Second Hospital. Medicine and Health (Luda Health Bureau) 1976 (2):76.

38. Pediatrics Department, Hepu County (Guangxi) People's Hospital. New Chinese Medicine 1975 (8):390.

39. Ye JH et al. Journal of Traditional Chinese Medicine 1955 (9):25.

40. Zhou LK. Acta Academiae Medicinae Anhui 1976 (2): 54.

41. Lung Department, First Teaching Hospital of Zhejiang Medical College. Xinyiyaoxue Zazhi (Journal of Traditional Chinese Medicine) 1973 (7):21.

42. Pediatrics Department, Fujian People's Hospital. Medical Information (Fuzhou Institute of Medical Sciences) 1975 (2):62.

43. Pediatrics Department, Changyi People's Hospital. Barefoot Doctor (Changwei District Health Bureau) 1977 (2):15.

44. Xishagou Production Brigade Health Post (Haogezhuang Commune, Changle County). Barefoot Doctor 1977 (2):17.

45. Pediatrics Department, Xiamen First Hospital. Medical Information (Fuzhou Institute of Medical Sciences) 1977 (1):111.

46. Pediatrics Department, Yuanling County People's Hospital. Hunan Yiyao Zazhi (Hunan Medical Journal) 1977 (4):39.

47. Zhonghe Health Centre (Shuilong District, Sandu County). Guizhou Pharmaceutical Bulletin 1976 (2):23.

48. Zhong CY. People's Military Medicine 1979 (3):39.

49. Children's Hospital of Jiangxi et al. Jiangxi Medical Information 1972 (2):15.

50. Shashi Second People's Hospital. Health Journal of Shashi — Special Issue on Combined Western and Traditional Chinese Medicine 1974:54.

51. Cooperative Medical Clinic of Anle Production Brigade (Tongxiang County). Notes on Science and Technology — Medicine and Health (Information Institute of Zhejiang Bureau of Science and Technology) 1972 (3):23.

52. Traditional Chinese Medicine Department, Zhanjiang District People's Hospital. Scientific and Technological Exchanges (Zhanjiang District People's Hospital) 1977 (1):25.

53. Internal Medicine Department, JiuJiang Second People's Hospital. New Medical Information (Jiangxi School of Pharmacy) 1971 (1):18.

54. Hangzhou Airforce Hospital of the Chinese PLA. Notes on Science and Technology — Medicine and Health (Information Institute of Zhejiang Bureau of Science and Technology) 1976 (12):18.

55. Zhang XZ. Guangxi Zhongyiyao (Guangxi Journal of Traditional Chinese Medicine) 1980 (3):43.

56. May 7 Cadre's School of the Ministry of Health of the People's Republic of China. Pharmaceutical Industry 1972 (2):19; 1972 (8):5.

57. Chinese Traditional and Herbal Drugs Communications 1977 (8):30.

58. Yangpu District Hospital of Traditional Chinese Medicine. Exhibition of the Achievements in Combined Western and Traditional Chinese Medicine. Shanghai Exhibition Group. 1974. p. 121.

59. Chen XB et al. Shanghai Zhongyiyao Zazhi (Shanghai Journal of Traditional Chinese Medicine) 1979 (3):14.

60. Si SZ et al. Xinyiyaoxue Zazhi (Journal of Traditional Chinese Medicine) 1975 (6):40.

61. Chenjia Commune (Zigui County) Health Centre et al. Health and Epidemic Prevention (Hubei Sanitation and Anti-epidemic Station) 1973 (2):11.

62. Liang YQ. Heilongjiang Yiyao (Heilongjiang Medical Journal) 1978 (5):22.

63. Chinese Traditional Drugs Department, Chengdu College of Traditional Chinese Medicine. Scientific Research Compilation. 4th edition. Chengdu College of Traditional Chinese Medicine. 1975. p. 6.

64. Hu SH et al. Xinyiyaoxue Zazhi (Journal of Traditional Chinese Medicine) 1977 (6):14.

65. Cao R. Journal of Barefoot Doctor 1976 (7):19.

66. Surgery Department, Qianyang Hospital. Hunan Yiyao Zazhi (Hunan Medical Journal) 1976 (5):28.

67. Lu ZJ. New Chinese Medicine 1972 (10):51.

68. Jiangxi Maternal and Child Health Centre et al. Jiangxi Medical Information 1972 (2):16.

69. Ji HK et al. Xinyiyaoxue Zazhi (Journal of Traditional Chinese Medicine)1975 (2):44.

70. Ji HK et al. Xinyiyaoxue Zazhi (Journal of Traditional Chinese Medicine) 1977 (7):34.

71. Ji HK et al. Xinyiyaoxue Zazhi (Journal of Traditional Chinese Medicine) 1979 (5):28.

72. Tokkai 53-50313, Nihon Kokai Senri Sen Dai 5 Satsu 1979 (3):15.

73. Changyang County Health Bureau. Xinyiyaoxue Zazhi (Journal of Traditional Chinese Medicine) 1973 (7):12.

74. Changyang County Health Bureau. Xinyiyaoxue Zazhi (Journal of Traditional Chinese Medicine) 1973 (11):38.

75. Mi AQ. Notes on Science and Technology — Medicine and Health (Information Institute of Zhejiang Bureau of Science and Technology) 1978 (4):43.

76. Shanghai No. 4 Pharmaceutical Factory. Compiled Information on Decanoyl Acetaldehyde. 1970.

77. Jiangxi Yaowu Yanjiu (Jiangxi Research of Materia Medica) (Jiangxi Institute of Materia Medica) 1976 (1):48.

78. Wang L et al. Zhongji Yikan (Intermediate Medical Journal) 1979 (12):66.

79. Chinese Traditional Drug Popularization Group, Fenghua County (Zhejiang) People's Hospital New Chinese Medicine 1973 (4):205.

80. He SS. Shaanxi Medical Journal 1979 (8):36.

81. He C et al. New Medical Communications (Hubei College of Traditional Chinese Medicine) 1974 (1):29.

82. Cen GQ. Xinzhongyi (Journal of New Chinese Medicine) 1979 (5):47.

83. Zhang YH et al. People's Military Medicine 1980 (4):73.

(Deng Wenlong)

ZEXIE 澤瀉

<Zexie> is the tuber of *Alisma orientalis* (Sam.) Juzep. (Alismataceae). The tuber has a sweet taste and a "cold" property, and is known to have diuretic and "damp-heat"-clearing actions. It is used as treatment for dysuria, edema, urinary tract infection, retention of fluid and phlegm, and vertigo.

CHEMICAL COMPOSITION

The tuber of *A. orientalis* contains triterpenes: alisol A, alisol B, and acetates of alisols A, B, and C. The stem and leaf also contain alisol A, alisol B and their acetates. The tuber also contains volatile oil, alkaloids, choline, lecithin, methionine, formyltetrahydrofolate, vitamin B_{12}, biotin, and stigmasterol.

PHARMACOLOGY

1. Antilipemic Effect

The lipid-soluble fraction of <Zexie> has distinct anticholesterolemic and antiatherosclerotic effects in rabbits with experimental hypercholesterolemia (1,2). The isolated constituent alisol A, the acetates of alisols A, B, and C were all found to have marked anticholesterolemic action. Addition of 0.1% of any of these active principles to feed given to rats with experimental hypercholesterolemia decreased blood cholesterol by over 50%; this effects was very prominent with alisol A-24-acetate (3). The antilipemic effect did not emanate from the constituents choline and lecithin (1,2). Experiments in China also proved that the ethanol extract of <Zexie>, the ethyl acetate extract of the ethanol extract and its acetic acid-water insoluble residue all possess anticholesterolemic action, with the last two agents showing pronounced effects. A marked decrease in the cholesterol level was also obtained by daily oral administration of 1 g/kg of the acetate extract to rats on a regular diet (4).

The antilipemic mechanism of <Zexie> has not yet been fully elucidated. Radioisotope tracing proved that alisol A inhibited the esterification of cholesterol in the mouse small intestine (6) and reduced the absorption of cholesterol in the rat small intestine by 34%, but failed to influence the absorption of linoleic acid (7). In addition, <Zexie> probably modified the metabolism of endogenous cholesterol (4).

Concomitant with the lowering of serum cholesterol seen during clinical application of the herb are triglyceride reduction, increase in high-density lipoprotein, and increase in the high-density lipoprotein cholesterol/total cholesterol ratio (8). These effects are doubtless beneficial to be prevention and treatment of atherosclerosis. The decremental effect of <Zexie> on triglycerides is probably related to the improvement of fat metabolism in the liver (8,9).

2. Lipotropic Effect

Administration of <Zexie> to rabbits fed with a high-cholesterol and high-fat diet decreased hepatic lipids, indicating that the herb has lipotropic effect (1). The herb was also shown to be effective in rats with fatty liver due to a low-protein diet and in those with liver damage due to carbon tetrachloride (8,9). The herb extract contains many lipotropic substances: choline, lecithin, methionine, formyltetrahydrofolate, vitamin B_{12}, biotin, and unsaturated fatty acids (10). However, the chief lipotropic principle is believed to be a new substance, the biological activity of which is different from that of choline and lecithin (1,2).

3. Effect on the Cardiovascular System

Intravenous injection of the <Zexie> extract into dogs or rabbits elicited a mild hypotensive effect, sustained for about 30 minutes (4,12). The agent exerted a slow, relaxant action on the isolated rabbit aorta strip contracted by epinephrine (4). The water-soluble fraction of the ethanol extract of the herb perfused into the isolated rabbit heart dilated the coronary vessels. Neither an increase in the ^{86}Rb uptake of the mouse myocardium nor antagonism to pituitrin-induced myocardial ischemia was observed after intraperitoneal injection of the herb extract at doses as high as 10 g/kg. The extract slightly inhibited cardiac contractility, but had no significant effect on the heart rate (4).

4. Diuretic Effect

Despite differences in experimental results, most investigators believe that the <Zexie> decoction and extract are diuretic in man and various animals, increasing the excretion of sodium, chloride, potassium and urea in the urine (12–18). In rabbits with uranium nitrate-induced nephritis, the retention of urea and cholesterol in the blood was reduced by intraperitoneal injection of the fluidextract of the herb (18). The diuretic effect of the herb was found to be largely influenced by the season of its collection. Herbs harvested in winter, which are considered to be authentic specimens, are superior to those collected in spring. No diuretic effect was obtained with the young tuber which paradoxically decreased the urine output (16). The method of processing the herb had also some bearing on its diuretic effect: the uncured herb, the wine-treated herb and the wheat bran-treated herb were efficacious, whereas the salt-treated herb was inactive (17).

5. Hypoglycemic Effect

Subcutaneous injection of the <Zexie> extract to rabbits produced a weak hypoglycemic effect. Lowest blood glucose level which was only about 16% lower than the predrug measurement (19) appeared 3–4 hours after the injection. However,there is a report stating that this is devoid of hypoglycemic action (20).

6. Miscellaneous Actions

<Zexie> cannot increase the tolerance of hypoxia (4). It antagonized acetylcholine-induced spasm of the isolated intestine.

7. Toxicity

The LD_{50} of the methanol extract of <Zexie> in mice were 0.98 g/kg IV and 1.27 g/kg IP. No death occurred after oral administration of 4.0 g/kg. Administration of feed containing 1% of the herb to rats over a period of 2.5 months did not result in significant toxicity (22).

Administration of the ethanol extract of <Zexie> to mice at 100 g/kg PO did not cause any death within 72 hours. When rats were given feeds mixed with the powdered extract of the herb 1 and 2 g/kg (corresponding to 20 and 40 times the clinical dose) for 3 months, the animals remained healthy in general, their body weights increased and there were no significant alterations in the SGPT activity and hemoglobin count relative to the control. Nevertheless, various extents of cloudy swelling and degeneration of the hepatocytes and proximal renal tubular cells were discovered in pathological examinations; these changes which were considered significant compared to the control were found to be more prominent in the high dosage group. The changes could have been triggered by the extract. No significant changes were seen in the cardiac tissue however (4).

CLINICAL STUDIES

1. Hyperlipidemia

Two hundred and eighty-one cases were treated with the <Zexie> tablet (each contained the ethanol extract 0.15 g and fine powder 0.15 g, corresponding to 2.5–2.8 g of the crude drug) at 3–4 tablets 3–4 times a day by mouth for a course of 1–3 months. Laboratory results in 154 of these cases showed a marked lowering of blood cholesterol and triglycerides in 89.6 and 74.7%, respectively; cholesterol was lowered by a mean of 44.84 mg% (16.86%), and triglycerides, by 32.5 mg% (14.13%). The efficacy of this tablet was generally similar to that of clofibrate. Many patients experienced improvement of symptoms: dizziness, distending sensation in the head, and chest discomfort (15,23). Another group of 20 cases of hyperlipidemia were treated with the tablet prepared from the <Zexie>

extract (each corresponding to 3 g of the crude drug), 3 tablets thrice daily. After 19 weeks, the serum total cholesterol and triglycerides were decreased, the serum high-density lipoprotein cholesterol was increased by 13.6±23.6 mg% (an increase of 51.7%±54.8%) and the high density density lipoprotein cholesterol/total cholesterol percentage by 11.5±7.2% (an increase of 84.8±70.3%) (8). The tablet was effective in hyperlipoproteinemia types IIa, IIb, IV and V, and was especially good for chronic liver diseases secondary to hypertriglyceridemia (24).

2. Acute Nephritis, Oliguria, and Edema

<Zexie> is usually decocted with the sclerotium of *Poria cocos* and the seed of *Plantago asiatica* (25).

ADVERSE EFFECTS

Out of more than 200 cases of hyperlipidemia, only one case developed allergic skin rash; some developed mild digestive reactions with soft stools and frequent defecation, normal measurements following two weeks of uninterrupted medication. No abnormalities in the blood and urine routine examinations were found (5,23,24).

REFERENCE

1. Koboyashi T. Journal of the Pharmaceutical Society of Japan (Tokyo) 1960 80(10):1460.
2. Koboyashi T. Journal of the Pharmaceutical Society of Japan (Tokyo) 1960 80(11):1617.
3. Tadakazu M. Chemical and Pharmaceutical Bulletin 1970 18:1347, 1369.
4. Institute of Materia Medica, Zhejiang People's Academy of Health. Chinese Traditional and Herbal Drugs Communications 1976 (7):26.
5. Zhejiang Research Group on Alisma orientalis et al. Chinese Traditional and Herbal Drugs Communications 1976 (7):31.
6. Tamura S et al. Chemical Abstracts 1971 74:41003z.
7. Imai Y et al. Chemical Abstracts 1971 74:52017h.
8. Coronary Disease Section, Jiangsu Institute of Traditional Chinese Medicine et al. Exchanged information. 1979.
9. Koboyashi T. Journal of the Pharmaceutical Society of Japan (Tokyo) 1960 80(11):1606.
10. Koboyashi T. Journal of the Pharmaceutical Society of Japan (Tokyo) 1960 80(11):1612.
11. Koboyashi T. Journal of the Pharmaceutical Society of Japan (Tokyo) 1960 80(11):1456.
12. Jing LB et al. Chinese Reports of the Institute of Physiology (National Peiping Research Institute) 1936 3(3):259.

13. Rao MR et al. Chinese Medical Journal 1959 45:67.

14. Deng ZF et al. Chinese Medical Journal 1961 47:7.

15. Wang LW et al. Acta Academiae Medicinae Dalian 1965 (1):40.

16. Xu WF. Fujian Zhongyiyao (Fujian Journal of Traditional Chinese Medicine) 1963 8(1):42.

17. Shi JL et al. Harbin Zhongyiyao (Harbin Journal of Traditional Chinese Medicine) 1962 5(1):60.

18. Jing LB et al. Chinese Reports of the Institute of Physiology (National Peiping Research Institute) 1936 2(10):211.

19. Jing LB et al. Chinese Reports of the Institute of Physiology (National Peiping Research Institute) 1936 3(1):1.

20. Tang RY et al. Chinese Medical Journal 1958 44(2):150.

21. Koboyashi T. Yakugaku Kenkyu 1960 32(5):350.

22. Alisma orientalis Research Unit, Jiangxi First People's Hospital. Xinyiyaoxue Zazhi (Journal of Traditional Chinese Medicine) 1975 (2):24.

23. Zhongshan Teaching Hospital of Shanghai First Medical College et al. Zhonghua Yixue Zazhi (National Medical Journal of China) 1976 (11):693.

24. Hunan College of Traditional Chinese Medicine. Clinical Handbook of Commonly Used Chinese Traditional Drugs. 1972. p. 117.

(Xue Chunsheng)

XIXIN 細辛

<Xixin> refers to the plant *Asarum heterotropoides* Fr. Schmidt var. *mandshuricum* (Maxim.) Kitag., or *A. sieboldii* Miq. (Aristolochiaceae). It is pungent. "warm", and slightly toxic. Its actions are considered to be "cold"-discutient, antirheumatic, antitussive, and analgesic. It is chiefly used to treat headache due to common cold, cough and dyspnea with excessive sputum, arthritis, nasal congestion, and toothache.

CHEMICAL COMPOSITION

<Xixin> contains volatile oil composed of methyleugenol, kakuol and safrole. It also contains N-isobutyldodecatetramine (N-IBDTA), and dl-demethylcoclaurine (higenamine) (1).

PHARMACOLOGY

1. Sedative and Analgesic Effects

Intraperitoneal injection of the volatile oil of <Xixin> produced a significant central depressant effect. Sleep was induced in mice 5 minutes after the medication, and the righting reflex was lost. In guinea pigs the the drug produced unsteady gait, sedation and markedly prolonged thiopental sodium-induced sleep (2). Administration of the volatile oil 0.5 ml/kg PO to rabbits produced analgesia against pain due to electrical stimulation of the dental nerve; the analgesic strength was equal to that of 0.5 g/kg of antipyrine (3). The herb decoction administered intragastrically also produced analgesia in mice (4).

2. Antipyretic and Anti-inflammatory Effects

An antipyretic effect was achieved by intragastric administration of the volatile oil to rabbits with fever induced by exposure to heat, typhoid vaccine, or tetrahydro-β-naphthylamine. The oil also lowered the body temperature of normal animals (5). *A. sieboldii* inhibited formaldehyde- and egg white-induced paw swelling in rats (6).

3. Local Anesthetic Effect

The ethanol extract of *A. sieboldii* exerted an anesthetic effect on the sciatic nerve plexus of frogs, the intradermal nerve endings of guinea pigs, and also the human glossal mucous membrane (7).

4. Effect on the Respiratory System

Intravenous injection of the ethanol extract of *A. sieboldii* to rabbits antagonized respiratory depression precipitated by morphine (7). Methyleugenol significantly relaxed the isolated guinea pig bronchi (8). The ethanol extract of *A. heterotropoides* caused a brief decrease, followed by a sustained increase of 15–30 minutes in the perfusion volume of the isolated lung; isoproterenol did not show an initial lowering effect though it increased the perfusion volume of the lung, and the duration of its effect was the same as that of the extract. Thus the aftereffect of the herb is similar to the response elicited by isoproterenol. These actions served as the pharmacological basis for the traditional treatment of "cough and dyspnea due to retention of phlegm" with <Xixin> (9).

1-Pipecolic acid, which was isolated from a related Japanese species, A. hexalobum, exhibited an antitussive effect on SO_2-induced cough in guinea pigs (8).

The leaf extract, or the flavones of a related species grown in Europe, *A. europaeum* injected intravenously abated or relieved bronchial spasm in cats induced by neostigmine; the extract was more effective than the crude flavones (10).

5. Effect on the Cardiovascular System

The volatile oil of <Xixin> produced stimulation at low dosage and inhibition at high dosage on the isolated frog heart, stopping the heart at the diastolic phase (11). The ethanol extract of *A. heterotropoides* had a marked stimulant effect on the isolated heart of rabbits and guinea pigs; it promptly increased the cardiac contractility and heart rate for 7–10 minutes, suggesting the presence of positive inotropic and chronotropic effects. The agent increased the coronary flow in the isolated guinea pig heart but not in the isolated rabbit heart (9).

Intravenous injection of the volatile oil 25 mg/kg antagonized pituitrin-induced myocardial ischemia in rabbits and increased tolerance of mice to hypobaric hypoxia (2). Vasodilation was achieved by perfusing the volatile oil into the toad splanchnic blood vessels (12). Intravenous injection of the oil to anesthetized dogs produced hypotension, stimulated the kidney, reduced the kidney volume, and transiently suppressed urination (7). Intravenous injection of the volatile oil to anesthetized cats also decreased the blood pressure, whereas the herb decoction produced a significant pressor effect (12). The action of the decoction was enhanced by cocaine, but reversed by ergotoxine; it also caused contraction of the cat nictitating membrane. These effects appear to be adrenergic. Since potassium salt and other ash components did not evoke these effects, it is inferred that an organic constituent with a pressor effect exists in the herb (13). The leaf extract of *A. europaeum* injected intravenously to anesthetized cats elevated the blood pressure, whereas the flavones of the leaf lowered it (10).

6. Enhancement of Metabolism

dl-Demethylcoclaurine (higenamine) has been shown to exert a wide variety of β-adrenergic effects including cardiotonic, vasodilatory, smooth muscle relaxant, lipid-metabolism enhancing, and hyperglycemic effects. It has successfully been isolated from traditional drugs with "cold"-eliminative properties such as this herb <Xixin>, the lateral root-tuber of *Aconitum carmichaeli*, and the ripe fruit of *Evodia rutaecarpa*. The aforesaid effects resemble those achieved with "cold"-eliminative medicines (1). Thus the effects of higenamine may serve as the basis for the pharmacological use of "cold"-eliminative. medicines. This is an example of employing modern pharmacological methods to elucidate the traditional classification of herbs on the basis of their character, taste and reputed actions.

7. Antihistaminic and Antiallergic Effects

From the insoluble fraction of the methanol extract of *A. heterotropoides*, four components — methyleugenol, kakuol, N-isobutyldodecatetramine, and higenamine — were found to markedly inhibit histamine-induced contraction of the isolated guinea pig ileum (1). An antiallergic activity was demonstrated by the aqueous or ethanol extract of <Xixin> which reduced by more than 40% the total amount of allergic mediators released in immediate hypersensitivity reaction (1,14).

8. Effect on Smooth Muscles.

Low concentrations of the volatile oil of <Xixin> initially increased the tension of the isolated uterus and intestine of rabbits, with aftereffects of decreased tension and increased contraction amplitude, whereas high concentrations produced inhibition (11,15). The agent was also shown to inhibit the isolated rat uterus (3,5).

9. Antibacterial Effect

In vitro studies proved that the ethanol extract and the volatile oil of <Xixin> inhibited gram-positive bacteria, *Bacillus subtilis*, and *Salmonella typhi*, and that the herb decoction was inhibitory against *Mycobacterium tuberculosis* and *Salmonella typhi* (16,17). The volatile oil of *A. europaeum* was also found to have potent inhibitory action against gram-positive bacteria (18).

10. Toxicity

The LD_{50} of *A. sieboldii* in mice were 12.375 g/kg PO and 0.778 g/kg IV (7). The MLD of the volatile oil of <Xixin> in mice was 200 mg/kg IP, and the LD_{50} was 247 mg/kg (2). The aqueous extract of the herb was more toxic than the decoction (19). Inhibition was induced in frogs, mice, and rabbits, after an initial excitation, by the volatile oil. Voluntary movement and respiration were slowed, reflexes were lost, and death due to respiratory paralysis occurred; the heart ceased to beat on failure of respiration (20). Safrole contained in the volatile oil had a higher toxicity; it was shown to be carcinogenic, and, when mixed with animal feed, induced hepatoma in 28% of test rats after two years (21).

CLINICAL STUDIES

1. Common Cold, Headache, and Cough

The decoction of 1–3 g of <Xixin> can be given by mouth (22).

2. Toothache and Gingivitis

The patent medicine, "Yatongshui" (Toothache Liquid) (containing Herba Asari, Fructus Piperis Longi, Rhizoma Alpiniae Officinarum, Borneolum, etc.) is applied locally with cotton (23).

3. Tooth Extraction

<Xixin> and the uncured tuber of *Arisaema consanguineum* provides an anesthetic effect which is useful in tooth extraction (23).

4. Local Anesthesia

An injection prepared from the 3% volatile oil of <Xixin> was used as a local infiltrative anesthesia and nerve blocker in 52 cases of otorhinolaryngological and ophthalmic operations with good effects in 33 cases, relatively good effect (occasional local pain during operation) in 17 cases, and no effect in 2 cases. The addition of 0.1% of epinephrine into this anesthetic solution prolonged the duration of anesthesia and reduced postoperative tissue swelling (24).

5. Aphthous Stomatitis

A plaster prepared from the herb powder 9–15 g, water and small amounts of glycerin or honey is applied with gauze over the umbilical area and fixed with adhesive tape. The plaster is retained for at least 3 days. Two applications may be required in intractable cases. An aggregate effective rate of 93.4% was achieved in 106 cases so treated (25). In addition, some compound formulae containing the herb, notably, "Guanxinling" and "Kuanxiong" aerosol, have been satisfactorily used in recent years to treat coronary disease (26).

ADVERSE EFFECTS

<Xixin> is nephrotoxic; hence, it must be used with caution in patients with renal insufficiency (26).

REFERENCE

1. Kosuge T. Kampo Kenkyu 1978 11:429.

2. Coronary Disease Research Group, Taixi Hospital. Notes on Medical Science and Technology (Qingdao Health Bureau) 1975 (5): 14.

3. Ishihara T. Japan Centra Revuo Medicina 1960 153:339.

4. Pharamcology Department, Nanjing College of Pharmacy. Acta Pharmaceutica Sinica 1966 13(2): 95.

5. Ishihara T. Folia Pharmacologica Japonica 1957 53(2):60.

6. Song ZY et al. Acta Pharmaceutica Sinica 1963 10(12):708.

7. Yan YJ. Acta Academiae Medicinae Qingdao 1959 (2):20.

8. Kuwa N et al. The Japanese Journal of Pharmacognosy 1977 31(2):175.

9. Wang HX et al. The effects of Herba Asari on the isolated heart and lung. In: Pharmacological Studies of Herba Asari I. Hunan Institute of Traditional Chinese Medicine. 1978.

10. Akhmetova BKh. Farmakologiia I Toksikologiia 1970 33(2):191.

11. Kondo. The Keijo Journal of Medicine 1930 1:223.

12. He JL et al. Proceedings of the 2nd National Congress of the Chinese Pharmaceutical Association. Vol. 2. 1956. p. 44.

13. He JL et al. Abstracts of the Chinese Pharmaceutical Association (Beijing Branch). 1957. p. 68.

14. Zhang BH. Chinese Pharmaceutical Bulletin 1979 14(5):224.

15. Li TZ. Japan Centra Revuo Medicina 1932 34:1021.

16. Wang Y et al. Acta Botanica Sinica 1953 2(2):312.

17. Xu Z et al. News of Agriculture 1947 1(16):17.

18. Gracza L. Chemical Abstracts 1965 62:11626d.

19. Harbin Zhongyi (Harbin Journal of Traditional Chinese Medicine) 1961 4(9):49; Encyclopedia of Chinese Materia Medica. Vol. l. Shanghai People' s Publishing House. 1977. p. 1477.

20. Kondo T. Choson Uihakhoe Chapchi 1928 88:44.

21. Jiang TL. Chinese Traditional and Herbal Drugs 1980 (9):425.

22. Zhongshan Medical College (editor). Clinical Applications of Chinese Traditional Drugs. Guangdong People' s Publishing House. 1975. p. 17.

23. Jiangxi College of Traditional Chinese Medicine (editor). Lectures on the Pharmacology of Chinese Traditional Drugs. 1974. p. 3.

24. First Teaching Hospital, Wuhan Medical College. Health Journal of Hubei 1972 (1):68.

25. He ES. Xinyiyaoxue Zazhi (Journal of Traditional Chinese Medicine) 1977 (1):13.

26. China' s Pharmacopoeia. Part I. People' s Medical Publishing House. 1977. P. 379.

(Chen Quansheng)

GUANZHONG 貫眾

<Guanzhong> refers to the rhizome and the base of the leaf stalk of *Dryopteris crassirhizoma* Nakai (Dryopteridaceae) or *Osmunda japonica* Thunb. (Osmundaceae). The herb derived from the first plant is also known as <Mianmaguanzhong> or <Dongbeiguanzhong>; that derived from the second is called <Ziqiguanzhong>.

<Guanzhong> has a bitter taste and slightly "cold" property. Its actions are regarded as being latent-heat-clearing, antipyretic, detoxicant, anti-inflammatory, hemostatic, and anthelmintic; it is able to remove pathogenic "heat" from the blood. Thus, the herb is mainly used in the treatment of common cold due to pathogenic "wind-heat", macular eruption in febrile diseases, hematemesis, epistaxis, bloody stool, metrorrhagia, taeniasis, and oxyuriasis.

The botanical source of <Guanzhong> used in China is rather complicated. According to a report the herb is derived from 29 species of five genera (1). Apart from *D. crassirhizoma*, the main species include *Lunathyrium acrostichoides* (SW.) Ching or <Emeijueguanzhong>; *Matteuccia stuthiopteris* (L.) Todaro or <Jiaguojueguanzhong or Xiaoyeguanzhong>; *Blechnum orientale* L. or <Wumaojueguanzhong>; *Brainia insignis* (Hook.) J. Sm. or <Sutiejueguanzhong>; *Woodwardia japonica* (L.f.) Sm. or <Goujiquanzhong or Dayeguanzhong>; *Cyrtomium fortunei* J. Sm. or <Hunjitou>.

CHEMICAL COMPOSITION

D. crassirhizoma contains filicic acids, flavaspidic acids, and traces of albaspidin and dryocrassin. It also contains fernene, pterosterone, tannin, volatile oil, and resin. Filicic acids and Flavaspidic acids are anthelmintics.

M. stuthiopteris contains ponasterone A, ecdysterone, pterosterone, and fatty acids (mainly arachidonic acid).

O. japonica contains ponasterone A, ecdysterone, and ecdysone.

B. orientale contains chlorogenic acid.

W. japonica contains tannin and large amounts of starch.

The aerial part of *C. fortunei* contains flavonoid glycosides isoquercitrin, astragalin, cyrtopterin and cyrtomin, but the rhizome and the base of the leaf stalk do not contain phenolic filicic acids.

PHARMACOLOGY

1. Antimicrobial Effect

<Guanzhong> has a strong inhibitory action against multiple viruses. In experiments with chicken embryos, the herb decoction exhibited a significant inhibitory action on Asian influenza virus PR_8

strain, type A Jingke 68–1 strain, 57–4 strain, new A$_1$ Lianfang 77–2 strain, influenza viruses type B (Lee), type C (1232), and type D (Xiantai) (2–5). Different degrees of inhibition were observed no matter whether the decoction was given before or after viral infection, and its potency was directly proportional to the concentration (5). The herb decoction has been reported to inhibit influenza virus at concentrations of 1:10,000–100,000 (2). In the monolayer primary cultures of the epithelial cells of human embryonic kidney and lung, <Guanzhong> was also shown to inhibit influenza virus Jingke 68–1 strain, parainfluenza Xiantai virus, adenovirus type III, poliomyelitis virus type II, ECHO virus type 9, Coxsackie virus, epidemic encephalitis B virus, and herpes simplex virus (6–8). Since <Guanzhong> did not significantly protect mice from infection by influenza virus instilled into the nose, whereas the tannin content in the herb used was 14.5%, the antiviral effect of the herb *in vitro* might be due to the tannin it contains (2) (*Error of the Chinese passage). Another paper reported that influenza virus and rhinovirus were inhibited by "Gui Guan Xiang" (Cinnamomum-Dryopteris Incense) or "Gui Guan Yin Xiang" (Cinnamomum-Dryopteris-Artemisia Incense) used for fumigation (9,10).

<Guanzhong> also provides a bacteriostatic effect. It was quite potent against *Shigella dysenteriae, Salmonella typhi, Escherichia coli, Pseudomonas aeruginosa* and *Proteus vulgaris*, and effective to some extent against *Staphylococcus aureus* (11,12).Fumigation with the Cinnamomum-Dryopteris Incense for 4–6 hours markedly reduced the bacteria flora in the air, but this might be due to the smoke itself (9,13). In addition, the herb inhibited some skin fungi (14).

2. Anthelmintic Effect

The filmarone subtances contained in *D. crassirhizoma* were extremely toxic to tapeworms, causing paralysis and detachment of worms from the intestinal wall and their expulsion by purgatives. Filicic acid was found to be more effective than flavaspidic acid. *D. crassirhizoma* can be used as a substitute for Dryopteris filix-mas Schott, a traditional drug for treating tapeworm infection, which is, however, rarely used nowadays because of its high toxicity (15).

Chinese investigators reported that <Guanzhong> was active against swine ascarides, earthworms, and leeches *in vitro* (16,17). The decoctions of *D. crassirhizoma, M. stuthiopteris, O. japonica, W. japonica*, and *C. fortunei* at a concentration of 16% exerted different degrees of inhibitory action on the head of swine ascaris; concentrations of 50–70% were required to inhibit the whole worm (17). The decoction of *D. crassirhizoma* was able to expel bovine liver fluke (18); its compound prescription was effective against flat flukes and broad sucker flukes in cows (19). *O. japonica* was reported to be capable of expelling human intestinal parasites such as *Ancylostoma duodenale, Ascaris lumbricoides*, and *Trichuris trichiura* (20). A recent paper claimed that an excellent therapeutic effect could be achieved with *D. crassirhizoma* in the experimental treatment of schistosomiasis in animals; in mice the crude herb powder could promote the migration of schistosomes to the liver. The petroleum ether dialysate and its acid precipitate as well as dryocrassin, which could markedly promote the migration of schistosomes to the liver in mice and rabbits, were also lethal to the parasites (21).

3. Effect on the Uterus

The <Guanzhong> decoction had a stimulant effect on the uterus. The refined decoction at 1:3000 increased the contractility of the isolated rabbit uterus, and given intravenously, it significantly increased the tension of the rabbit uterus *in situ* (22). <Guanzhong> obtained from *D. crassirhizoma* stimulated the isolated guinea pig uterus, increased the frequency of contraction and tonicity, and decreased the contraction amplitude. Spastic contraction induced by increasing the dosage was reversed by washing away the herb solution. A similar action was demonstrated in the isolated uterus of nonpregnant rabbits (23).

A mixture of filicic acids obtained from <Guanzhong> at concentrations as low as 25–35 μg/ml caused tonic contraction of the isolated guinea pig uterus. At the concentration of 8.9 μg/ml it caused spastic contraction. Compared with ergometrine, the duration of action of the filicic acids was more prolonged, and their effect stronger; excitation was sometimes sustained for as long as one hour. Intravenous injection of this mixture to guinea pigs at 1 mg/animal resulted in marked excitation of the uterus *in vivo* (24).

Clinically, the injection preparation of *C. fortunei* also showed a marked contractile effect on the uterus, usually appeared within 3–5 minutes after injection (25). On the other hand, *L. acrostichoides* had no significant action on the uterus (23).

4. Termination of Early Pregnancy and Abortifacient Effect

The <Guanzhong> extract can terminate early pregnancy and has an abortifacient effect. In mice, subcutaneous injection of 2 or 3 mg thrice starting from the 7th day of pregnancy, or one intravaginal application of 50 mg, or one intragastric administration of 10 or 15 mg of the extract, could significantly terminate pregnancy at the early stage. The same effect was achieved in rats by subcutaneous injection of 15 mg 5 times. Subcutaneous injection to rabbits of the herb extract at 75 mg/animal 3 times, or 50 mg/animal 5 times, starting from the 10th day of pregnancy was combined with intravaginal application of 450 mg; dissection carried out on the 18th day of pregnancy revealed almost complete expulsion of the placenta in most of the animals. An abortifacient effect was obtained with the extract at 500 mg/kg PO on the 16th day of pregnancy; the fetuses were completely expelled in 24 to 41 hours, while the mother mice remained healthy (24).

5. Estrogenic Activity

Experiments showed that intragastric administration of the <Guanzhong> extract to young mice at 2 mg/day for 3 days resulted in a marked increase of the uterus weight. Vaginal smears of adult mice receiving the drug also showed certain estrogenic activity of the herb (24).

6. Hemostatic Effect

The 1:1 decoction of *O. japonica* significantly shortened the coagulation time of rabbits. A compound prescription which chiefly contains *O. japonica* also tended to shorten bleeding and coagulation times (26).

7. Miscellaneous Actions

The <Guanzhong> decoction significantly inhibited the isolated toad heart (27). Intramuscular injection of the herb preparation excited the smooth muscles of the urinary bladder and intestine (12).

8. Toxicity

<Guanzhong> derived from different plant species varies considerably in toxicity. Intravenous injection of *D. crassirhizoma* 2 ml to anesthetized rabbits did not affect respiration and blood pressure; its LD_{50} in mice was 1.7 ± 0.021 g/kg. Injection of large doses to rabbits for several days did not produce any significant influence on the main organs (23).

The acute LD_{50} of the acid-precipitated substance of *D. crassirhizoma* in mice was 560 mg/kg, and that of dryocrassin, 640 mg/kg. Reactions are chiefly referrable to the gastrointestinal tract. Large doses of the acid-precipitated substance caused paralysis of the hind limbs, followed by death of the animals (21). The LD_{50} of the mixture of filicic acids from *D. crassirhizoma* in 18–22-g mice was 420 mg/kg SC or 670 mg/kg PO. In most of the pregnant mice weighing over 40 g, however, no toxic symptoms developed after administration of 500 mg/kg PO. These results indicate that this mixture apparently produced different degrees of toxicity in animals of different ages. Oral administration of this mixture 100 or 200 mg/kg twice to dogs given at interval of days, or intramuscular injection of 75 or 200 mg/kg daily for 12 days, resulted in slight impairment of hepatic and renal functions, mild to moderate cloudy swelling of the renal convoluted tubular epithelium, interstitial congestion and cloudy swelling of liver cells, and mild blood stasis in a minority of animals; in most of the animals there were no abnormalities in the blood picture, liver and kidney functions, heart, liver, spleen, lungs, kidneys, stomach, intestine, uterus, optic nerve, adrenal, thyroid and pituitary gland, and vision. Signs of abortion were also observed in the uterus and placenta of pregnant dogs (24).

A related species *D. filix-mas* was found to be very toxic. Daily administration of magnesium filicate to dogs at 40 mg/kg PO induced spermatocytic changes, diarrhea, and weight loss, while administration of large doses from 40 to 80 mg/kg for 10–15 days damaged the optic nerve resulting in blindness, and also damaged cerebral white matter. The LD_{50} of *D. filix-mas* intragastric administration in mice was 298 mg/kg, in rats 1076 mg/kg, and in guinea pigs 273 mg/kg (28). Fat accelerates its absorption and thereby increasing its toxicity.

CLINICAL STUDIES

1. Respiratory Tract Infections Such as Common Cold and Influenza

Treatment of drinking water with <Guanzhong> is a folk practice for the prevention of common cold (29). Numerous reports on the clinical use of the herb and its compound formulae for the prevention and treatment of common cold and influenza are available (9,30–39). For instance, the incidence of common cold was only 12% in 306 persons who took the herb granule infusion for prophylaxis twice weekly in comparison to 33% in 340 controls (30). In approximately 800 persons who were given the "Fufang Guanzhong Pian" (Compound Dryopteris Crassirhizoma Tablet) (Rhizoma Dryopteris Crassirhizomae (chief herb), Folium Isatidis, Radix Glycyrrhizae) to prevent influenza, the incidence rate of influenza was reported to be 2–3.8% compared to 78.4% in 130 controls. This tablet also had a curative effect (31). Optimal effects could be obtained by fumigation with the incense prepared from <Guanzhong> and the leaf of *A. argyi* in the prevention of influenza (9,40). <Guanzhong> has also been used to treat epidemic meningitis (41), measles (42), and pneumonia in children caused by adenovirus (43).

2. Obstetrical and Gynecological Hemorrhages

<Guanzhong> plus the dried feces of *Trogopterus xanthipes* was reported to be effective in the treatment of menorrhagia (44). The injection preparation of *C. fortunei* was effective in hemorrhages following therapeutic abortion, delivery, and dilatation and curettage; uterine contraction was usually initiated 3–5 minutes after the injection, along with reduction or cessation of bleeding (25). The injection of *D. crassirhizoma* also had a good contractile effect on the uterus, usually detectable 10 minutes after the medication, and it stopped bleeding. Forty-four out of 48 cases treated with this injection benefitted (24). Excellent effects were also achieved in 120 cases including menorrhagia, missed abortion, profuse bleeding after therapeutic abortion, retention of placenta, and severe postpartum hemorrhage. A rapid and more pronounced effect could be obtained by intracervix injection rather than intrauterine or intramuscular injection (45). The oral hemostatic preparation of *O. japonica* was tried in 78 cases of different types of gynecological hemorrhage, and 37 were cured, 35 ameliorated, and 6 unchanged (26).

3. Hemostasis

The *C. fortunei* decoction at 60 g divided into 3–4 doses, or the fluidextract 15 ml 4 times daily, was administered to 102 cases of hemorrhage of various origins such as pulmonary tuberculosis, bronchiectasis, and upper gastrointestinal bleeding,. Amelioration of bleeding was achieved on the first day of treatment; for 52 cases, bleeding stopped in 2–3 days, and for 32 cases in 4–5 days. Concurrent sedative and hypnotic effects were also achieved (46). In addition, a preparation, "Zhixuejing", consisting of <Guanzhong> and the rhizome of *Polygonum bistorta*, etc. applied externally was found to have hemostatic, analgesic and anti-inflammatory actions (47).

4. As Anthelmintics

The *O. japonica* tablet was reported to be superior to diethylcarbamazine citrate in the treatment of ancylostomiasis, ascariasis, and trichuriasis (20). A compound <Guanzhong> prescription was effective in biliary ascariasis (48). Although the herb and its compound prescriptions have been used to treat ancylostomiasis (49), their therapeutic effect requires further validation.

5. Miscellaneous

Excellent therapeutic effects of <Guanzhong> plus earthworm and licorice in the management of tropical eosinophilia have been reported (50). The *O. japonica* tablet and a compound <Guanzhong> prescription were effective in chronic bronchitis (51,52). The decoction of <Guanzhong> and the rhizome of *Dioscorea hypoglauca* was used to treat 11 cases of lead poisoning; 8 cases showed marked improvement and 3 cases were ameliorated (53). Six cases of chyluria were cured with carbonized <Guanzhong>; one relapsed in one year but was cured again with the same drug (54). In addition, this herb had been employed as a quick water purifier (55).

ADVERSE EFFECTS

D. crassirhizoma is highly toxic; oral administration of it could cause gastrointestinal irritation, and in severe cases, vomiting and diarrhea. Overdosage or concomitant ingestion of a large amount of fat would enhance absorption of the herb and consequently cause poisoning which could lead to optic nerve damage and even blindness, central disturbances, tremor, convulsion, etc. Therefore, it is rarely used nowadays. The herb is contraindicated in pregnant women, asthenic patients, young children, patients with organic disease, and peptic ulcer. The other <Guanzhong> species are less toxic.

REFERENCE

1. Beijing Institute for the Control of Drugs and Biological Products et al. Handbook for Identification of Chinese Medicinal Materials. Vol. 1. Science Press. 1972. p. 303.

2. Shanghai Sanitation and Anti-epidemic Station. Shanghai Zhongyiyao Zazhi (Shanghai Journal of Traditional Chinese Medicine) 1960 (2):68.

3. Laboratory of Xi'an Centre of Influenza. Shaanxi Journal of Medicine and Health 1959 (1):14.

4. Guiyang Medical College. Medical Information (Guizhou Health Bureau) 1972 (4):2.

5. Lianyungang Sanitation and Anti-epidemic Station. Weishengwuxue Tongbao (Bulletin of Microbiology) 1979 (2):20.

6. Virus Section, Institute of Chinese Materia Medica of the Academy of Traditional Chinese Medicine. New Chinese Medicine (Reference Information) 1972 (4):4.

7. Guangzhou Institute of Medicine and Health. The References of Traditional Chinese Medicine 1973 (2):14.

8. 302nd Hospital of the Chinese PLA. Health Bulletin — Supplement (Health Division of the Logistics Department of the Chinese PLA) 1972 (9):49.

9. "Ganmaoxiang" Coordinating Research Group. Selected Medical Information (General Hospital of the Chinese PLA) 1975 (9):26.

10. "Ganmaoxiang" Coordinating Research Group. Selected Medical Information (General Hospital of the Chinese PLA) 1975 (9):29.

11. Hu JY. Jiangxi Zhongyiyao (Jiangxi College of Traditional Chinese Medicine) 1960 (5):37.

12. Ob-Gyn Department, Yichun District People's Hospital. Xinyiyao (Modern Chinese Medicine) (Yichun District, Jiangxi) 1974 (6):23.

13. "Ganmaoxiang" Coordinating Research Group. Selected Medical Information (General Hospital of the Chinese PLA) 1975 (9):33.

14. Cao RL et al. Chinese Journal of Dermatology 1957 (4):286.

15. Goodman LS et al. The Pharmacological Basis of Therapeutics. 3rd edition. 1965. p. 1058.

16. Wu YR et al. Chinese Medical Journal 1948 34(10):437.

17. Nanjing College of Pharmacy. Experimental Data 1973 (11); Nanjing College of Pharmacy. Chinese Traditional Pharmacy. Vol. 2. Jiangsu People's Publishing House. 1976. p. 54.

18. Zheng ZJ. Journal of Chinese Zootechnics and Veterinary Medicine 1956 (1):17.

19. Zheng ZJ et al. Journal of Chinese Zootechnics and Veterinary Medicine 1958 (10): 474.

20. Zhao XG et al. Jiangsu Zhongyi (Jiangsu Journal of Traditional Chinese Medicine) 1962 (10):14.

21. Pharmacology Department, Institute of Parasitology of the Chinese Academy of Medical Sciences. Proceedings of the 4th Symposium of the Chinese Pharmaceutical Association. Vol. 2. Chinese Pharmaceutical Association (Shanghai Branch). 1979.

22. Takenaga S et al. Japan Centra Revuo Medicina 1943 84:451; 1944 86:13.

23. Pharmaceutical Factory of Changchun Health School. New Pharmaceutical Communications (Shenyang College of Pharmacy) 1971 (4–5):18.

24. Chen Q et al. Tianjin Medical Journal 1980 (8):488.

25. Chongzuo County (Guangxi) People's Hospital. Chinese Traditional and Herbal Drugs Communications 1970 (5–6):35.

26. Scientific Research Compilation. 59171 Unit of the Chinese PLA. 1976. p. 80.

27. Kimura M et al. Japan Centra Revuo Medicina 1944 88:221.

28. Georges A et al. Chemical Abstracts 1970 73:54474h.

29. Paotong (Henan) Coordinating Research Group on Chronic Bronchitis. Prevention and Treatment of Chronic Bronchitis (Henan Health Bureau) 1975 (9):1.

30. Hangzhou Sanitation and Anti-epidemic Station. Hangzhou Yiyao (Hangzhou Medical Journal) 1972 (1):6.

31. Jinghong County (Yunnan) Centre for the Popularization of Ethnomedicine. Xinyiyaoxue Zazhi (Journal of Traditional Chinese Medicine) 1978 (12):40.

32. Ge ZS. People's Military Medicine 1979 (3):14.

33. Zhuang Autonomous Region (Guangxi) Sanitation and Anti-epidemic Station et al. Chinese Traditional and Herbal Drugs Communications 1977 (12):32.

34. Beilan Production Brigade Health Post (Wulajie People's Commune, Yongji County, Jilin). Journal of Barefoot Doctor 1975 (1):38.

35. Hangzhou First Cotton Textile and Dye Factory. Chinese Traditional and Herbal Drugs Communications 1973 (6):40.

36. Xushuirongcheng County. Journal of Traditional Chinese Medicine 1959 (1):45.

37. Ping' an Health Centre (Taoan County). Jilin Yiyao (Jilin Medical Journal) 1973 (2):36.

38. Qiongshan County Health Bureau et al. Guangdong Medical Information 1975 (Supplement):1.

39. Hongqi Commune (Tonggu County) Health Centre. New Medical Information (Jiangxi School of Pharmacy) 1971 (3):24.

40. Chronic Bronchitis Unit, Staff Hospital of Gansu No. 1 Bureau of Construction Engineering. Chinese Journal of Internal Medicine 1978 (5):329.

41. Nanchang Sanitation and Anti-epidemic Station. Jiangxi Yiyao (Jiangxi Medical Journal) 1962 (1):8.

42. Wenling County Sanitation and Anti-epidemic Station. Notes on Science and Technology — Medicine and Health (Information Institute of Zhejiang Bureau of Science and Technology) 1973 (11):6.

43. Pediatrics Department, First Teaching Hospital of Hubei Medical College. Health Journal of Hubei 1976 (3):39.

44. Ren XW. Journal of Traditional Chinese Medicine 1961 (6):24.

45. Sun HY et al. Guizhou Pharmaceutical Bulletin 1978 (4):23.

46. Zhao DH. Zhejiang Zhongyiyao (Zhejiang Journal of Traditional Chinese Medicine) 1977 3(1):19.

47. First Laboratory of 236 Unit of the Chinese PLA. Studies on "Zhixuejing". 1971.

48. Tong JD et al. Heilongjiang Zhongyiyao (Heilongjiang Journal of Traditional Chinese Medicine) 1966 2(5):36.

49. Pest and Disease Eradication Supervisory Group, Changde County (Hunan) Revolutionary Committee. Chinese Pharmaceutical Bulletin 1959 7(4):184.

50. Chinese Traditional and Herbal Drugs Communications 1977 (12):19.

51. Bronchitis Group et al. Tuberculosis (Beijing Institute of Tuberculosis) 1973 (3):8.

52. Huang YQ. Fujian Medicine and Health 1978 (4):50.

53. Sanatorium of Shenyang Ironworks Factory et al. Xinyiyaoxue Zazhi (Journal of Traditional Chinese Medicine) 1975 (1):39.

54. Liu SH et al. New Chinese Medicine 1980 (4):215.

55. 157th Hospital of Guangzhou Military Region. Health Bulletin — Supplement (Health Division of the General Logistics Department of the Chinese PLA) 1971 (4):18.

(Deng Wenlong)

ZHIQIAO AND ZHISHI 枳殼與枳實

<Zhiqiao> is the almost ripe fruit of *Citrus aurantium* L., *C. aurantium* L. var *amara* Engl., or *C. wilsonii* Tanaka (Rutaceae). It has a bitter and sour taste and slightly "cold" property. <Zhishi> is the young fruit of *C. aurantium* and *C. wilsonii*. It is bitter and has a "cold" property.

<Zhiqiao> disperses stagnant vital energy ("poqi"), produces an expectorant effect and acts as a digestant. It is mainly used to treat excessive accumulation of phlegm, thoracic distress, distention of the costal region, dyspepsia, eructation, vomiting, dysentery with tenesmus, and prolapse of the uterus or rectum.

<Zhishi> also disperses stagnant vital energy, relieves the sensation of fullness, eliminates phlegm and acts as a digestant. It is a remedy for abdominal and thoracic distention, chest pain, sensation of fullness and pain, accumulation of phlegm in the hypochondriac region, edema, dyspepsia, constipation, gastroptosis, and prolapse of the uterus of rectum.

CHEMICAL COMPOSITION

The fruit contains volatile oil mainly composed of limonene and linalool. It also contains flavonoids (poncirin, hesperidin, rhoifolin, and naringin). The flower also contains volatile oil, and the almost ripe fruit contains synephrine and N-methyltyramine (1).

PHARMACOLOGY

1. Effect on the Cardiovascular System

The decoctions of either <Zhiqiao> or <Zhishi> perfused into the isolated frog heart increased the cardiac contractility and contraction amplitude, but higher concentration (>20%) caused inhibition (2). These decoctions, or the ethanol extract of <Zhiqiao> injected intravenously into anesthetized rabbits or dogs elicited a marked pressor effect (2,3). The <Zhishi> injection 1.5 g/kg administered intravenously to anesthetized dogs increased the blood pressure to equal to that achieved with 0.1 mg/kg of norepinephrine. However, the effect of the former agent appeared faster and lasted longer than the latter, registering a double peak elevation followed by a slow descent, but no hypotensive aftereffect like that of epinephrine. During elevation of blood pressure, no transient respiratory depression and tachycardia, which are characteristic features of norepinephrine, developed. No tachyphylaxis developed after continuous medication with the herb (4,5). The pressor principle was determined to be synephrine and N-methyltyramine (1); the latter was found to produce tachyphylaxis (6). Experiments proved that the <Zhishi> injection, synephrine. and N-methyltyramine markedly increased the contractility of the papillary muscles of the isolated cat heart and induced its automaticity. N-methyltyramine exhibited the most pronounced effect, followed by the <Zhishi> injection; the effect of synephrine was weakest (7). These three agents also significantly increased the speed of intraventricular pressure change (dp/dt) and the common peak isovolumic systolic pressure CPIP, and accelerated the myocardial contraction (Vce). However, the effect of <Zhishi> injection was more prominent than those of the other two agents, and it also constricted the renal and cerebral blood vessels as well as increasing the resistance of these vasculatures (8). Increased sensitivity to <Zhishi> was observed in reserpinized dogs. When the α-receptor was blocked by phentolamine <Zhishi> caused hypotension, and when the β-receptor was blocked by alprenolol it produced a pressor effect. These events indicate the association of the pressor effect of <Zhishi> with the stimulation of the α-receptor (4,5). In the case of reserpinized dogs, however, intravenous injection of N-methyltyramine did not elicit a pressor reaction, but the 3:1 mixture of synephrine and N-methyltyramine produced a marked pressor effect. Thus, the supersensitivity of reserpinized dogs to the <Zhishi> injection is presumed to be due to synephrine, a direct α-agonist (9). The extent of blood pressure elevation in reserpinized rats and dogs was significantly less, and the renal vascular resistance in reserpinized dogs was also markedly reduced after intravenous injection of tyramine or N-methyltyramine. Intraperitoneal injection of N-methyltyramine 20 mg/kg to rats decreased the norepinephrine content of the myocardium (6). These events suggest that like tyramine, N-methyltyramine releases endogenous sympathetic transmitters (9,10). Experiments on the isolated guinea pig atrium and *in situ* rabbit heart proved that the positive inotropic effect of N-methyltyramine was weakened by premedication with the β-blocker alprenolol (10). The cardiotonic action of N-methyltyramine and synephrine was also weakened by premedication with phentolamine or tolazoline blocking the α-receptors of the isolated guinea pig atrium and heart. The radioimmunoassay proved that N-methyltyramine markedly increased the plasma and myocardial cGMP in mice (11). These experimental results indicate that: the cardiotonic, pressor and the peripheral vascular effects of <Zhishi> were due to stimulation of the α- and β-adrenergic receptors and release of endogenous sympthatic transmitters, and that the interaction of synephrine and N-methyltyramine, which respectively directly and indirectly stimulate the α- and β-receptors, can decrease tachyphylaxis to the pressor effect.

2. Diuretic Effect

Intravenous injection of <Zhishi>, or N-methyltyramine induced a diuretic effect concurrent with marked increases in the blood pressure and renal vascular resistance. Under the experimental condition where renal blood flow was fixed by means of constant perfusion, the diuretic effect of <Zhishi> and N-methyltyramine did not correlate with the changes in renal blood flow and filtration volume. Hence, it is postulated that diuresis is probably caused by the inhibition of renal tubular reabsorption and other actions (12).

3. Effect on the Gastrointestinal Smooth Muscles

The decoction of <Zhiqiao> and that of <Zhishi> partially inhibited the isolated mouse intestinal tract and completely inhibited that of the rabbit. This effect was antagonized by acetylcholine (13). In contrast, intragastric admistration of 10 ml of the 100% decoction of either herb to dogs with gastric and intestinal fistulae produced stimulation, thereby increasing gastrointestinal motility (14). These effects may be considered as the pharmacological basis for the use of <Zhishi> and <Zhiqiao> in the treatment of gastric dilation, gastric retention, indigestion due to gastrointestinal asthenia, prolapse of the rectum, and hernia in traditional Chinese medicine.

4. Effect on the Uterus

In the case of isolated and *in situ* uteri of nonpregnant and pregnant rabbits and in uterine fistulae of nonpregnant rabbits, both of the decoctions of <Zhiqiao> and <Zhishi> initiated a significant stimulant effect by increasing rhthmic contraction (14). However, the herbs partially inhibited the isolated uteri of pregnant or nonpregnant mice, (13).

5. Toxicity

<Zhishi> has a low toxicity and a wide safety range. Intravenous injection of 2 g/kg in total within 30 minutes to anesthetized dogs caused no serious reactions. Gastrointestinal distention and profuse salivation may occur in a minority of animals given large doses (2). The LD_{50} of the <Zhishi> injection was determined be 71.8 ± 6.5 g/kg IV in mice (15).

CLINICAL STUDIES

1. Shock

The <Zhishi> injection, synephrine, and N-methyltyramine were used with therapeutic benefit in 152 cases of infectious, anaphylactic or cardiogenic shock and shock due to other causes. They were effective when given intravenously, but not orally. It was not applicable in shock of the low-output and high-resistant type. For the <Zhishi> injection, an initial dose of about 20 g was considered appropriate followed by intravenous infusion of 20–60 g/100 ml.

   Dosage and administration of synephrine and N-methyltyramine: According to the severity of shock, synephrine and N-methyltyramine 20–60 mg each, diluted with normal saline or glucose solution, are given by intravenous push; blood pressure is monitored within 10 minutes of medication. Then intravenous infusion of synephrine and N-methytyramine each 20–100 mg/100 ml at the speed of 30–40 drops per minute is given. If the blood pressure is still not ideal, the intravenous push can be repeated every 30 minutes until the blood pressure gradually increases. The dose is adjusted according to the level of ameliorated or stabilized, drug concentration and infusion speed can be gradually reduced (15–17).

2. Cardiac Failure

The <Zhishi> injection was used with therapeutic benefit in 20 cases of cardiac failure (18). It, however, should be contraindicated in heart failure since it stimulates α- and β-adrenergic receptors, increases cardiac output, constricts blood vessels, increases the total peripheral resistance, and increases cardiac load.

3. Prolapse of the Postapartum Uterus and Rectal Prolapse in Chronic Diarrhea

The <Zhiqiao> decoction can be given thrice daily for 5–10 days (19). <Zhishi> has also been used in hernia (20).

REFERENCE

1. Hunan Institute of Medical and Pharmaceutical Industry. Chinese Research on Traditional Drugs for Cardiovascular Diseases. 1976. p. 14.

2. Yan YJ. Chinese Medical Journal 1955 (5):437.

3. Wang JM. Jiangxi Zhongyiyao (Jiangxi Journal of Traditional Chinese Medicine) 1955 (2):41.

4. Internal Medicine Section, Hunan Medical College. Hunan Information on Science and Technology — Medicine and Health 1974 (1):12.

5. Internal Medicine Section, Second Teaching Hospital of Medical College. Hunan Yiyao Zazhi (Hunan Medical Journal) 1974 (1):37.

6. Chen X. Proceedings of the 1980 Symposium of the Chinese Society of Physiology (Hunan Branch). 1980. p. 6.

7. Jia HJ et al. Abstracts of the First National Symposium of the Society of Pharmacology. 1979. p. 39.

8. Chen X et al. Acta Pharmaceutica Sinica 1980 15(2):71.

9. Pharmacology Department, Hunan Medical College et al. Chinese Traditional and Herbal Drugs Communications 1978 (4):29.

10. Chen X et al. Medical Research Information (Hunan Medical College) 1978 (2):5.

11. Yan YF et al. Abstracts of the First National Symposium on Cardiovascular Pharmacology. 1980. p. 101.

12. Chen X. Abstracts of the First National Symposium of the Society of Pharmacology. 1979. p. 41.

13. Yan YJ. Chinese Medical Journal 1955 (5):433.

14. Zhu SM. Chinese Medical Journal 1955 42(10):946.

15. Internal Medicine Section, Second Teaching Hospital of Hunan Medical School. Xinyiyaoxue Zazhi (Journal of Traditional Chinese Medicine) 1978 (3):25.

16. Pediatrics Section, Second Teaching Hospital of Hunan Medical College et al. Chinese Traditional and Herbal Drugs Communications 1977 (10):34.

17. Internal Medicine Section, Second Teaching Hospital of Hunan Medical College. Chinese Traditional and Herbal Drugs 1980 (9):406.

18. Cardiovascular Unit of the Internal Medicine Department, Second Teaching Hospital of Hunan Medical College. Chinese Traditional and Herbal Drugs 1980 (4):171.

19. Ye XM. Medicine 1951 4(6):233.

20. Ye JQ. Beijing Zhongyi (Beijing Journal of Traditional Chinese Medicine) 1953 2(7):17.

(Yuan Wei)

GOUQIZI 枸杞子

<Gouqizi> is the ripe fruit of *Lycium chinese* Miller of *Lycium barbarum* L. (Solanaceae). Sweet and "mild", the herb is vital-essence-nourishing, hematinic, "jing" (essence of life)-tonifying, and Vision-improving. It is, therefore, used in deficiency of the liver and "kidney", pain and weakness of the low-back and limbs due to insufficiency of the essence of life and blood, dizziness, tinnitus, and spermatorrhea.

CHEMICAL COMPOSITION

<Gouqizi> contains about 1% of betaine (1). It also contains zeaxanthine, physalein and traces of carotene, thiamine, riboflavine, nicotinic acid, ascorbic acid, calcium, phosphate, and iron (2).

PHARMACOLOGY

1. Enhancement of Nonspecific Immunity

The 100% aqueous extract of *L. barbarum* administered intragastrically to mice at 0.4 ml once daily for 3 days, or a single intramuscular injection of the 100% ethanol extract at 0.1 ml, markedly increased the reticuloendothelial phagocytosis of Indian ink (3). An electuary, Codonopsis-Lycium Linctus, prepared from the extracts of the root of *Codonopsis pilosula* and the *Lycium* fruit in the proportion of 2:1, also markedly increased the phagocytic ability of mice peritoneal macrophages (4).

2. Hematopoietic Effect

Administration of the 10% *L. chinense* decoction to normal mice at 0.5 ml/day PO for 10 days enhanced hematopoiesis, leading to lymphocytic leukocytosis. It antagonized the inhibition of leukocytes by cyclophosphamide, in particular lymphocytes (5).

3. Growth Stimulant Effect

Betaine is a biostimulator. When 4–6 kg this agent was added to each ton of chicken feed, the body weight of the fowls was increased relative to the control, i.e., in the case of hens, by 12–13%, and for cocks by 17–18%. Egg production was boosted by 24.3% relative to the control when 8 kg was added to the feed (6).

Intragastric administration of the 1:10 Codonopsis-Lycium Linctus to mice at 0.2 ml for 4 days markedly increased the body weight of the animals to more than twofold that of the control; the linctus-fed animals had glossy hair, were fleshy, and had bright red blood (4).

4. Antilipemic, Liver-Protective and Lipotropic Effects

L. chinense decreased blood cholesterol in rats (1). It slightly inhibited the formation of experimental atherosclerosis in rabbits. Prolonged feeding (75 days) with animal feed containing the aqueous extract of the herb (0.5% and 1%), or betaine (0.1%), protected the animals from carbon tetrachloride-induced liver damage, inhibited the fatty change in the serum and liver, shortened thiopental sodium-induced sleep, reduced bromsulphalein (BSP) retention, and decreased GOT (1,7). The aqueous extract of the herb slightly inhibited fat deposition in the hepatocytes due to liver damage induced by carbon tetrachloride and fostered the regeneration of the hepatocytes (8). Betaine aspartate also afforded protection against toxic hepatitis due to carbon tetrachloride (9). The liver-protective effects of betaine is probably due to its being a methyl donor (1,7).

5. Hypoglycemic Effect

The *L. barbarum* extract caused a marked and sustained decrease of the blood glucose level in rats and increased the animals' tolerance to carbohydrates. The hypoglycemic actions was presumed to have been contributed by the guanidine derivatives (10). Early studies also reported the hypoglycemic action of *L. chinense* (11).

6. Miscellaneous Actions

The aqueous extract of *L. chinense* initiated cholinergic effects including hypotension, cardiac depression and intestinal excitation, whereas betaine was devoid of these actions (12). The *L. chinense* extract also fostered the growth of lactobacillus and its production of acid (13).

7. Toxicity

The toxicity of *L. chinense* is very low. Betaine was excreted unchanged; injection of 2.4 g/kg IV to rats did not result in toxic reactions (14). Injection of 25 g/kg IP to mice triggered generalized spasm and respiratory arrest within 10 minutes (12). The LD_{50} of the aqueous extract of *L. chinense* in mice was 8.32 g/kg SC, and that of betaine was 18.74 g/kg, suggesting that the toxicity of the former was more than double that of the latter (15).

CLINICAL STUDIES

1. "Kidney" Deficiency and Insufficiency of Life-Essence and Blood

Lumbar soreness, weakness of the lower extremities, dizziness, diminished vision, fever due to "yin" deficiency, spontaneous sweating, tinnitus, nocturnal emission and neurasthenia due to "kidney" deficiency and insufficiency of the life-essence and blood may be treated with the Lycium fruit in combination with the flower of *Chrysanthemum morifolium*, the cured rhizome of *Rehmannia glutinosa*, the pulp of *Cornus officinalis*, the tuber of *Dioscorea opposita*, and the tuber of *Alisma orientalis* as in the Lycium-Chrysanthemum-Rehmannia Pill, or in combination with the cured rhizome of *Rehmannia glutinosa*, the tuber of *Dioscorea opposita*, the bark or root bark of *Cinnamomum cassia*, the lateral root-tuber or *Aconitum carmichaeli*, the tuber of *Colocasia esculenta*, the bark of *Eucommia ulmoides*, and the root of *Angelica sinensis* as in the "Yougui Pill". The herb is contraindicated in patients with "exogenous sthenic heat", deficiency of "spleen" with damp, and diarrhea.

2. Chronic Liver Diseases

In recent years, 131 cases of various chronic liver diseases (liver cirrhosis, chronic hepatitis, toxic or metabolic liver disease, and hepatic insufficiency due to biliary tract diseases) were treated with betaine citrate (16). Determination of transaminase, alkaline phosphatase, neutral fat, cholesterol and total lipid, total protein, albumin/globulin ratio, serum bilirubin, and serum iron level showed that this drug was efficacious.

REFERENCE

1. Kajimato Y et al. Folia Pharmacologica Japonica 1961 57(6):105.

2. Xie HZ. Chinese Pharmaceutical Bulletin 1956 4(2):71.

3. Coordinating Research Group on Drugs and Pharmacology, Hui Autonomous Region (Ningxia) Office for Chronic Bronchitis Prevention and Treatment. Ningyi Tongxun (Communications of Ningxia Medical College) 1974 (9):56.

4. Zhu CW et al. Studies on Chinese Proprietary Medicine 1979 (5):46.

5. Tumor Group, Pharmacology Department of Neimenggu Medical College. Acta Academiae Medicinae Neimenggu 1974 (4):76.

6. Li AI et al. Chemical Abstracts 1976 85:31872v.

7. Kajimato Y et al. Yakugaku Kenkyu 1962 34(4):274.

8. Lu ZZ et al. Abstracts of the Symposium of the Chinese Society of Physiology (Pharmacology). 1964. p. 123.

9. Dormard Y et al. Excerpta Medica. Sec 30. 1974 31:3410.

10. Lapinina LO et al. Chemical Abstracts 1967 66:1451e. (Erratum: In the abstract Lycium barbatum should read Lycium barbarum).

11. Jing LB et al. Chinese Reports of the Institute of Physiology, National Beiping Research Institute 1936 3(1):1.

12. Kajimato Y et al. Folia Pharmacologica Japonica 1980 56(4):151.

13. Nishiyama R. Chemical Abstracts 1966 64:20530b.

14. Sollmann T. A Manual of Pharmacology. 8th edition. Saunders. 1957. p. 414.

15. Kurokawa S. Chemical Abstracts 1962 57:11822c. (Erratum: In the abstract 83.2 g/kg should read 8.32 g/kg).

16. Dameris W. Excerpta Medica. Sec 30. 1974 30:2785.

(Ye Songbai)

JINGJIE 荆芥

<Jingjie> is the aerial part of the plant *Schizonepeta tenuifolia* (Benth.) Briq. (Labiatae). A related species, *Schizonepeta multifida* (L.) Briq., is also used as a source of <Jingjie>.

<Jingjie> is pungent and slightly "warm". It has a diaphoretic action and has the ability to induce eruption of measles at the early stage of the disease. The charred herb is hemostatic. The crude <Jingjie> is prescribed for headache due to common cold, pharyngolaryngitis, early stage of measles, non-eruptive measles, sores, and scabies; the charred herb is a remedy for bloody stool and metrorrhagia. The effects of the fruit-spike of the plant are similar to those of <Jingjie>, but the former has a more pronounced diaphoretic effect.

CHEMICAL COMPOSITION

The aerial part contains 1.8% of volatile oil, the fruit-spike 4.11%. The major components of the volatile oil are d-menthone and dl-menthone. The volatile oil also contains small amounts of d-limonene.

PHARMACOLOGY

1. Antipyretic Effect

Intragastric administration of the decoction or ethanol extract of *S. multifida* 2 g/kg to rabbits with fever induced by mixed typhoid vaccine produced only a very weak antipyretic effect (1).

2. Antimicrobial Effect

In vitro, the <Jingjie> decoction showed a strong activity against *Staphylococcus aureus* and *Corynebacterium diphtheriae* and was active to some extent against *Bacillus anthracis*, beta streptococcus, *Salmonella typhi*, *Shigella dysenteriae*, *Pseudomonas aeruginosa* (2,3) and *Mycobacterium tuberculosis* var. *hominis* (4). Treatment of chicken embryos with 0.1 ml of the 50% <Jingjie> decoction produced no inhibitory effect on influenza virus type A PR$_8$ strain (5).

3. Hemostatic Effect

The hemostatic effects of the crude and charred <Jingjie> (stir-fried over low heat) were compared by determining the bleeding time in mice by means of Akopov's method, and the coagulation time in rabbits by means of the capillary method. The drugs were reconstituted with normal saline and administered intragastrically at 2 g/kg to rabbits and at 5 g/kg to mice; control animals were given the vehicle. The results of the experiment showed that the crude herb did not significantly shorten the bleeding time, whereas the charred herb shortened it by 72.6%; the former shortened the coagulation time by 30%, the latter by 77.7% (6). Thus, only the stir-fried herb has hemostatic action.

4. Miscellaneous Actions

In vitro, <Jingjie> exhibited a weak inhibitory action on cancer cells (7).

CLINICAL STUDIES

1. Common Cold

"Jing Fang Baidu Powder" (Herba Schizonepetae, Radix Ledebouriellae, Rhizoma et Radix Notopterygii, Radix Angelicae Pubescentis, Radix Bupleuri, Radix Peucedani, Rhizoma Chuanxiong, Radix Platycodi, Fructus Aurantii, Herba Menthae, Radix Glycyrrhizae, Rhizoma Zingiberis Recens), "Yin Qiao San" (Lonicera-Forsythia Powder) (8,9), the "Jing Fang Heji" (Schizonepeta-Ledebouriella Mixture) (10), or the "Biaolishuangjie Tang" (Diaphoretic-Purgative Decoction) (11) was used in the treatment of influenza. The symptoms abated in 1–2 days in most cases and a cure was achieved in 4–6 days.

2. Skin Diseases

The fine powder of the fruit-spike was applied evenly to skin lesions and rubbed until the skin became hot. Mild urticaria was cured after 1–2 applications and severe cases after 2–4 applications (12). Moreover, compound formulae such as "Jing Fang Baidu Decoction", and "Wuwei Xiaodu Yin" (Five-Herb Detoxicant Decoction), modified to suit the patients' needs, were also efficacious in the treatment of allergic dermatitis, pruritus, urticaria, exanthema desquamativum, eczema, and psoriasis (13,14).

REFERENCE

1. Sun SY. Chinese Medical Journal 1956 42(10):964.
2. Lingling District Sanitation and Anti-epidemic Station. Hunan Yiyao Zazhi (Hunan Medical Journal) 1974 (5):56.
3. Microbiology Department. Journal of Nanjing College of Pharmacy 1960 (5):10.

4. Research Laboratory of Liaoning Institute of Tuberculosis. Liaoning Medical Journal 1960 (7):29.

5. Microbiology Laboratory. Hubei Sanitation and Anti-epidemic Station. Chinese Medical Journal 1958 44(9):888.

6. Pharmacology Section, Shandong Institute of Chinese Materia Medica. Chinese Pharmaceutical Bulletin 1965 11(12):562.

7. Sato A. Kampo Kenkyu 1979 (2):51.

8. Guo ZQ. Zhejiang Journal of Traditional Chinese Medicine 1959 (11):28.

9. Ye JH. Shanghai Journal of Traditional Chinese Medicine 1958 (5):14.

10. Wang ZZ. Harbin Zhongyi (Harbin Journal of Traditional Chinese Medicine) 1959 (11):17.

11. Fan ZM. Medicine and Health (Shaoxing District Centre of Medical and Health Information, Zhejiang) 1979 (2):15.

12. Ma YJ. Journal of Traditional Chinese Medicine 1965 (12):18.

13. Wu SM. Xinyiyaoxue Zazhi (Journal of Traditional Chinese Medicine) 1978 (6):26.

14. Han ZY. Weifang Yiyao (Weifang Medical Journal) (Health Research Laboratory of Weifang Health Bureau et al.) 1977 (2):23.

(Gong Xuling)

NANGUAZI 南瓜子

<Nanguazi> refers to the seeds obtained from the pumpkin *Cucurbita moschata* Duch., *C. moschata* var. *toonas*, and *C. moschata* var. *melonaeformis* Makino (Cucurbitaceae). It is sweet and "warm" and is credited with anthelmintic activity. It is a remedy for taeniasis, schistosomiasis, whooping cough, and postpartum edema of the hands and feet.

CHEMICAL COMPOSITION

<Nanguazi> contains an anthelmintic cucurbitine, fixed oil, proteins and vitamins B_1 and B_2.

PHARMACOLOGY

1. Anthelmintic Effect

In vitro studies showed that the 40% decoction of the defatted *Cucurbita* kernel, or the 30% normal saline solution of the crystal extracted from the kernel produced a paralyzing effect on the middle and terminal proglottides of beef and pork tapeworms (*T. saginata* and *T. solium*). The decoction caused thinning, widening, and sagging of the end and especially the central proglottides. However, the decoction was inactive on the scolex and immature proglottides (1). *In vitro* studies indicated that 1:500 cucurbitine was unable to paralyze dog tapeworms. Nevertheless, on account of its stimulant action, cucurbitine caused spastic contraction of the worms. This drug synergized with arecoline hydrobromide (2). An anthelmintic effect was achieved in dogs with *T. marginata*, *T. pisiformis* and *T. mansoni* after intragastric administration of 1–5 g of cucurbitine, cucurbitine perchlorate, or cucurbitine hydrobromide (2–3).

2. Antischistosomal Effect

2.1 *Effect on cercariae schistosomes.* Starting from the first day of cercarial infection in mice, daily intragastric administration 1–3 g of <Nanguazi> for 28 days greatly reduced the growth rate of the young worms; the worm reduction rate was 85.3–95.7%. The effect was dose-dependent. The effect was poorer if treatment was started one or two weeks after cercarial infection (4–7).

Satisfactory results were also achieved with daily intragastric administration of 265.5 g of the defatted powder of pumpkin seeds for 28 days in cercaria-infected pigs (7). Intragastric administration to mice of 46 kinds of extracts of pumpkin seeds, obtained by different methods, revealed that only the defatted powder and the aqueous extract exhibited good antischistosomal effect (8). Seeds from

C. moschata var. *melonaeformis* had a better prophylactic effect than those from *C. melonaeformis* var. *toonas*, whereas the pumpkin powder itself was inactive (9).

Intragastric administration of cucurbitine 100–500 mg/kg daily for 28 days markedly reduced the number of worms (10). Like pumpkin seeds, cucurbitine inhibited sexually immature cercariae. Furthermore, in mice with experimental schistosomiasis the intragastrically administered pumpkin seeds killed some cercariae in the host liver, as shown by inflammatory reaction and degeneration of the worms (4,10).

2.2 *Effect on adult schistosomes.* Doses of 3, 4, and 5 g of pumpkin seeds were intragastrically administered to separate groups of mice for 28 days after 4 weeks of schistosomal infection; the survival rates of worms in the treatment groups were not much different from those of the control (4–6,11–12). But the concurrent use of these doses with antimony preparations markedly increased the therapeutic effect (4–5,7,10). The pumpkin seed decoction 0.6 ml (corresponding to 8 g of the crude drug) administered intragastrically to animals for 28 days afforded a worm survival rate which was significantly lower than that of the control group, indicating that at high dosage the decoction was both inhibitory and lethal (6). Starting from the 35th day of cercarial infection, intragastric administration of pumpkin seeds 4 g to mice for 35 days produced no significant inhibition on the ovulation of female worms (4,13). Two hours after intraperitoneal injection of cucurbitine 1 g/kg to mice on the 36th day of cercarial infection, a marked migration of the parasites to the liver was observed, compared with the control (10). In experimental treatment of mice with small doses of pumpkin seeds, histology of the host liver and mesenteries showed that except for some diminution in the intestinal pigment granules of the adult worms, no significant changes in the gross appearance, reproductive organs, and internal structures of the worms were found, whereas high doses caused atrophy of the worms, degeneration of the reproductive organs, degeneration and reduction or even disappearance of ova in the uteri. Female worms were more sensitive to the herb than male worms. However, these changes were usually reversed soon after discontinuation of the drug. Cucurbitine had no significant effect on the level and distribution of RNA and phosphatase of the worms (4–5,10,12,15).

3. Miscellaneous Actions

Intravenous injection of cucurbitine to rabbits at doses of 150–250 mg/kg caused hypertension as well as deep and rapid breathing. Cucurbitine salts at the concentration range of 1:3300–1:20,000 markedly inhibited contractions of the isolated ileum of guinea pigs and rabbits (10).

4. Pharmacokinetics

Four or 24 hours after administration of ^{14}C-cucurbitine 100–200 mg/kg PO or IP to mice, the highest drug level appeared in the liver and kidneys, but after 24 hours, drug levels in various tissues did not significantly differ, irrespective of the route of administration. The blood concentration of cucurbitine in mice given 100 mg/kg of pumpkin seeds intravenously rapidly dropped to one-fifth of the initial level at the end of 5 minutes, and after 1 hours only traces were detected. The drug was excreted mainly in the urine and marginally in the stool. Analysis of the urinary metabolites showed that 97% were cucurbitine. It was also reported that though the drug could penetrate the body of the worm, it was not incorporated into the tissue protein (14).

5. Toxicity

The LD_{50} of cucurbitine perchlorate and cucurbitine hydrochloride in mice were 1.25 and 1.10 g/kg PO, respectively. Thirty minutes after injection of cucurbitine perchlorate at 1.2–2.4% g/kg IP to mice, unsteady gait and hypersensitivity to external stimuli appeared. In the group dosed with 1.6–2.0 g/kg, excitation and paroxysmal spasm convulsion and death occurred; the surviving animals eventually recovered about 1 week after discontinuation of the medication (10). Pathological examinations showed the following results: In normal mice both pumpkin seeds and cucurbitine induced transient pathological changes of the liver, lungs, kidneys, and duodenum, a decrease in the liver glycogen and an increase in the fat content of the liver; recovery was rapid on discontinuation of the drugs (4,10,15). No encapsulation of worms by host tissue or inflammation was observed during the treatment (10).

CLINICAL STUDIES

1. Taeniasis

A cure rate of 70% was achieved in 85 cases treated with the aqueous extract of pumpkin seeds (16). A paper reported the cure of 6 cases of *T. saginata* infection with raw pumpkin seeds at 300 g (17). Only one out of 9 cases of T. saginata infection benefitted from a single dose of 120 g of pumpkin seeds, whereas an effective rate of 95.19% was achieved in 96 cases treated with pumpkin seeds plus the seeds of *Areca catechu*. While 2 cases of *T. solium* infection did not benefit from 120 g of pumpkin seeds, all 4 cases treated with this herb and the seed of *Areca catechu* did (1). Hence, this herb is usually used nowadays in combination with the seed of *Areca catechu* to achieve a better therapeutic effect.

2. Schistosomiasis

In 362 cases of acute and chronic schistosomiasis, the short-term therapeutic effect was 17–64% (3 successive negative stool examinations), and the long-term therapeutic effect after discontinuing the drug for 1–3 months was 22–35%. The rate of negative stool examination was higher in children than in adults; a good antipyretic effect was achieved in acute cases.

Dosage and administration: Four dosage forms are available, viz., powder, decoction (10 g/ ml), aqueous extract (4 g) and kernel paste powder (the crude kernel ground with water and the juice dried). A course of 30 days is recommended. Optimal prophylactic and curative effects were achieved with the extract preparation (6,18–21). For the time being, pumpkin seed is deemed less effective than antimony and furapromide; hence, further evaluation evaluation is necessary.

3. Filariasis

A mixture of an emulsion prepared from 60 g of pumpkin seeds and a decoction of 30 g of the seed of *Areca catechu* can be taken by mouth on an empty stomach (22).

4. Whooping Cough

The fine powder of browned pumpkin seeds may be taken with brown sugar solution several times a day (23).

ADVERSE EFFECTS

A few patients experienced dizziness, nausea, vomiting, gastric distention, anorexia, diarrhea, and borborygmus, but these symptoms were controlled without discontinuing the treatment (6,20).

REFERENCE

1. Feng LZ. Chinese Medical Journal 1956 42(2):138.

2. Pharmacology Department, Wenzhou Medical College. Abstracts of the Symposium of the Chinese Society of Physiology (Pharmacology). 1964. p. 86.

3. Chen ZK et al. Acta Pharmacologica Sinica 1980 1(2):124.

4. Xiao SH. Acta Pharmaceutica Sinica 1959 7(8):300.

5. Zhou HR. Proceedings of the 1958 National Symposium on Parasitic Diseases. People's Medical Publishing House. 1958. p. 115.

6. National Committee on Schistosomiasis Research, Ministry of Health of the People's Republic of China. Research Literature on Schistosomiasis Prevention and Treatment. Shanghai Sci-Tech Literature Publishing House. 1960. p. 335.

7. No. 3 Parasitology Research Division, Zhejiang People's Academy of Health. Studies on Schistosomiasis. Shanghai Sci-Tech Literature Publishing House. 1958. p. 329.

8. Institute of Parasitology, Chinese Academy of Medical Sciences. Studies on Schistosomiasis. Shanghai Sci-Tech Literature Publishing House. 1958. p. 339.

9. Institute of Parasitology, Chinese Academy of Medical Sciences. Studies on Schistosomiasis. Shanghai Sci-Tech Literature Publishing House. 1958. p. 338.

10. Xiao SH. Acta Pharmaceutica Sinica 1962 9(6):327.

11. Institute of Parasitology, Chinese Academy of Medical Sciences. Studies on Schistosomiasis. Shanghai Sci-Tech Literature Publishing House. 1958. p. 334.

12. No. 3 Parasitology Research Division, Zhejiang People's Academy of Health. Zhejiang Journal of Traditional Chinese Medicine 1958 (5):2.

13. Institute of Parasitology, Chinese Academy of Medical Sciences. Studies on Schistosomiasis. Shanghai Sci-Tech Literature Publishing House. 1958. p. 335.

14. Liang YY. Yuanzineng Kexue Jishu (Scientific Technology of Atomic Energy) 1964 (11):1257.

15. Institute of Parasitology, Chinese Academy of Medical Sciences. Studies on Schistosomiasis. Shanghai Sci-Tech Literature Publishing House. 1958. p. 341.

16. Colora Do Iris R et al. Chinese Journal of New Medicine 1952 3(2):116.

17. Xie JR. Neimenggu Weisheng Tongxun (Inner Mongolia Health Communications) — Supplement 1957 (2):37.

18. Zhou XZ. Chinese Journal of Internal Medicine 1959 7(8):764.

19. Zhou XZ. Journal of Traditional Chinese Medicine 1959 (2):547.

20. Zhenze County Centre of Schistosomiasis. Studies on Schistosomiasis. Shanghai Sci-Tech Literature Publishing House. 1958. p. 642.

21. Pediatrics Department, Shanghai Second Medical College. Studies on Schistosomiasis. Shanghai Sci-Tech Literature Publishing House. 1958. p. 645.

22. Anhui Health Bureau. Chinese Materia Medica of Anhui. Anhui People's Publishing House. 1974. p. 567.

23. Ye JQ. Jiangxi Zhongyiyao (Jiangxi Journal of Traditional Chinese Medicine) 1953 (3):20.

(Zheng Zhenyuan)

QIANCAOGEN 茜草根

<Qiancaogen> is derived from the root and stem of *Rubia cordifolia* L. (Rubiaceae). It is also obtained from *R. cordifolia* L. var. *longifolia* Hand.-Mazz, *R. chinensis* Reg. et Maack., *R. truppeliana* Loes, and *R. cordifolia* L. var. *pratensis* Maxim. Bitter tasting and "cold", it removes pathogenic "heat" from the blood, and exerts hemostatic, stasis-eliminative and channel-deobstruent actions. It is chiefly used to treat hematemesis, epistaxis, metrorrhagia, amenorrhea, as well as wounds and injuries, and strains.

CHEMICAL COMPOSITION

<Qiancaogen> contains anthraquinones such as alizarin, munjistin, purpuroxanthin, purpurin, and pseudopurpurin. *R. tinctorum* contains an extra component rubiadin.

PHARMACOLOGY

1. Hemostatic Effect

In the experiment on rabbits with severed femoral artery, bleeding was readily stopped by local application of R. cordifolia Powder applied on gauze and pressed for 35 seconds (1). Oral administration of 0.1 g/20 g of the charred herb from *R. cordifolia* to mice with tail wounds was more effective in shortening the bleeding time than the same dosage of the crude herb (2). The infusion of <Qiancaogen> also shortened the coagulation time in rabbits (3). In man, oral intake of the <Qiancaogen> decoction resulted in some shortening of the bleeding and coagulation time, indicating the presence of a weak hemostatic action. However, *in vitro* studies showed that the weak anticoagulant effect of the decoction was due to alizarin which combined with calcium ions in the blood (4).

2. Antitussive and Expectorant Effects

In cough induced by ammonia solution spray and through the phenol red method, the orally administered <Qiancaogen> decoction was shown to produce marked antitussive and expectorant effects in mice at 75 g/kg, whereas the supernatant obtained after alcohol precipitation was inactive (5).

3. Effect on Smooth Muscles

The <Qiancaogen> decoction had a spasmolytic action, antagonizing acetycholine-induced spasm of the isolated rabbit intestine (5). Another report, however, claimed that alizarin and purpurin had no significant spasmolytic action on the isolated small intestine of mice (6). The aqueous extract of Qiancaogen> excitated the isolated guinea pig uterus. When orally administered to women during labor, it strengthened uterine contraction (7).

4. Antibacterial Effect

In vitro studies proved that the aqueous extract of <Qiancaogen> was inhibitory against *Staphylococcus aureus*, and to a lesser extent against pneumococcus, *Hemophilus influenzae*, and some skin fungi, but that it was inactive against *Escherichia coli*, and alpha and beta streptococci (5,8).

5. Effect on Urolithiasis

Feeding of mice with the 20% *R. tinctorum* was effective in preventing the formation of experimental renal and urinary bladder stones, particularly calcium carbonate stones. Other studies indicated that, despite its dissolving effect on calcium or magnesium stones, *R. tinctorum* had little effect on bladder stones. Its lithagogic action was attributed to the stimulation of the bladder muscles (10).

6. Miscellaneous

The infusion of <Qiancaogen> caused vasodilation in frog webs (3). Like rutin, alizarin suppressed the permeability of rat cutaneous connective tissues, but its inhibitory effect on the depolymerization of hyaluronic acid was weaker (11).

7. Toxicity

No mortality was reported in mice given the *R. cordifolia* decoction 150 g/kg, but one of the 5 test animals died when the dose was increased to 175 g/kg (5). Purpurin and alizarin were toxic to earthworms, cysticerci and snails but non-toxic to mammals and human subjects (12).

CLINICAL STUDIES

1. Hemorrhagic Diseases

Forty-one patients with profuse bleeding after tooth extraction were treated with the powder of *R. cordifolia* extract applied locally; bleeding stopped altogether after 1–2 minutes. A good hemostatic effect was also achieved by local application of the *R. cordifolia* powder in individual patients with nasal bleeding due to injury of the middle turbinate, in those with profuse bleeding due to eschar sloughing following electrocauterization of the uterine cervix (13), and in some patients with bleeding from residual teeth roots due to hepatic insufficiency as well as in others with traumatic injuries (1).

Hemostasis was achieved in over 10 cases of menorrhagia 2 days after daily treatment with a decoction of 90 g of the herb derived from *R. cordifolia*, added with yellow wine and brown sugar (14).

2. Chronic Bronchitis

The decoction of *R. cordifolia* and the peel of *Citrus sinensis* was efficacious in 123 cases of chronic bronchitis; it was slightly more effective in the asthmatic than in the simple type. Dry and moist rales as well as wheezing decreased or disappeared after medication.

ADVERSE EFFECTS

The pigment of *R. cordifolia* may cause pink discoloration of the urine (15). In clinical trials, prolonged nausea and mild elevation of blood pressure appeared after oral administration of the <Qiancaogen> decoction (4).

REFERENCE

1. Chen YC. Journal of Barefoot Doctor 1975 (6):39.

2. Chinese Materia Medica Processing Section, Shandong Institute of Traditional Chinese Medicine and Materia Medica. Studies on Traditional Chinese Medicine (Shandong Institute of Traditional Chinese Medicine and Materia Medica) 1975 (8):69.

3. Notsu T. Nihon Yakubutsugaku Zasshi 1943 38(2):114.

4. Hangzhou Second People's Hospital. Preliminary studies on the pharmacological activity of <Qiancaogen>. April 1971.

5. Guangdong Health Bureau. Guangdong Selected Information on Senile Chronic Bronchitis. 1972. p. 78.

6. Shibata S. Journal of the Pharmaceutical Society of Japan (Tokyo) 1960 80:620.

7. Indian Journal of Medical Research 1948 36(1):47; Jiangsu College of New Medicine. Encyclopedia of Chinese Materia Medica. Vol. 2. Shanghai People's Publishing House. 1977. p. 1967.

8. Gaw HZ et al. Science 1949 110(1):11.

9. Madaus G et al. Chemical Abstracts 1944 38:2728(9).

10. Keller J et al. Chemical Abstracts 1946 40:4479(5).

11. Fabianek J et al. Chemical Abstracts 1966 65:9444g.

12. Lagrange E. Chemical Abstracts 1948 42:667h.

13. Mianyang District Research Group on Chinese Traditional Drugs. Medical and Health Communications (Mianyang District, Sichuan) 1974 (1):54.

14. Wenzhou District (Zhejiang) Health Bureau. A New Edition of South Zhejiang Herbal. 1975. p. 339.

15. Zhao S. Fangyuan Yixue Cankao Ziliao (References on Preventive Medicine of Atomic Radiation) 1973 (15):15.

(Zhang Zunyi)

CAOWU 草烏

<Caowu> refers to the root tuber derived from *Aconitum chinense* Paxt., *A. kusnezoffii* Reichb, *A. delavayi* Franch., and *A. vilmorinianum* Komar. (Ranunculaceae). It is pungent, "warm" and highly toxic. It has antirheumatic and analgesic effects and is used to treat rheumatism, paralysis due to apoplexy, carbuncle, furuncle, and deep-rooted ulcer at the early stage.

CHEMICAL COMPOSITION

The root tuber contains aconitine, hypaconitine, mesaconitine, isoaconitine, deoxyaconitine, jesaconitine, and a large amount of starch. A new alkaloid, temporarily named beiwutine, was isolated from the root of *A. kusnezoffii* (1). The leaf of *A. kusnezoffii* contains alkaloids aconitine, hypaconitine and mesaconitine, flavonoids, carbohydrates, and sterols (2). The aerial part of *A. delavayi* contains alkaloids from which crystalline delvaconitine was isolated.

PHARMACOLOGY

<Caowu> and <Chuanwu> (the root tuber of *A. carmichaeli*) shared similiar actions; the former contains 0.425% of alkaloids and the latter, 0.5991% The pharmacological actions of aconitine are described under the monograph of <Chuanwu>.

1. Analgesic Effect

The intraperitoneally injected 70% ethanol extract of <Caowu> produced marked analgesia in rats with electrically stimulated tail; the effect achieved with doses of 0.19, 0.095 and 0.048 g/kg exceeded that of 12, 6 and 3 mg/kg of morphine, respectively. At these doses, however, <Caowu> caused various degrees of toxic reaction, and its therapeutic index (3.91) was much lower than that of morphine (48.58) (3). The hot plate experiment on mice showed that 20 mg/kg of delvaconitine elevated the pain threshold by 45% (P<0.05), but its analgesic index was only one-fifth that of morphine (4). Analgesia was also provided by beiwutine and hypaconitine (1). The <Caowu> injection prepared from hydrolyzed alkaloids of *A. vilmorinianum* (1 mg/ml in terms of the crude alkaloids) given to mice at 15 ml/kg IP also exhibited a marked analgesic effect; within 2 hours of medication, drug effect peaked, with the elevation of the pain threshold by 2.2 times (5). The toxicity of <Caowu> was reduced upon processing with licorice and black beans, but beans, but its analgesic effect was unchanged (6).

2. Local Anesthetic Effect

Local surface anesthesia was provided by 1% delvaconitine, the potency of which was twice that cocaine. In experiments on rabbit cornea, the anesthetic effect lasted for at least 40–60 minutes, and on the web of spinal frogs, 15–60 minutes. Human subjects experienced numbness and tingling sensation of the tongue; the former effect lasted from 4 to 5 hours and the latter 1.5 hours. The anesthetic effect was not abolished by heat (boiling for 6 minutes) or by long storage at room temperature for 2–3 months (7). Injection of delvaconitine or isoaconitine around the sciatic nerves of mice blocked nerve conduction. Isoaconitine, however, caused local irritation and poisoning due to its rapid absorption (4). Beiwutine also had a local anesthetic action in animals (1).

3. Effect on the Heart

Using the ECG changes as parameters, it was found that the crude alkaloid of *A. kusnezoffii* administered to rabbits at 5–10 μg/kg was able to reinforce the action of epinephrine, antagonize calcium chloride-induced T wave inversion and antagonize initial ST elevation and subsequent ST depression caused by pituitrin. It also enhanced the toxicity of ouabain (8).

4. Miscellaneous Actions

Although a single dose of *A. kusnezoffii* decoction 5 g/kg PO failed to inhibit the development of egg white-induced paw swelling in rats, it promoted the subsidence of the swelling 6 hours after the egg white injection (9). The <Caowu> injection exerted an antipyretic action in rabbits with fever induced by the mixed vaccine (cholera, typhoid, paratyphoids A and B, and tetanus toxoid) (5). The crude alkaloid of *A. kusnezoffii* had an antihistaminic effect (8).

5. Toxicity

The LD_{50} of the 70%-ethanol extract of <Caowu> was 0.38 g/kg IP in mice (3); the LD_{50} of delvaconitine nitrate and isoaconitine nitrate in mice was 112 and 0.26 mg/kg SC, respectively (4). The LD_{50} of delvaconitine in house mice were 106 mg/kg SC and 28 mg/kg IV; death occurred after intravenous injection of 5–10 mg/kg to rabbits; after intravenous injection of 10–12 mg/kg to anesthetized dogs the heart rate and blood pressure were decreased, and death ensued with respiratory arrest (7). The LD_{50} of the <Caowu> decoction (decocted for 6 hours) in mice was 41.59±2.118 g/kg IP (10).

CLINICAL STUDIES

1. Rheumatic Arthritis, Arthralgia, Low-Back and Leg Pain, and Neuralgia

Good therapeutic effects were reported in the treatment of 64 cases with the <Caowu> injection (5).

2. Anesthesia with Chinese Traditional Drugs

<Caowu> and the flowers of *Datura metel*, the root of *Angelica sinensis* and the rhizome of *Ligusticum chuanxiong* are usually prepared as a decoction, a granule infusion, and as an injection to be used in general anesthesia. Good results were achieved in more than 1000 cases receiving these preparations. Systematic analysis performed in 973 of them revealed an aggregate effective rate of 92.9% (11). Refer to the monograph on <Yangjinhua> for the dosage. Since aconitine produced bradycardia and salivation which could offset tachycardia and xerostomia caused by the flowers of *D. metel*, the combination of these two agents successfully cancelled the opposing toxic reactions and side effects, thus potentiating the anesthetic effect (12).

The crude <Caowu>, the tuber of *Arisaema consanguineum*, the tuber of *Pinellia ternata*, and the plant *Asarum forbesii* made into a tincture may be used as surface anesthetic.

3. Miscellaneous

The <Caowu> injection was effective in 8 out of 10 febrile cases of common cold (3). "Sanwu Linctus" (Radix Polygoni Multiflori, Radix Aconiti, Radix Aconiti Kusnezoffii) was in the treatment of 50 cases of facial paralysis; 45 cases were cured and 5 basically cured (13).

ADVERSE EFFECTS

<Caowu> is an extremely toxic drug with a narrow safety range; clinical fatality due to this herb has been reported. The toxic symptoms are: salivation; nausea; vomiting; diarrhea; dizziness; blurred vision; numbness of the mouth, tongue, extremities and whole body; dyspnea; jerking of the extremities; unconsciousness; urinary and fecal incontinence; hypotension; hypothermia; and arrhythmia. The causes of death are depression of the respiratory center and ventricular fibrillation. Therefore, the herb must be used with great caution. The antidotes for poisoning include atropine, lidocaine, procainamide, and propranolol. Honey, green beans, and rhinoceros horn may also be used (3,12,14–16).

REFERENCE

1. Wang YG et al. Acta Pharmaceutica Sinica 1980 15(9):526.
2. Gu WZ. Zhongyiyao Tongxun (Communications on Traditional Chinese Medicine) (Neimenggu Autonomous Region Institute of Traditional Chinese and Mongolian Medicine) 1979 (5):71.
3. Su XR et al. Scientific Research Compilation (Shenyang Medical College) 1959 (3):6.
4. Tang XC et al. Acta Pharmaceutica Sinica 1966 13(3):227.
5. Pharmaceutical Factory, 58th Hospital of the Chinese PLA. Chinese Traditional and Herbal Drugs Communications 1972 (3):36.

6. Zhang ZW et al. Chinese Pharmaceutical Bulletin 1964 (4):186.

7. Jin GZ et al. Acta Pharmaceutica Sinica 1957 5(1):39.

8. Liu SF et al. Acta Pharmaceutica Sinica 1980 15(9):520.

9. Zhang SC et al. Xinyiyaoxue Zazhi (Journal of Traditional Chinese Medicine) 1974 (7):43.

10. Clinical Pharmacology Department. Bulletin of Chinese Materia Medica Research (Beijing Institute of Chinese Materia Medica) 1978 (2):5.

11. Xuzhou Coordinating Research Group on Chinese Traditional Anesthesia. Proceedings of the National Workshop on Chinese Traditional Anesthetics. 1971. p. 25.

12. Pharmacy of the First Teaching Hospital, Zhejiang Medical College. Proceedings of the National Workshop on Chinese Traditional Anesthetics. 1971. p. 315.

13. Lu HB et al. Liaoning Yiyao (Liaoning Medical Journal) 1978 (1):52.

14. Li BX et al. Chinese Journal of Paediatrics 1962 (7):450.

15. Ta XZ. Yunnan Medical Journal 1964 (4):18.

16. Sun NK et al. Chinese Medical Journal 1962 (10):661.

(Liu Changwu)

YINCHEN 茵陳
(APPENDIX: BEIYINCHEN 附: 北茵陳)

<Yinchen> refers to the shoot of *Artemisia capillaris* Thunb. (Compositae). It has a bitter and pungent taste and a slightly "cold" property. The herb is for its "damp-heat" clearing, cholagogic, choleretic and anti-jaundice effects. It is therefore used as a remedy for jaundice, hepatitis, and oliguria with yellow urine.

CHEMICAL COMPOSITION

The shoot of *A. capillaris* contains 6,7-dimethoxycoumarin. The amount of 6,7-dimethoxycoumarin is small in the shoot but can reach 1.98% during the flowering season.

The whole plant contains about 0.23% of volatile oil, which is composed of β-pinene, capillin, capillone, capillene, and capillarin.

The shoot contains chlorogenic acid, caffeic acid capillarisin (1,2), methylcapillarisin (2), four phenoxychromone derivatives, and four flavonoids (1).

PHARMACOLOGY

1. Cholagogic and Choleretic Effects

The following preparations of <Yinchen> fostered bile secretion and excretion decoction (3,4), aqueous extract, volatile oil-free aqueous extract (5), volatile oil (4,6), ethanol extract (6), 6,7-dimethoxycoumarin (8,9), chlorogenic acid and caffeic acid (9,10). Intravenous injection of the aqueous extract 0.25 g/kg or the refined extract (with or without the volatile oil) 1 g/kg to dogs with acute gallbladder intubation, or intragastric administration of the refined extract 1 g/kg to dogs with chronic gallbladder fistulae, produced a cholagogic effect whether the animals were healthy or had liver damage due to carbon tetrachloride (5). The dry weight of the bile was increased with an increase of its secretion (8).

One of the choleretic and cholagogic principles of the herb is 6,7-dimethoxycoumarin (8,9); infusion of this compound at 0.2 and 0.3 g/kg into the duodenum of anesthetized rats increased bile secretion 0.5 later by a mean of 50 and 180%, respectively. In dogs with chronic gallbladder fistulae, administration of 6,7-dimethoxycoumarin at 0.3 g/kg PO increased the production of bile by a mean of 73.86% in 3 hours (11). The use of this agent in combination with genipin obtained from the fruit of *Gardenia jasminoides* in rats produced a synergistic effect in promoting bile secretion (12).

The <Yinchen> decoction also decreased the tone of the Oddi's sphincter in anesthetized dogs (13). Two other choleretic and cholagogic principles, capillarisin and methylcapillarisin, have been isolated recently from the herb; they have a more powerful action than 6,7-dimethoxycoumarin (2,14).

2. Liver-Protective Effect

After daily injection of the <Yinchen> decoction 0.61 g SC to rats with carbon tetrachloride-induced liver damage, histological examination on the 8th day revealed that swelling of hepatocytes, vacuolization, fatty degeneration, and necrosis were mild, compared with the control group. The liver glycogen and RNA content were normalized or almost recovered, and the SGPT activity was markedly reduced. This evidence suggests that the drug possesses a liver-protective action (15).

The increase of serum bilirubin in rabbit after ligation of the common bile duct could be diminished by intragastric administration of the <Yinchen> extract (16). The food intake of rabbits with carbon tetrachloride-induced liver damage could be augmented by administration of the volatile oil or 6,7-dimethoxycoumarin. However, another paper reported that the decoction or volatile oil had no effect on the elevated transaminase level (4).

3. Antilipemic, Coronary Dilatory, and Fibrinolytic Effects

Administration of the <Yinchen> decoction in experimental hypercholesterolemic rabbits at 3 g/kg PO for 2 and 3 weeks lowered serum cholesterol level by 19.2 and 30 mg%, respectively, and also significantly reduced β-lipoprotein. Atherosclerosis was milder and the cholesterol content of the aortic wall was much lower in the treatment group than in the control. These results suggest that the herb has an antiatherosclerotic action (17).

Both the <Yinchen> injection and 6,7-dimethoxycoumarin increased the coronary flow of the isolated rabbit heart (7,18). Through determination of recalcification time, observation of antithrombin action, protein electrophoresis, fibrinolysis test, staphylococci aggregation test, and determination of fibrin fibrinogen degradation products, it was proved that <Yinchen> has anticoagulant and fibrinolytic activities (18).

4. Hypotensive Effect

The aqueous extract, ethanol-water extract, volatile oil, and 6,7-dimethoxycoumarin exhibited hypotensive activity (7,19–21). The latter agent given intravenously or intraduodenally to rats, cats, and rabbits under general or local anesthesia at the dose range 0.4–10 mg/kg produced a significant hypotensive effect which was neither blocked by hexamethonium and atropine nor potentiated by phentolamine. It did not antagonize the pressor effect of epinephrine. The hypotensive effect produced by intravertebroarterial injection of one-fiftieth to one-tenth of the intravenous dose was largely equipotent to that of the full intravenous dose, suggesting a central action (7,21).

In addition, 6,7-dimethoxycoumarin enhanced the contractility of the rabbit and cat hearts *in situ* (7).

5. Antibacterial Effect

In vitro studies showed that the <Yinchen> decoction inhibited to various extents *Staphylococcus aureus, Corynebacterium diphtheriae, Bacillus anthracis Salmonella typhi, Salmonella paratyphi A, Pseudomonas aeruginosa, Escherichia coli, Shigella flexneri, Shigella shigae, Neisseria meningitidis*, and *Bacillus subtilis* (22–28). The 10% decoction completely inhibited the growth of *Mycobacterium tuberculosis* var. *hominis* (29). At 1:100 concentration, it inhibited both the bovine and human *Mycobacterium tuberculosis* (30).

The high boiling point volatile oil of <Yinchen> 60–135°C, p=1 mmHg) exhibited a very strong inhibitory action against fungi such as *Trichophyton gypseum*. The MIC against *Epidermophyton floccosum* and *Microsporum audouini* was 1:64,000. On the other hand, the low boiling point volatile oil (50°C, p=1 mmHg) had a weaker effect (31).

In addition, the 1:100 volatile oil plaster applied locally could completely cure experimental epidermophytosis in rats caused by *E. floccosum* (31). The volatile oil also exhibited a strong inhibitory action against pathogenic cutaneous mycelia. The antibacterial potency of the volatile oil was not attenuated by prolonged heat treatment at over 100°C. Further studies showed that capillin, diluted 4,000,000 times, could still completely inhibit the growth of *Trichophyton rubrum* (32).

6. Antileptospiral Effect

In vitro studies showed that at high concentrations the <Yinchen> decoction produced inhibitory and lethal effects against *Leptospira pomona* (33). Acting over a period of 3 days, the 5% decoction completely liquefied 10 types of leptospirae (*L. interrogans, L. javanica, L. canicola, L. byrens, L. pyrogenes, L. autumnalis* B, *L. grippotyphosa* and *L. hebdomadis*) (34).

7. Ascaricidal Effect

The 1:2 <Yinchen> decoction paralyzed and killed 8 out of 15 swine ascarides *in vitro* (35). The volatile oil exhibited a paralyzing effect against swine and human ascarides (36).

8. Antipyretic Effect

Administration of the ethanol extract of <Yinchen> at 2 g/kg PO produced a significant antipyretic effect in rabbits with artificial fever. The effect appeared half an hour after medication, and when it peaked, body temperature dropped below normal (37).

9. Effect on Smooth Muscles

The decoction and the ethanol extract of <Yinchen> produced weak excitation of isolated rabbit intestine (3). Another paper reported that the aqueous extract of the herb inhibited the motility of the canine intestine *in situ* and the isolated rabbit intestine. The motility and tone of isolated frog and rabbit intestines were reduced by the volatile oil (36).

The refined extract had a stimulant effect on the isolated uterus of nonpregnant rabbits and that of postpartum guinea pigs (5). The stimulant effect on the uterus of nonpregnant guinea pigs could be antagonized by diphenhydramine (3).

10. Miscellaneous Actions

Diuresis of various degrees was elicited by the aqueous extract, refined aqueous extract, volatile oil, chlorogenic acid, caffeic acid, and 6,7-dimethoxycoumarin (4,5,10,11). The latter agent also had an antiasthmatic effect (9). <Yinchen> administered orally was inhibitory and lethal to Erhlich ascites carcinoma cells (38).

11. Toxicity

Daily intragastric administration of the 50% decoction 5 ml for 2 weeks to rats did not alter the appetite and body weight of the animals compared with the control group (3). The LD_{50} of 6,7-dimethoxycoumarin in mice was 497 mg/kg PO. Death mostly occurred within 4 hours of medication, and was usually preceded by paroxysmal convulsion. The dose 30–50 mg/kg IV produced transient atrioventricular and intraventricular conduction block on the ECG of some cats and rabbits (7). The acute LD_{50} of capillin in mice was determined to be 6.98 mg/kg (39).

CLINICAL STUDIES

1. Hepatitis

A rapid subsidence of jaundice and fever as well as marked decrease in the size of the liver were observed in 32 cases of icteric hepatitis given 30–45 g of <Yinchen> PO for a mean course of 7 days (40). The decoction of <Yinchen> plus the root and rhizome of *Glycyrrhiza uralensis*, and the fruit of *Ziziphus jujuba* var. *inermis* was reported to be effective against infectious hepatitis in young children (41). There is also a report on infectious hepatitis effectively treated with <Yinchen> plus the bark of *Phellodendron amurense*, the fruit of *Gardenia jasminoides*, and the root of *Isatis tinctoria* (42). Other workers achieved a prophylactic effect against viral hepatitis with <Yinchen> used in combination with the root of *Salvia miltiorrhiza*, the leaf of *Isatis tinctoria* and the fruit of *Ziziphus jujuba* (43), or with the plants *Serissa serissoides*, *Hypericum japonicum*, *Patrinia scabiosaefolia*, and the root and rhizome of *Glycyrrhiza uralensis* (44).

2. Biliary Tract Infection and Cholelithiasis

Lithagogue Decoction (Nos. 1–6) (45), modified from the A. capillaris Decoction the Major Tricosanthes Decoction and the Major Bupleurum Decoction, was used in 598 cases, with good effects in 86.5%; 64.4% cases passed stones, and the mortality rate was 1.7% (46). Lithagogue Decoction No. 2 (Herba Artemisiae, Herba Lysimachiae, Tuber Curcumae Aromaticae, Flos Lonicerae, Fructus Forsythiae, Radix et Rhizoma Rhei, Radix Aucklandiae, Fructus Aurantii, Mirabilitum Dehydratum) was employed in 127 cases of cholelithiasis of the "damp-heat" type, of which 115 cases (90.5%) successfully passed stones. The calculus passing rate was 90.5% Eight cases had remission, and 44 cases were operated on. Out of 29 cases of toxic cholelithiesis treated with the decoction, 19 passed stones, 3 had remission and 7 had surgery (47).

3. Biliary Acariasis

Oral administration of the <Yinchen> decoction, plus analgesia by acupuncture of the "Neiguan" point and other anthelmintic measures, was used for 70 cases; 67 achieved a clinical cure and 2 cases were improved. Cure was achieved in 3.72 days and pain was remitted in 1.47 days, on average. The therapeutic course was much shorter than that with Western medicines, or with Anti-ascaris Decoction of P. mume Fruit (13).

4. Hyperlipidemia and Coronary Disease

A. capillaris Tablet (corresponding to 24 g of the crude drug), 7 tablets thrice daily for 30 days, was used in 21 cases of hyperlipidemia. Serum cholesterol in 10 cases with hypercholesterolemia was reduced by a mean of 96.86 mg%; serum triglycerides in 18 cases with hypertriglyceridemia was lowered by a mean of 63.58 mg% (48). Treatment of 30 cases of hyperlipidemia with the herb <Yinchen> in combination with the tuber of *Alisma orientalis*, and the root and rhizome of *Glycyrrhiza uralensis* for one month, decreased the cholesterol level by an average of 36.9 mg% (49) and the triglycerides by 9.25 mg% (49). <Yinchen> used with the tuber of *Alisma orientalis* and the root tuber of *Pueraria lobata* produced significant antilipemic effect (50).

Seventy-four cases of coronary disease were treated with a basic prescription consisting of <Yinchen>, the rhizome of *Atractylodes lancea*, the vine of *Spatholobus suberectus*, and the rhizome of *Curcuma zedoaria*; cases with "yang" deficiency were given, in addition, the lateral root-tuber of *Aconitum carmichaeli* and those with "yin" deficiency, the root of *Scrophularia ningpoensis*. Different degrees of improvement and remission on the ECG and anginal pain were achieved (18).

6,7-Dimethoxycoumarin 25 and 50 mg thrice daily for 4 weeks was employed to treat angina pectoris in two groups of 18 and 23 cases, respectively; anginal pain was remitted to various extents and the ECG also improved (51).

5. Influenza and Common Cold

The decoction and the ethanol extract of <Yinchen> was used prophylactically in 44,000 person-times during epidemic periods of influenza; no single person contracted the disease. These agents also have therapeutic value in influenza and common cold (52).

6. Superficial Dermatophytosis

The 5% volatile oil spirit Nos. I–II were prepared by adding 95% ethanol to 5 ml of each fraction of the volatile oil of <Yinchen> with boiling points of 88–103°C (p=0.4 mmHg) and 93–134°C (p=1 mmHg), respectively. A third preparation (No. III) was similarly prepared from 5 ml of the aqueous residue left behind after volatile oil was distilled off. These three preparations were used to treat tinea corporis and tinea pedis twice daily for 4 weeks. The No. II preparation cured 5 out of 7 cases and improved the other 2. With the No. I preparation 2 out of 4 cases were cured and the other 2 were improved, and with the No. III preparation only 2 out of 9 cases were cured (31). These clinical results proved that the antifungal principle of <Yinchen> resides mainly in the volatile oil fraction with high boiling point.

When griseofulvin 7.5 mg/kg (i.e., 50% the regular dose for tinea favosa and 70% the dose for tinea albus) was given with <Yinchen> fluidextract 25 g (crude drug) daily to 18 cases of tinea favosa, 15 of the patients were cured. On the other hand, 46 out of 48 cases of tinea favosa and all 12 cases of tinea albus receiving 30 mg/kg of hydroxyacetophenone daily instead of the extract were cured. <Yinchen> fluidextract or hydroxyacetophenone synergized griseofulvin in the clinical treatment of tinea capitis (53).

7. Miscellaneous

A report recommended a decoction of the following herbs for the treatment of leptospirosis: the shoot of *Artemisia capillaris*, talc, root of *Scutellaria baicalensis, Mentha haplocalyx, Pogostemon cablin*, fruit of *Forsythia suspensa*, vine of *Aristolochia mandshuriensis*, and fruit of *Ammomum cardamomum* (34). The <Yinchen> extract lowered the blood glucose level in diabetic patients dose-dependently (54). The <Yinchen> Oral use of the <Yinchen> decoction produced weak contraction of the human gallbladder (55).

ADVERSE EFFECTS

After daily administration of 24 g of <Yinchen> by mouth, 7 out of 21 patients developed dizziness, nausea, upper abdominal distention and heartburn; these symptoms usually appeared on the first day of medication and they gradually disappeared. Two other cases had mild diarrhea and one experienced transient palpitation (48). All 6 cases taking 6,7-dimethoxycoumarin 250 mg thrice daily developed transient dizziness, with or without nausea and vomiting. When 5 cases took the reduced dosage of 100 mg for 3 days, transient dizziness and fatigue as well as slight T wave depression on some leads of ECG were seen in individual cases (51). The decoction of <Yinchen> plus the tuber of *Alisma orientalis*, and the root of *Pueraria lobata* each 15 g given for 26–279 days produced xerostomia, malaise, or indigestion in a few patients, but no abnormalities in the urine and blood routine examinations, platelet count, and liver function tests (50). Two adult women developed arrhythmia and Adams-Stokes syndrome on the first and fourth days respectively, after taking Artemisia-Ziziphus Decoction (Herba Artemisiae 60 g, Fructus Ziziphi Jujubae 18 pieces, decocted and given once in the morning and again in the evening); they were saved by emergency treatment (56). The use of <Yinchen> in cases of "yellowing" not due to "damp-heat" but caused by anemia and parasitic infection is discouraged by some workers (57).

(APPENDIX: BEIYINCHEN 附: 北茵陳)

<Beiyinchen> refers to the shoot of *Artemisia scoparia* Waldst et Kit. (Compositae). Also known as <Binhao>, this herb is used as <Yinchen>. It shares similar characteristics, properties, actions and indications with the latter. It is usually employed in compound prescriptions for the treatment of icteric hepatitis.

PHARMACOLOGY

1. Choleretic and Cholagogic Effects

Intraduodenal administration of hydroxyacetophenone 25–50 mg/kg to rats produced a significant choleretic effect. At 50 mg/kg, it increased the solid content, cholic acid, and bilirubin of the bile. It also enhanced bile secretion in rats with hepatic damage due to carbon tetrachloride (58).

2. Antiviral Effect

The tissue culture experiment proved that the 1:10 herb decoction was inhibitory to $ECHO_{11}$ virus. Whether given during or after viral infection of the tissue cells, it significantly delayed cellular damage. However, the decoction was inactive against herpes virus, influenza virus, and adenovirus (59).

3. Toxicity

The LD_{50} of hydroxyacetophenone in mice was 0.5 g/kg IP; the acute LD_{50} in rats was 2.2 g/kg PO.

When hydroxyacetophenone was given to rats at 400, 200, and 50 mg/kg PO, respectively, for 3 months, no significant changes were found in the blood and urine routine examinations performed every half a month, in the monthly histological examination of some animals from each dose group, and in the liver function tests carried out at the end of 3 months. Intraduodenal injection of hydroxyacetophenone 50 mg/kg to anesthetized cats did not effect the respiration, blood pressure and heart rate of the animals. When the dose was boosted to 250 mg/kg, except for a fall in the blood pressure by 40 mmHg, the respiration and heart rate were not significantly modified. Administration of hydroxyacetophenone at 250–500 mg/kg PO to conscious cats triggered vomiting in 10–40 minutes, suggesting irritation of the gastrointestinal tract by large doses (58).

REFERENCE

1. Komiya T et al. Journal of the Pharmaceutical Society of Japan (Tokyo) 1976 96(7):841,859.
2. Oshio et al. Kokai Tokkyo Koho 1976 51:9709.
3. Pharmacology Department, Shandong Medical College. Academiae Medicinae Shandong 1961 (1):19.
4. Chen L et al. Journal of Nanjing College of Pharmacy 1961 (6):42.
5. Yang ZW et al. Abstracts of the Symposium of the Chinese Society of Physiology (Pharmacology). Chinese Society of Physiology. 1964. p. 120.
6. Tianjin Institute for Drug Control and Tianjin Institute of Chinese Materia Medica. Tianjin Medical Journal 1976 4(6):287.
7. Xiyuan Hospital of the Academy of Traditional Chinese Medicine Prevention and Treatment of Coronary Disease and Hypertension. Xiyuan Hospital of the Academy of Traditional Chinese Medicine. 1972. p. 64.
8. Mashimo K et al. Chemical Abstracts 1965 62:3302g.
9. Chinese Medical Journal 1973 53(8):471.
10. Tu GR et al. Abstracts of the 1964 Symposium of Beijing Society of Physiology. Beijing Society of Physiology. 1964. p. 147.
11. Zhou SQ et al. Abstracts of the 1962 Symposium of the Chinese Pharmaceutical Association. 1963. p. 331.
12. Yuda M et al. Journal of the Pharmaceutical Society of Japan (Tokyo) 1976 96(2):147.
13. Dalian Airforce Hospital of the Chinese PLA. People's Military Medicine 1974 (5):54.
14. Deng HZ (abstract translator). Chinese Traditional and Herbal Drugs Communications 1976 (5):47.
15. Han DW et al. Chinese Traditional and Herbal Drugs Communications 1976 (8):23.
16. Yang WY et al. Scientific Papers — Special Issue on Basic Medical Sciences (Fourth Military Medical College) 1959 (12):35.
17. Cardiovascular Pharmacology Unit, Sichuan Institute of Chinese Materia Medica. Research Information on Chinese Traditional Drugs (Sichuan Institute of Chinese Materia Medica) 1973 (10):39.

18. Cardiovascular Diseases Research Unit, Second Teaching Hospital of Zhejiang Medical College. Preliminary report on Artemisia therapy of coronary disease. In: Proceedings of the 1979 National Symposium on Coronary Disease. Shanghai: 1979.

19. Li GC et al. Abstracts of the 1956 Academic Conference of the Chinese Academy of Medical Sciences. 1956. p. 70.

20. Zhu Y. Pharmacology and Applications of Chinese Medicinal Materials. People's Medical Publishing House. 1958. p. 178.

21. Fourth Research Department, Institute of Chinese Materia Medica of the Academy of Traditional Chinese Medicine. Proceedings of the Symposium on Hypertension and Cardiovascular Diseases (Internal Medicine). 1964. p. 252.

22. Cheng H et al. New Chinese Medicine 1970 (8):35.

23. Xu Z. News of Agriculture 1947 1(6):17.

24. Medical Laboratory, 178th Hospital of the Chinese PLA. Medical Information (Fuzhou Military Region) 1976 (3):54.

25. Lingling District Sanitation and Anti-epidemic Station. Hunan Yiyao Zazhi (Hunan Medical Journal) 1974 (4):50 and (5):49.

26. Microbiology Department, Nanjing College of Pharmacy. Journal of Nanjing College of Pharmacy 1960 (5):10.

27. Traditional Chinese Medicine and Materia Medica Research Unit of the Internal Medicine Department, First Teaching Hospital of Chongqing Medical College. Acta Microbiologica Sinica 1960 (1):52.

28. Zhang WX. Chinese Medical Journal 1949 67:648.

29. Chen YY et al. Jiangxi Yiyao (Jiangxi Medical Journal) 1961 (12–13):31.

30. Guo J et al. Chinese Journal of Prevention of Tuberculosis 1964 5(3):481.

31. Microbiology Section, Pharmacology Department of Sichuan Institute of Chinese Materia Medica. Sichuan Communications on Chinese Traditional and Herbal Drugs 1976 (3):28.

32. Kanai T. Journal of the Pharmaceutical Society of Japan (Tokyo) 1956 76(4):397, 400, 405.

33. Fujian Sanitation and Anti-epidemic Station. Medicine and Health (Fujian) 1972 (3):46.

34. Leptospirosis Research Group of Jiangsu College of New Medicine. Selected Information (Jiangsu College of New Medicine) 1974 (12):78.

35. Parasitology Department, Tianjin Medical College. Xinyiyaoxue Zazhi (Journal of Traditional Chinese Medicine) 1974 (2):31.

36. Yamamoto. Nihon Kagaku Soran Dai 2 Shu 1952 26(5):480.

37. Sun SX. Chinese Medical Journal 1956 (10):964.

38. Fujian Institute for Drug Control. Selected Articles on Medical Achievements in Fujian. 1962. p. 71.

39. Kanai T. Japan Centra Revuo Medicina 1956 132:724.

40. Huang YC. Fujian Zhongyiyao (Fujian Journal of Traditional Chinese Medicine) 1959 4(7):42.

41. Production and Construction Corps of Xinjiang Military Region. Corps Information on Science and Technology 1962 (4):16.

42. Liver Diseases Unit, Teaching Hospital of Hubei College of Traditional Chinese Medicine. Wuhan Journal of New Traditional Chinese Medicine 1973 3(1):25.

43. Zibo District (Shandong) Sanitation and Anti-epidemic Station. New Chinese Medicine 1973 (8):391.

44. Xiangtan District Sanitation and Anti-epidemic Station. Hunan Yiyao Zazhi (Hunan Medical Journal) 1975 (2):45.

45. Pei DK. Communications on Combined Western and Traditional Chinese Therapy of Acute Abdomen 1977 (2):61.

46. Nankai (Tianjin) Hospital and Zunyi Medical College. New Perspectives on Acute Abdomen. Ist edition. People' s Medical Publishing House. 1977 p. 296.

47. Qingdao Municipal Hospital. Cholelithiasis. Shandong People' s Publishing House. 1973. p. 103.

48. Coronary Disease Therapy Unit, Luzhou Medical School. Luyi Ziliao (Journal of Luzhou Medical School) 1975 (2):59.

49. Liang RL. Medical Exchanges (Shanghai) 1975 (6):46.

50. Coronary Disease Unit, Shantou (Guangdong) Second People' s Hospital. Xinzhongyi (Journal of New Chinese Medicine) 1976 (3):36.

51. Xiyuan Hospital of the Academy of Traditional Chinese Medicine. Prevention and Treatment of Coronary Disease and Hypertension. Xiyuan Hospital of the Academy of Traditional Chinese Medicine. 1972. p. 42.

52. Health Team of 5804 Unit of the Chinese PLA. New Medical Communications (Guangzhou Health Bureau) 1973 (2):23.

53. Jiangsu Institute of Dermatology. Chinese Traditional and Herbal Drugs Communications 1977 (7):38.

54. Kadomoto E et al. Japan Centra Revuo Medicina 1955 118:397.

55. Jiang WX et al. Shanxi Medical Journal 1963 7(3):1.

56. Shi GS. Chinese Journal of Internal Medicine 1961 9(7):439.

57. Editorial Group (Zhongshan Medical College) of "Clinical Applications of Chinese Traditional Drugs". New Chinese Medicine 1972 (3):36.

58. Hunan Institute of Medical and Pharmaceutical Industry. Chinese Medical Journal 1974 54(2):101.

59. Virus Section, Institute of Chinese Materia Medica of the Academy of Traditional Chinese Medicine. Xinyiyaoxue Zazhi (Journal of Traditional Chinese Medicine) 1973 (1):26.

(Wu Chongrong)

FULING 茯苓

<Fuling> is the sclerotium of *Poria cocos* (Schw.) Wolf (Polyporaceae). It is known by various by various names depending on the part used, its color, and the way it is processed. Thus, the black skin removed from the sclerotium is known as <Fulingpi>, the inner white portion is called <Baifuling> and the reddish variety, <Chifuling>. <Fushen> refers to the sclerotium that encircles the root of the pine tree.

<Fuling> is sweet, bland, and "mild". It has "spleen"-invigorative, stomach-tonifying, sedative, tranquilizing, diuretic and "damp"-clearing actions. It is mainly used to treat retention of phlegm and fluid, dysuria, edema, poor appetite with watery stool, palpitation, and insomnia.

CHEMICAL COMPOSITION

The sclerotium contains β-pachyman, pachymic acid, ergosterol, choline, histidine, and potassium salts.

PHARMACOLOGY

1. Diuretic Effect

Injection of the 25% ethanol extract of <Fuling> to rabbits at 0.5 g/kg IP daily for 5 days resulted in marked diuresis equipotent to mersalyl at 0.1 mg/kg IM. The diuretic action was unrelated to the potassium salt, suggesting the existence of other diuretic components (1). Intragastric administration of "Wuling San" or ethanol extract of <Fuling> to normal rats also produced a diuretic effect (2); no such action was achieved by the decoction or ethanol extract of <Fuling> administered orally to rabbits.

In acute experiments on dogs with ureteral fistulae, intravenous injection of <Fuling> did not cause diuresis (3). In acute diuretic experiments on rats, no significant modification of the urine output and urinary sodium excretion was noted (4). These inconsistent reports are attributable to the differences in experimental conditions. Oral administration of the decoction to 5 volunteers at 15 g resulted in a slight increase in the urine output in 4 of them (5).

The mechanism of the diuretic action of <Fuling> has not yet been elucidated. Experiments indicated that the decoction used by itself, or in combination with desoxycorticosterone, fostered sodium excretion but did not antagonize the action of aldosterone. Further study is required for the elucidation of the active natriuretic principle and the mechanism of action (6). According to one report, the 30% <Fuling> decoction contained 0.186 mg/ml of sodium and 11.2 mg/ml of potassium, thus its natriuretic effect appeared unrelated to its sodium content, but its high potassium content might contribute to the increase in potassium excretion (6). Reviewing material on "Wuling San" in the ancient Chinese medical documents "Shang Han Lun" (Treatise on Febrile Diseases) and "Jin Kui Yao Lue" (Synopsis of Prescriptions of the Golden Chamber), Japanese workers suggest that "Wuling San" syndrome is due to downward-setting of osmotic pressure homeostasis and that "Wuling San" increases the setting. Diuresis is achieved through a direct action on the osmoreceptor, neurosecretory cells and no the neurons in the thirst center, and consequent modification of the afferent nerve impulses of these structures. It also lowers the antidiuretic hormone level (ADH). The diuretic and thirst-quenching effects were thus achieved (7).

2. Sedative Effect

Intraperitoneal injection of "Fushen Decoction" to mice markedly reduced the spontaneous activity of the animals; it also antagonized over-excitation due to caffeine. Significant synergism with pentobarbital sodium was demonstrated by intraperitoneal injection of the <Fuling> decoction to mice (8).

3. Antineoplastic Effect

Pachymaran, which was obtained by structural transformation of pachyman, produced an inhibition rate of 96.88% against sarcoma in mice (9).

4. Effect on Immunologic Function

Oral administration of the compound formula decoction (Radix Codonopsis Pilosulae, Rhizoma Atractylodis Alba, Poria) significantly increased the spontaneous rosette formation and phytohemagglutinin-induced lymphocyte transformation rate. It also increased serum IgG. These evidences indicate that the agent promotes cellular and humoral immunity (10).

5. Effect on Digestive System

<Fuling> exerted a direct stimulant effect on the isolated rabbit intestine (11). It inhibited gastric ulcer provoked by ligation of the pylorus in rats and decreased gastric secretion and free acidity (12). <Fuling> also protected rats against carbon tetrachloride-induced liver damage, markedly decreasing GPT activity and preventing necrosis of hepatocytes (13).

6. Miscellaneous

The aqueous, ethanol, or ether extract of <Fuling> enhanced myocardial contractility and increased the heart rate (14,15). Another report, however, claimed that the aqueous extract or the tincture of

<Fuling> at high concentrations depressed the isolated frog heart (16). In rabbits, the ethanol extract first increases blood glucose level, and then reduces it (17,18). *In vitro* antibacterial assays showed that <Fuling> inhibited *Staphylococcus aureus, Mycobacterium tuberculosis*, and *Proteus vulgaris* (18,19); the ethanol extract killed leptospirae (20) whereas the decoction was inactive (21). <Fuling> could not relieve emesis in pigeons due to digitalis (22).

CLINICAL STUDIES

1. Edema and Oliguria

One of the useful prescriptions is "Wuling San". There is also "Fuling Daoshui Tang", (Diuretic Decoction of Poria cocos) (Poria, Rhizoma Alismatis, Cortex Mori, Pericarpium Citri Reticulatae, Radix Aucklandiae, Fructus Chaenomelis, Fructus Amomi, Rhizoma Atractylodis Macrocephalae, Folium et Fructus Perillae, Semen Arecae, Radix Ophiopogonis, Medulla Junci, Pericarpium Arecae), which was used with good therapeutic effects in 3 cases of nephritic edema, cardiac edema and postpartum jaundice and edema (23). In addition, out of 17 cases of hydramnios treated with the herb, 14 were cured; it was more effective in single-fetus pregnancy than in twin pregnancy, and more effective in chronic than in acute conditions (24).

2. Neurasthenia, Insomnia and Others

<Fuling> is usually used in combination with the kernel of *Ziziphus jujuba*, 9–18 g each time as a decoction (25).

3. Indigestion due to Asthenia of "Spleen and Stomach" and Diarrhea due to Deficiency of "Spleen"

<Fuling>, which is reputed to invigorate the "spleen" and eliminate the "damp" pathogenic factor, is useful for indigestion and diarrhea. One of the useful prescriptions is "Weiling Tang" (Gastric Decoction of Poria) (25).

REFERENCE

1. Gao YD et al. Chinese Medical Journal 1955 41(10):963.
2. Zhu Y. Proceedings of the 1962 Symposium of the Chinese Pharmaceutical Association. 1963. p. 327.
3. Wang LW et al. Abstracts of the Symposium of the Chinese Society of Physiology (Pharmacology). 1964. p. 133.
4. Wang LW et al. Chinese Traditional and Herbal Drugs 1980 (5):222.

5. Internal Medicine Department, Beijing Medical College. Chinese Medical Journal 1961 47(1):7.

6. Luo HW et al. Journal of Nanjing College of Pharmacy 1964 (10):69.

7. Ito Y. The Journal of Society for Oriental Medicine in Japan 1978 28(3):1.

8. Hu CJ. Acta Academiae Medicinae Wuhan 1957 (1):125.

9. Shanghai Institute of Materia Medica. Progress in the Research of Phytogenic Antineoplastic Constituents during the Last Decade Outside China. 1972.

10. Song FJ et al. Xinyiyaoxue Zazhi (Journal of Traditional Chinese Medicine) 1979 (6):61.

11. Tomizawa S. Japan Centra Revuo Medicina 1962 180:710.

12. Tomizawa S. The Journal of Society for Oriental Medicine in Japan 1962 13(1):5.

13. Han DW et al. Chinese Journal of Internal Medicine 1977 2(1):13.

14. Takahashi S et al. Yakugaku Kenkyu 1968 39(8):281.

15. Nakamura H. Yakugaku Kenkyu 1967 39(8):281.

16. Wang WX et al. Selected Papers of Dalian Railways Medical College. 1960. p. 41.

17. Read BE. Chinese Medical Journal 1925 39:314.

18. Nanjing College of Pharmacy. Chinese Traditional Pharmacy. Vol. 2. Jiangsu People's Publishing House. 1976. p. 15.

19. Wang SY et al. Kexue Tongbao (Science Bulletin) 1958 (12):379.

20. Microbiology Department, Xuzhou Medical College. New Medical Information (Xuzhou Medical College) 1971 (1):27.

21. Li XX et al. Chinese Medical Journal 1955 41(10):952.

22. Zhou JG. Tianjin Medical Journal 1960 2(2):131.

23. Ma CX. Notes on Medical Sciences and Technology (Information Unit of Qingdao Health Bureau) 1977 (6):15.

24. Zhao JS. Zhongji Yikan (Intermediate Medical Journal) 1979 (5):24.

25. Zhongshan Medical College. Clinical Applications of Chinese Traditional Drugs. Guangdong People's Publishing House. 1975. p. 137.

(Chen Quansheng)

HOUPO 厚朴

<Houpo> refers to the dried bark and root bark of *Magnolia officinalis* Rehd, et Wils. and *M. officinalis* Rehd. et Wils. var. *biloba* Rehd. et Wils. (Magnoliaceae); the flowers and fruits of these plants are also used as medicine.

<Houpo> is bitter, pungent and "warm". It is "damp"-clearing, digestant, laxative, vital-energy-stimulant (or carminative) and antiasthmatic. It is, therefore, used in the treatment of distention and pain of the abdomen, dyspepsia, and asthmatic cough. The flower, which has a slightly bitter taste and a "warm" property, relieves chest congestion, and is carminative. It is used for thoracic distress.

The Japanese <Houpo> is obtained from the species *M. obovata* Thunb.

CHEMICAL COMPOSITION

The root bark contains 1% of volatile oil which is mainly composed of machilol. The volatile oil also contains magnolol, honokiol, tetrahydromagnolol and traces of magnocurarine (mulanjiandujian). A soluble alkaloid also called "magnocurarine" (houpojian) (chemical structure not elucidated) was isolated from the bark (1).

PHARMACOLOGY

1. Muscle Relaxant Effect

A water-soluble alkaloid magnocurarine (houpojian), isolated by Chinese workers from the herb, had a relaxant effect on striated muscles; 13.8 mg/kg IV of this substance caused head drop in rabbits. Repeated administration to rabbits of the same dosage did not attenuate the muscle relaxant effect, indicating the absence of tachyphylaxis. In experiments with the phrenic nerve-muscle specimen of albino rats, the 30% magnocurarine decreased the contraction amplitude of the phrenic muscle by about 40%; increasing the drug concentration to 40% almost stopped the contraction. As with tubocurarine (0.5 mg/animal IV), intravenous injection of magnocurarine to chickens at doses over 40 mg/kg resulted in flaccid paralysis. These events indicate that magnocurarine is probably a nondepolarizing muscle relaxant. The activity of magnocurarine was markedly enhanced after methiodization (2).

A curariform alkaloid, probably the crude extract of magnocurarine (mulanjiandujian), obtained from the bark of *M. obovata*, injected into the lymphatic sac of frogs at 1 mg/animal blocked the neuromuscular transmission; intravenous injection of this agent to rabbits at 30 mg/kg produced curariform paralysis (3). The same agent successfully isolated from *M. obovata* was proved to have a relaxant effect on striated muscles though it was found to be weaker than tubocurarine (4).

In recent years magnolol and isomagnolol isolated from *M. obovata* were discovered to have central muscle relaxant action; large doses of these agents abolished the righting reflex in mice. In assays on the spinal reflexes of chicken, intraperitoneal injection of either magnolol or isomagnolol conspicuously inhibited the extensor reflex; the action could be antagonized by large doses of strychnine. These drugs are therefore considered to be noncurariform muscle relaxants more potent than mephenesin. Both magnolol and isomagnolol had specific and prolonged muscle relaxant effect (5).

2. Effect on Smooth Muscles

The <Houpo> decoction exerted a stimulant effect on the isolated intestines and bronchi of rabbits (6). The decoction stimulated isolated intestines of mice at the concentration of 1:166 and inhibited them at the concentration of 1:100. The action of the decoction on isolated guinea pig intestines was essentially identical to that on mice; however, the inhibitory effect was more pronounced than the stimulant effect. Intravenous injection of magnocurarine (houpojian) to anesthetized cats caused a decrease in the tension of the small intestines *in vivo* (7).

3. Central Depressant Effect

Intraperitoneal injection of the ether extract of <Houpo> to mice inhibited the spontaneous activity of the animals and antagonized stimulation due to methamphetamine or apomorphine (8). Magnolol and isomagnolol also exhibited a marked central depressant effect. Administration of the ether extract of the herb to rats caused spontaneous high amplitude slow waves on the EEG, and elevation of the level of serotonin and its metabolites in the brain a few hours later, without altering catecholamine levels. Complete inhibition of the spinal reflexes of chickens was obtained after magnolol medication (8).

4. Prevention of Peptic Ulcer

Magnolol inhibited gastric ulcers caused by Shay's pyloric ligation and by stress due to drowning and to some extent histamine-induced duodenal spasm. Gastric secretion produced by intravenous injection of tetragastrin and bethanechol in anesthetized rats was inhibited by gastric perfusion of magnolol (9).

5. Effect on the Heart and Blood Vessels

The water-soluble substance of the magnolia flower tincture intravenously or intramuscularly injected to anesthetized rabbits or cats triggered hypotension and tachycardia (10). The hypotensive action of magnocurarine (houpojian) was not causally related to histamine release since it could be antagonized by promethazine (2).

6. Antibacterial Effects and Others

The <Houpo> decoction is a broad-spectrum antibacterial agent, with an antibacterial principle that is heat-stable and resistant to acid alkaline (11). *In vitro*, the decoction inhibits *Staphylococcus aureus* (12–13), *Streptococcus hemolyticus, Corynebacterium diphtheriae, Bacillus subtilis, Shigella dysenteriae*, and common pathogenic skin fungi (11,13–16). In guinea pigs artificially infected with *Bacillus anthracis*, daily intraperitoneal injection of the decoction 0.5 ml per animal for 4 days significantly delayed the death of the animals (11). Certain improvement on the parenchymal lesions of mice with experimental viral hepatitis was also achieved with the decoction (17). Furthermore, the decoction could also kill swine ascaris *in vitro* (18).

7. Toxicity

A single intragastric administration of the <Houpo> decoction 60 g/kg to mice did not result in any fatality over a period of three days. The oral dosage was less toxic since magnocurarine (mulanjiandujian), the chief toxic conponent, was poorly absorbed from the gastrointestinal tract, and once absorbed, was disposed of by the kidneys; thus its blood level was low (19,20). The LD_{50} of the <Houpo> decoction in mice was 6.12 ± 0.038 g/kg IP (7); the LD_{50} of magnocurarine (mulanjiandujian) was 45.55 mg/kg IP (21). The MLD of the <Houpo> decoction in cats was 4.25 ± 1.25 g/kg IV (7). The common muscle relaxant dosage of the decoction did not influence the ECG of experimental animals, but large doses caused death due to respiratory depression (7).

CLINICAL STUDIES

1. Constipation, Abdominal Distention and Pain

<Houpo> and the unripe citrus fruit each 9 g, and rhubarb 6 g, decocted together can be given by mouth (6). The flower and fruit of the *Magnolia* plant are chiefly used as stomachic; they are less effective in eliminating "dampness" than <Houpo> and are indicated in mild indigestion or epigastric discomfort (22).

2. Acute Enteritis, Bacillary or Amebic Dysentery

The powdered <Houpo> 3 g/dose, or pills prepared from this herb and flour 4.5–9 g/dose can be given 2–3 times daily. The herb may also be made into injections (1 g crude drug/ml) to be given intramuscularly, 2 ml 2–3 times a day (6).

Forty-six cases of amebic dysentery were treated orally with the <Houpo> decoction at 10 ml (corresponding to 6 g of the crude drug) twice daily; 43 of these cases were cured after 3–9 days, 2 were improved and one case was unresponsive. Whether it is lethal to ameba requires confirmation by future studies (23).

3. Uses in Gynecological and Obstetrical Operations

The <Houpo> powder has been used in recent years to suppress meteorism during panhysterectomy under acupuncture anesthesia. Dosage: 5–7.5 g in patients weighing less than 50 kg and 7.5–10 g for those over 50 kg. A significant difference in the improvements of intestinal volvulus was observed between the powder-treated group and others given remedies. The powder did not alter the respiration, blood pressure, and heart rate (24).

4. Furuncle

The 25% ointment of the <Houpo> powder and vaseline is recommended for topical use (25).

REFERENCE

1. Fujita R. Journal of the Pharmaceutical Society of Japan (Tokyo) 1973 93 (4):415.
2. Pharmacology Department, Shanghai College of Traditional Chinese Medicine. Xinyiyaoxue Zazhi (Journal of Traditional Chinese Medicine) 1974 (5):41.
3. Zhu Y. Pharmacology and Applications of Chinese Medicinal Materials. 1st edition. People's Medical Publishing House. 1958. p. 123.
4. Ogyu K. Japan Centra Revuo Medicina 1954:112–669.
5. Watanabe K. The Japanese Journal of Pharmacology 1975 25(5):605.
6. Harbin Medical College. Research Papers on Combined Western and Traditional Chinese Medicine (Harbin Medical College) 1961 2:112.
7. Basic Medical Sciences Department, Faculty of Pharmacy of Shanghai First Medical College. Xinyiyaoxue Zazhi (Journal of Traditional Chinese Medicine) 1973 (4):31.
8. Watanabe M. Folia Pharmacologica Japonica 1976 72(3):11.
9. Watanabe M. Folia Pharmacologica Japonica 1976 72(2):60.
10. Pharmacology Department, Hunan Medical College. Bulletin of Hunan Medical College (Special Issue on Traditional Chinese Medicine and Materia Medica) 1958:129.
11. Liao YX. Acta Pharmaceutica Sinica 1954 2(1):5.
12. Hsuch-Chieu. Chemical Abstracts 1953 47:8175d.
13. Zhao ZQ et al. Journal of Beijing Medical College 1959 (1):75.

14. Xu ZL et al. Chinese Medical Journal 1947 33(3–4):71.

15. Liu GS et al. Chinese Journal of New Medicine 1950 1:95.

16. Chen LF et al. Drug Control Work Bulletin 1980 (4):209.

17. Pharmacology Department, Shanghai Medical School. Proceedings of the National Symposium on Combined Western and Traditional Chinese Medicine. 1961. p. 304.

18. Kato Y. Japan Centra Revuo Medicina 1954:110–130.

19. Fan ZQ. Xinyiyaoxue Zazhi (Journal of Traditional Chinese Medicine) 1975 (3):42.

20. Murakami M et al. Yakuriteki Shoyakugaku 1933 p. 50.

21. Ogyu K et al. Folia Pharmacologica Japanica 1953 48(2):72.

22. Zhongshan Medical College (editor). Clinical Applications of Chinese Traditional Drugs. Guangdong People's Publishing House. 1975. p. 211.

23. Sun XC. Zhongji Yikan (Intermediate Medical Journal) 1960 (7):453.

24. Teaching Hospital of Obstetrics and Gynecology, Shanghai First Medical College. Xinyiyaoxue Zazhi (Journal of Traditional Chinese Medicine) 1973 (4):25.

25. Nanjing College of Pharmacy. Chinese Traditional Pharmacy. Vol. 2. Jiangsu People's Publishing House. 1975. p. 316.

(Chen Quansheng)

WEILINGXIAN 威靈仙

<Weilingxian> comes from the rhizome and root of *Clematis chinensis* Osbeck (Ranunculaceae). It is also derived from other *Clematis* plants such as *C. hexapetala* Pall., also called <Miantuantiexianlian>, mainly used in the northeastern and northern parts of China, Shandong, and Jiangsu; *C. armandi* Franch. in Yunnan, Hunan, Guangxi, and Zhejiang; *C. uncinata* Champ. ex Benth. in Guangdong, Guangxi, Guizhou, Sichuan, Fujian, Zhejiang, and Jiangxi; *C. meyeniana* Walp. in Guangxi, Fujian, and Hunan; *C. henryi* Oliv. in Guangxi, Jiangxi, Anhui, and Zhejiang; *C. finetiana* Lévl. et Vant. in Guangxi, Jiangxi, Zhejiang, and Anhui; *C. manshurica* Rupr. in northeastern China; and *C. paniculata* Thunb. in Jiangsu and Zhejiang.

The herb tastes pungent and slightly bitter and has a "warm" property. It is reputed to be antirheumatic, channel-deobstruent and analgesic. It is mainly used as a remedy for rheumatism, arthralgia, poor joint movement, numbness of the limbs, wounds and injuries, and for the release of bones lodged in the throat.

CHEMICAL COMPOSITION

The whole plant of *C. chinensis* contains protoanemonin, the amounts of which in the root, leaf and stems are 0.25, 0.2 and 0.12%, respectively. Protoanemonin can readily polymerize into anemonin. The root also contains anemonol, sterols, carbohydrates, and saponins.

PHARMACOLOGY

1. Effect on Smooth Muscles

Intensification of esophageal peristalsis and increase in its frequency and amplitude were produced in anesthetized dogs after intragastric administration of the <Weilingxian> decoction. The herb relaxed pharyngeal or upper esophageal spasm caused by a fish bone lodged in the throat; it enhanced peristalsis, allowing the bone to dislodge. The herb had an antihistaminic action on the isolated smooth muscle of rabbit intestines. A related species, *C. angustifolia* Jacq., (*= *C. hexapetala*. See Encyclopedia of Chinese Materia Medica Vol. 2. 1977. p. 1633. Shanghai Sci-Tech Literature Publishing House) which is used as <Weilingxian> in some areas, exerted a marked stimulant action on the isolated intestines of mice (1). The 1% protoanemonin antagonized the bronchospastic effect of 0.01% histamine.

2. Induction of Labor

Injection of the dilute-ethanol extract of <Weilingxian> 15 g(crude drug)/kg IM for 5 days to mice at mid-term pregnancy induced labor; over 80% of the animals had complete delivery (2).

3. Antibacterial Effect

The paper-disk method showed that the 100% decoction of the root was inhibitory against *Staphylococcus aureus* and *Shigella shigae*, and that the 1:3 aqueous preparation inhibited *Microsporum audouini in vitro*. Protoanemonin exhibited a strong inhibitory action against gram-positive and gram-negative bacteria as well as against fungi; the MIC against streptococci was determined to be 1:60,000 *Escherichia coli* 1:83,000–33,000, and *Candida albicans* 1:100,000 (3).

4. Miscellaneous Actions

The decoction and extract of a related species *C. angustifolia* produced an initial inhibition, succeeded by stimulation, of the isolated toad heart; the potency of the extract was greater than that of the decoction. The preparation also decreased the blood pressure and renal volume of anesthetized dogs. In mice, rats, and guinea pigs, no significant antidiuretic effect was observed. The antidiuretic efficacy of 0.2 ml of the 50% decoction approximated that of 0.1 unit of pituitrin but the decoction had a longer duration of action (1).

5. Toxicity

Contact with the mucus of the stem or protoanemonin causes irritation, blistering and mucosal congestion.

CLINICAL STUDIES

1. Fish Bone Lodged in the Esophagus

<Weilingxian> 30 g (or together with the root of *Angelica dahurica*, the unripe fruit of *Prunus mume*, the root and rhizome of *Glycyrrhiza uralensis*) made into a concentrated decoction, or used with vinegar, was given slowly by mouth (30 min–1 h) 1–2 doses a day to over 100 cases of choking caused by fish bone lodged in the pharynx and esophagus; the effective rate was 87.6% (4–7).

2. Hypertrophic Spondylitis and Lumbar Muscular Strain

Injection of the steam distillate preparation of <Weilingxian> into the "Huatojiaji" acupoints of the hypertrophic paravertebral area, 1 ml to each of the 2–4 points daily or on alternate days, was used to treat over 100 cases of hypertrophic spondylitis; responsive cases accounted for 83–93.81%. Out of 32 cases of lumbar muscular strain treated with the herb, 14 had prominent effects, and 18 moderate effects (8,9).

3. Filariasis

The fresh root of *C. chinensis* 500 g was decocted for 30 minutes; the resulting liquid was boiled with white wine 60 g and brown sugar 500 g for a short period. The medicine was divided to be taken twice daily, morning and evening over a 5-day period. In 34 cases of filariasis so treated, 75–100% became worm-free (10).

4. Psoriasis

The decoction of <Weilingxian> 90 g, taken by mouth once every morning and evening until desquamation disappeared, was effective in 6 cases (11).

5. Esophageal Cancer

Out of 300 cases of esophageal cancer treated with <Weilingxian> together with the root of *Isatis tinctoria*, the aerial part of *Euphorbia lunulate*, the cured tuber of *Arisaema consanguineum*, artificial bovine bezoar, and sal ammoniac, 33 cases (11%) had short-term remission, 53 (18%) marked effects, 180 (60%) moderate effects, and 34 (11.3%) no response (12).

6. Induction of labor

The following procedure to induce labor has been reported: The fresh root of *C. chinensis* is washed with clean water, then sterilized with iodine tincture and 75% alcohol. It is gradually introduced into the uterine cavity until resistance is felt; 2 cm of the root is left outside the cervix and fixed with gauze. This method was applied in 149 cases of pregnancy of different duration, resulting in an effective rate of 95.6% (67.8% had complete abortion and 14.6% incomplete abortion). Abortion usually occurred 24–48 hours after medication (13). However, this method is not scientific and should be discarded. Further studies are required to improve the dosage from and route of administration.

7. Miscellaneous

<Weilingxian> was reported to be effective in acute mastitis (14), chronic cholecystitis (15), acute tonsillitis (16), and balanitis in young children (17).

REFERENCE

1. Pi XP. Acta Academiae Medicinae Qingdao 1971 (1):9.

2. Zhou SQ et al. Selected Information on Family Planning. Northeastern Sichuan Coordinating Group on Family Planning. 1979. p. 59.

3. Baer H et al. Journal of Biological Chemistry 1946 162:65.

4. EENT Department, 157th Hospital of the Chinese PLA et al. New Chinese Medicine 1973 (3):144.

5. EENT Department, Gejiu People's Hospital. Yunnan Yiyao (Yunnan Medical Journal) 1976 (2):38.

6. Pharyngolaryngology Department, Luzhou Medical School. Luyi Ziliao (Journal of Luzhou Medical College) 1976 (1):64.

7. Class 1971 of Traditional Chinese Medicine for Doctors Trained in Western Medicine, Guangxi College of Traditional Chinese Medicine. Teaching of Traditional Chinese Medicine (Guangxi College of Traditional Chinese Medicine) 1973 (1):23.

8. Traditional Chinese Medicine Department, Huashan Teaching Hospital of Shanghai First Medical College. Medical Exchanges 1975 (1):60.

9. Shanghai First People's Hospital. Shanghai Exhibition on Achievements in Combined Western and Traditional Chinese Medicine. 1974. p. 16.

10. Dean County Sanitation and Anti-epidemic Station. New Medical Information (Jiangxi School of Pharmacy) 1971 (3):36.

11. Hospital of Datonggou Coal Mine (Jixi). Jixi Bulletin of Science and Technology 1973 (4):13.

12. Anhui People's Hospital. Chinese Traditional and Herbal Drugs Communications 1972 (2):14.

13. Wenjiang District Committee on Science and Technology. Wenjiang Science and Technology (Seismology Group of Wenjiang District Production Management Unit, Sichuan) 1972 (3):17.

14. Shimen Commune (Huangpi County) Health Centre. Health Journal of Hubel 1973 (2):54.

15. Zhang CC. Xinzhongyi (Journal of New Chinese Medicine) 1974 (5):11.

16. Mashan People's Hospital (Suburbs of Wuxi, Jiangsu). Xinyiyaoxue Tongxun (Bulletin of New Chinese Medicine) 1971 (3):56.

17. Li YR. Xinzhongyiyao (Modernized Traditional Chinese Medicine) 1958 (4):33.

(Wu Tingkai)

YADANZI 鴉膽子

<Yadanzi>, also known as <Kushenzi>, refers to the ripe fruit of *Brucea javanica* (L.) Merr. (*B. sumatrana* Roxb. or *B. amarissima* Desv.) (Simaroubaceae). It is extremely bitter, has a "cold" property and is toxic. It produces latent-heat-clearing, antipyretic, detoxicant, anti-inflammatory, antimalarial, antidysenteric effects and has a necrotizing effect on warts. Hence, the herb is a remedy for chronic diarrhea, dysentery, and externally, for corns and simple warts. In other countries, the bark or root bark of the Brucea plant is a folk remedy for dysentery, verrucous tumor or cancer.

CHEMICAL COMPOSITION

The major active constituents of <Yadanzi> are bitter substances, from which brusatol, bruceolide and bruceines A, B, C, D, E, F, and G were isolated. <Yadanzi> also contains glycosides such as yatanoside, kosamine, brucealin and yatanin; these are crude preparations lacking in detailed chemical studies. Bruceosides A and B were recently reported to have antineoplastic activity (1–3); these are actually glucosides of bruceines. Alkaloids such as yatanine were reported as constituents, but they were not further confirmed. <Yadanzi> contains 36.8–56.2% of oil of which oleic acid was reported to have antineoplastic activity *in vitro* (4).

PHARMACOLOGY

1. Antiamebic Effect

1.1 *In vitro studies.* Ameba in feces was killed on contact with the aqueous extract or ether extract of the defatted <Yadanzi> (5). But with the 1:1000 aqueous extract 48-hour contact was required to kill two of three kinds of amebae in the culture medium (6). <Yadanzi> oil was inactive (5).

The amebicidal effect of yatanoside in the culture medium was about one-fifth to one-tenth that of emetine (7). The purified product yatanoside A had a weaker amebicidal effect, i.e., only one-fourth that of yatanoside and one-fortieth that of emetine. The crude glycoside yatanin at the concentration of 1:20,000 killed amebae within 48 hours of contact (8). Another crude glycoside, brucealin, was slightly more potent than yatanin (8). When refined these two glycosides were markedly weakened. These findings indicate that the active principle is probably not a glycoside, but the water-soluble bitter substances as reported by Japanese investigators (9). The active principle, therefore, has been not determined (10). The bitter substances were recently identified by the late in Lin Qishou as the real antiamebic constituent (11). However, the basis of the document was not clear.

1.2 *Experimental therapy.* In cats, puppies, adult dogs, and monkeys naturally or artificially infected with amebae, oral administration or injection of the preparation of the kernel of the herb and its extract was effective (7,8,12); however, the radical cure rate of <Yadanzi> in amebiasis was not high. In experiments with dogs, all the tested animals died within a short period irrespective of the result of the stool examination. Death also occurred in cats and monkeys during the treatment period. It is worth noting that, with yatanoside therapy, the mortality rate was markedly increased and the cure rate markedly decreased, suggesting that it was not the active principle of this herb (8).

2. Antimalarial Effect

Experiments on chickens with malaria indicated that both the orally administered kernel and the intramuscularly injected crude noncrystalline powder had a marked antimalarial action, causing the rapid reduction or even disappearance of the plasmodium from the blood; radical cure, however, has not been confirmed. In contrast, the pure crystal showed a weaker antimalarial activity (13). The antimalarial principle is highly soluble in water, heat-stable and has antiplasmodial effect; the asexual bodies were more sensitive to it than the gametocytes. The MED of the kernel decoction was 0.02 g/kg which was equivalent to that of quinine but smaller than that of the root of *Dichroa febrifuga* (14).

Further studies proved that when the infusion of <Yadanzi> was orally ingested, or when the bitter mixture was injected intramuscularly, it was necessary to increase the dosage to one-half of the LD_{50}, or even to approximate the LD_{50} in order to be effective. In the experiment, some of the chickens died within a short time, and the survivors relapsed upon discontinuation of the drug and eventually died. Therefore, the therapeutic value of the herb is doubtful (15,16). It was proved that the antimalarial potency was greatly influenced by the variation in the sources of the herb and by the duration of storage. The conflicting experimental results were thus attributed to these differences (14). This, however, does not appear to be the case.

3. Antiparasitic Effect

Kosamine, the crude extract of <Yadanzi>, had an anthelmintic activity in dogs with pinworms (*Enterobius vermicularis*) and tapeworms (18). It was discovered during the treatment of dysentery that <Yadanzi> was also active against whipworms (*Trichuris trichiura*) and roundworms (Ascaris) (7). A strong anthelmintic activity against hookworms has also been reported (17). A bitter glycoside extracted from the kernel at the concentration of 1:10,000 was lethal to the adult *Paragonimus westermani in vitro* within 24 hours. the kernel itself was inactive against experimental paragonimiasis in dogs (18). <Yadanzi> was found to be lethal to *Trichomonas, Paramecium*, and *Protozoa urosonus*. Mosquito larvae and eggs were completely killed on contact with the 5–10% extract of the herb for 18–48 hours. Treatment of stagnant water by the stem and leaves was also effective (18).

4. Antineoplastic Effect

In mice with skin cancer (epithelioma) and papilloma induced by "methylcholanthrene acetone", the paste and aqueous preparation of the kernel locally applied caused regressive degeneration and necrosis of the tumor cells; however, a similar action was also seen in normal tissue (19).

Injection of the methanol extract of <Yadanzi> markedly inhibited Ehrlich ascites carcinoma, Walker carcinoma 256 and P-388 lymphocytic leukemia. Prominent therapeutic effect were obtained against P-388 leukemia by daily administration of bruceoside A 6 mg/kg (1). A similar antineoplastic activity was also exhibited by bruceoside B (2). *In vitro*, brusatol, bruceine D, and another bitter substance exhibited antineoplastic activity (20), but that of bruceine B was only marginal (21). An antineoplastic action was also shown by the oil of <Yadanzi>; the active principle was determined to be oleic acid (4).

<Yadanzi> derived from *B. antidysenteria* Mill. grown in Ethiopia is used as a folk remedy for dysentery and cancer. The ethanol extract of its bark produced a conspicuous inhibitory action on human nasopharyngeal carcinoma KB cells, Walker carcinoma 256, and P-388 lymphocytic leukemia. At a very low dosage, i.e., a few μg/kg, bruceantin, isolated from the Ethiopian herb, demonstrated a marked antineoplastic action on P-388 lymphocytic leukemia; the cytotoxic concentration (EC_{50}) against KB cells *in vitro* was 1 ng/ml. A moderate activity was exhibited by another principle — bruceantarin (21,22). Neither bruceantin nor bruceantarin has ever been isolated from the plant *B. javanica* that grows in China.

5. Effect on the Cardiovascular System

Intravenous injection of the extract of the defatted <Yadanzi> and of the its other crude extracts caused a transient fall in the blood pressure of dogs. Their effect on the *in situ* and isolated hearts was characterized by inhibition which was not abolished by vagotomy or atropine injection. They produced vasodilation but this effect was unstable; in frogs vasoconstriction was produced. The effect of yatanoside on the heart and blood vessels was inconspicuous (8,23).

6. Effect on Smooth Muscles

Various extracts of the kernel stimulated the isolated uterus and small intestine as well as the small intestine *in situ* (23). Yatanoside had no effect on isolated organs but small doses by intravenous injection initiated strong intestinal contraction 20 minutes after the medication (7).

7. Miscellaneous Actions

<Yadanzi> had no marked inhibitory or lethal actions against *Shigella dysenteriae, Salmonella typhi, Vibrio cholerae*, and other common pathogenic bacteria (24,25). Yatanoside at 1:500 did not

influence the ciliary movement of the frog pharynx and mice bronchus, indicating the absence of inhibition on the cellular protoplasmic movement (7).

8. Toxicity

<Yadanzi> has marked toxic effects. The toxic component resides in the water-soluble bitter substances, whereas the fixed oil has no significant toxicity; the volatile oil could cause local irritation (7,26). Toxic manifestations include nausea, vomiting, diarrhea, bloody stool, gastrointestinal hyperemia and bleeding, liver congestion and fatty degeneration, renal congestion and degeneration, and in severe cases somnolence, convulsion, and death. The MLD of the defatted <Yadanzi> in cats was about 0.1 g/kg PO (26). The LD_{50} of the <Yadanzi> decoction in chicks was determined to be 0.25 g/kg IM or 0.4 g/kg PO. No death occurred after injection of the shell at 2 g/kg IM (15). Long-term medication resulted in cumulative toxicity (6). Apart from gastrointestinal symptoms, the crude extract injection caused shortness of breath, hypothermia, myasthenia, coma, and death (7).

CLINICAL STUDIES

1. Amebic Dysentery

Oral ingestion of the <Yadanzi> kernel, the crushed kernel, and the powder of the defatted kernel, respectively, had therapeutic value in acute or chronic amebic dysentery and in carriers. Better effects could be obtained when the extract was administered orally and as an enema concurrently. Like emetine, it could rapidly control the symptoms, but the radical cure rates as reported by different investigators are very inconsistent (5,8,27). No one has yet reported on its efficacy in extraenteric amebiasis.

2. Malaria

The first report on the use of <Yadanzi> for the treatment of malaria involved 27 cases (10 quartan, 10 tertian and 7 subtertian or malignant). Capsules prepared from 5–15 kernels were given by mouth thrice daily after meals for a course of 5 days. After treatment, 85.2% either suffered no further malarial attacks or at the most had one attack. The blood smears became negative in 25 cases, while 2 cases were still positive for gametocytes (14). Another group of 89 cases were reportedly treated with the herb. Of these, 58 (95.1%) out of 67 cases with tertian malaria were cured; 6 of 13 subtertian cases were cured, as were 7 out of 9 quartan cases. No severa adverse reaction was seen (28).

However, another report claimed that the herb was ineffective in quartan malaria (29); susceptibility to relapse and a high incidence of toxic reactions of up to 78.3% were reported (30).

3. Trichomonas Vaginitis

Eighty-eight percent of the cases treated by local perfusion of the <Yadanzi> decoction registered negative in the test for trichomonas after madication (31).

4. Schistosomiasis

A few patients were treated with <Yadanzi> alone, or in combination with the powder of the peel of *Zanthoxylum bungeanum* fruit. The stool examination for the ova became negative in 100% of these cases; the therapeutic course was, however, rather long (20 or 40 days) (17,32).

5. Cancer

Forty-three advanced cases of squamous carcinoma of the cervix were given intratumor or parauterine injection of <Yadanzi> oil concomitant with the intramascular dose. Short-term remission was achieved in 21 cases, and marked effects in 8 cases. Intratumor injection of the <Yadanzi> oil induced dissolution, necrosis and sloughing of the tumor mass. No relapse or cancer cells were observed in 21 cases with short-term remission, followed-up from 2 to 5 years upwards, whereas in those cases with marked effects, conspicuous degenerated and organized cancer cells enclosed by the surrounding tissues were discovered during operation (33,34). The herb was also effective in esophageal cancer (35).

6. Wart, Papilloma, Corn, and Keloid

Local application of the <Yadanzi> oil was very effective in the treatment of papilloma of the external ear canal (36,37), papilloma of the throat (38), verruca vulgaris, verruca juvenilis, and verruca acuminata (36). But the oil was irritating and destructive to normal tissues. The topically applied crushed kernel was also quite effective on wart lesions (39). It was also useful in the treatment of corns (40) and keloids (41).

ADVERSE EFFECTS

Locally, <Yadanzi> caused strong irritation of the skin and mucous membrane. The oral dosage caused abdominal discomfort, nausea, vomiting, abdominal pain, diarrhea, "bearing down distention", dizziness, and lassitude (8). The incidence of reactions which were usually mild in nature was as high as 78.3% (30). For 200 years no single death has been reported due to poisoning with this herb; only one case of cerebral congestion due to overdosage was known (8). Occasional allergic reactions from external application of the herb have been reported, wherein 20 minutes after medication, dyspnea developed followed by the patient slipping into a semiconscious state. These reactions were reversed after emergency measures (42).

REFERENCE

1. Lee KH et al. Journal of the Chemical Society — Chemical Communications 1977 (2):69.

2. Lee KH et al. Journal of Organic Chemistry 1979 44(13):2180.

3. Li R et al. Chinese Traditional and Herbal Drugs 1980 11(12):530.

4. Xu HX et al. Chinese Traditional and Herbal Drugs 1980 11(12):529.

5. Liu XL. Chinese Medical Journal 1937 52(1):89.

6. Quan CG. Chinese Medical Journal (Shanghai) 1944 63(2):89.

7. Zhang YD. Chinese Medical Journal 1951 37(6):480.

8. Quan CG. Chinese Journal of New Medicine 1951 2(5):358.

9. Utohei K. Journal of the Pharmaceutical Society of Japan (Tokyo) 1943 63(11):579.

10. Geissman TA. Annual Review of Pharmacology 1964 4:305.

11. Lin QS. Chemical Studies on Chinese Traditional Drugs. Science Press. 1977. p. 638.

12. Zhou TC et al. Chinese Medical Journal 1948 66:359.

13. Wang JY et al. Chinese Medical Journal 1950 36(11):469.

14. Zhang SS et al. Acta Pharmaceutica Sinica 1954 2(2):85.

15. Li GC et al. Abstracts of the 1956 Academic Conference of the Academy of Medical Sciences. Vol. 1. 1956. p. 28.

16. Xue AZ et al. Journal of Military Medicine 1958 1:369.

17. Mobile Medical Team of Changshan County Hospital. Notes on Science and Technology — Medicine and Health (Information Institute of Zhejiang Bureau of Science and Technology) 1971 (2):5.

18. Chen ZK et al. Acta Academiae Medicinae Zhejiang 1958 1(2):117.

19. Zhang JZ. Chinese Journal of Dermatology 1965 11(5):328.

20. Li X et al. Chinese Traditional and Herbal Drugs Communications 1979 10(11):14.

21. Kupchan SM et al. Journal of Organic Chemistry 1973 38(1):178.

22. Kupchan SM et al. Cancer Chemotherapy Reports 1962 25:1.

23. You SS et al. Chinese Journal of Physiology 1941 16(1):13.

24. Ding XZ. Peking Natural History Bulletin 1949 17(4):229.

25. Microbiology Department, Shandong Medical College. Acta Academiae Medicinae Shandong 1958 (8):4.

26. Zheng WS et al. Chinese Medical Journal (Chengdu edition) 1944 62A(4):133.

27. Wu ZZ. Chinese Medical Journal (Washington edition) 1943 61(4):337.

28. Foziling Antimalaria Medical Team, Shanghai First Medical College. Yiwu Shenghuo (Medical Life) 1953 (6):10.

29. Zhejiang People's Academy of Health. Second Annual Report of Zhejiang People's Academy of Health. 1951. p. 61.

30. Chen X. Chinese Medical Journal 1959 (9):721.

31. Bao JY. Zhongji Yikan (Intermediate Medical Journal) 1956 (11):6.

32. Yu HM. Shanghai Zhongyiyaoxue Zazhi (Shanghai Journal of Traditional Chinese Medicine) 1957 (12):22.

33. Tumor Group of the Ob-Gyn Department, Western Hospital of Ankang Steel Works. Short-Term Effects of the Chinese Traditional Drug, Oleum Bruceae, in Thirty-three Cases of Uterine Carcinoma (Internal Information). 1976.

34. Li JD. Anshan Yiyao (Anshan Medical Journal) 1978 (2):86.

35. Changwei District Health Bureau. Barefoot Doctor 1970 (2):28.

36. Li BS. Chinese Medical Journal 1950 68(3–4):103.

37. Gao SC. Journal of Traditional Chinese Medicine 1958 (2):112.

38. Li Z. Chinese Journal of Otorhinolaryngology 1959 (3):186.

39. Xia MH. Chinese Journal of Dermatology 1957 (4):360.

40. Zhang ZY. Chinese Medical Journal 1955 (10):966.

41. Li XT. Shanghai Zhongyiyaoxue Zazhi (Shanghai Journal of Traditional Chinese Medicine) 1958 (6):20.

42. Fei XZ. Jilin Yiyao (Jilin Medical Journal) 1976 (1):53.

(Xue Chunsheng)

GOUTENG 鈎藤

<Gouteng> comes from the hook-bearing branch and stem of *Uncaria rhyncophylla* (Miq.) Jackson (Rubiaceae). It is also obtained from other *Uncaria* species such as *U. lancifolia* Hutch., *U. macrophylla* Wall., *U. hirsuta* Havil., *U. sessifructus* Roxb., and U. scandens (Smith) Hutch. It is sweet with a bitter aftertaste and a slightly "cold" property. It has latent-heat-clearing, "pinggan" (hepatic-depressant), sedative, anticonvulsant, muscle-relaxant, antidinic and antiflatulent actions. Thus, the herb is chiefly used in paralysis due to stroke, facial paralysis, general numbness, hemiplegia, abnormal fetal movements, high fever (*with slight chills, dry mouth, yellowish tongue coating, and floating pulse, etc.), vertigo, dizziness, infantile convulsion, and colic.

CHEMICAL COMPOSITION

<Gouteng> contains alkaloids rhynchophylline, isorhynchophylline, corynoxeine, isocorynoxeine, corynantheine, dihydrocorynantheine, hirsutine, and hirsuteine. The root and stem each contains about 0.041% of alkaloids.

PHARMACOLOGY

1. Hypotensive Effect

Whether administered intravenously or intragastrically, the ethanol extract of <Gouteng>, the total alkaloids, and rhynchophylline all elicited a hypotensive response in anesthetized or unanesthetized animals, and in normal or hypertensive animals; they did not produce tachyphylaxis. Injection of the <Gouteng> decoction 2–3 g/kg IV to anesthetized rabbits or 0.05 g/kg to anesthetized dogs lowered the blood pressure by 30–40% of the original level; the action lasted 3–4 hours or longer (1). Intravenous injection of the <Gouteng> decoction 6.25 g/kg, the chloride of the total alkaloids 20 mg/kg, or rhynchophylline hydrochloride 20 g/kg to anesthetized cats produced a triphasic change in the blood pressure: an initial fall followed by quick rise, and then a secondary fall; the changes in the blood pressure during the three phases ranged from 30–70%, 13.9–23.2%, and 11.7–41.7%, respectively; the hypotensive effect was sustained for 3–4 hours (2,3). However, the hypotensive action of the herb was attenuated by prolonged decoction; a decocting time shorter than 20 minutes was deemed appropriate (4). The potency of the ethanol extract 3 g/kg was similar to that of the decoction 2 g/kg (1). In rats with renal hypertension, daily intragastric administration of the <Gouteng> decoction 8 g/kg, the total alkaloids 50 mg/kg, or rhynchophylline 50 mg/kg for 15–20 days resulted in the lowering of blood pressure starting from the third to fifth day, with the lowest level attained between the 7th–15th day; the decrements obtained by these three agents were 16.9, 12, and 18 mmHg, respectively. Blood pressure fell the day rhyncophylline 20 mg/kg IP was administered, and an average reduction of 24 mmHg was obtained after 8 days of medication (2).

However, reports in other countries claimed that the hypotensive action of the ethanol extract of <Gouteng> in rabbits was weak (5). Rhyncophylline produced a sustained pressor effect in rabbits after a brief hypotensive episode (6,7).

The stem and branch (including the tender ones) with or without hooks of *U. macrophylla, U. hirsuta,* and *U. sessifructus* exhibited a hypotensive effect which was weaker than that of *U. rhynchophylla* (8). The hypotensive effect produced by the stem and branch was equipotent to that of the hooks but had a shorter duration; the old branches has a weak and transient effect (9).

1.1 *Mechanism of the hypotensive effect.* The pressor response to the blockade of blood flow of the bilateral common carotid arteries could be inhibited by the decoction and the ethanol extract of the <Gouteng> to different extents. These agents did not modify the actions of pituitrin, epinephrine, norepinephrine, acetylcholine, and nicotine on the blood pressure. Bilateral vagotomy, or vagal blockade with local anesthetics weakened the hypotensive effect, whereas atropine or atropine plus subdiaphragmatic vagotomy had no effect on it. These findings suggest the association of the hypotensive effect with the function of the afferent fibers of thoracic vagal nerves.

These <Gouteng> preparations were inactive when perfused into isolated rabbit auricular vessels, but caused vasodilation of isolated rabbit ears with intact nerves. Therefore, their hypotensive action is intimately related to the inhibition of the vasomotor center (1,2). Also, some investigators were able to prove that the <Gouteng> preparations could lower the blood pressure of hypertensive animals with bilaterally sectioned depressor nerves and sinus nerves, thus suggesting a direct inhibitory action on the vasomotor center. On the other hand, when the blood pressure of animals with bilaterally sectioned carotid vagal nerves and depressor nerves was lowered by administration of the decoction or ethanol extract of <Gouteng>, sectioning of the sinus nerves elevated the blood pressure. Procaine blockade of the cardiovascular receptors weakened the hypotensive effect. Thus, the hypotensive action of the <Gouteng> decoction and ethanol extract relates to the sinus nerve and receptors at various sites.

Based on these findings it is postulated that the hypotensive action of the decoction and ethanol extract of <Gouteng> was consequent to direct and indirect inhibition of the vasomotor center, causing peripheral vasodilation and lowering of peripheral resistance (1). Rhynchophylline shares the same action mechanism with these preparations: it inhibited the pressor reflex triggered by bilateral blockade of the common carotid artery but did not significantly modify the hypotensive action of acetylcholine. It inhibited or interrupted hypotension due to electrical stimulation of the efferent vagal nerve, but was incapable of antagonizing the pressor response to epinephrine, norepinephrine, and amphetamine. Paradoxically, it greatly reinforced the pressor response to epinephrine and norepinephrine. Also, it caused vasodilation of the isolated rabbit ear (2), implying a direct action on the peripheral blood vessels.

Therefore, apart from the inhibition of the vasomotor center, of the transmitter release from nerve ganglions and nerve endings, and of intravascular baroreceptors, another contributing factor in the drop of blood pressure is direct peripheral vasodilation (1,2).

2. Sedative and Anticonvulsant Effects

Injection of the decoction or the ethanol extract of <Gouteng> to albino mice at 0.1 g/kg IP inhibited the spontaneous activity of the animals for 3–4 hours and also antagonized caffeine-induced hyperactivity. However, no potentiation of the hypnotic effect of pentobarbital sodium was observed even after increasing the dosage of the agents by 25 times (2.5 g/kg), but delayed the death of the animals by high dosage of pentobarbital sodium. Further increasing the dosage to 50 to 100 times the initial dose (5–10 g/kg) still failed to abolish the righting reflex of the animals (1).

The decoction of the hooks and stems of *U. rhyncophylla* at 1 g/kg IP decreased the cerebral cortical excitability and weakened the integration of impulses in rats. In some rabbits, it delayed the positive conditioned reflexes. However, it had no significant effect on the inhibition of differentiation and on non-conditioned reflexes (10).

The ethanol extract of <Gouteng> at 2 g/kg SC in guinea pigs with experimental epilepsy had prophylactic and therapeutic effects; it suppressed epileptic attacks, though these recurred 3 days after discontinuation of the drug. The extract also prevented sudden death in guinea pigs caused by clipping the hair at the epileptic focus (11).

A paper reported that injection of the <Gouteng> decoction 40 g/kg IP to albino mice did not antagonize convulsions induced by pentylenetetrazole, caffeine, or strychnine. However, the ethanol extract of the genuine <Gouteng> was proved in another experiment to antagonize pentylenetetrazole-induced convulsions, and the <Gouteng> injection was shown to antagonize convulsions caused by electrical shock. Therefore, it is imperative to carry out active investigation in order to elucidate the presumed anticonvulsant action as well as the active principle of the herb (8).

3. Effect on Smooth Muscles

The <Gouteng> decoction at 17 mg/ml briefly decreased the tone of the isolated ileum and concurrently caused a rapid increase in the contraction amplitude. It also exhibited antihistaminic action, but no antinicotinic and antiserotonergic actions (8). Rhynchophylline inhibited the isolated rabbit intestinal tract and stimulated the isolated rat uterus (6,7). *In vivo* antihistamine test on guinea pigs revealed that a single injection of the <Gouteng> decoction 2–4 g/kg IP had a spasmolytic effect. Whether *in vitro* or *in vivo*, larger doses were required to obtain a marked effect, as well as to increase the contraction amplitude of the normal intestinal muscle. Therefore, the herb has no clinical value; these results simply indicate a direct action on the smooth muscle fibers (8).

4. Miscellaneous Actions

Experiments proved that rhynchophylline inhibited the heart of frogs and rabbits *in vivo* and *in vitro*, and that it inhibited respiration and caused miosis in mice (6,7).

5. Toxicity

The LD_{50} of the <Gouteng> decoction in mice was determined to be 26.1±4.3 g/kg IP (8), or 29.0±0.8 g/kg IP (1), and that of the decoction of the young branches was 35.2±5.4 g/kg (8). The LD_{50} of the chloride of the total alkaloids in mice were 514.6±29.1 mg/kg PO and 144.2±3.1 mg/kg IP (2). The LD_{50} of rhynchophylline in mice were 162.3 mg/kg IP (2) and 165 mg/kg SC (6,7).

Administration of the <Gouteng> decoction to rabbits at 5 g/kg PO twice daily for 50 days did not result in any significant toxic symptoms. The chloride of the total alkaloids administered to young rats at 50 mg/kg PO (the therapeutic dose) once daily did not produce pathological changes in the internal organs as shown by autopsy after 14 days. Doubling the dose elicited only minimal inflammatory changes in the liver which were quickly reversed after discontinuation of the drug; on other alterations were found (2,4). In experiments weaned rats were orally given 50–100 mg/kg/day of the chloride of the total alkaloids for 2 months. Postmedication observations carried out over one month revealed that low dosage (50 mg/kg) did not initiate significant modifications in the growth, development, hepatic and renal functions, and blood picture, with the exception of some mild trophic disorders of the kidneys on pathological examination, whereas high dosage (100 mg/kg) was fatal to the animals. Marked pathological changes were observed in the heart, liver, and kidneys of the dead animals (2,4).

CLINICAL STUDIES

<Gouteng> if often effectively used in traditional prescriptions, and in combination with other herbs in the management of hypertension. The known prescriptions include "Tianma Gouteng Yin" (Ganoderma-Uncaria Decoction), "Lingyang Gouteng Tang" (Saiga-Uncaria Decoction), etc. The total alkaloids of <Gouteng> has therapeutic value in hypertension: 245 cases of hypertension were treated with the tablet preparation at 60 mg (20–40 mg per tablet) thrice daily (for adults); a total of 77.2% of the cases showed a decrease in blood pressure and marked effects were achieved by 38.2%. The drug was most effective in hypertension of the "yin deficiency and yang hyperactivity" type. It caused remission of headache, insomnia, palpitation, tinnitus, constipation, and numbness of the extremities. Its action was stable and prolonged, and side effects mild (12).

REFERENCE

1. Yuan WX et al. Acta Pharmacologica Sinica 1962 25(6):162.

2. Tianjin Institute for Drug Control and Tianjin Institute of Materia Medica. Chinese Traditional and Herbal Drugs Communications 1974 (4):8.

3. Zhang TX et al. National Medical Journal of China 1978 58(7)408.

4. Guo XX. Shanghai Zhongyiyao Zazhi (Shanghai Journal of Traditional Chinese Medicine) 1959 (1):46.

5. Tsurumi S. Folia Pharmacologica Japonica 1958 54:124.

6. Katsusuke U. Chemical Abstracts 1962 56:1222Td.

7. Usui S. Folia Pharmacologica Japonica 1959 55(4):123.

8. Fan YJ et al. Information on Medical Sciences and Technology (Guangxi Institute of Medical and Pharmaceutical Sciences) 1975 (1):19.

9. Peng H et al. Chinese Pharmaceutical Bulletin 1965 11(12):563.

10. Che XP et al. Acta Academiae Medicinae Xi' an 1965 (7):44.

11. Kuang AK. Chinese Medical Journal 1958 44(6):582.

12. Editorial Group. Chinese Traditional and Herbal Drugs Communications 1976 (7):45.

(Du Deji)

XIANGFU 香附

<Xiangfu>, also known as <Xiangfuzi>, is the tuber obtained from *Cyperus rotundus* L. (Cyperaceae). Pungent, slightly bitter and "mild", it is credited with vital-energy-regulative (or carminative), menstruation-corrective and analgesic actions. This herb is, therefore, used in the treatment of digestive disorders due to the depressed vital energy of the liver, retention of phlegm and fluid, chest and costal pain, irregular menstruation, dysmemorrhea, and for various ailments during the perinatal period. It is the chief drug used in various affections of the vital energy, and an important remedy for gynecological diseases.

In India, the herb is a folk remedy used for fever, dysentery, urticaria, pain, vomiting and various hematological diseases (1), it is also prescribed for irregular menstruation (2).

CHEMICAL COMPOSITION

<Xiangfu> contains 0.3–1% of volatile oil, the content of which varies with the source. The volatile oil produced in China contains cyperene and patchoulenone, whereas that produced in Japan contains cyperol, cyperene, α-cyperone, cyperotundone and cyperolone. Cyperene is not a pure substance, it consists of cyperene I and cyperene II; both are terpenes. This herb also contains alkaloids, cardiac glycosides, and flavonoids (3).

PHARMACOLOGY

1. Estrogenic Effect

The volatile oil of <Xiangfu> has a mild estrogenic activity in ovariectomized rats; subcutaneous injection of 0.2 ml every 6 hours resulted in complete keratinization of the vaginal epithelium 48 hours later; three doses of 0.3 ml each precipitated the appearance of many white blood cells among a large number of keratinized cells. The appearance of white blood cells was probably due to stimulation by the volatile oil. Of the isolated constituents of the volatile oil, cyperene I was the most potent though it was not comparable to the volatile oil itself. The volatile oil, cyperene I, and cyperolene administered intravaginally caused epithelial keratinization, whereas cyperol and cyperene II did not. The effective systemic dose did not exceed the doubled local dose. These constituents are believed to be proestrogenic compounds which exhibit high bioactivity after biotransformation. This estrogenic effect is considered to be one of the important bases for the use of <Xiangfu> in the treatment of irregular menstruation (2).

2. Effect on the Uterus

The 5% <Xiangfu> fluidextract was inhibitory to the isolated uteri of pregnant or nonpregnant guinea pigs, cats, and dogs; it decreased the contractility and tension. Its action was similar in nature to that of angelicone, but weaker (4).

3. Anti-inflammatory Effect

Significant inhibition of carrageenin- and formaldehyde-induced paw swelling in rats was achieved with the use of the ethanol extract of <Xiangfu> at 100 mg/kg IP. The effect was found to be more pronounced than that achieved with 5–10 mg/kg of hydrocortisone (1). The anti-inflammatory constituents were determined to be triterpenes, one of which was IV-B. Its inhibitory effect on carrageenin-induced paw swelling was 8 times stronger than that of hydrocortisone, and its safety range 4 times wider. It also inhibited formaldehyde-induced paw swelling. The efficacy ratio of the intragastric and intraperitoneal dose was 1:3, indicating partial absorption from the gastrointestinal tract (5).

4. Antipyretic and Analgesic Effects

Subcutaneous injection of the 20% ethanol extract of <Xiangfu> markedly elevated the pain threshold in mice (6). The analgesic effect of triterpene IV-B at 5 mg/kg was equal to that of acetylsalicylic acid at 30 mg/kg (5). Antipyresis was achieved with the <Xiangfu> ethanol extract administered to rats with fever due to injection of yeast. Its efficacy was found to be 6 times that of sodium salicylate (1). The active antipyretic principles were also triterpenes (5).

5. Central Effect

The ethanol extract of <Xiangfu> has a tranquilizing action in mice: it decreased spontaneous activity, inhibited passive activity due to cage transfer, and enhanced the anesthetic effect of phenobarbital. It also abolished the conditioned avoidance of rats. The extract prevented emesis induced by anhydrous morphine. It afforded no protection to mice against convulsions elicited by electric shock and pentylenetetrazole (1).

6. Effect on the Cardiovascular System

Systolic cardiac arrest in frogs was triggered by subcutaneous injection of the aqueous, or water-alcohol extract of <Xiangfu>. At lower concentrations, the extracts exerted cardiotonic and bradycardic effect on the isolated frog heart and the frog, rabbit and cat hearts *in situ*. These effects, as well as a significant hypotensive effect, were also observed with the aqueous solution of the total alkaloids, glycosides, flavonoids, and phenolic compounds (7). Injection of the ethanol extract of the herb to anesthetized dogs at 20 mg/kg IV caused a progressive fall in the blood pressure for 0.5–1 hour. This extract did not modify the action of epinephrine and acetylcholine on the blood pressure, but it partially blocked the response to histamine (1).

7. Effect on the Intestines and Bronchi

The ethanol extract, at the concentration of 20 μg/ml, directly inhibited the isolated ileal smooth muscle of rabbits. It protected guinea pigs from bronchospasm induced by histamine spray (1).

8. Antibacterial Effect

In vitro studies showed that the <Xiangfu> oil inhibited *Staphylococcus aureus*; it was inactive against other bacteria. The bacteriostatic actions of cyperenes I and II were stronger than that of the volatile oil itself. In addition, they were active against *Shigella sonnei*, and hydrogenation did not modify their efficacy. On the other hand, cyperolone was completely inactive (8). The herb extract was also inhibitory on some fungi (9).

9. Toxicity

<Xiangfu> has a low toxic profile. Rats tolerated feed containing less than 25% of this herb, but their growth inhibited by feed containing 30–50% of the herb (10). The acute LD_{50} of the ethanol extract of the herb in mice was about 1500 mg/kg IP (1). The LD_{50} in mice of triterpene IV-B, which has the most pronounced anti-inflammatory effect, was 50 mg/kg IP (5).

CLINICAL STUDIES

1. Irregular Menstruation and Dysmenorrhea

The decoction of <Xiangfu> 6–9 g, alone or in combination with the root of *Angelica sinensis* and the leaves of *Artemisia argyi*, may be taken. It can regulate menstruation and stop bleeding (2,11).

2. Gastritis of the "Gold" Stasis and Vital-Energy Stagnation Type, and Gastric Spasm

Rhizoma Cyperi 120 g and Rhizoma Alpiniae Officinarum 90 g ("Liang Fu Wan", Apinia-Cyperus Pill, from the medical treatise "Liangfang Jiye"), were ground to fine powder. Dosage: 3 g once every morning. An 80% effective rate was achieved in 30 cases (12).

3. Intolerable Epigastric and Abdominal Pain (Except Acute Inflammation)

<Xiangfu> is usually prescribed with the leaf of *Artemisia argyi* (13).

4. Fever, Diarrhea, and Other Gastrointestinal Disorders

The extract or decoction of adequate amounts of <Xiangfu> may be taken by mouth (2).

5. Filariasis

Five cases were treated with a decoction of fresh <Xiangfu> 30–60 g in two doses, one to be taken in the morning, and the other, in the evening. Fever, acute lymphadenitis and lymphangitis were controlled (14). No blood smears were carried out in these cases.

ADVERSE EFFECTS

Rare. According to the experience of Chinese herbalists, caution should be exercised when using this herb in patients with deficiency of "yin" and weakness of the vital energy.

REFERENCE

1. Singh N et al. Indian Journal of Medical Research 1970 58(1):103.
2. Indira M et al. J Sci Indust Res 1956 15C:202.
3. Akperbekova BA. Farmatsiia 1967 16(3):36.
4. Zhang FC et al. The National Medical Journal of China 1935 12:1351.
5. Gupta MB. Indian Journal of Medical Research 1971 59:76.
6. Deng SZ et al. Acta Academiae Medicinae Guiyang (National Day Commemorative Papers) 1959:113.
7. Akperbekova BA. Chemical Abstracts 1966 65:20702d.
8. Radomir S et al. Cur Sci 1956 25:118.
9. Meguro M et al. Chemical Abstracts 1972 76:95653w.
10. Wu JYP et al. American Journal of Pharmacy 1952 124:48.
11. Chengdu College of Traditional Chinese Medicine (editor). Lectures on Chinese Traditional Pharmacy. 1961. p. 225.
12. Luda Health Bureau. Applications of Chinese Traditional Prescriptions. 1976. p. 101.
13. Zhu Y. Pharmacology and Applications of Chinese Medicinal Materials. People's Medical Publishing House. 1958. p. 239.
14. Ye XQ. Zhejiang Zhongyiyao (Zhejiang Journal of Traditional Chinese Medicine) 1958 (12):30.

(Xue Chunsheng)

DUHUO 獨活

<Duhuo> is derived from the root and rhizome of the following plants of the families Umbelliferae and Araliaceae: *Angelica pubescens* Maxim. f. *biserrata* Shan et Yuan, *A. pubescens* Maxim., *A. dahurica* (Fisch. ex Hoffm.) Benth. et Hook. f. ex Franch et Sav., *A. prophyrocaulis* Nakai et Kitag., *Heracleum hemsleyanum* Diels, *H. lanatum* Michx., and *Aralia cordata* Thunb. There are a few other species from the genera *Angelica, Heracleum* and *Aralia* that are also used as sources of <Duhuo> is some localities in China.

<Duhuo> has a pungent, bitter taste and a "warm" property. It is reputed to be antirheumatic, "cold"-discutient and analgesic. It is chiefly used in the treatment of rheumatism, heaviness of the low-back and knee, and contracture of limbs.

CHEMICAL COMPOSITION

The chemical composition varies with the genera and species from which the herb is obtained.

The root of *A. pubescens* contains angelol, angelicone (glabralactone), bergapten, osthol, umbelliferone, scopoletin, angelic acid, tiglic acid, palmitic acid, flavonoids, and small amounts of volatile oil.

The root of *A. dahurica* contains byak-angelicin, byak-angelicol, oxypeucedanin, imperatorin, isoimperatorin, phellopterin, isobyakangelicol, neobyakangelicol, scopoletin, alloisoimperatorin, angelicotoxin, xanthotoxin, marmesin, and 5-methoxy-8-hydroxypsoralen.

The root of *H. lanatum* contains furanocoumarins angelicin, pimpinellin, bergapten, xanthotoxin, sphondin, isopimpinellin, and isobergapten.

The root of *A. cordata* contains alkaloids volatile oil and diterpene carboxylic acids, 1-kaur-16-en-19-oic acid, 16, 17-dihydroxy-16-β-1-kauran-19-oic acid, 1-pimara-8(14), 15-dien-19-oic acid, 7-keto-1-pimara-8(14), 15-dien-19-oic acid, 7 α-hydroxy-1-pimara-8(14), 15-dien-19-oic acid, 7 β-hydroxy-1-pimara-8(14), 15-dien-19-oic acid, and 1-pimara-8(14), 15-dien-19-ol.

PHARMACOLOGY

1. Analgesic, Sedative, and Anti-inflammatory Effects

In the plate experiment with mice, injection of the <Duhuo> decoction 2 g/kg IP markedly prolonged the reaction time of the animals to pain, indicating a strong analgesic effect. Analgesia was also achieved with "Duhuo Jisheng Tang" (Decoction of A. pubescens-V. coloratum). Sedation and hypnosis were achieved with the fluidextract and the <Duhuo> decoction, and "Duhuo Jisheng Tang" intragastrically or intraperitoneally administered to mice or rats. Subcutaneous injection of the <Duhuo> extract to frogs prevented convulsion due to strychnine, but not death associated with the latter. Intragastric administration of "Duhuo Jisheng Tang" inhibited formaldehyde-induced paw swelling, reducing the inflammation and making the subsidence of swelling rapid (1,2).

2. Effects on the Cardiovascular System and Respiration

Intravenous injection of the tincture or decoction of <Duhuo> to anesthetized dogs produced a significant hypotensive effect of short duration; the tincture had a more pronounced effect than the decoction. Bilateral vagotomy did not modify the hypotensive effect but atropine could either partially or completely block it.

<Duhuo> also markedly depressed the isolated frog heart; cardiac arrest was precipitated by high dosage (2).

Perfusion of the <Duhuo> decoction into the frog hind limb vessels caused vasoconstriction dose-dependently (1). Byak-angelicin, isopimpinellin, and 5-methoxy-8-hydroxypsoralen had coronary dilatory action similar to but weaker than that of khellin. The potency of these agents was rated follows: isopimpinellin > byak-angelicin > 5-methoxy-8-hydroxypsoralen (3,4). The aminoethyl derivatives of angelicin had adrenergic blocking effect (5).

Intravenous injection of the <Duhuo> extract stimulated respiration, making it deeper and faster; the action was not weakened by procaine blockade of the vascular chemoreceptors (2).

3. Spasmolytic Effect

Bergapten, xanthotoxin, isopimpinellin, and alloisoimperatorin exerted a significant spasmolytic action on the rabbit ileum. Isopimpinellin, pimpinellin, and angelicin conspicuously antagonized barium chloride-induced spasm of the rat duodenal segment (6,7). Scopoletin relieved estrogen- or barium chloride-induced spasm of the rat uterus *in vivo* or *in vitro*, the ED_{50} was 0.09 mg/kg (8).

4. Photosensitivity

The furanocoumarins bergapten, xanthotoxin, and alloisoimperatorin were found to be "photoactive substances" (9). Once inside the body, they could cause dermatitis solaris with resultant reddening, swelling, pigmentation, and even thickening of the epidermis of the sites exposed to sunlight or ultraviolet rays (10). Enteral use of <Duhuo> also caused dermatitis solaris. Of the psoralen derivatives, xanthotoxin produced the most pronounced phototoxicity followed in descending order by bergapten and alloisoimperatorin, whereas isopimpinellin and the others were devoid of such activity (11). If the photosensitizing activity of psoralen were to be rated as 100, then that of xanthotoxin would be 71, and bergapten, 61 (12). Photosensitizing activity could be useful in the treatment of vitiligo. Patients treated with the photosensitizing substances such as psoralen and xanthotoxin showed increases in skin pigmentation (13) as well as in cutaneous RNA and DNA

(14). Daily administration of 0.01 mg of psoralen to toads for 60 days resulted in increases in cutaneous and hepatic melanin, and tyrosinase activity (15). Xanthotoxin also increased plasma copper in patients with vitiligo, and in rats (16).

5. Antibacterial Effect

Escherichia coli, Shigella dysenteriae, Proteus vulgaris, Salmonella typhi, Pseudomonas aeruginosa, Vibrio cholerae, and *Mycobacterium tuberculosis* var. *hominis* were found to be susceptible to the decoction of *A. dahurica* (17,18). The MIC of the <Duhuo> decoction against *Mycobacterium tuberculosis in vitro* was determined to be 1:100 (19). The MIC of xanthotoxin against *Mycobacterium tuberculosis* var. *hominis* $H_{37}RV$ was 100 µg/ml (20). Umbelliferone was a potent inhibitor of *Brucella* organisms, the MIC being 1:2500 (21,22). The furanocoumarins such as xanthotoxin generally had no significant antibacterial activity; however, when exposed to light together with *Staphylococcus aureus*, and *Escherichia coli*, they produced a photosensitizing effect which killed the bacteria (23–25).

6. Miscellaneous Actions

The furanocoumarins have an anti-gastric ulcer action. Experiments with rats showed that bergapten and pimpinellin afforded reasonable protection against experimental gastric ulcer, whereas isopimpinellin and xanthotoxin were weak (26). Breast cancer in rats caused by chemicals was apparently inhibited by scopoletin; in contrast, umbelliferone was ineffective (27). Xanthotoxin and bergapten were lethal to Ehrlich ascites carcinoma cells (28). In addition, <Duhuo> contracted the isolated abdominal straight muscle of frogs (2).

7. Toxicity

The LD_{50} of xanthotoxin in rats was 160 mg/kg IM, that of isoimperatorin 335 mg/kg, and bergapten 945 mg/kg (29). Angelicin or imperatorin administered to young rats at a dose of 2.5 mg/75 kg for 60 days did not markedly affect the growth of the animals, but caused liver damage (30). Xanthotoxin at 400 mg/kg killed guinea pigs, in which adrenal hemorrhage was observed; at doses of 200–300 mg/kg it caused cloudy swelling, fatty degeneration, and acute hemorrhagic necrosis of the liver, severe renal congestion, and hematuria. Administration of 1–2 mg/kg to young rats for 5 months caused necrosis of the liver. Imperatorin was less toxic, its lethal dose being 800 mg/kg; the 600-mg dose caused fatty degeneration and necrosis of the liver but caused no fatality (31).

Another report claimed that the stimulation of the spinal cord and medulla centers-vasomotor, respiratory and vagal — by small doses of angelicotoxin caused elevation of the blood pressure, slowing of the pulse, deep respiration, salivation, and emesis. Large doses caused tonic-clonic convulsions followed by general paralysis (32).

CLINICAL STUDIES

1. Rheumatic Syndrome

<Duhuo> is often used in compound formulae to treat rheumatic syndrome due to "wind, cold, and damp pathogenic factors". A representative prescription is "Duhuo Jisheng Tang" (Decoction of A. pubescens-V. coloratum). A volatile oil injection prepared from the plant *Heracleum lanatum* Michx. was used in 112 cases of soft tissue damage with a marked effective rate of 76.5%; pain was markedly reduced, swelling subsided, and functions recovered (33).

2. Vitiligo

Along with phototherapy, xanthotoxin 20 mg (adult) may be given by mouth once daily. This agent can also be applied locally to the skin (34).

3. Chronic Bronchitis

Antitussive and antiasthmatic effects were achieved in 422 cases treated with the <Duhuo> decoction; 6.9% had marked effects while 66.8% showed some response (35).

ADVERSE EFFECTS

Numbness of the tongue, nausea, vomiting, and gastric discomfort occurred during treatment of bronchitis with the herb (35).

REFERENCE

1. Feng GH. Jiangxi Yiyao (Jiangxi Medical Journal) 1961 (6):26.

2. Zheng YL et al. Acta Academiae Medicinae Shandong 1957 (1):43.

3. Yakugaku Kenkyu 1958 29:824.

4. Valenti P et al. Chemical Abstracts 1980 92:22410k.

5. Montanari P et al. Chemical Abstracts 1980 92:22411m.

6. Novak I et al. Planta Medica 1965 13(2):226.

7. Khadzhai YI et al. Farmakologiia I Toksikologiia 1966 29(2):156.

8. Jarboe CH et al. Journal of Medicinal Chemistry 1967 10(3):488.

9. Watt JM. Medicinal and Poisonous Plants of Southern and Eastern Africa. 2nd edition. 1962. p. 920.

10. Fowlks WL. Journal of Investigative Dermatology 1959 32:233.

11. Khadzhai YI et al. Chemical Abstracts 1966 64:41255.

12. Caporale G et al. Experientia 1967 23(12):985.

13. Becker SW. Science 1958 127:878.

14. Abidov MM. Chemical Abstracts 1966 64:13275h.

15. Chakraborty DP et al. Chemical Abstracts 1961 55:15734c.

16. El-Mofty AM. Chemical Abstracts 1962 56:13436h; 1964 61:15111d.

17. Liu KS et al. Chinese Medical Journal 1950 68:307.

18. Wang Y et al. Acta Botanica Sinica 1953 2(2):312.

19. Liaoning Hospital of Tuberculosis. Liaoning Medical Journal 1960 (7):29.

20. Rodghiero G. Chemical Abstracts 1957 51:10736a.

21. Greib E et al. Chemical Abstracts 1954 48:10999a.

22. Duquenois P. Chemical Abstracts 1957 51:2115b.

23. Oginsky E et al. Journal of Bacteriology 1959 78:821.

24. Fowlks WL et al. Nature 1958 181:571.

25. Dadak V et al. Experientia 1966 22(1):38.

26. Khadzhai YI et al. Chemical Abstracts 1965 63:7530h.

27. Wattenberg LM et al. Cancer Research 1979 39(5):1651.

28. Musajo L et al. Experientia 1967 23(5):335.

29. Sherif MAF et al. Chemical Abstracts 1961 55:22588h.

30. Mukherrji A. Chemical Abstracts 1961 55:5773h.

31. Anwar MF. Chemical Abstracts 1951 45:4362a.

32. Zhu Y. Pharmacology and Applications of Chinese Medicinal Materials. People's Medical Publishing House. 1958. p. 116.

33. Orthopedics Department, Xining First People's Hospital. Qinghai Yiyao (Qinghai Medical Journal) 1979 (1−2):64.

34. Goodman LS et al. The Pharmacological Basis of Therapeutics. 4th edition. 1971. p. 996.

35. Wuhan Fourth Hospital. Wuhan Journal of New Traditional Chinese Medicine 1971 (3):24.

(Deng Wenlong)

JIXINGZI 急性子

<Jixingzi> refers to the seed of *Impatiens balsamina* L. (Balsaminaceae). It has a bitter and pungent taste and a "warm" property; it is slightly toxic. <Jixingzi> is a hemostasis discutient and digestant and has a softening effect on hard masses ("ruanjian"). It is, therefore, used to treat amenorrhea, lump or obstruction in the abdomen, sensation of obstruction in the esophagus, and choking caused by inadvertent swallowing of bones.

CHEMICAL COMPOSITION

<Jixingzi> contains saponins and fixed oil. The oil contains balsaminasterol, parinaric acid, volatile oil, quericetin, kaempferol derivatives, and naphthaquinones.

PHARMACOLOGY

1. Effect on the Uterus

The <Jixingzi> syrup had a prominent stimulant effect on isolated mice uteri; similarly, the decoction, tincture, and aqueous extract of the herb caused stimulation of the isolated uteri of nonpregnant rabbits and those of pregnant or nonpregnant guinea pigs. These preparations increased the frequency of contraction and enhanced the tone of the uterus, to the extent of producing tonic contraction. Injection of the aqueous extract to anesthetized rabbits at 0.05–0.3 g/kg IV or IM also produced excitation of the uterus (1,2).

2. Antifertility Effect

When male and female mice, dosed for 10 days with the <Jixingzi> decoction 3 g/kg, were caged together on the 5th day of medication and dissected after 35 days, a contraceptive rate of 100% was found achieved. This effect is probably related to the suppression of ovulation, and to atrophy of the uterus and ovaries (3). An anti-implantation rate of 33% was obtained with the decoction at a dose of 80 g/kg (4), and a rate of 65% with the 65% ethanol extract at 40 g/kg (5). However, exceedingly small doses, for instance, the water-ethanol extract at 0.5–1.0 g(crude drug)/mouse (about 0.02–0.04 g/kg), or the mixture of ethanol and ether extracts at 0.36 g(crude drug)/mouse (about 0.014 g/kg), were devoid of anti-implantation and anti-early pregnancy actions (5). Another paper reported that administration of the aqueous extract of the herb 3 g/kg PO thrice at hourly intervals to pregnant guinea pigs produced neither abortion nor toxicity (2).

3. Miscellaneous Actions

The aqueous extract or tincture of <Jixingzi> inhibited the isolated rabbit intestine (2).

CLINICAL STUDIES

1. Contraception, Induction of Menstruation, and Termination of Pregnancy.

Pills were made from <Jixingzi>, the seed of *Areca catechu*, the plant *Campsis grandiflora*, and the stem and leaf of *Eupatorium fortunei*, ground to find powder and mixed with honey. Dosage: Orally 20 g twice daily, morning (on an empty stomach) and evening (after meals) to be taken for 10 days. The contraceptive rate in 160 cases was 68.2%; however, if medication was started on the third day of menstruation, the contraceptive rate could be increased to 80%, and if started on the second postpartum day, a 62.5% contraceptive rate was achieved (6). One paper reported the induction of menstruation and termination of pregnancy by the following recipe: <Jixingzi>, *Mylabris phalerata*, the kernel *of Prunus persica*, the flower of *Carthamus tinctorius*, the tuber of *Sparganium stoloniferum*, the rhizome of *Curcuma zedoaria, Anoplophora chinensis, Hirudo nipponica, Eupolyphaga sinensis*, twigs of *Cinnamomum cassia*, the root and rhizome of *Rheum palmatum*, and the flower of *Campsis grandiflora*. Six of 14 treated cases had uterine hemorrhage, menstruation or tissue expulsion, whereas the other 8 cases were unresponsive (7).

2. Cancer of the Upper Digestive Tract and Other Malignant Tumors

Thirty cases of esophageal cancer and 26 cases of gastric cancer, treated with a pill prepared from <Jixingzi> and honey, obtained symptomatic improvements particularly in dysphagia; some effects were also obtained in respect of vomiting, and pain of the thorax and epigastrium (8). The compound tablet "Diai Pian" (Anticancer Tablet) composed of this herb and other herbal medicines was beneficial to various malignant tumors such as nasopharyngeal cancer, hepatoma, cancer of the rectum, tongue and breast, and leukemia (9).

ADVERSE EFFECTS

Some patients developed xerostomia, nausea, and anorexia after prolonged use of this herb, but these ill effects usually disappeared after reduction of the dosage or discontinuation of medication for 2-3 days (8).

REFERENCE

1. Shanghai First Medical College et al. Screening of Chinese Traditional Contraceptives. 1971.

2. Xia BN et al. Acta Academiae Medicinae Guiyang 1958 1(1):29.

3. Gao YD et al. Abstracts of the Symposium of the Chinese Society of Physiology (Pharmacology). 1964. p. 69.

4. Contraceptive Group, Sichuan Institute of Chinese Materia Medica. Studies on the anti-implantation and anti-early pregnancy actions of the seed of Impatiens balsamina. 1978.

5. Reference Materials on Contraceptive Drug Research (Action Unit of the Shanghai Supervisory Group on Contraceptive Drug Research) 1975 (4):141, 151.

6. Reference Materials on Contraceptive Drug Research (Action Unit of the Shanghai Supervisory Group on Contraceptive Drug Research) 1975 (4):51.

7. Reference Materials on Contraceptive Drug Research (Action Unit of the Shanghai Supervisory Group on Contraceptive Drug Research) 1975 (4):115.

8. Huang YR et al. Scientific Research Information on Traditional Chinese Medicine (Fujian Institute of Traditional Chinese Medicine et al.) 1963 (5):10.

9. Foshan (Guangdong) Hospital of Traditional Chinese Medicine. National Exhibition of Chinese Traditional Drugs and New Therapeutic Methods. 1971. p. 406.

(Chen Zizhang)

YANGJINHUA 洋金花

<Yangjinhua> refers to the flower of *Datura metel* L. and *D. innoxia* Mill. (Solanaceae). Also known as <Mantuoluohua> or <Jiuzuihua>, it has a pungent taste, a "warm" property, and is toxic. <Yangjinhua> is noted for its antiasthmatic, antirheumatic, anesthetic and analgesic effects. Hence, it is employed in asthma, convulsion or epilepsy induced by fright, and in rheumatism. It is also used as an anesthetic in surgery. The "Ben Cao Gang Mu" (Compendium of Materia Medica) records that "Three qian of <Yangjinhua> mixed with warm wine is enough to make one tipsy so that when given to a person before a boil operation or moxibustion it makes him oblivious to the pain".

CHEMICAL COMPOSITION

<Yangjinhua> contains 0.3−0.43% of alkaloids, about 85% is scopolamine and 15% is hyoscyamine and atropine. The proportion of scopolamine to hyoscyamine varies tremendously with the growing location and season of harvest, anywhere from 3:1 to 18:1 (1). A crystalline methyl compound was isolated from the soluble alkaloids of <Yangjinhua>; it has a relaxant effect on striated muscles (2).

PHARMACOLOGY

Atropine and scopolamine contained in the herb are muscarinic receptor blockers with extensive pharmacological actions.

1. Effect on the Central Nervous System

1.1 *Behavioural Effects.* In persons receiving intramuscular injection or intravenous infusion of the total alkaloids of <Yangjinhua>, dizziness, heaviness of the eyelids, uncommunicativeness, weakness of the extremities, unsteady gait, and drowsiness developed, followed by euphoretic manifestations, such as a wide stare, head raising, and delirium, then an anesthetized condition (1,3−5).

Oral administration of scopolamine at a dose of 0.65 mg in man resulted in decreased mental activity, while 20 mg caused amnesia, and 45 mg initiated hallucination, amnesia, and disorientation. Coma was precipitated by the intramuscular dose of 5−50 mg. Scopolomine also prolonged the anesthetic effect of ether and barbiturates (6,7). Injection of scopolamine at 6 mg/kg to the lateral ventricle of rabbits made the animals close their eyes, lie on their side, and lose their righting reflex, but they recovered after about 40 minutes of reduced activity (8). The combined use of scopolamine and "Dongmian Heji" (Hibernation Mixture) in man, monkeys, and dogs produced general anesthesia (9,10). Combined with meprobamate or pentobarbital, scopolamine also significantly reduced the activity of mice, indicating synergism with central depressants. However, a paper reported that: small doses of scopolamine (0.1–0.2 mg/kg) increased the spontaneous activity of mice; at 4 mg/kg IP it enhanced the actions of central stimulants (amphetamine, methamphetamine and caffeine), increasing the animals' activity, and the drug offset the decremental effect of reserpine and chlorpromazine on activity. These findings show that it has central stimulant effect. Consequently, it is believed that the central action of scopolamine is dual (11).

1.2 *Effect on the EEG.*   In conscious cats with implanted electrodes, five minutes after injection of scopolamine hydrobromide 0.05–0.1 mg/kg IP low-amplitude fast waves on the EEG were transformed into irregular high-amplitude slow waves. Despite their quietness, the animals' arousal reaction was intact. Increasing the dosage to 0.25–0.5 mg/kg produced highly synchronized and irregular high-amplitude slow waves on the EEG, abolished the arousal reaction of the animals and made them excited and manic (12). The EEG responses of monkeys, dogs, rabbits and rats to scopolamine were very similar. The drug blocked the arousal reaction to various physiological stimuli (7,8,13). During intravenous anesthesia in man with the <Yangjinhua> total alkaloids or scopolamine, combined with the muscle relaxant carbachol, the EEG revealed: prompt suppression of the alpha wave and appearance of low-amplitude beta waves; appearance of theta waves after 1–2 minutes; and gradual emergence of a complex pattern primarily composed of slow waves with predominant theta waves after about 15 minutes. During the whole period of anesthesia, the EEG pattern was characterized by these irregular theta waves with low to medium amplitudes. These EEG features of Chinese herbal anesthetics were rather specific in that they were unmodified by stimulation due to operation. After administration of the analeptic physostigmine, quite regular alpha waves usually emerged within 4 minutes along with the disappearance of slow waves. Compared with the EEG before anesthesia, the patterns 1–4 hours after arousal still consisted of less regular alpha waves with lower amplitudes, interpersed with a few theta waves. Clinically, the patients were under sedation yet they were able to answer questions directly and correctly. The EEG changes were essentially consistent with the clinical and pharmacological effects, indicating that physostigmine was able to abolish the EEG-desynchronizing effect of scopolamine (14). On the other hand, desynchronization by physostigmine could also be antagonized by scopolamine (7,8,15).

1.3 *Effect on conditioned reflexes.*   Injection of scopolamine 0.05–100 mg/kg SC to rats blocked the conditioned avoidance reflex and the secondary conditioned reflex to different extents; the extent of blockage paralleled the dosage (16). During inhibition of the conditioned avoidance in rats, the effect of scopolamine on the secondary conditioned reflex and the conditioned reflexes was particularly strong, whereas that of atropine was weaker (12).

1.4 *Effect on pain perception.*   The potassium method in rabbits and the hot plate method in mice proved that scopolamine could produce analgesia and enhance the analgesic action of pethidine. The lowering of the pain threshold and the attenuation of pethidine analgesia by intra-lateral ventricular injection of norepinephrine could be antagonized by scopolamine (17). The pain threshold of mice to radiant heat was increased by 54.7% fifteen minutes after intraperitoneal injection of the total alkaloids of <Yangjinhua> 0.2 mg per animal (18). However, a paper reported that scopolamine displayed antagonism to the central analgesic action of tremorine, and that its action was stronger than that of atropine (12).

1.5 *Interaction with neurotransmitters.* Perfusion of scopolamine 1:100,000 to the lateral ventricle of the cat brain increased the release of acetylcholine, but no further increases were achieved after addition of 1 mg/kg by intravenous injection during perfusion (19). On the other hand, intraperitoneal injection of scopolamine 0.63 mg/kg to rats caused a 31% reduction in the cerebral acetylcholine; the action peaked 60 minutes after medication and disappeared in 120 minutes (20,21). These findings suggest that administration through routes other than the lateral ventricle also facilitated acetylcholine release, thereby decreasing the level of cerebral acetylcholine. The mechanism of the decremental effect of scopolamine on the cerebral acetylcholine is not quite clear. This could have been triggered by blockade of the postsynaptic muscarinic receptors, leading to an increase in the compensatory physiological release of acetylcholine from the central cholinergic nerve endings, or it could have been due to blockade of presynaptic cholinergic receptors, relieving the cholinergic nerve endings of negative feedback, consequently, accelerating the release of acetylcholine from the central cholinergic nerve terminals (22,23).

Intravenous injection of reserpine 0.5–1.0 mg/kg or intracerebroventricular injection of p-chlorophenylalanine (PCPA) 5.0 mg/animal to rabbits prolonged anesthesia produced by lateral ventricular injection of scopolamine 2–3 mg/kg. Intracerebroventricular injection of serotonin 250 μg/animal and intravenous injection of pargyline 50 mg/kg significantly shortened the anesthestic period of scopolamine, whereas intracerebroventricular injection of norepinephrine 200 μg/animal had no such effect (24).

In conclusion, scopolamine primarily depressed some sites of the cerebral cortex and subcortical region, causing symptoms such as loss of consciousness and anesthesia. These effects are believed to be causally related to the blocked of muscarinic receptors in the cerebral cortex and in the reticular formation of the brain stem, and probably to its antagonism to the central norepinephrine (8,25). However, scopolamine initiated stimulant effects in different degrees on the medulla oblongata and spinal cord, particularly the medullary respiratory center (5). Thus, scopolamine increased the respiratory rate in conscious dogs and cancelled the respiratory depressant effect of drugs that induce artificial hibernation (pethidine and chlorpromazine) (26).

2. Effect on the Circulatory System

2.1 *Heart.* Scopolamine relieved vagal inhibition of the heart, producing predominant sympathetic effects, manifested in the increase in the heart rate which depended on the extent of vagal control on the heart. The action of scopolamine was most pronounced in young and robust persons with strong vagal control, in whom the heart rate could reach 120–160 beats/minute after onset of anesthesia with Chinese herbs and could gradually stabilize at 100 beats/minute after 15 minutes. To preclude this undesirable effect, propranolol was used as a premedication. On the other hand, scopolamine had no significant effect on the heart rate of old persons (5,27–30). A similar but stronger action was achieved with atropine (31). In normal rabbits and anesthetized dogs, intravenous injection of atropine 2–4 mg/kg, or scopolamine 4 mg/kg antagonized arrhythmia (atrial or ventricular premature beat, ventricular tachycardia, etc.) induced by epinephrine or norepinephrine 50 μg/kg, but not the accompanying tachycardia (32,33). The antiarrhythmia mechanism is not yet clear. It is postulated that large doses of atropine and scopolamine can also produce quinidine-like effects on the myocardium (4). But, atropine and its congeners, in excessive doses, could also induce arrhythmia; for instance, it was reported that the incidence of arrhythmia was increased with the use of atropine and scopolamine during fluothane and cyclopropane anesthesia (6,34). After intravenous injection of the total alkaloids of <Yangjinhua> or scopolamine, patients' EEG showed sinus tachycardia, ST depression and flat T waves in some, and in rare cases T wave inversion, These might be due to prolonged tachycardia and increased cardiac load. However, these aberrant patterns recovered successively (1).

2.2 *Blood vessels.* Scopolamine 20 mg perfused into the blood vessel of isolated rabbit ears antagonized the vasoconstricting effect of norepinephrine 20 μg/0.1 ml, but scopolamine was much weaker than atropine (32). During clinical initiation of Chinese herbal anesthesia, vasodilation occurred, evidenced by the widening of the amplitude of the finger pulse, flushing, hot and dry skin, and excellent blood flow in the nail bed occurred (35). Hemodromogram of the lower extremities in 36 cases receiving Chinese anesthetics revealed 33 cases with a mean increase of 5.9% in the constriction amplitude (36). Meanwhile, the effect of scopolamine on terminal circulation depended upon the functional state, i.e., the amplitude of finger pulses may be wide, large or small, and the skin temperature may be decreased or elevated (37).

2.3 *Hemodynamics.* In dogs with hemorrhagic shock, intravenous injection of the total alkaloids of <Yangjinhua> did not increase the cardiac output unless the blood volume was first replenished by transfusions. Hence, the effect of the herb on cardiac output was dependent on the blood volume (4,38). Clinically, scopolamine was observed to further lower the stroke volume by about 15% on top of the 25% reduction by prior administration of Artificial Hibernation Mixture (Chlorpromazine, etc.). However, cardiac output was not greatly changed because of the marked increase in the heart rate (39).

Injection of scopolamine 10–20 mg/kg IV to anesthetized rabbits antagonized the pressor response to epinephrine or norepinephrine 5 μg/kg, but the action was weaker than that of atropine because the dosage used was 2.5–5.0 times greater (32). Furthermore, when using Chinese anesthetics such as <Yangjinhua> during operations on patients in the prone position, the blood pressure should be carefully monitored for changes in order to preclude accidents (40). However, other investigators believe that the effect of scopolamine on the blood pressure is minimal, as the dose of 20 mg/kg IV was found to decrease the blood pressure of rats by a mean of 10 ± 2.5 mmHg only, and the drug was shown to antagonize acetylcholine-induced hypotension (32). Experiments also showed that scopolamine improved the microcirculation in dogs with blood loss (4,38,41); this action was confirmed in clinical trials (36,37).

3. Effects on the Respiratory System and Smooth Muscles

3.1 *Respiratory system.* Low dosage of <Yangjinhua> injection completely antagonized acetylcholine-induced contraction of the isolated bronchial smooth muscle of guinea pigs, while only high dosage antagonized contraction induced by histamine (42). The herb inhibited the bronchial mucous glands of rats with experimental bronchitis, significantly reducing the number of cup-shaped cells; the action resembled that achieved by unilateral vagotomy (43). Clinically, scopolamine was able to dilate the bronchi and inhibit the respiratory tract glandular secretion, resulting in xerostomia which is essential for good ventilation during anesthesia using Chinese traditional drugs (5). Marked anoxia, carbon dioxide accumulation, and P_{CO_2} increase were not observed during the anesthesia induction period or operation. Oxygen saturation before and after the operation was improved, and the acid-base equilibrum stabilized (44,45).

3.2 *Smooth muscles.* Scopolamine decreased gastrointestinal peristalsis and tone; it blocked the cholinergic nerves, relaxed the detrusor muscle, and constricted the sphincter of the urinary tract, thus causing urinary retention (5).

4. Effect on Body Temperature

During anesthesia with the total alkaloids of <Yangjinhua> or scopolamine, peripheral vasodilation and higher skin temperature relative to preanesthetic reading occurred. However, the body temperature in most cases went down by 1 to $3°C$, and in a very few cases, by 4 to $5°C$. Not a single case has elevated body temperature. These events are attributed to peripheral vasodilation and increased heat dissipation (46). Nevertheless, the body temperature rose again $2-6$ hours after operation, usually to $37.8-38.5°C$; in exceptional cases, it rose to 39 and $39.1°C$. Hence, the development of hyperpyrexia should always be watched during anesthesia using Chinese traditional drugs (47). Some workers, however, reported that Chinese anesthetics have very little influence on the body temperature, and that anesthesia could be initiated during the hot summer season in Hainan Island, even in patients with fever (48,49).

5. Effect on Cholinesterase Activity

In psychotic patients, the effect of <Yangjinhua> anesthesia on the blood cholinesterase activity the following morning was related to the route of administration. The mean cholinesterase level was markedly elevated by the intravenous injection, in contrast to the inconspicuous effect of the intramuscular dose (50). Three hours after the induction of anesthesia with 10 mg of the total alkaloids in psychotic patients, 3 or 4 mg of physostigmine gave the best analeptic effect. At this time the depletion of the blood cholinesterase activity was most conspicuous. However, there were no significant changes in the blood electrolytes (Na^+, K^+, Cl^-, Ca^{++}) in the course of anesthesia (50).

6. Pharmacokinetics

The intragastrically administered ^3H-scopolamine appeared in the plasma of rats 15 minutes after administration. In rats with ligated common bile duct, the ^3H-scopolamine solution injection into the intestine disappeared rapidly and completely; the highest drug concentration was found in the kidneys, the next highest in the liver (51). Following intravenous injection of ^3H-scopolamine to rats, the highest concentration was found in the lungs, followed by the kidneys, liver, stomach, intestine, heart, brain, testes, plasma, and fat. The mean drug concentration in the brain 30 minutes after the intravenous dose was estimated to be about 3 times that in plasma. The corpora striata, cerebral cortex, and hippocampi showed high concentrations, followed by the septal area; the diencephalon, the inferior brain stem and cerebellum had lower concentrations. The pharmacodynamics of ^3H-scopolamine fitted into a two-compartment model (51). The amount of radioactivity excreted in the urine of rats 48 hours after the ^3H-scopolamine injection accounted for 62% of the administered dose; 12% was in the original form. While most of the dose was excreted within 8 hours, about one-half the total dose was disposed of during the first hour. The 48-h biliary excretion represented 25% of the administered dose, indicating considerable reabsorption by the intestine. The amount of radioactivity excreted in the urine and feces accounted for 87% of the original dose, indicating a rather complete disposal. Within one hour of the intravenous injection, the amount of the original drug recovered in the urine, feces or bile represented only one-fifth to one-fourth of the radioactivity excreted, suggesting rapid and extensive metabolism of the drug (51). Experiments with incubated isolated tissues indicated that the metabolism of scopolamine in rats was primarily carried out by the liver which has a very high metabolic activity. The extent of the metabolism of scopolamine varied greatly in different species; it was extensive in rabbits, poor in cats, and least in dogs (51).

7. Toxicity

The LD_{50} of the <Yangjinhua> injection in mice was 8.2 mg/kg IV (42). The MLD of the total alkaloids of the herb was about 75–80 mg/kg IV; three days after a single injection of 2.5 mg/kg IV to dogs, no significant changes in the morphology of 13 important organs were found, relative to the control (9). According to available statistics, the MLD of scopolamine in adults was about 100 mg and in young children about 10 mg. The anesthetic dose of scopolamine did not depress the respiratory and circulatory centers or impair the hepatic and renal functions in the course of anesthesia (5).

CLINICAL STUDIES

1. Anesthesia

<Yangjinhua> can be used as the chief agent in combination with chlorpromazine and pethidine in intravenous compound anesthesia. Since the anesthetic principle of <Yangjinhua> is scopolamine (52), scopolamine hydrobromide is now used in lieu of the total alkaloids in anesthetic procedures employing Chinese traditional drugs (53,54). This kind of compound anesthesia was found to be applicable to patients of different ages (55) and in various major and medium operations. It was also suitable in oral and faciomaxillary operations (56–58), osteoarthritic operations (59), pediatric surgery (60–63), and gynecological and obstetrical operations (64,65). The drug has also been successfully used in visual intracardiac surgery with extracorporeal circulation (66–68), in severe arrhythmia (69), and in cranial and brain surgery (70–72). It has been used as an anesthetic in emergency operations in earthquake and war (73,74). Incomplete statistics reporting hundreds of thousands of surgical operations using Chinese anesthetics were published in many medical journals such as "Zhongma Tongxun" (Communications on Chinese Traditional Anesthesia) between 1974 and 1978. There is general agreement that Chinese anesthetics have certain advantages: consistent results, wide applicability, relative safety, portability and easy storage. Another merit of Chinese anesthetics, absent in all other anesthetics, is their anti-shock effect during anesthesia in patients with surgical shock (55,75). However, Chinese anesthetics have certain drawbacks such as shallow anesthetic effect, incomplete muscle relaxation, and acceleration of the heart rate. Complications such as psychotic symptoms, elevation of body temperature, visual disturbances, superficial nodules, and bleeding from operation wounds in some patients have been reported (76–79).

Apart from intravenous infusion of the total alkaloids 0.08–0.1 mg/kg or scopolamine hydrobromide 0.06–0.1 mg/kg, other routes of administration including oral, rectal, intramuscular, acupoint injection (ear and nose acupoints), and earlobe non-acupoint injection may also be used to obtain similar anesthetic effects (80–82).

Chinese anesthetics are contraindicated in patients with glaucoma, and should be used with caution in patients with tachycardia, cardiopulmonary insufficiency, severe hepatic and renal damage, and hyperpyrexia (4). Owing to the prolonged effect of the Chinese anesthetics, slow intravenous injection of physostigmine 2–4 mg may sometimes be necessary to arouse the patient (83–86), or the more effective and less toxic "Cuixingning" may be used intravenously instead (71).

2. Psychosis

Forty-eight cases of psychosis were treated with the total alkaloids or the 0.5% scopolamine hydrobromide injection intramuscularly once on alternate days thrice weekly for a total of 5–17 times. Marked therapeutic effects were obtained in 22 cases, amelioration in 16 cases and no effect in 10 cases (87). Another paper (88) reported that very unstable therapeutic effects were achieved in 86 cases of psychosis (divided into three groups) treated with <Yangjinhua> preparations combined with chlorpromazine and other tranquilizers. Other investigators (4,89) reported that 204 cases were effectively treated with intramuscular <Yangjinhua> and small doses of chlorpromazine; better results were obtained in manic patients. The herb could reduce the dose of chlorpromazine, side effects, and accidental complications. The mechanism of action in psychotic diseases has not been clarified yet. It is postulated that the action is probably linked with regulation of the dynamic equilibrium of acetylcholine in the CNS.

3. Intractable Pain

The <Yangjinhua> preparations had optimal effects in cases of severe pain in advanced malignancy refractory to pethidine, morphine, or fentanyl. *Dosage and administration*: Scopolamine 2 mg plus Artificial Hibernation Mixture No. 4, one-fourth the usual dose, to be given by a bolus intravenous injection; or scopolamine 2 mg intramuscularly or combined with chlorpromazine 12.5–25 mg once daily or once every 2–3 days (3).

4. Shock

Atropine and scopolamine have been employed with satisfactory therapeutic results during the last 10 years to treat shock due to infection and toxin (3,90–93). Chinese anesthetics were effective in shock patients requiring operation, saving many critical patients (94–101). The anti-shock mechanisms of <Yangjinhua> can be summarized as follows: (1) Relief of vasospasm due to the liberation of large quantities of catecholamines during shock, thus improving microcirculation and increasing blood flow into the vital organs. (2) Increase in minute stroke volume of the heart. (3) Improvement of renal function. (4) Stimulation of the respiratory hydrobromide *Dosage and administration*: Atropine 0.03–0.05 mg/kg or scopolamine hydrobromide 0.01–0.02 mg/kg may be given by intravenous injection every 10–30 minutes until the face is flushed, the extremities are warm, the blood pressure has increased, and the pupils are dilated (3,4).

5. Thromboangiitis Obliterans

Ten cases of third-degree angiitis were treated with scopolamine 1–3 mg IM or IV, or the total alkaloids 5 mg for anesthesia, in combination with chlorpromazine 12.5–50 mg. Some patients received, in addition, tetrandrine 60 mg, and when necessary, analeptics. Analgesia was achieved in all 10 cases receiving 60 doses of the Chinese anesthetic. The effect was better in mild and moderate pain; however, severe pain could also be relieved by the medication. Pain was abated for two days usually after one medication; gradual remission or disappearance of pain depended on the number of treatments (102).

6. Chronic Bronchitis

The <Yangjinhua> injection was highly efficacious in over 900 cases of chronic bronchitis; the clinical control rate was over 70%. However, the incidence of side effects, particularly of psychotic symptoms, was up to 55%. In over 600 cases of chronic bronchitis treated with various preparations of <Yangjinhua> (injection, liquor, tablet, herb cigarette, and suppository) where the dose of <Yangjinhua> was maintained at approximately 0.01 mg/kg, the psychotic side effects were significantly reduced, achieving a clinical control rate of 50–60% (103). Another paper reported on 114 cases of chronic bronchitis treated with the <Yangjinhua> tablet 0.01 mg/kg once daily at bed time for 5 courses (10 days per course). Amelioration to various degrees, recovery or near normalization of various symptoms and laboratory results compared with the pretreatment condition were achieved; the clinical control rate was 63% (104).

7. Miscellaneous

Satisfactory effects were obtained in 86 children with pneumonia given scopolamine as adjuvant. This agent could stimulate the respiratory center, depress the cerebral cortex and relieve spasm; the drug had a high specificity for pneumonia in children. It was markedly effective during the acute stage of the various types of disease, improving microcirculation of the lungs, heart, and brain (105). Resuscitation efforts in two cases of meningococcal septicemia treated with scopolamine were reported to be successful (106).

ADVERSE EFFECTS

The effects of the oral and the parenteral administration of <Yangjinhua> in psychotic patients are nausea and vomiting. In one patient gastric bleeding was discovered, and in another, dyspnea due to laryngeal spasm. In 47 cases, indications of myocardial damage of various degrees appeared on the ECG of 4 cases (107). Chinese anesthetics given with fentanyl and ketamine, or with carbachol precipitated sudden cardiac arrest; one case for each drug combination was reported (108,109). Also, circulatory collapse occurred in one case receiving the analeptic "Cuixingning" (106). One patient with hepatoma developed postoperative phlebitis of the extremities and abdominal wall following hepatic lobectomy under Chinese anesthetics (110).

REFERENCE

1. Teaching Hospital of Xuzhou Medical College. Chinese Traditional Anesthetics. People's Medical Publishing House. 1971.

2. Teaching Hospital of Xuzhou Medical College. Zhongma Tongxun (Communications on Chinese Traditional Anesthesia) 1976 (2):56.

3. Xuzhou Medical College. Clinical Uses of and Discussions on Chinese Traditional Anesthetics. Shanghai People's Medical Publishing House. 1973.

4. Bian CP. Zhongma Tongxun (Communications on Chinese Traditional Anesthesia) 1977 (4):58.

5. Internship Department, Guangzhou Military Medical College. Compiled Information 1977 (11):80.

6. Eger EIJ. Anesthesiology 1962 23(3):365.

7. Longo VG. Pharmacology 1966 18(2):965.

8. Pharmacology Department. Xuzhou Medical College. Xinyiyaoxue Zazhi (Journal of Traditional Chinese Medicine) 1976 (1):27.

9. Chinese Traditional Anesthesia Research Unit, Xuzhou Medical College. Xinyiyaoxue Zazhi (Journal of Traditional Chinese Medicine) 1974 (11):44.

10. Anesthesia Unit, Teaching Hospital of Nantong Medical College. Zhongma Tongxun (Communications on Chinese Traditional Anesthesia) 1974 (1):33.

11. Niu XY et al. Acta Physiologica Sinica 1965 28(1):50.

12. Neuropharmacology Section, Institute of Chinese Materia Medica of the Chinese Academy of Medical Sciences. Zhongma Tongxun (Communications on Chinese Traditional Anesthesia) 1975 (4):10.

13. Zhang CS et al. Progress in Pharmacology. Shanghai Sci-Tech Literature Publishing House. 1962. p. 141.

14. Chinese Traditional Anesthesia Unit, Shanghai Second Hospital of Tuberculosis. Zhongma Tongxun (Communications on Chinese Traditional Anesthesia) 1975 (4):14.

15. Shanghai Coordinating Research Group on Chinese Traditional Anesthesia. Zhongma Tongxun (Communications on Chinese Traditional Anesthesia) 1974 (1):52.

16. Niu XY et al. Acta Physiologica Sinica 1965 28(1):42.

17. Bian CP et al. Zhongma Tongxun (Communications on Chinese Traditional Anesthesia) 1978 (3–4):6.

18. Jin GZ. Zhongma Tongxun (Communications on Chinese Traditional Anesthesia) 1975 (2):41.

19. Polak RL. Journal of Pharmacology 1965 (181):317.

20. Giaman NJ et al. British Journal of Pharmacology 1962 (19):226.

21. Giaman NJ et al. British Journal of Pharmacology 1964 (23):123.

22. Pepeu G. Progress in Neurobiology 1973 2(3):259.

23. Zou G. Medical References 1974 (10):404.

24. Sun JN et al. Zhongma Tongxun (Communications on Chinese Traditional Anesthesia) 1978 (2):1.

25. White RP et al. Journal of Pharmacology 1959 (125):239.

26. New Chinese Medicine Department, Shanghai Second Medical College. Zhongma Tongxun (Communications on Chinese Traditional Anesthesia) 1978 (3-4):1.

27. Chinese Traditional Anesthesia Group, Hospital of Zhengzhou Textile Factory. Zhongma Tongxun (Communications on Chinese Traditional Anesthesia) 1976 (2):24.

28. Chinese Traditional Anesthesia Unit, Rugao County People's Hospital. Zhongma Tongxun (Communications on Chinese Traditional Anesthesia) 1974 (1):68.

29. Chinese Traditional Anesthesia Unit, Rugao County People's Hospital. Zhongma Tongxun (Communications on Chinese Traditional Anesthesia) 1976 (2):41.

30. Chinese Traditional Anesthesia Unit, Rugao County People's Hospital. Zhongma Tongxun (Communications on Chinese Traditional Anesthesia) 1976 (4):29.

31. Goodman LS et al. The Pharmacological Basis of Therapeutics. 4th edition. New York: 1971. p. 528.

32. Pharmacology Department, Xuzhou Medical College. Chinese Medical Journal 1976 56(11):697.

33. Jiang WD et al. Acta Physiologica Sinica 1963 26(2):172.

34. Averill KH et al. American Journal of Medical Sciences 1959 237:304.

35. Anesthesia Department, Friendship Hospital of Beijing. Zhongma Tongxun (Communications on Chinese Traditional Anesthesia) 1976 (3):6.

36. Operating Room, 234th Hospital of the Chinese PLA. Zhongma Tongxun (Communications on Chinese Traditional Anesthesia) 1978 (2):24.

37. Zhou ZD et al. Zhongma Tongxun (Communications on Chinese Traditional Anesthesia) 1978 (1):13.

38. Xuzhou Medical College. New Medical Information 1973 (3):14.

39. Shen YT et al. Zhongma Tongxun (Communications on Chinese Traditional Anesthesia) 1978 (2):5.

40. Da YT et al. Zhongma Tongxun (Communications on Chinese Traditional Anesthesia) 1978 (3-4):60.

41. Chinese Traditional Anesthesia Research Unit, Xuzhou Medical College. Zhongma Tongxun (Communications on Chinese Traditional Anesthesia) 1976 (3):1.

42. Pharmacology Department, Baotou Medical School. Baotou Yixue (Baotou Medical Journal) 1977 (4):61.

43. Norman Bethune Hospital for International Peace. Information on Combined Western and Traditional Chinese Medicine 1975 (14):4.

44. Medical Laboratory and Anesthesia Department, First Teaching Hospital of Zhongshan Medical College. Zhongma Tongxun (Communications on Chinese Traditional Anesthesia) 1978 (3-4):38.

45. Zhang J et al. Zhongma Tongxun (Communications on Chinese Traditional Anesthesia) 1978 (3-4): 46.

46. Staff Hospital of Dadun Coal Mine (Shanghai). Zhongma Tongxun (Communications on Chinese Traditional Anesthesia) 1977 (4):38.

47. Xuzhou First People's Hospital. Zhongma Tongxun (Communications on Chinese Traditional Anesthesia) 1978 (1):21.

48. 26th Hospital of the Chinese PLA. Zhongma Tongxun (Communications on Chinese Traditional Anesthesia) 1978 (2):43.

49. Anesthesia Department, Hospital of Nongken Seaport (Hainan, Guangdong). Zhongma Tongxun (Communications on Chinese Traditional Anesthesia) 1978 (1):19.

50. Shanghai Psychiatric Hospital. Zhongma Tongxun (Communications on Chinese Traditional Anesthesia) 1974 (1):94.

51. Yue TL et al. Zhongma Tongxun (Communications on Chinese Traditional Anesthesia) 1977 (4):1.

52. Proceedings of the National Symposium on Chinese Traditional Anesthetics. 1976. p. 268.

53. Xuzhou Coordinating Research Group on Chinese Traditional Anesthesia. Zhongma Tongxun (Communications on Chinese Traditional Anesthesia) 1975 (1):10.

54. Friendship Hospital of Beijing. Zhongma Tongxun (Communications on Chinese Traditional Anesthesia) 1974 (1):5.

55. 'General anesthesia successfully induced by traditional medicine in China'. In: Report on the National Seminar on Chinese Traditional Anesthesia. People's Daily October 8, 1974.

56. Ningbo Second Hospital. Zhongma Tongxun (Communications on Chinese Traditional Anesthesia) 1975 (1):20.

57. You LF et al. Zhongma Tongxun (Communications on Chinese Traditional Anesthesia) 1976 (4):27.

58. Mandibulomaxillofacial Surgery Department, Teaching Hospital of Beijing Medical College. Zhongma Tongxun (Communications on Chinese Traditional Anesthesia) 1976 (1):55.

59. Chinese Traditional Anesthesia Unit, Second Teaching Hospital of Xi'an Medical College. Zhongma Tongxun (Communications on Chinese Traditional Anesthesia) 1976 (1):52.

60. 222nd Hospital of the Chinese PLA. Zhongma Tongxun (Communications on Chinese Traditional Anesthesia) 1975 (2):63.

61. Anesthesia Department, Xinhua Teaching Hospital of Shanghai Second Medical College. Zhongma Tongxun (Communications on Chinese Traditional Anesthesia) 1976 (1):32.

62. Anesthesia Unit, Children's Hospital of Nanjing. Zhongma Tongxun (Communications on Chinese Traditional Anesthesia) 1976 (1):44.

63. Surgery Department, Xinhua County (Guangdong) People's Hospital. Zhongma Tongxun (Communications on Chinese Traditional Anesthesia) 1976 (4):33.

64. Taixing (Jiangsu) People's Hospital. Zhongma Tongxun (Communications on Chinese Traditional Anesthesia) 1974 (1):48.

65. Yang LJ et al. Zhongma Tongxun (Communications on Chinese Traditional Anesthesia) 1975 (1):14.

66. Ruijin Teaching Hospital, Shanghai Second Medical College. Zhongma Tongxun (Communications on Chinese Traditional Anesthesia) 1976 (1):19.

67. Anesthesia Department, Fuwai Teaching Hospital of the Chinese Academy of Medical Sciences. Zhongma Tongxun (Communications on Chinese Traditional Anesthesia) 1976 (1):24.

68. Anesthesia Department, Second Teaching Hospital of Jiangxi Medical College. Zhongma Tongxun (Communications on Chinese Traditional Anesthesia) 1976 (1):29.

69. Anesthesia Department, Xinhua Teaching Hospital of Shanghai Second Medical College. Zhongma Tongxun (Communications on Chinese Traditional Anesthesia) 1976 (1):69.

70. Anesthesia Department, Liaodun Teaching Hospital of Shenyang Medical College. Zhongma Tongxun (Communications on Chinese Traditional Anesthesia) 1976 (4):24.

71. Anesthesia Department, General Hospital of the Chinese PLA. Zhongma Tongxun (Communications on Chinese Traditional Anesthesia) 1978 (1):23.

72. Anesthesia Department, General Hospital of the Chinese PLA. Zhongma Tongxun (Communications on Chinese Traditional Anesthesia) 1978 (2):10.

73. 353rd Hospital of Shenyang Military Region of the Chinese PLA. Zhongma Tongxun (Communications on Chinese Traditional Anesthesia) 1976 (1):18.

74. Anesthesia Department, 59th Hospital of the Chinese PLA. Zhongma Tongxun (Communications on Chinese Traditional Anesthesia) 1976 (1):15.

75. National Seminar on Chinese Traditional Anesthetics. Zhongma Tongxun (Communications on Chinese Traditional Anesthesia) 1976 (1):4.

76. Chinese Traditional Anesthesia Unit, Teaching Hospital of Xuzhou Medical College. Zhongma Tongxun (Communications on Chinese Traditional Anesthesia) 1974 (4):48.

77. Anesthesia Department, First Teaching Hospital of Yunnan Medical College. Zhongma Tongxun (Communications on Chinese Traditional Anesthesia) 1976 (3):42.

78. Anesthesia Unit, Zhuang Autonomous Region (Guangxi) People's Hospital. Zhongma Tongxun (Communications on Chinese Traditional Anesthesia) 1976 (2):39.

79. Chinese Traditional Anesthesia Group, Suzhou Third People's Hospital. Zhongma Tongxun (Communications on Chinese Traditional Anesthesia) 1976 (2):37.

80. Chinese Traditional Anesthesia Group, Teaching Hospital of Qinghai Medical College. Zhongma Tongxun (Communications on Chinese Traditional Anesthesia) 1974 (3):40.

81. Operating Room, Yinxian (Zhejiang) People's Hospital. Zhongma Tongxun (Communications on Chinese Traditional Anesthesia) 1975 (3):39.

82. Wenling County (Zhejiang) People's Hospital. Zhongma Tongxun (Communications on Chinese Traditional Anesthesia) 1975 (3):49.

83. Xinyang District (Henan) People's Hospital. Zhongma Tongxun (Communications on Chinese Traditional Anesthesia) 1974 (1):63.

84. Tianjin Region (Hebei) People's Hospital. Zhongma Tongxun (Communications on Chinese Traditional Anesthesia) 1974 (1):66.

85. Chinese Traditional Anesthesia Group, Teaching Hospital of Qinghai Medical College. Zhongma Tongxun (Communications on Chinese Traditional Anesthesia) 1974 (2):63.

86. Shanghai Coordinating Research Group on Chinese Traditional Anesthetics. Zhongma Tongxun (Communications on Chinese Traditional Anesthesia) 1974 (1):52.

87. Neuropsychiatry Department, 102nd Hospital of the Chinese PLA. Zhongma Tongxun (Communications on Chinese Traditional Anesthesia) 1974 (1):81.

88. Shanghai Psychiatric Hospital. Zhongma Tongxun (Communications on Chinese Traditional Anesthesia) 1974 (1):88.

89. 215th Hospital of the Chinese PLA. Zhongma Tongxun (Communications on Chinese Traditional Anesthesia) 1976 (3):30.

90. Qian C et al. Chinese Journal of Paediatrics 1964 13(5):363.

91. Zhu SH. Chinese Journal of Internal Medicine 1966 14(1):19.

92. Ma YX et al. Acta Academiae Medicinae Wuhan 1965 2(4):218.

93. Ouyang XM et al. Chinese Journal of Paediatrics 1975 14(1):7.

94. Ningbo District (Zhejiang) Coordinating Group on Chinese Traditional Anesthesia. Zhongma Tongxun (Communications on Chinese Traditional Anesthesia) 1974 (2):1.

95. Chinese Traditional Anesthesia Coordinating Research Unit, Xuzhou Medical College. Zhongma Tongxun (Communications on Chinese Traditional Anesthesia) 1974 (2):9.

96. Chinese Traditional Anesthesia Unit, Hongqiao District (Tianjin) First Hospital. Zhongma Tongxun (Communications on Chinese Traditional Anesthesia) 1974 (2):18.

97. Daxing County People's Hospital. Zhongma Tongxun (Communications on Chinese Traditional Anesthesia) 1974 (2):20.

98. Anesthesia Department, Xinhua Teaching Hospital of Shanghai Second Medical College. Zhongma Tongxun (Communications on Chinese Traditional Anesthesia) 1974 (4):26.

99. Yudong (Henan) Coordinating Group on Chinese Traditional Anesthesia. Zhongma Tongxun (Communications on Chinese Traditional Anesthesia) 1975 (1):23.

100. Xiangshan County (Zhejiang) People's Hospital. Zhongma Tongxun (Communications on Chinese Traditional Anesthesia) 1975 (1):42.

101. Taizhou District People's Hospital. Zhongma Tongxun (Communications on Chinese Traditional Anesthesia) 1975 (3):46.

102. Vasculitis Group, Ruijin Teaching Hospital of Shanghai Second Medical College. Zhongma Tongxun (Communications on Chinese Traditional Anesthesia) 1974 (1):103.

103. General Hospital of the Chinese PLA. Medical Information 1975 (9):1.

104. General Hospital of the Chinese PLA. Medical Information 1975 (9):10.

105. Xu XW et al. Zhongma Tongxun (Communications on Chinese Traditional Anesthesia) 1976 (3):33.

106. Internal Medicine Department, Linhai County (Zhejiang) Second People's Hospital. Zhongma Tongxun (Communications on Chinese Traditional Anesthesia) 1976 (3):35.

107. Han WB. Zhongma Tongxun (Communications on Chinese Traditional Anesthesia) 1978 (3–4):72.

108. Zhang TH. Zhongma Tongxun (Communications on Chinese Traditional Anesthesia) 1978 (2):67.

109. Zhang YJ et al. Zhongma Tongxun (Communications on Chinese Traditional Anesthesia) 1977 (4):34.

110. Anesthesia Group of the Operating Room, 255th Hospital of the Chinese PLA. Zhongma Tongxun (Communications on Chinese Traditional Anesthesia) 1978 (3–4):73.

(Bao Dingyuan)

QIANHU 前胡

<Qianhu> is the root of *Peucedanum praeruptorum* Dunn, or *P. decursivum* Maxim. (Umbelliferae). Bitter, pungent and slightly "cold", it is credited with latent-heat-clearing, antipyretic, antitussive and mucolytic actions. It is, therefore, chiefly used in the treatment of cough with thick sputum and dyspnea, upper respiratory infections (*with fever, chest pain, yellow viscous sputum, etc.), and nonproductive cough.

CHEMICAL COMPOSITION

The root of *P. praeruptorum* contains volatile oil and peucedanins A, B, C and D (seselin derivatives).

The root of *P. decursivum* contains volatile oil, nodakenin, nodakenetin (marmesin), decursidin, and umbelliferone. The volatile oil mainly contains estragol and limonene.

Peucordin, a furanocoumarin, was recently isolated from *P. arenarium* (1).

PHARMACOLOGY

1. Expectorant Effect

In studies where secretions from the respiratory tract of anesthetized cats were collected, oral administration of 1 g/kg of the <Qianhu> decoction produced a prolonged expectorant effect demonstrated by the increase in respiratory tract secretion (2). In cats with cough induced by intrapleural injection of 1–1.5 ml of 1% iodine, no significant antitussive effect was demonstrated after 0.8–2.0 g/kg PO of the decoction (3).

2. Antibacterial Effect

Blood coagulation tests on the allantoic fluid obtained from the allantois of the chicken embryo, inoculated with the 1:1 herb decoction and the Asian influenza virus type A and incubated for 72 hours, showed that the herb inhibited the said virus (4).
Umbelliferone and marmesin were shown to have antibacterial and antifungal actions (5).

3. Coronary Dilatory Effect

Peucedanin C increased the coronary flow but did not modify the heart rate and cardiac contractility (6). Peucordin at a concentration of 2×10^{-5} increased the coronary flow in the isolated rabbit heart by over 165%. Injection of 10 mg/kg IV increased the coronary flow by 82% and decreased the myocardial oxygen consumption in anesthetized pigs. Peucordin also antagonized pituitrin-induced coronary constriction but exerted marginal effect on the blood pressure; hence, it is believed to be a highly specific coronary dilator (1).

CLINICAL STUDIES

1. Common Cold with Cough

<Qianhu> is often prescribed concomitantly with other herbal medicines in the management of common cold, cough, bronchitis, and hiccups.

2. Virulent Swelling of Various Origins

The crushed fresh root may be applied locally (1–3).

REFERENCE

1. Petkov V (Wei JJ, translator). Guowai Yixue (Medicine Abroad) — Traditional Chinese Medicine and Materia Medica 1980 (3):12.
2. Gao YD et al. Chinese Medical Journal 1954 40(5):331.
3. Huang QZ. Chinese Medical Journal 1954 40(11):849.
4. Microbiology Section, Shandong Institute of Traditional Chinese Medicine and Materia Medica. The References of Traditional Chinese Medicine 1975 (8):51.
5. Chakraborty DP et al. Chemical Abstracts 1962 56:1835b.
6. Yan ZH et al. Chinese Traditional Pharmacy. 1st edition. Beijing College of Traditional Chinese Medicine. 1979. p. 149.

(Wang Jingsi)

CHUANSHANLONG 穿山龍

<Chuanshanlong>, also called <Guoshanlong>, refers to the rhizome of *Dioscorea nipponica* Makino (Dioscoreaceae). It is sweet with a bitter aftertaste and a "warm" property. The herb has antirheumatic, muscle-relaxant, circulation-activating, antitussive and mucolytic actions. It is mainly used to treat rheumatism, wounds and injuries, low-back sprain, and cough with dyspnea. The plant, *D. caucasia* Lipsky, has similar actions (1,2).

CHEMICAL COMPOSITION

<Chuanshanlong> contains many steroid saponins such as dioscin. Hydrolysis of the total saponins yields 1.5–2.6% of diosgenin. It also contains small amounts of 25-D-spirosta-3,5-diene.

PHARMACOLOGY

1. Effect on the Cardiovascular System

The <Chuanshanlong> preparations (water-ethanol extract chiefly containing the total saponins) at concentrations of 1:4000–1:1000 had cardiotonic effects on the isolated frog heart. The highly concentrated preparation (1:1000) caused cardiac arrest but the heart recovered after the drug was washed away. Intraintestinal injection of the 4% <Chuanshanlong> solution 0.2 ml to frogs increased contraction amplitude of the *in situ* hearts by more than 50% and also prolonged their activity (3,4). Intravenous injection of the total saponins of *D. nipponica* to anesthetized rabbits, dogs, and cats primarily caused hypotension, bradycardia, and respiratory excitation. The total saponins of *D. caucasia* also decreased the blood pressure, 140–150 mmHg, in rabbits with experimental atherosclerosis by 40–60 mmHg (1,3,5).

The total saponins of *D. nipponica* at concentrations of 1:100,000 and 1:200,000 increased the perfusion volume of the isolated normal rabbit ear by only 4–5.8% in contrast to 23.6–34.5% in rabbits with experimental atherosclerosis (2,6). Perfusion of the <Chuanshanlong> solution at 1:100,000–1:250 to isolated rabbit ears caused vasoconstriction in some and vasodilation in others; however, exceedingly high concentrations (>1:250) elicited only constriction (3,4).

Premedication with the saponins of *D. niponnica* 180 mg/kg PO or IV improved the ECG of rabbits with myocardial ischemia induced by pituitrin, the improvement rate being 57% in the oral group and 80% in the intravenous group, in contrast to the natural improvement rate of only 25% in the control (3). The ^{86}Rb tracing method indicated that <Chuanshanlong> increased the coronary blood flow in mice by 61.5% (5). Injection of the 10% *D. nipponica* preparation 0.4–0.8 ml/kg IV to anesthetized cats markedly increased the coronary flow, reduced the myocardial oxygen consumption and lowered the arteriovenous oxygen difference. In particular, the effect on the myocardial oxygen consumption of the group receiving 0.8 ml/kg was most significant (3,4).

2. Effect on Blood Lipids and Atherosclerotic Plaques

Daily oral administration of the saponins of *D. caucasia* 5–10 mg/kg for 15–20 days lowered the plasma cholesterol level in cats from 360–500 mg% to 50–90 mg% (2). Likewise, in rabbits with experimental hyperlipidemia the drug reduced blood cholesterol from 1040±271 mg% to 310±78 mg% (1). Injection of the total saponins of *D. nipponica* to rabbits with experimental atherosclerosis at 5 mg/kg IV daily for 74 days also decreased lipid infiltration into the aortic wall and cornea, apart from decreasing plasma cholesterol (6,7). Prophylactic and therapeutic effects against atherosclerotic plaques were obtained by daily oral administration of the <Chuanshanlong> preparation for 10 weeks in rabbits (8).

3. Anticoagulant Effect

Dioscin prolonged the coagulation and prothrombin times and decreased the prothrombin index of rabbit blood (7).

4. Tolerance to Hypoxia

Determination of the oxygen consumption within a given period as well as of the time of death by asphyxia revealed that a single intraperitoneal injection, or 3 intragastric doses of the <Chuanshanlong> preparation decreased the oxygen consumption of intact rats and enhanced their tolerance to hypoxia (3,4).

5. Effect on Smooth Muscles

The primary effect of the water-soluble saponins of <Chuanshanlong> on isolated rabbits uteri at low concentration (4–30 mg/ml) was stimulation, and at high concentration (150 mg/100 ml), inhibition. Contractions were slowly restored to normal after washing off the drug (3). Experiments on isolated intestinal muscles showed that low concentrations of the herb preparation (1–7 mg/100 ml) increased the tension of some intestinal segments, but the number of hypertonic segments progressively decreased when drug concentration was increased. Large doses (over 16 mg/kg) reduced the tension of most intestinal segments. The herb increased the *in situ* intestinal activity of anesthetized dogs dose-dependently (3).

6. Antitussive, Antiasthmatic, and Expectorant Effects

6.1 *Antitussive effect.* It was proved that, in cough induced by ammonia water in mice, the oral administration of the total saponins, the water soluble or water-insoluble saponins, molecular sieve No. I, or intragastric or intraperitoneal administration of the decoction of *D. nipponica* had a significant antitussive effect, whereas diosgenin was ineffective. The bioactive principle primarily resided in the portion with the greatest polarity. Likewise, the steroid saponins were also effective in large doses (9,10).

6.2 *Expectorant effect.* The phenol red method indicated that the orally administered total saponins, water-insoluble saponins molecular sieve No. I, or the intraperitoneally injected decoction had a significant expectorant effect in mice, whereas the water-soluble saponins had none (9,10). The capillary method also proved that the herb preparations had expectorant activity in rats (12).

6.3 *Antiasthmatic effect.* The histamine spray method in guinea pigs showed that the <Chuanshanlong> preparations at 0.15 and 0.25 g/kg suppressed asthma in 70 and 100% of treated cases, respectively (11,12).

7. Miscellaneous Actions

The decoction of *D. nipponica* 2 g(crude drug)/ml, preparations of *D. nipponica* and *D. caucasia*, all, increased the 24-hour urine output in mice and rabbits (1,2,7). After 7–10 days of medication with the D. nipponica preparation, the survival rate of mice exposed to a total dose of 750 rads of ^{60}Co radiation was found to be 35–39% higher than that of the control, indicating an antiradiation effect (13).

8. Toxicity

The toxicity of the water-soluble saponins of *D. nipponica* varied with the methods of processing. The oral tolerant dose in mice was 15.6 g/kg; the No. II preparation was more toxic with an LD_{50} of 11.5 g/kg. The LD_{50} of the water-soluble saponins of *D. nipponica* in mice was 750 mg/kg IV (3) and that of the pure agent was 406–425 mg/kg (3,4). In subacute toxicity tests, No. I and II water-soluble saponins administered at 60–180 mg/kg/day PO for 7 weeks did not produce significant effects on the leukocyte count, hemoglobin, routine urinalysis, hepatic and renal functions, or any gross or microscopic pathological changes in the heart, liver, spleen, lungs, kidneys and adrenal glands of the animals (4). Rare instances of diarrhea occurred after a doubled dose.

CLINICAL STUDIES

1. Coronary Disease

The <Chuanshanlong> preparation (sold under the trademark: Chuanlong Guanxinning), 160 mg per tablet, is to be given two tablets thrice daily. In 216 cases treated with the No. I preparation and

269 cases treated with the No. II preparation, the remission rates for angina pectoris were 91 and 93.5%, respectively; the ECG improvement rates at rest and given exercise were 41 and 60% for the No. I preparation, and 38.6 and 70.8% for the No. II preparation, respectively; cases with reduced cholesterol accounted for 42 and 61.3%, and those with reduced triglycerides, 46 and 55%, respectively. The medication reduced blood pressure in hypertensive patients; 69% of treated cases benefitted (14–16). The saponins from *D. nipponica* have been used abroad with good effects in angina pectoris, myocardial infarction, heart failure, and hypertension complicated with arteriosclerosis; they also improved the ECG patterns (1,2). *D. nipponica*, the root tuber of *Hemsleya macrosperma*, and the flower bud of *Sophora japonica* afforded good therapeutic results in 276 cases of coronary disease by improving angina pectoris and ECG aberrations; an antilipemic effect was also achieved (5).

2. Cerebral Arteriosclerosis

Two hundred cases of cerebral arteriosclerosis of 2–15 years' duration were treated with the tablets of the saponins of *D. caucasia* 0.02–0.2 g daily. Observation carried out over 2–3 months revealed normalization of the blood cholesterol level in most patients, recovery from neuropsychotic symptoms, lowering of blood pressure, relief of headache and dizziness, improvement of memory and increase of working capacity (2).

3. Chronic Bronchitis

Thirty-seven cases benefitted from the decoction of *D. nipponica* (17). The tablets and decoction consisting of *D. nipponica* as the chief ingredient plus the root of *Scutellaria baicalensis*, the root of *Platycodon grandiflorum*, the root and rhizome of *Aster tataricus*, the root tuber of *Stemona japonica*, and the fruit of *Schisandra chinensis* were effective in 464 cases of chronic bronchitis; 287 cases also benefitted from the tablet and other preparations derived from the root of *Scutellaria baicalensis*, the bulb of *Fritillaria cirrhosis*, and *D. nipponica* (18,19).

4. Rheumatic Arthritis

The medicinal wine prepared with *D. nipponica* is reputed to have antirheumatic, tendon-relaxant, blood-stimulant and analgesic effects in patients with rheumatic arthritis (20). A 92.7% effective rate achieved in 222 cases of rheumatic and rheumatoid arthritis treated with <Chuanshanlong> and dog bones (21–23).

5. *Miscellaneous*

Patients with chronic brucellosis were reported to be responsive to *D. nipponica* decoction (24,25). Likewise, the *D. nipponica* decoction benefitted cases with acute suppurative arthritis (26), and the *D. nipponica* extract had therapeutic value in thyroid adenoma and hyperthyroidism (27).

ADVERSE EFFECTS

The side effects of <Chuanshanlong> are mild and most disappear spontaneously without special management; diarrhea is commonly associated with its use (14).

REFERENCE

1. Sokolova LN. Rast Resur 1968 4(1):43.
2. Sokolova LN. Med Prom SSSR 1961 (7):43.
3. Pharmacology Department, Sichuan Medical College et al. Preliminary studies on the pharmacology of the total saponins of Dioscorea nipponica. 1978.
4. Yang ZW et al. Abstracts of the First National Symposium on Cardiovascular Pharmacology. 1980. p. 92.
5. Sichuan Institute of Chinese Materia Medica. Experimental Data and Clinical Uses of "Jin Huai Guanxin Tablet", 5. 1973. p. 19.
6. Sokolova LN. Provlemy Dolcholemiia. 1959. p. 34.
7. Sokolova LN. Farmakologiia I Toksikologiia 1959 22(1):42.
8. Pharmacology and Pathology Sections, Sichuan Medical College et al. Proceedings of the 1973 National Seminar on Coronary Disease. People's Medical Publishing House. 1973. p. 327.
9. Jiangsu College of New Medicine. Enyclopedia of Chinese Materia Medica. Vol. 2. Shanghai People's Medical Publishing House. 1977. p. 1726.
10. Sokolova LN et al. Chemical Abstracts 1968 69:42740w.
11. Pharmacology Department, Shenyang Medical College. Medical Research (Shenyang Medical College) 1972 (1):15.
12. Hunan Institute of Medical and Pharmaceutical Industry. Preliminary report of the antiradiation effect of Dioscorea nipponica. 1973.
13. Sichuan Institute of Industrial Health. Preliminary report of the antiradiation effect of Dioscorea nipponica. 1973.
14. Sichuan Institute of Biology et al. Zhonghua Yixue Zazhi (National Medical Journal of China) 1977 57(8):520.
15. Dioscorea nipponica Group, Sichuan Institute of Biology. Pharmaceutical Industry 1977 (2):3.
16. Internal Medicine Department, Teaching Hospital of Occupational Diseases of Sichuan Medical College. Internal information. 1980.

17. Pharmacology and Chemistry Departments, Shenyang Medical College et al. Medical Research (Shenyang Medical College) 1977 (3):14.

18. General Hospital of Jinan Military Region of the Chinese PLA et al. Selected Information on Senile Chronic Bronchitis. 1971. p. 41.

19. Academy of Traditional Chinese Medicine. Selected Information on Chronic Bronchitis. 1971. p. 32.

20. Daqing Commune (Tieling Country, Liaoning) et al. Liaoning Yiyao (Liaoning Medical Journal) Supplement 1975 (2):28.

21. Shandong Coordinating Research Group on Dog Bone Gelatin Medicinal Liquor. Chinese Traditional and Herbal Drugs Communications 1976 (12):12.

22. Shandong Medicinal Materials Company. Chinese Traditional and Herbal Drugs Communications 1976 (8):45.

23. Shandong Medicinal Materials Company. Chinese Traditional and Herbal Drugs Communications 1977 (5):21.

24. Gansu Bureau of Science and Technology. Scientific and Technological Development in Gansu 1975 (1):1.

25. Weinan District (Shaanxi) Scientific Research Group on Combined Western and Traditional Chinese Medicine. Information on Medical Sciences and Technology. 1974. p. 48.

26. Third Military Medical College of the Chinese PLA. Cailiao Huibian (Compiled Data) 1971 (1):23.

27. Qinghai Second People's Hospital et al. Clinical study of Dioscorea nipponica therapy of thyroid diseases and hyperthyroidism. 1971.

(The Editors of Chinese edition)

CHUANXINLIAN 穿心蓮

<Chuanxinlian> comes from the leaf or aerial part of *Andrographis paniculata* (Burm.f.) Nees (Acanthaceae). Also called <Yijianxi> or <Lanhelian>, the herb is bitter and "cold". It is considered to be latent-heat-clearing, antipyretic, detoxicant, anti-inflammatory, and detumescent and is thought to remove pathogenic "heat" from the blood. It is prescribed in pharyngolaryngitis, diarrhea, dysentery, cough with thick sputum, carbuncle, sores, and snake bites. <Chuanxinlian> is usually imported from the countries in southeast Asia, but today it is widely cultivated in many regions in China. In India and other countries, the herb is used as stomachic, antipyretic, alterative, and anthelmintic and is an effective remedy for dysentery, gastroenteritis, and diabetes.

CHEMICAL COMPOSITION

A. paniculata contains lactones and flavonoids. Four kinds of lactones were isolated from the aerial part in China, named chuanxinlian A (deoxyandrographolide), chuanxinlian B (andrographolide), chuanxinlian C (neoandrographolide), and chuanxinlian D (14-deoxy-11,12-didehydroandrographolide). Homoandrographolide was also isolated outside China. The flavonoids mainly exist in the root; these are polymethoxyflavones andrographin, panicolin, mono-0-methylwightin, and apigenin-7, 4' -dimethyl ethers. In China, flavonoids were also isolated from the leaf. The aerial part also contains alkanes, ketones, and aldehydes.

PHARMACOLOGY

1. Antibacterial Effect

Early studies (1) showed that the aqueous extract of <Chuanxinlian> was inactive against *Staphylococcus aureus* and *Escherichia coli*, but many reports in China later claimed that the <Chuanxinlian> decoction inhibited *Staphylococcus aureus, Pseudomonas aeruginosa, Proteus vulgaris, Shigella dysenteriae*, and *Escherichia coli* (2–8). Furthermore, it was found that the water-soluble fraction of the herb containing flavones had a strong inhibitory action against *Shigella dysenteriae* (9). However, this fraction was clinically ineffective in dysentery (10). On the other hand, the water-insoluble lactones, which were found to be devoid of antibacterial activity, had clinical value in many infections.

Deoxyandrographolide, andrographolide, neoandrographolide, 14-deoxy-11,12-didehydroandrographolide, and many of their soluble derivatives showed no significant antibacterial effect *in vitro*. Blood assays at various intervals after administration of large doses of the lactones and their derivatives to animals did not reveal any evidence of transformation of these compounds into active metabolites. Experimental therapy using these compounds afforded no significant protection from pneumococcus, *Staphylococcus aureus, Escherichia coli*, and leptospirae (11,12). In rabbits with pneumococcal keratitis, intravenous injection of andrographolide sulfonate (AS Injection), total andrographolide sulfonate (Xiyanping Injection), or andrographolide sodium hydrogen sulfite adduct (Deoxyandrographolide Compound Injection) for one week markedly controlled inflammation and accelerated its subsidence; of these, AS Injection was the most effective (11,13).

2. Effect on the Immunologic Function

The <Chuanxinlian> decoction increased leukocytic phagocytosis of *Staphylococcus aureus in vitro* (14). Oral administration of the herb to patients with tumor or other afflictions, or to healthy subjects, augmented the delayed cutaneous hypersensitivity to not quite fresh tuberculin (15). Successive administration of AS Injection to rabbits or mice markedly increased peripheral phagocytosis of pneumococcus or *Staphylococcus aureus*. Likewise, deoxyandrographolide injection and Xiyanping Injection enhanced the phagocytic function. *In vitro* studies showed that various injection preparations of the soluble derivatives of the herb, such as AS Injection, inhibited PHA-induced increase of ^{3}H-thymidine incorporation into lymphocytes (13). 14-Deoxy-11,12-didehydroandrographolide hemisuccinate (DAS) also inhibited the delayed hypersensitivity of mice to 2,4-dinitrochlorobenzene (16).

3. Antipyretic Effect

Deoxyandrographolide, andrographolide, neoandrographolide, and 14-deoxy-11,12-didehydroandrographolide had an antipyretic effect in rabbits with fever induced by typhoid and paratyphoid vaccines, and in albino rats with fever caused by 2,4-dinitrophenol. Their rank in terms of potency was as follows: 14-deoxy-11,12-didehydroandrographolide > deoxyandrographolide and neoandrographolide > andrographolide (17,18). In rabbits with fever induced by typhoid vaccine, antipyretic action in various degrees was achieved with: DAS (16) and its sodium hydrogen sulfite adduct (Yanning-4 Injection) (19); Yanning-3 (the mixture of DAS and Yanning-4) (20); AS Injection; Deoxyandrographolide Injection; the open ring product of alkaline hydrolysis of andrographolide; and deoxyandrographolide sodium hydrogen sulfite adduct (21). Intraperitoneal injection of the suspensions of deoxyandrographolide and neoandrographolide to rabbits with fever induced by concurrent subcutaneous injection of *Diplococcus pneumoniae* or *Streptococcus hemolyticus* delayed and modulated the rise in body temperature (22).

4. Anti-inflammatory Effect

Deoxyandrographolide, andrographolide, neoandrographolide, and 14-deoxy-11,12-didehydroandrographolide each produced and anti-inflammatory effect different in degree; 1 g/kg

PO administered to mice inhibited the increase in cutaneous or peritoneal capillary permeability induced by xylene or acetic acid, and reduced acute exudation in Selye granulocysts induced by cotton oil, without modifying granular tissue hyperplasia. They also inhibited egg white-induced paw swelling in rats, but the action disappeared after adrenalectomy. Among the four lactones, 14-deoxy-11,12-didehydroandrographolide exerted the most potent anti-inflammatory action, followed by neoandrographolide and deoxyandrographolide; andrographolide was found to be the weakest (18). Injection of the soluble derivatives of the <Chuanxinlian> lactones also produced anti-inflammatory effect in various degrees; for instance, injection of DAS 125–250 mg/kg SC or IP markedly inhibited the increase in cutaneous or peritoneal capillary permeability in mice induced by xylol, histamine, or acetic acid, as well as egg white-induced paw swelling and croton oil-induced inflammatory exudation in rat granuloma. The anti-inflammatory action of DAS on paw swelling induced by egg white also disappeared after bilateral adrenalectomy (23). It is therefore evident that the anti-inflammatory effect of the four lactones and DAS was mediated by the adrenal glands. In addition, the anti-inflammatory potencies of AS Injection, DAS Injection, and 250–500 mg/kg of Deoxyandrographolide Injection were similar (21).

5. *Effect on the Pituitary-Adrenocortical Function*

High dosage of the four lactones caused thymic atrophy in young mice, suggesting intensification of the adrenocortical function (18). Likewise, DAS caused thymic atrophy in young mice, and also markedly decreased the vitamin C content of the rat adrenal gland. No tachyphylaxis occurred after five days of medication, at which time the ACTH content in the anterior pituitary was found to be slightly higher than that in the control. Hypophysectomy totally abolished the decremental effect of DAS on the vitamin C content of the rat adrenals; it did not prolong the survival period of adrenalectomized young rats. These results suggest that DAS does not exert an adrenocorticoid effect but is capable of markedly activating the anterior pituitary gland, promoting the synthesis and release of ACTH, and consequently enhancing the adrenocortical function. Since DAS still decreased the adrenal vitamin C of rats anesthetized with pentobarbital sodium, and since under pentobarbital sodium anesthesia, morphine, dexamethasone and chlorpromazine could completely block this effect, the site of DAS action (activation of the pituitary-adrenocortical function) is inferred to be at the subcortical region (23). Apart from DAS, Yanning[-4] Injection (19), Xiyanping Injection and Deoxyandrographolide Injection also activated the pituitary-adrenocortical function, because all of them were found to reduce the vitamin C content in the rat adrenal (24).

6. *Antivenin and Muscarinic Effects*

Intraperitoneal injection of the ethanol extract of <Chuanxinlian> to mice poisoned with cobra venom very markedly delayed the occurrence of respiratory failure and death. This extract lowered the blood pressure of dogs; this effect was reinforced by physostigmine and blocked by atropine but unmodified by antihistamines and β-blockers. It also inhibited the frog heart *in situ*, and its action was blocked by atropine. The extract caused contraction of the guinea pig ileum, which was intensified by physostigmine and blocked by atropine but unchanged by antihistamines. It had no effect on the musculi rectus abdominis of frogs. These findings indicate that the herb does not modify the activity of nicotinic receptors but produces significant muscarinic action which accounts for its antivenin effect (25).

7. Termination of Pregnancy

A contraceptive effect was achieved in mice fed with <Chuanxinlian> (26); administration of the herb to pregnant rabbits resulted in abortion (27). Intraperitoneal injection of the <Chuanxinlian> decoction to albino mice prevented implantation and caused abortion at different gestational periods. Early pregnancy was also terminated by <Chuanxinlian> given by the intramuscular, subcutaneous, intravenous and oral routes; the best effects were obtained by the intrauterine, intraperitoneal and intravenous routes, although good effects were also achieved with small doses by the intrauterine route. Similar results were observed in rabbits in early pregnancy. Progesterone or luteinizing hormone releasing hormone (LHRH) completely or markedly antagonized the abortifacient effect of <Chuanxinlian>, suggesting antagonism between the herb and the endogenous progesterone. In addition, <Chuanxinlian> suppressed the growth of human placental chorionic trophoblastic cells *in vitro* (28). Some semisynthetic derivatives of andrographolide also exhibited anti-early pregnancy actions of different strengths (29). The sodium salt of andrographolide hemisuccinate was deleterious to the placental chorionic trophoblastic cells (30).

8. Miscellaneous Actions

<Chuanxinlian> had a choleretic action in rats; it also increased the weight of the animals' liver and shortened cyclobarbital-induced sleep (31). The extract of the stem and leaf of *A. paniculata*, or andrographolide did not modify the blood glucose level in normal or diabetic rats (32). 11-Deoxy-11,12-didehydroandrographolide hemisuccinate inhibited transplanted Walker carcinoma 256.

9. Pharmacokinetics

Experiments with the ^{35}S-labelled adduct of andrographolide sodium hydrogen sulfite revealed a quick fall of the drug level in the blood after intravenous injection; the drug rapidly crossed the blood-brain barrier to gain access to the various sites of the CNS. The highest concentration was found in the spinal cord, and showed significant descending localization. Among the visceral organs, the kidney had the highest drug level, but 6 hours later the highest drug level was found in the rectum. The drug was rapidly excreted in the urine mainly unchanged (33). Experiments with ^{3}H-andrographolide showed that the intravenous dose of 0.33 mg had a rapid distribution and slow elimination in mice. The distribution constant was 0.189 minute^{-1} and the elimination constant 0.0026 minute^{-1}. The intragastric dose in mice (0.66 mg) also had a rapid absorption and distribution; peak absorption was recorded at 30.75 minutes; the peak blood level was 16 µg/ml, and the bioavailabilty was 44.06%. The absorbed drug rapidly gained access to the organs; the highest level appeared in the stomach and small intestine in 30 minutes, and in other organs in 60 minutes. The highest radioactivity was detected in the gallbladder, stomach, liver and small intestine, next in the uterus, kidneys, ovaries, and lungs, while radioactivity was low in the rectum, spleen, heart, and brain. Radioactivity in various organs gradually declined but some was still detectable even after 48 hours; the radioactivities in the various organs in terms of the respective peak concentrations were heart 11.1%, liver 5.6%, spleen 14.9%, lungs 10.9%, kidneys 7.9%, brain 20.9%, small intestine 3.2%, rectum 8.6%, uterus 5.1%, and ovaries 5.1%. The amount of the drug excreted in the urine and feces 24 hours after the oral dose accounted for 89.7%, and after 48 hours, 94.25%, of which urinary excretion represented 48.97% and fecal excretion, 45.28%. Thin-layer chromatographic analysis of the urine and liver showed that ^{3}H-andrographolide accounted for a mere 11 and 10.7%, whereas the fat-soluble metabolites constituted 87 and 77%, respectively (34).

10. Toxicity

<Chuanxinlian> has a low toxicity. The LD$_{50}$ of the lactones and their major derivatives in mice are listed in the following table:

Preparation	Composition	Route of administration	LD$_{50}$ (g/kg)	Reference
Total lactones		PO	13.4	35
Deoxyandrographolide		PO	> 20	18
Andrographolide		PO	> 40	17
Neoandrographolide		PO	> 20	18
14-Deoxy-11,12-didehydroandrographolide		PO	> 20	18
AS Injection	Andrographolide sulfonate	IV	2.47 – 2.94	36
Deoxyandrographolide Injection	Andrographolide sodium hydrogen sulfite adduct	IV	1.075 – 1.145	37
A$_{104}$ Injection	Andrographolide sodium sulfite adduct	IV	1.95 – 2.09	38
BC$_{104}$ Injection	Deoxyandrographolide and the adduct of neoandro-grapholide and sodium sulfite	IV	2.2	39

(cont' d)

Table (cont' d)

Preparation	Composition	Route of administration	LD$_{50}$ (g/kg)	Reference
Chuanhuning (DAS) Injection	14-deoxy-11,12-dide-hydroandrographolide hemisuccinate	IV IP	0.600±0.020 0.675±0.030	40
Yanning^{-4} Injection	Adduct of sodium hydrogen sulfite and 14-deoxy-11, 12 didehydroandrographo-lide hemisuccinate	IV IP	2.12±0.08 3.92±0.10	19
Yanning^{-3} Injection	Mixture of 14-deoxy-11, 12-didehydroandrograp-holide hemisuccinate and its sodium hydrogen sulfite adduct	IV IP	0.693–0.900 1.344–1.390	20

In subacute toxicity tests, administration of andrographolide to albino rats or rabbits at 1 g/kg PO once daily for 7 days not significantly change the body weight, blood picture, hepatic and renal functions and histology of important organs (17). Similar results were obtained with deoxyandrographolide (18). DAS Injection administered to rats at 84 mg/kg IP for 10 days also produced no toxic effects (40). In healthy volunteers, oral administration of andrographolide 0.5 g four times daily (the first dose 1.0 g) for 4 days caused a transient elevation of SGPT in some. Upon discontinuation of the medication, however, normal levels were gradually recovered. Hepatic and renal functions were not impaired with the 0.3 g dose given thrice daily for 5 days (17).

CLINICAL STUDIES

Various preparations of <Chuanxinlian> have been widely used to treat many kinds of infectious and non-infectious diseases. The following table shows a summary of the clinical results (12,14–42).

1. Enteric Infections

Many preparations of <Chuanxinlian> had therapeutic value in acute bacillary dysentery and enteritis. For example, 121 out of 137 cases of acute bacillary dysentery, and 523 out of 573 cases of acute gastroenteritis were cured by the tablet of the ethanol extract of the herb, the cure rate being 88.3 and 91.3%, respectively (43). Out of 122 cases of acute bacillary dysentery treated with andrographolide, 111 achieved clinical cure, 7 were ameliorated and only 4 unresponsive (44). The neoandrographolide tablet was even more effective; it cured 55 out of 66 cases; most of the unresponsive cases were the fulminant or toxic type (10). The new Compound A. paniculata Glycoside Tablet, which contains andrographolide and neoandrographolide in the proportion of 7:3 was also effective, i.e., 119 out of 131 cases of bacillary dysentery so treated were cured, achieving a cure rate of 91.1% which was higher than that obtained with furazolidine or chloramphenicol (45). The andrographolide-free fluidextract tablet was also very effective against bacillary dysentery (46). Deoxyandrographolide Injection cured 173 and improved 50 out of 228 cases of bacillary dysentery, the effective rate being 94.9%; the same agent benefitted 86 out of 92 cases of enteritis; the effective rate was 96.6% (37). According to a report, 200 cases of acute bacillary dysentery were given acupoint injection of <Chuanxinlian>; 72.8% were cured after one injection, and 96.2% after two injection (47). Moreover, there were reports on the efficacy of compound formulae containing <Chuanxinlian> as the chief ingredient in the treatment of typhoid fever (48,49), and of the <Chuanxinlian> decoction used as an enema in intestinal trichomoniasis (50).

Disease	No. of cases	No. of effective cases	Effective rate %
Bacillary dysentery	1611*	1471	91.3
Enteritis	955	872	91.3
Typhoid fever	31	29	93.6*
Respiratory tract infection	2717	2430	89.4
Tuberculosis	321	280	87.2
Leptospirosis	185	160	86.5
Leprosy	112	105	93.7
Skin infection	359	347	96.1
Hepatitis	112	93	83.0
Fulminant hepatitis	26	20	
Acute pyelonephritis	64	62	
Otitis media	55	51	92.6*
Pelvic inflammation	186	183	98.4
Choriocarcinoma and malignant hydatidiform mole	60	47	78.3*
Induction of labor	331	296	89.4
Thromboangiitis obliterans	108	101	93.5

(*From reference 12.)

2. Respiratory Tract Infections

The <Chuanxinlian> preparations were of therapeutic value in differing degrees in respiratory tract infections caused by virus and bacteria, such as upper respiratory tract infection, acute tonsillitis, influenza, bronchitis, lobar pneumonia, and viral pneumonia. The aggregate effective rates of the pills made from powdered whole plant of *A. paniculata* with water, and of the tablets of the aqueous extract of the herb, in upper respiratory tract infection were significantly different; 88 and 61%, respectively (51). Deoxyandrographolide and neoandrographolide were more effective than andrographolide against influenza and other respiratory tract infections (52,53). A paper reported the treatment of 129 cases of acute tonsillitis with the adduct of andrographolide and sodium hydrogen sulfite; a marked effective rate of 65% and a moderate effective rate of 27% were achieved. This drug was used to treat 49 cases of pneumonia; 35 cases had marked effects and 9, moderate effects (37). AS Injection had very good effects in lung infection; for instance, an aggregate effective rate of 91.2% was achieved in 131 cases (111 cases of pneumonia and 20 cases of chronic bronchitis complicated with pneumonia); fever disappeared in 72.3% within 3 days, inflammation subsided in 40% within 1 week, and the disease was absorbed in 79% within 2 weeks. It was also quite effective against pneumonia of the shock type (36). DAS Injection had optimal effects against pneumonia in infants and children, and in upper respiratory tract infections of viral origin; the effective rate in 455 cases was 90.2%; 72.3% of the cases were relieved of fever after 3.1 days (54). Salutary effects were also obtained from the total lactone sulfonates used to combat respiratory tract infections (55). In addition, <Chuanxinlian> and formulae containing this herb as the principal ingredient have been used with various degrees of efficacy against common cold (56), parotitis (57), pharyngolaryngitis (58,59), epidemic asthmatic pneumonia (60), and asthmatic bronchitis (61). These preparations were also injected into acupoints to treat acute tonsillitis (62), and chronic bronchitis of aged persons, with various therapeutic results (63).

3. Leptospirosis

Thirty-one out of 35 cases were cured with the tablet of the total lactones (64). Following therapy with deoxyandrographolide, andrographolide and neoandrographolide, 40 out of 46 cases were cured (65). There were also reports on the effective treatment of leptospirosis with some injection preparations or tablets of <Chuanxinlian> (54,66–68).

4. Tuberculosis and Leprosy

<Chuanxinlian> had therapeutic value in pulmonary tuberculosis, especially in the exudative type (69–71). It appeared to synergize with isoniazid (72). Seventy cases of tuberculous meningitis were treated with the open ring product of andrographolide (by alkaline hydrolysis). There were only 6 deaths, indicating a marked decrease in the mortality rate (73). The herb was also reported to be effective in 112 cases of leprosy (74).

5. Hepatitis and Biliary Tract Infection

<Chuanxinlian> had therapeutic value in hepatitis (9,75,76). The treatment of 26 cases of fulminant hepatitis with <Chuanxinlian> in concert with Western drugs showed the following results: 8 clinically cured, 12 improved, 1 unchanged, and 5 deceased (41). The compound formulae of <Chuanxinlian> were reportedly effective in biliary tract infection (77,78).

6. Acute Pyelonephritis

Fifty-eight cases were cured and 4 improved out of 64 cases treated with the <Chuanxinlian> tablet. The effects of this tablet for chills, fever, bladder irritation, tenderness over the kidney area upon percussion, and the recovery time of routine urinalysis were similar to those of nitrofurantoin, but the former had fewer side effects (42).

7. Choriocarcinoma, Malignant Hydatidiform Mole and Early- and Mid-term Abortifacient Effect

<Chuanxinlian> had specific action on malignant trophoblasts. Out of 60 cases of choriocarcinoma (chorioepithelioma) and malignant hydatidiform mole, of which 41 had metastasis prior to admission, 47 cases obtained short-term remission after treatment with <Chuanxinlian> and other therapeutic agents; 12 of these cases were managed with <Chuanxinlian> solely; 4 cases with malignant hydatidiform mole were conceived or delivered (79). The use of the herb preparations to induce labor showed good prospects (27,80,81).

8. Thromboangiitis Obliterans

Intra-arterial and retrograde intravenous injections (with pressure on the proximal end) of the herb were effective in thromboangiitis obliterans. Better results were achieved in the "heat toxic type" (82).

9. Viper Bites

Ten cases of viper bites (4 of bamboo pit viper, 5 mountain pit viper, and 1 many-banded krait) were all cured, mostly in 3 to 5 days, by a compound formula which has <Chuanxinlian> as the chief herb (83).

10. Miscellaneous

Many reports are available regarding the effectiveness of preparations and compound formula of <Chuanxinlian> in a variety of infectious and non-infectious diseases such as epidemic encephalitis B (84), suppurative otitis media (85), neonatal subcutaneous annular ulcer (2), vaginitis (86), cervical erosion (87), pelvic inflammation (88), herpes zoster, chicken pox, mumps (89,90), neurodermatitis, eczema (91), and burns (92). These preparations were also employed by veterinarians in treating gastroenteritis and bacillary dysentery in pigs and cows, and white dysentery in piglets and chickens (93).

ADVERSE EFFECTS

<Chuanxinlian> has few toxic and side effects. Large oral doses may cause gastric discomfort and loss of appetite. Emesis may be caused by the bitter andrographolide. One should be aware of

reports on the occurrence of anaphylactic shock due to the injection of the crude extract of this herb (94–102). Acute amniotic fluid embolism in induction of labor by exchanging the amniotic fluid with <Chuanxinlian> extract has been reported (103).

REFERENCE

1. Osborn EM. British Journal of Experimental Pathology 1943 24:227.

2. Qiu WC. Fujian Zhongyiyao (Fujian Journal of Traditional Chinese Medicine) 1965 (4):32.

3. Ninghua Hospital (Fujian). Medicine and Health (Fujian Health Bureau) 1971 (1):49.

4. Zhejiang People's Academy of Health. In vitro bacteriostatic tests of more than 200 kinds of Chinese traditional drugs. 1971.

5. Shandong Institute for Drug Control. Shandong Pharmaceutical Industry 1973 (1):27.

6. Wuhan Sanitation and Anti-epidemic Station. Hubei Science and Technology — Medical Series 1972 (6):37.

7. Pathological-Microbiology Section, Baise Medical School. Health Bulletin (Baise District Health Bureau, Guangxi) 1972 (6):15.

8. Anshun Coordinating Research Group for Chronic Bronchitis. Medical Information (Guizhou Health Bureau) 1973 (4):30.

9. Clinical Antibiotics Research Unit, Huashan Teaching Hospital of Shanghai First Medical College. Summary of the clinical studies on <Yijianxi> (Andrographis paniculata). 1970.

10. Shanghai Institute of Chinese Materia Medica et al. Xinyiyaoxue Zazhi (Journal of Traditional Chinese Medicine) 1973 (9):23.

11. Clinical Antibiotics Research Unit, Huashan Teaching Hospital of Shanghai First Medical College. Chinese Traditional and Herbal Drugs Communications 1978 (8):30.

12. Deng WL. Chinese Traditional and Herbal Drugs Communications 1978 (10):27.

13. Zhang ZL et al. Abstracts of the First National Symposium of the Society of Pharmacology. 1979. p. 96.

14. Hangzhou Second Hospital. Hangzhou Yiyao (Hangzhou Medical Journal) — Compiled Information (Centre of Medical and Health Information of Hangzhou Health Bureau) 1977:62.

15. Chinese Traditional Drugs Unit, Hangzhou Second People's Hospital. Notes on Science and Technology — Medicine and Health (Information Institute of Zhejiang Bureau of Science and Technology) 1978 (4):36.

16. Deng WL et al. Studies on the pharmacological effects of 14-deoxy-11,12-didehydroandrographolide hemisuccinate. II. Antipyretic effect and influence on the immunologic function. 1980.

17. Pharmacology Department, Sichuan Institute of Chinese Materia Medica. Sichuan Communications on Chinese Traditional and Herbal Drugs 1975 (1):21.

18. Deng WL et al. Comparative pharmacological studies of deoxyandrographolide, andrographolide, neoandrographolide, and 14-deoxy-11,12-didehydroandrographolide. 1980.

19. Deng WL et al. The pharmacological and clinical studies of the water-soluble Andrographis paniculata preparation Yanning⁻⁴ Injection. 1979.

20. Deng WL et al. Chinese Traditional and Herbal Drugs Communications 1978 (8):26.

21. Deng WL et al. Pharmacological studies of thirteen kinds of Andrographis paniculata injections. I. Antipyretic and anti-inflammatory actions and toxicity. 1979.

22. Li KH. Chinese Traditional and Herbal Drugs Communications 1974 (3):46.

23. Deng WL et al. Acta Pharmaceutica Sinica 1980 15(10):590.

24. Deng WL et al. Pharmacological studies of thirteen kinds of Andrographis paniculata injections. II. Effect on the pituitary-adrenocortical function. 1980.

25. Nazimudeen SK et al. Indian Journal of Pharmaceutical Sciences 1978 40(4):132.

26. Shamsuzzoha M et al. Lancet 1978 II:900.

27. Ob-Gyn Department, Guangdong People's Hospital et al. Guangdong Medical Information 1977 (1):28.

28. Physiology Department, Beijing Medical College. Acta Physiologica Sinica 1978 30(1):75.

29. Lin QS et al. Pharmaceutical abstracts. In: Proceedings of the Shanghai Regional Symposium on Pharmacy. Chinese Pharmaceutical Association (Beijing Branch). 1978. p. 243.

30. Sun MZ et al. Journal of Beijing Medical College 1979 (2):79.

31. Chaudhuri SK. Indian Journal of Experimental Biology 1978 16(1):830.

32. Moniruddin A et al. Chemical Abstracts 1968:158484h.

33. Wuxi Institute of Medical Sciences et al. Studies on Chinese Proprietary Medicines 1978 (2):15.

34. Zheng ZY et al. Absorption, distribution, excretion and metabolism of 3H-andrographolide. 1981.

35. Deng WL et al. Toxicity experiments of the tablet of the total lactones of Andrographis paniculata. 1978.

36. Shanghai Coordinating Research Group on Andrographis paniculata. Chinese Traditional and Herbal Drugs Communications 1976 (3):10.

37. Shanghai No. 2. Chinese Medicines Factory. Pharmaceutical Industry 1976 (1):24.

38. Suzhou Chinese Medicines Factory et al. Chinese Traditional and Herbal Drugs Communications 1976 (11):6.

39. Meng ZM et al. Chinese Traditional and Herbal Drugs Communications 1979 (7):6.

40. Deng WL et al. Studies on the pharmacological effects of 14-deoxy-11,12-didehydroandrographolide Hemisuccinate. III. General pharmacology and toxicity. 1980.

41. Infectious Diseases Department, Meixian District People's Hospital. Xinzhongyi (Journal of New Chinese Medicine) 1977 (6):31.

42. Gao WW. Journal of Bethune University of Medical Sciences 1979 (4):72.

43. Shantou Pharmaceutical Factory. Chinese Traditional and Herbal Drugs Communications 1970 (1):24.

44. Infections Diseases Department, 39th Army Hospital of the Chinese PLA. People's Military Medicine 1977 (6):77.

45. Chen XD et al. Studies on Chinese Proprietary Medicines 1978 (2):8.

46. Pharmaceutics Department, Shanghai Institute of Pharmaceutical Industry. Studies on Chinese Proprietary Medicines 1979 (4):1.

47. Li GD. Chinese Medical Journal 1975 (2):140.

48. Internal Medical Department, Baoan County People's Hospital. New Chinese Medicine 1972 (8): 29.

49. Internal Medical Department, Shantou District Hospital. Shantou Yiyao (Shantou Medical Journal) 1976 (1):10.

50. Health Team of the 8th Regiment of the 3rd Division of the Chinese PLA. Selected Information on Military Medicine and Health. Vol. 2. Logistics Department of the Production and Construction Corps of Guangzhou Military Region. 1974. p. 61.

51. Wang CF et al. Xinyiyaoxue Zazhi (Journal of Traditional Chinese Medicine) 1976 (10):25.

52. Sichuan Institute of Chinese Materia Medica. Sichuan Communications on Chinese Traditional and Herbal Drugs 1973 (2):16.

53. Sichuan Institute of Chinese Materia Medica. Sichuan Communications on Chinese Traditional and Herbal Drugs 1973 (2):14.

54. Sichuan Coordinating Clinical Research Group on Andrographis paniculata. Chinese Traditional and Herbal Drugs Communications 1978 (8):32.

55. Pharmaceutical Factory, Hospital of Bayi Herbal Nursery. Medical Information (Ganzhou District Health Bureau, Jiangxi) 1973 (2):23.

56. Chaoan (Guangdong) Pharmaceutical Factory. Chinese Traditional and Herbal Drugs Communications 1970 (5,6):48.

57. Yicheng Hospital of Yixing County (Jiangsu). Compiled information on the identification of deoxyandrographolide. Shanghai No. 2 Chinese Medicines Factory et al. 1976. p. 45.

58. EENT Department, General Hospital of Fuzhou Military Region. Medical Information (Fuzhou Institute of Medical Sciences) 1976 (2):45.

59. Jing ZH. Jiangsu Yiyao (Jiangsu Medical Journal) 1978 (2):45.

60. Anji County First Hospital. Notes on Science and Technology — Medicine and Health (Information Institute of Zhejiang Bureau of Science and Technology) 1972 (5):17.

61. Internal Medicine Department, OPD of the Nitrogenous Fertilizer Area of the Staff Hospital of Nanjing Chemical Industry Company. Jiangsu Yiyao (Jiangsu Medical Journal) 1978 (1):44.

62. Zhai F. Zhejiang Zhongyi Xueyuan Xuebao (Journal of Zhejiang College of Traditional Chinese Medicine) 1979 (3):22.

63. Haizhu District (Guangzhou) Coordinating Research Group on Senile Chronic Bronchitis. New Medical Communications (Guangzhou Institute of Medicine and Health) 1971 (2):35.

64. Sichuan Institute of Chinese Materia Medica et al. Sichuan Communications on Chinese Traditional and Herbal Drugs 1972 (3):12.

65. Sichuan Institute of Chinese Materia Medica et al. Xinyiyaoxue Zazhi (Journal of Traditional Chinese Medicine) 1973 (7):7.

66. Daxian District (Sichuan) Sanitation and Anti-epidemic Station. Medical Trends (Information Section of the Chinese Academy of Medical Sciences) 1971 (8):4.

67. Chengdu College of Traditional Chinese Medicine. Chinese Traditional and Herbal Drugs Communications 1972 (2):30.

68. Internal Medicine Department, Jiutai County Hospital. Jilin Yiyao (Jilin Medical Journal) 1974 (6):35.

69. Shantou Pharmaceutical Factory. Chinese Traditional and Herbal Drugs Communications 1970 (1):26.

70. Shanghai Second Hospital of Tuberculosis et al. Chinese Traditional and Herbal Drugs Communications 1973 (3):49.

71. Internal Medicine Department, 167th Hospital of the Chinese PLA. Yixue Xueshu (Medicine). Medical Research Department of 103 Guangzhou Unit of the Chinese PLA. 1974.

72. 31st Field Hospital of the Chinese PLA. Studies on the efficacy of Andrographis paniculata plus isoniazid in eighty-nine cases of pulmonary tuberculosis. In: Andrographis paniculata. Health Division of the Logistics Department of Guangzhou Military Region. 1974. p. 58.

73. Infectious Diseases Department, Shantou District People's Hospital. New Chinese Medicine 1977 (1):14.

74. 31st Field Hospital of the Chinese PLA et al. Dermatological Research Communications 1975 (2):158.

75. Hengyang Hospital of Infectious Diseases. Proceedings of the Hengyang Symposium on Medical and Health Research. Science and Technology Group of the Hengyang Production Management Unit. 1972. p. 82.

76. Infectious Diseases Department, Southwestern Teaching Hospital of the Third Military Medical College of the Chinese PLA. Summary of the treatment of acute infectious hepatitis with the tablet of the total lactones of Andrographis paniculata. 1978.

77. Jieyang County People's Hospital. Information on Medical Sciences and Technology (Guangdong Institute of Medicine and Health) 1973 (10):40.

78. Guangzhou Institute for Drug Control. Chinese Traditional and Herbal Drugs Communications 1977 (12):21.

79. Ob-Gyn Department, Meixian District People's Hospital. Zhonghua Yixue Zazhi (National Medical Journal of China) 1977 (12):755.

80. Ob-Gyn Department, Zhongshan Medical College et al. Clinical efficacy of Andrographis paniculata solution in 231 cases of induced abortion at mid-term pregnancy. 1977.

81. Family Planning Unit, First Teaching Hospital of Beijing Medical College. Preliminary studies on the clinical applications of the bitter component of Andrographis paniculata. In: Pharmaceutical Abstracts (Proceedings of the 1978 Shanghai Regional Symposium on Pharmacy). Chinese Pharmaceutical Association (Beijing Branch). 1978. p. 253.

82. 141st Hospital of the Chinese PLA. New Chinese Medicine 1977 (1):8.

83. Zhainan Commune Health Centre (Liannan County, Guangdong). Journal of Barefoot Doctor 1975 (4):16.

84. Luoding County People's Hospital. Trends on Medical Sciences and Technology (Guangdong Institute of Medicine and Health) 1971 (4):6.

85. Baoan County Hospital. New Chinese Medicine 1971 (2):13.

86. Lingtand Commune (Gaoyou County) Health Center. Jiangsu Yiyao (Jiangsu Medical Journal) 1975 (6):45.

87. Ding GH. Zigong Yiyao (Zigong Medical Journal) 1980 (2):30.

88. 169th Hospital of the Chinese PLA. Yixue Xueshu (Medicine). Medical Research Department of 103 Guangzhou Unit of the Chinese PLA. 1974. p. 112.

89. Huang QZ. Health Journal of Guangxi 1974 (5):43.

90. Huang QZ. Guangxi' s Barefoot Doctor 1978 (9):21.

91. Traditional Chinese Medicine Department, Jiangsu Institute of Dermatology et al. Dermatological Research Communications 1972 (2):130.

92. Cooperative Medical Clinic of Zuoqiao Production Brigade (Sanchagang Commune, Douchang County, Jiangxi). Journal of Barefoot Doctor 1975 (4):11.

93. Danyang Hospital of Veterinary Medicine (Jiangsu). Zootechnics and Veterinary Medicine 1973 (1):30.

94. Fenjie Commune Health Centre (Gaozhou County, Guangdong). New Chinese Medicine 1971 (5):46.

95. Yiyuan Health Clinic (Maodian Commune, Ganxian, Jiangxi). New Chinese Medicine 1972 (3):47.

96. Health Clinic of Wuxi No. 5 Pharmaceutical Factory. New Chinese Medicine 1972 (7):34.

97. Zhang XY. New Chinese Medicine 1972 (11):53.

98. Xixi Commune (Wuxing County) Health Centre. Notes on Science and Technology — Medicine and Health (Information Institute of Zhejiang Bureau of Science and Technology) 1972 (12):34.

99. He XF. Fuzhou Yiyao (Fuzhou Medical Journal) 1974 (2–3):15.

100. Xiao WC et al. Hunan Yiyao Zazhi (Hunan Medical Journal) 1976 (4):30.

101. Internal Medicine Department, Eshan Branch of Fengcheng District Hospital. Zaozhuang Yiyao (Zaozhuang Medical Journal) 1978 (2):19.

102. Li D. Henan Zhongyi Xueyuan Xuebao (Journal of Henan College of Traditional Chinese Medicine) 1979 (2):63; Zhongji Yikan (Intermediate Medical Journal) 1979 (2):43.

103. Ob-Gyn Department, Huiyang District People' s Hospital. Guangdong Medical Information 1978 (1):35.

(Deng Wenlong)

MEIRENJIAO 美人蕉

<Meirenjiao> comes from the rhizome and flower of *Canna indica* L. (Cannaceae). Also known as <Fengweihua>, the herb is sweet and bland to the taste and has a "cool" property. It is considered to be "damp-heat"-clearing, tranquilizing, and hypotensive, and is a well-known remedy for the treatment of icteric hepatitis, chronic dysentery, hemoptysis, metrorrhagia, leukorrhea, and for external use in wounds and injuries, as well as for acne vulgaris.

CHEMICAL COMPOSITION

Six phenolic substances, 2 terpenes and 4 coumarins, were isolated from the underground part of *C. indica* (1). The underground part also contains starch, glucose, fat, alkaloids, and gum.

PHARMACOLOGY

1. Liver-Protective Effect

The 1:5 injection of <Meirenjiao> or its compound formula (Rhizoma Cannae, Radix Sambuci, Herba Lespedezae) administered to carbon tetrachloride-intoxicated mice at a daily dose of 15 ml/kg PO for 10 days decreased the serum BSP retention. The herb alone given prophylactically for 5 days was also effective. These results indicate that <Meirenjiao> protects the liver from carbon tetrachloride-induced injuries (2).

2. Cholagogic and Choleretic Effects

In anesthetized dogs with ligated gallbladder and catheterized common bile duct, injection of the 1:5 <Meirenjiao> preparation or its compound formula 1 ml/kg IV produced a significant choleretic action, increasing bile flow by 167.5% of the pretreatment level. The herb had a fast onset, and maximal effect was seen 30 minutes after medication, sustained for about one hour (2). Intravenous injection of the 1:10 <Meirenjiao> extract, containing six types of phenolic substances, to anesthetized dogs at a dose of 1 ml/kg promptly and very significantly increased bile flow from 0.41 ml/min 30 minutes before treatment to an average of 1.13 ml/min. This fact indicates that the choleretic activity of <Meirenjiao> resides in the phenolic substances; the phenolic substances were shown to have a choleretic action in anesthetized dogs with unligated cystic ducts, and this action was unaltered by atropine, suggesting that it was not mediated by vagal stimulation. Since the bilirubin content in bile was slightly increased following the use of the <Meirenjiao> extract, <Meirenjiao> is not a hydrocholeretic agent (1).

Thus, the actions of <Meirenjiao> to protect the liver, increase bile flow and promote bilirubin excretion are the pharmacological basis for its use in the treatment of acute icteric hepatitis.

3. Effect on Intestinal Musculature

Either <Meirenjiao> or its compound formula reduced the tonicity and contraction amplitude of the isolated rabbit intestine and antagonized intestinal contraction induced by barium chloride or acetylcholine. Hence, the herb has a direct relaxant effect on the intestinal muscle (2).

4. Effect on Blood Pressure

Hypotension promptly developed in anesthetized dogs given the 1:10 <Meirenjiao> solution 1 ml/kg IV; the lowest level was reached in 1–4 minutes and was restored gradually in about 10 minutes. Perfusion into the isolated rabbit ear vein preliminarily showed that this herb caused vasodilation; its acute hypotensive effect was probably due to peripheral vasodilation (2).

5. Toxicity

Intragastric administration of <Meirenjiao> or its compound formula to mice at doses as high as 400 g(crude drug)/kg (200 times the clinical dose) produced no toxic reactions. Intraperitoneal injection of the same dosage did not kill the animals within 24 hours. Intragastric administration of the 1:2 and 1:5 herb solutions or the 1:5 compound formula solution to albino rats at a dose of 7 ml/kg (12 times the clinical dose) for 4 weeks did not result in significant changes in the body weight, activity, hemoglobin, leukocyte and differential count, hepatic and renal functions, and histology of the heart, liver, spleen, kidneys, brain, adrenal glands and duodenum, relative to the control (2).

CLINICAL STUDIES

Out of 63 cases of acute icteric hepatitis treated with the oral decoction of the root of *C. indica* 60–120 g (maximal dose: 250 g) daily divided into 2 doses (morning and evening) for 20 times, 58 were cured and 3 improved. Cure was generally achieved in about 20 days, at most in 47 days. C indica Mixture (300-ml concentrated decoction of Rhizoma Cannae 90 g, Radix Sambuci 30 g, Herba Lespedezae 30 g; the amounts used are to be reduced by half when the dried herbs are used) may be given thrice daily to adults at 100 ml, children under 5 years 40 ml, 6–10 years 60 ml, and 11–19 years 80 ml. In 100 cases, 92 were cured and 8 basically cured. Symptoms and signs were rapidly improved and liver function was either improved or restored to normal. The average time for normalizing the icterus index was 12.8 days; in 67% of the cases, it was 10 days.

GPT was normalized in 22.8 days on average; normal GPT was achieved in 65% of the cases within 20 days. In comparison, the glucose control group had normal icterus index and GPT in 18.2 and 35.3 days, respectively. These results indicate a shorter therapautic course with <Meirenjiao> than with glucose (3–7).

REFERENCE

1. General Hospital of Chengdu Military Region of the Chinese PLA. Studies on Canna indica. 3rd edition. 1980.

2. Infectious Diseases Department, General Hospital of Chengdu Military Region et al. Chinese Traditional and Herbal Drugs Communications 1979 (12):22.

3. Infectious Diseases Department, General Hospital of Chengdu Military Region. Chinese Traditional and Herbal Drugs Communications 1972 (4):37.

4. Dangtu County (Anhui) Hospital. Chinese Traditional and Herbal Drugs Communications 1972 (4):38.

5. Dangtu County (Anhui) Hospital. Wuhu Yiyao (Wuhu Medical Journal) 1974 (1):5.

6. Infectious Diseases Department. Compiled Medical Information (64th Hospital of the Chinese PLA) 1975 (2):102.

7. Qiongzhong County People's Hospital. Health Journal of Hainan 1976 (4):21.

(Liao Nengge)

ZUSHIMA 祖師麻

<Zushima> refers to the bark or root bark of *Daphne giraldii* Nitsche (Thymelaeaceae). Other species from which the herb is derived are *D. retusa* Hemsl. and *D. tangutica* Maxim. (1).

<Zushima> is bitter, pungent, "warm", and slightly toxic. It is antirheumatic, blood-stimulative and analgesic. It is mainly used to treat wounds and injuries, rheumatism, numbness the of limbs, epigastric pain, and stomachache.

CHEMICAL COMPOSITION

<Zushima> contains daphnetin (7,8-dihydroxycoumarin), daphnin (7,8-dihydroxy-coumarin-7-β-D-glucoside) and syringin (2–4). Twelve compounds were isolated from the ether extract of <Zushima> including daphnetin, 7, 8-dimethoxy-coumarin, 7-hydroxy-coumarin, 7-hydroxy-8-methoxycoumarin, 7-methoxy-8-hydroxycoumarin, 4', 5-dihydroxy-7-methoxyflavone, 3, 4, 5-trimethoxybenzoic acid and β-sitosterol (5). It also contains zushima saponin (probably a triterpene, saponin content may reach 10%) and daphnetoxin (6).

Daphnetin also exists in other plants of the same genus; for example, *D. koreana* Nakai (7). Synthesis of daphnetin is in progress(8).

PHARMACOLOGY

1. Analgesic and Sedative Effects

<Zushima> has a pronounced analgesic effect, and daphnetin is its chief bioactive principle. Daphnetin demonstrated a marked analgesic effect in the hot plate method and hot-water tail flick test in mice, as well as in the electrical stimulation method in mice and dogs. The ED_{50} of the daphnetin determined in mice by the hot plate method was 174.3 ± 11.4 mg/kg PO and that by the electrical stimulation method was 296.2 ± 20.6 mg/kg (9). However, in one experiment also using the hot plate method, daphnetin 40 mg/kg IP produced a moderate and prolonged analgesic action in mice (6), while another paper reported maximal analgesia which was attained 15 minutes after 100 mg/kg IP but started to weaken after 30 minutes. The effect obtained was slightly weaker than that of 15 mg/kg of pethidine (10). Injection of 50–100 mg/kg IV to dogs also produced significant analgesia, markedly increasing the pain threshold to electrical stimulation. It has a fast onset but short action (11).

In patients receiving herbal and acupuncture anesthesia various methods, including spatial discrimination threshold, contact pain threshold, pain tolerance threshold, and skin electrical resistance determination, proved that intravenous infusion of daphnetin 5–10 mg/kg had a significant analgesic effect; the pain threshold started to rise 5 minutes after medication, peaked in 10–25 minutes, then slowly declined, and recovered in 60–70 minutes (12).

In addition, daphnetin has a marked sedative effect. The treadmill method proved that daphnetin at 100 mg/kg IP markedly decreased the spontaneous activity of mice, but did not synergize with the subthreshold hypnotic dose of pentobarbital sodium (9,10). However, another report claimed that daphnetin 40 mg/kg significantly synergized with pentobarbital sodium in depressing the CNS (6).

7,8-Dimethoxycoumarin and 7-hydroxy-8-methoxycoumarin were shown in the hot plate test to have a slightly more potent analgesic action than daphnetin in mice; daphnetin had a marked sedative effect and synergized with the subthreshold hypnotic dose of pentobarbital sodium (5).

The ED_{50} of the synthetic daphnetin dimethyl ether in mice determined by the hot plate method was 94.9 ± 7.5 mg/kg PO, and by electrical stimulation method, 146 ± 7.8 mg/kg. This derivative also produced a sedative effect. Possibly due to the increase in its lipid solubility after methylation, the drug was able to cross the blood-brain barrier with relative ease and had reinforced central depressive effect (13). Some of the recently synthesized daphnetin derivatives also had analgesic and hypnotic actions, but their structure-activity relationship has not yet been established (14).

Apart from daphnetin, the zushima saponin 2 g/kg IP also initiated definite analgesic effect in mice; daphnetoxin 40 mg/kg markedly potentiated CNS depression by pentobarbital sodium, and markedly increased the LD_{50} of strychnine in mice, but decreased the LD_{50} of caffeine (6).

2. Anti-inflammatory Effect

Inhibition of egg white- and dextran-induced paw swelling in rats was achieved with the 70% ethanol extract of <Zushima> 1.5 or 2 g/kg IP given 3 hours and 1 hour prior to the induction of inflammation. The anti-inflammatory effect closely resembled that of sodium salicylate 0.5 g/kg. Daily injection of the 70% ethanol extract of the herb 0.5 g/kg IP to rats also markedly inhibited formaldehyde-induced paw swelling and hyperplasia of granulation tissue induced by cotton pledget in rats; its action was stronger than that of butazolidine 0.1 g/kg PO (15). Daphnetin 400 mg/kg PO inhibited egg white- and dextran-induced rat paw swelling with a potency similar to or even slightly greater than that of the same dosage of sodium salicylate (9). Likewise, the dose 20 mg/kg IP inhibited egg white-, dextran- and formaldehyde-induced paw swelling in rats. The anti-inflammatory action disappeared after bilateral adrenalectomy. The drug markedly decreased the vitamin C content of the adrenal glands, but this effect was abolished by hypophysectomy. These results indicate that the anti-inflammatory effect of daphnetin was related to the stimulation of the pituitary-adrenocortical axis. Further experiments proved that pentobarbital sodium blocked the decremental effect of daphnetin on the adrenal vitamin C. After intraperitoneal injections of daphnetin daily for 5 days, the adrenal vitamin C level continued to decrease but this was unaccompanied by significant changes in the ACTH of the anterior pituitary relative to the control. These results suggest that in activating the pituitary-adrenocortical axis daphnetin does not act on the pituitary gland itself, but probably facilitates ACTH release from the pituitary gland through the neurosecretory mechanism of the hypothalamus. And, by accelerating ACTH biosynthesis daphnetin maintains the dyanamic equilibrium of ACTH in the pituitary (16).

However, daphnetin at 20 mg/kg IP did not significantly inhibit egg white-induced paw swelling in rats, whereas the zushima saponin 0.8 g/kg had an anti-inflammatory activity which was as potent as cortisone acetate 30 mg/kg (6). 7,8-Dimethoxycoumarin and 7-hydroxy-8-methoxycoumarin also inhibited egg white-induced paw swelling in rats, though the effect was weaker than that obtained by daphnetin (5).

3. Effect on the Cardiovascular System

Injection of daphnetin to rabbits at 10 mg/kg IV offered protection against pituitrin-induced acute myocardial ischemia. In the isolated rabbit heart and the cat heart *in situ*, daphnetin markedly dilated the coronary vessels and increased the coronary flow. Daphnetin also dilated the blood vessels of isolated rabbit ears and increased the perfusion flow by 1–2 times. Perfusion of D. koreana Injection chiefly composed of daphnetin into the blood vessels of the rat lower limb also markedly increased the blood flow, indicating terminal vasodilation. In mice with myocardial oxygen consumption increased by isoproterenol, daphnetin increased the animals' tolerance to hypobaric hypoxia. Thes results suggest that the mechanisms of the protective effect of daphnetin against pituitrin-induced acute myocardial ischemia involve coronary dilation, increase of coronary flow, peripheral vasodilation, reduction of peripheral vascular resistance, and decrease of myocardial oxygen consumption. In addition, daphnetin significantly protected mice from the deleterious effects of hypobaric as well as normobaric hypoxia, reducing the mortality and prolonging the survival period of the animals (17).

Injection of daphnetin 20–40 mg/kg IV to anesthetized cats produced a hypotensive effect which was blocked neither by bilateral vagotomy nor scopolamine but partially blocked by diphenhydramine. Only a weak action was obtained with the slow intravenous injection. Likewise, injection of daphnetin 40 mg/kg IV to anesthetized rabbits resulted in a transient and weak hypotensive effect (10,17).

4. Miscellaneous Actions

Daphnin was reported to have an anticoagulant action. Thus, administration of this drug to rabbits at 50 mg/kg PO decreased the coagulability of the blood, prolonged the thromboplastin time, lowered the sensitivity of blood to heparin, decreased the activity of factors II, VII and X, and prolonged the reaction time and clotting time in the clot elasticity graph. These results indicate that daphnin is a vitamin K antagonist (18). Daphnin was also a uricosuric (19). At concentrations of 1:2500–10,000 daphnetin markedly inhibited the motility of the isolated rabbit intestine, reducing its tension and contraction amplitude (13). Moreover, daphnetin antagonized pituitrin-induced contraction of isolated rat uterine smooth muscle (17).

Plating tests showed that daphnetin markedly inhibited *Staphylococcus aureus, Escherichia coli, Shigella flexneri*, and *Pseudomonas aeruginosa*, at the MIC of 1:10,000, 1:2000, 1:2000, and

1:1000, respectively. The agent was slightly stronger than the structurally similar fraxetin B (3). Syringin was found to have a hemostatic action (4).

5. *Toxicity*

The LD$_{50}$ of the 70% ethanol extract of <Zushima> in mice were 2.97±0.51 g/kg IP and 3.67±0.75 g/kg PO, while that in rats was 3.91±1.26 g/kg IP (15). The LD$_{50}$ of daphnetin in mice were 3.66±0.28 g/kg PO, 0.48 g/kg IP, and 0.33 g/kg IV (9,10). In another report the LD$_{50}$ were 5.37 g/kg PO and 0.375 g/kg IV (17). Injection of Daphnetin Injection 1.25 g/kg IV to 10 mice killed one of the animals (11). After daily administration of daphnetin 40 and 80 mg/kg for 18 days, autopsies carried out 24 hours as well as 5 days after cessation of treatment showed no significant changes in the heart, liver, spleen, lungs, and kidneys (17). Likewise, injection of this agent to dogs at 20 mg/kg IV daily for 3 days did not cause significant toxic effects, but salivation, vomiting and diarrhea occurred at higher dosages (9). Daily injection of daphnetin 75–94 mg/kg IV to monkeys for 2 weeks did not produce significant changes in routine blood tests, thymol turbidity, zinc turbidity, GPT, and renal function determined at Weeks 1 and 2 of treatment, and one week after cessation of medication. However, bradycardia was observed. Large doses resulted in depression of the J point of the ST segment on the ECG and a slight decrease in food intake during the treatment period. After the intravenous injection, occasional vomiting, reduced spontaneous activity, and slight weight reduction occurred (17).

CLINICAL STUDIES

1. *Analgesia*

In the northwestern and southwestern part of China <Zushima> is commonly used to treat traumatic injuries, hence the Chinese saying: "When knocked down, find <Zushima> quickly". Daphnetin, which has been the subject of chemical and pharmacological studies in recent years, is now used as a new type of analgesic in herbal and acupuncture anesthesia. It has reliable analgesic and mild hypnotic action with low side effects. In some instances, it can replace pethidine (20).

Daphnetin was used clinically to induce anesthesia in 212 cases of surgery (including 107 cases of herbal anesthesia, 44 acupuncture anesthesia, 56 continuous epidural block, 4 intravenous compound anesthesia, and 1 lumbar anesthesia) and in 29 non-operative cases (including 6 thromboangiitis obliterans, 4 peptic ulcer, and 14 operation-wound pain). Analgesia and sedation were achieved in all cases. Doses of 10–15 mg/kg given by intravenous infusion or by a slow single intravenous injection during anesthesia were deemed sufficient. Analgesia usually appeared in 20–30 minutes, peaked in 30 minutes, and started to attenuate after 1 hour; it lasted for 2–3 hours, or in some cases, 4–5 hours (21).

2. Arthritis

The 20% <Zushima> spirit, ointment, or plaster was applied locally to induce blisters. The exudate was aspirated and the blister allowed to from eschars. A total of 111 cases including 50 cases of rheumatic arthritis, 38 cases of benign arthritis, 7 cases of traumatic arthritis, 5 cases of rheumatoid arthritis, 11 cases of lumbago and myalgia were so treated several time with these medications. Sixty-six cases were cured and 38 ameliorated, the aggregate effective rate being 93.7% (22).

Daphnetin was effective in rheumatic and rheumatoid arthritis. Dosage: Oral 150 mg thrice daily increased three days later to 300–450 mg for 3 weeks; medication is then discontinued for one week (23). One hundred and fifty-eight cases of simple arthritis were treated with D. koreana Injection. The effective rate of one therapeutic course was 79% and the aggregate effective rate after two courses was 93% (24).

3. Coronary Disease

D. koreana Injection has therapeutic value in coronary disease and angina pectoris. Out of 72 cases treated, 55 obtained symptomatic improvement, and 35 had improved ECG. The medication also benefitted 35 out of 63 cases with ECG patterns of coronary insufficency and myocardial strain. In addition, it had an anticholesterolemic and β-lipoprotein-lowering effects (25).

4. Thromboangiitis Obliterans

In 72 cases treated with D. koreana Injection and 28 cases treated with daphnetin, an aggregate effective rate of 86% was obtained; 38% had excellent effects. The medications achieved better results in the "cold stasis transformed to heat type" of the first degree third stage. They were less satisfactory in the "extreme heat type" of the second degree third stage, and ineffective in cases complicated with infection. The efficacy of daphnetin has been attributed to the following actions; prevention or amelioration of frostbite, anti-inflammation, terminal vasodilation, and anticoagulation (26).

ADVERSE EFFECTS

<Zushima> produces strong local irritation. Direct local application of the crude drug may cause reddening and blistering of the skin probably due to daphnetoxin; this may be relieved by fresh ginger and licorice (6). In a minority of patients, daphnetin may cause generalized pruritus, rapid intravenous injection may cause a drop in the blood pressure and a rapid pulse rate. The resultant hypotension may be reversed in 15 minutes by rapid fluid infusion, or intravenous infusion of hypertonic glucose solution (27).

REFERENCE

1. Hu ZH. Medical Information (Nanjing College of Pharmacy) 1977 (1):42.

2. Wang MS et al. Chinese Traditional and Herbal Drugs Communications 1976 (10):15.

3. Chinese Traditional Anesthesia Research Unit, Nanjing College of Pharmacy. Xinyiyaoxue Zazhi (Journal of Traditional Chinese Medicine) 1977 (4):40.

4. Wang MS. Chinese Traditional and Herbal Drugs 1980 (8):389.

5. Wang MS et al. Chinese Traditional and Herbal Drugs 1980 (2):49.

6. Gansu Institute for Drug Control et al. Chinese Traditional and Herbal Drugs Communications 1978 (2):25.

7. Phytochemistry Section, Chinese Materia Medica Department of Jilin Institute of Traditional Chinese Medicine and Materia Medica. Xinyiyaoxue Zazhi (Journal of Traditional Chinese Medicine) 1977 (4): 13.

8. Wen Z et al. Traditional Chinese Medicine Research (Jilin Institute of Traditional Chinese Medicine and Materia Medica) 1979 (2):42.

9. Liu GQ et al. Chinese Traditional and Herbal Drugs Communications 1977 (3):21.

10. Chinese Traditional Anesthesia Research Unit, Nanjing College of Pharmacy. Pharmaceutical Information (Nanjing College of Pharmacy) 1977 (1):17.

11. Pharmaceutical Factory, Second Teaching Hospital of Xi' an Medical College. Shaanxi Medical Journal 1976 (4):53.

12. Anesthesia Research Department, Gulou Hospital of Nanjing. Pharmaceutical Information (Nanjing College of Pharmacy) 1977 (1):33.

13. Chinese Traditional Anesthesia Research Unit, Nanjing College of Pharmacy. Pharmaceutical Information (Nanjing College of Pharmacy) 1977 (1):21.

14. Yang ZX. Journal of Nanjing College of Pharmacy 1979 (2):1.

15. Pharmacology Department, Ningxia Medical College. Development of Science and Technology in Ningxia — Medicine and Health 1975 (7):1.

16. Qu SY et al. Xinyiyaoxue Zazhi (Journal of Traditional Chinese Medicine) 1977 (3):46.

17. Qu SY et al. Journal of Traditional Chinese Medicine 1980 21(6):43.

18. Lakini KM et al. Farmakologiia I Toksikologiia 1968 31(1):72.

19. Ishihara T et al. Folia Pharmacologica Japonica 1959 55(2):46.

20. Pharmaceutical Information (Nanjing College of Pharmacy) 1977 (1):1.

21. Nanjing First Municipal Hospital et al. Chinese Traditional and Herbal Drugs Communications 1978 (2):29.

22. Health Division of the Logistics Department of the Chinese PLA. Medical Techniques 1972 (14):55.

23. Traditional Chinese Orthopedics Department, Baixia District (Nanjing) Hospital. Pharmaceutical Information (Nanjing College of Pharmacy) 1977 (1):40.

24. Wang JF et al. Traditional Chinese Medicine Research (Jilin Institute of Traditional Chinese Medicine and Materia Medica) 1979 (2):54.

25. Wang AT et al. Traditional Chinese Medicine Research (Jilin Institute of Traditional Chinese Medinice and Materia Medica) 1979 (2):45; Xinyiyaoxue Zazhi (Journal of Traditional Chinese Medicine) 1977 (4):11.

26. Chen FL et al. Traditional Chinese Medicine Research (Jilin Institute of Traditional Chinese and Materia Medica) 1979 (2):49.

27. Pharmaceutical Information (Nanjing College of Pharmacy) 1977 (1):4.

(Deng Wenlong)

JIANGHUANG 薑黃

<Jianghuang> is the rhizome of *Curcuma longa* L. (*C. domestica* Valeton) (Zingiberaceae). The plant is often used interchangeably with *C. aromatica* Salisb.

The herb has a pungent and bitter taste, a "warm" property, and is nontoxic. Blood- and vital-energy-stimulant, emmenagogue and analgesic actions are ascribed to it. It is mainly used to treat distention of the chest and abdomen, frozen shoulder, obstruction or lump in the abdomen, amenorrhea due to blood stasis, postpartum abdominal pain due to stasis, wounds and injuries, carbuncle, and jaundice. In foreign countries, it is used to treat certain types of hepatitis.

CHEMICAL COMPOSITION

The rhizome of *C. longa* contains 0.3–4.8% of curcumin and 4.5–6% of volatile oil. The volatile oil is composed of turmerone 58%, zingiberene 20%, and small amounts of phellandrene, sesquiterpence alcohols and borneol. Unlike *C. longa*, the major component in the volatile oil of *C. aromatica* is curcumene.

PHARMACOLOGY

1. Antilipemic Effect

The ethanol or ether extract of <Jianghuang>, curcumin, and the volatile oil of the herb administered intragastrically to rats and rabbits with experimental hyperlipidemia significantly lowered serum cholesterol and β-lipoprotein levels. They also reduced liver cholesterol and corrected the imbalanced ratio of α- and β-lipoproteins, but did not affect the endogenous cholesterol (1–4). It was discovered recently that the decremental effect of <Jianghuang> on plasma triglycerides was even more prominent. The herb also reduced the aortic triglyceride and cholesterol levels in rats with experimental hyperlipidemia, suggesting an antiatherosclerotic action (4). Incubation of the liver homogenate with curcumin using ^{14}C-acetic acid as precursor preliminarily revealed that curcumin inhibited the synthesis of fatty acids but not that of cholesterol (5).

2. Effect on Experimental Myocardial Ischemia

Experiments showed that the intragastric dose of the <Jianghuang> extract antagonized ST segment and T wave changes in the rat ECG (6), induced by intravenous injection of pituitrin. Curcumin intragastrically administered to mice increased the myocardial blood flow (7).

3. Anti-platelet Aggregation and Fibrinolytic Effects

It is a well-known medical fact that platelet aggregation and fibrinolytic activity are closely related to the pathogenesis of atherosclerosis, angina pectoris, and myocardial infarction. Experiments showed that both the <Jianghuang> extract and curcumin enhanced the fibrinolytic activity and inhibited platelet aggregation; the volatile oil was devoid of these actions (4).

4. Cholagogic and Choleretic Effects

The <Jianghuang> extract, curcumin, the volatile oil, turmerone, zingiberene, borneol, and sesquiterpenol were found to have cholagogic and choleretic actions, increasing bile formation and secretion, and promoting gallbladder contraction (2,8–12); of these curcumin was the most potent (11), whereas the decoction and extract were found to be weaker (13). Curcumin and the volatile oil also have a very strong antibacterial action (12,14); thus, they are useful in cholecystitis and cholelithiasis (9). It has been reported that the choleretic effect of the herb is related to its antilipemic action (2).

5. Anti-inflammatory Effect

Curcumin was shown in experiments to have a significant anti-inflammatory effect on carrageenin-induced paw swelling in rats and mice. The effect was greatly weakened in the adrenalectomized animals. Curcumin, however, did not decrease the cholesterol and vitamin C contents of the adrenal glands or stimulates the adrenal cortex. Hence, the anti-inflammatory mechanism is not yet clear (15).

6. Antifertility Effect

The petroleum-ether extract of <Jianghuang>, the 95% ethanol extract, and the aqueous extract administered to female rats pregnant for 1–7 days at 100 mg/kg PO produced abortion rates of 100, 70 and 100%, respectively; no deformities were found in the aborted fetuses. These extracts had no influence on copper sulfate-induced ovulation in rabbits (16). The intraperitoneal or subcutaneous doses of the <Jianghuang> decoction afforded an abortion rate of 90–100% in pregnant mice and rabbits at different stages of gestation, but the oral doses were ineffective. The abortifacient effect of <Jianghuang> in mice at early term was antagonized by progesterone. <Jianghuang> also markedly inhibited the growth of traumatic decidual tumor in pseudopregnant mice. Consequently, the early-term abortifacient mechanism of this herb is probably due to the antagonization of progesterone and uterine contraction. Neither estrogenic nor anti-estrogenic activity could be confirmed by checking the increase in weight of the uterus of immature mice (17).

7. Effect on the Uterus

The decoction and the extract of <Jianghuang> had a stimulant effect on the isolated uteri of mice and guinea pigs as well as on the uterine fistulae of rabbits. They intensified paroxysmal contraction of the uterine fistula for 5–7 hours (13).

8. Cardiovascular Effects

The ethanol extract of <Jianghuang> depressed the isolated and *in situ* frog hearts. Hypotension and respiratory stimulation were produced by the intravenous injection. The hypotensive effect was not modified by atropine and vagotomy. High doses caused prostration and death. Pretreatment by injection with ergot fluidextract reversed the hypotensive effect in a fashion similar to the "reversal of berberine action". However, the ether extract had a very weak hypotensive action (18). The decoction and extract had no pronounced effects on the blood pressure and respiration. Administration of large doses by rapid intravenous injection caused hypotension and respiratory depression (13). Curcumin as an intravenous injection had no effect on the blood pressure and did not alter the effect of epinephrine, histamine, and acetylcholine on blood pressure. It did not affect contraction of the nictitating membrane induced by stimulation of the preganglionic sympathetic nerves. In other words, it had no ganglionic blocking action (15).

9. Antimicrobial Effect

At a concentration of 1:1,000,000, curcumin was shown *in vitro* to be an inhibitor of *Micrococcus pyogenes* var. *aureus* (14). The volatile oil had a strong antifungal action (12). <Jianghuang> prolonged the survival period of mice inoculated with virus and mitigated liver damage (19).

10. Miscellaneous Actions

<Jianghuang> was found to be lethal to files (18). It precluded the elevation of SGPT and SGOT in rats with formaldelyde-induced paw swelling. It also had antipyretic and analgesic actions (15).

11. Toxicity

In literature on the subject of traditional Chinese medicines and work published abroad it is reported that <Jianghuang> is nontoxic. The ethanol extract 40–100 g (crude drug) PO did not kill test mice observed over 3 days. The <Jianghuang> extract mixed in rat feed at doses of 5, 2 and 0.5 g/kg (equivalent to 50, 20 and 5 times the clinical dose) for 3 days produced no significant pathological changes in the heart, liver, kidney, aorta, or adrenal glands of the animals (6). The LD_{50} of curcumin in mice was over 2 g/kg PO (15).

CLINICAL STUDIES

1. Hyperlipidemia

In 16 cases of hyperlipidemia treated with Rhizoma Curcumae Longae Extract Tablet (equivalent to 3.5 g(crude drug)/tablet) 5 tablets thrice daily for 12 weeks, the blood cholesterol was reduced by a mean of 49 mg% of the pretreatment level, whilst the triglyceride level was down by 62 mg%. Its therapeutic effect was at least equal to that of the control drug, clofibrate (20). In a recent report on 90 cases of hyperlipidemia treated with this herb, cholesterol and triglyceride were reduced in 95.5 and 100%, respectively; again the effect on the triglycerides was more prominent (21).

2. Angina Pectoris

The Chinese herbal classic "Ben Cao Shu" states that the <Jianghuang> powder "cures intolerable precordial pain". According to "Yang Shi Jia Cang Fang" (Secret Prescriptions of the Yang Family), the <Jianghuang> powder "cures nine types of attacks of precordial pain. The herb has apparently been used by Chinese herbalists since early times to treat angina pectoris. The "Sheng Ji Zong Lu" (Imperial Encyclopedia of Medicine) lists the composition of the <Jianghuang> powder as follows: Rhizoma Curcumae Longae, Radix Angelicae Sinensis, Radix Aucklandiae and Radix Linderae. In recent years, it has been reported that the use of <Jianghuang> in hyperlipidemia also ameliorated angina pectoris (20,21).

3. Miscellaneous

<Jianghuang> was used to treat stomachache, cholelithiasis, jaundice and postpartum abdominal pain, in the form of powder or decoction given at 1–6 g daily in divided doses (10).

ADVERSE EFFECTS

<Jianghuang> had no untoward effects on hepatic and renal functions and in the routine urinalysis (20). Frequent bowel movement and mild gastric discomfort may occur in individual patients (21).

REFERENCE

1. Srinivasan M et al. Indian Journal of Experimental Biology 1964 2:104.
2. Rao DS et al. Journal of Nutrition 1970 100:1307.
3. Pachauri SR et al. Journal of Research on Indian Medicine 1970 5(1):27.
4. Xue CS et al. Xinyiyaoxue Zazhi (Journal of Traditional Chinese Medicine) 1978 (9):59.
5. Xue CS et al. Abstracts of the First National Symposium on Cardiovascular Pharmacology. 1980. p. 62.

6. He GQ et al. Abstracts of the First National Symposium on Cardiovascular Pharmacology. 1980. p. 21.

7. He GQ et al. Acta Academiae Medicinae Chongqing 1979 (1):86.

8. Jentzsch K et al. Pharm Acta Helv 1959 34:181.

9. Robbers H. Archives of Experimental Pathology and Pharmacology 1936 181:328.

10. Ramprasad C et al. Chemical Abstracts 1957 51:16946f.

11. Ramprasad C et al. J Sci Industr Res 1956 15c:262.

12. Sawada T et al. The Japanese Journal of Pharmacognosy 1971 25:11.

13. Zhang YZ. Chinese Medical Journal 1955 (5):400.

14. Ibragimov FI. Osnovye Lekarstvennye Sredstva Kitaiskoi Meditsina. Medgiz. 1960. p. 116

15. Srimal RC et al. Journal of Pharmacy and Pharmacology 1973 25(6):447.

16. Gray SK. Planta Medica 1974 26(3):225.

17. Zhang YG et al. Chinese Pharmaceutical Bulletin 1980 (10):40.

18. Jiangsu College of New Medicine. Encyclopedia of Chinese Materia Medica. Shanghai People's Publishing House. 1975. p. 1735.

19. Wang JM. Shanghai Zhongyiyao Zazhi (Shanghai Journal of Traditional Chinese Medicine) 1956 (1):36.

20. Coronary Disease Group of the Internal Medicine Department, First and Second Teaching Hospitals. Acta Academiae Medicinae Chongqing 1979 (1):88.

21. He LY et al. People's Military Medicine 1980 (9):42.

(Xue Chunsheng)

CHUCHONGJU 除蟲菊

<Chuchongju> is the flower of *Pyrethrum cinerariifolium* Trev. (*Chrysanthemum cinerariaefolium* Vis.) (Compositae). The whole plant is used as medicine. <Chuchongju> is bitter, "cool" and toxic. It is an insecticide and is useful in the treatment of scabies.

CHEMICAL COMPOSITION

The main insecticidal components in the flower of *P. cinerariifolium* are pyrethrins I and II. Cinerins I and II also have insecticidal properties (1). The flower also contains pyrethrosin (chrysanthin), β-cyclopyrethrosin, chrysanthene and pyrethrone. Hydrolysis of the last yields pyrethol (2). The insecticidal components are sensitive to light, easily inactivated by hydrolysis, and readily biodegradated.

Since the plants has a very low toxicity to mammals, leaves hardly any residue after use and dose not pollute the environment, many derivatives of pyrethrin have been synthesized recently. These derivatives have a much stronger insecticidal effect and are more stable (1).

PHARMACOLOGY

1. Insecticidal Effect

<Chuchongju> is lethal to many insects such as the mosquito, fly, bedbug, and cockcroach, causing overexcitation, ataxia, and paralysis within 1–2 minutes of contact. Some insects may recover after one day. Concomitant use of sesamin, asarinin, or piperine with this herb produced a synergistic effect (3). But pyrethrosin etc. had no insecticidal activity.

Pyrethrin is a typical neurotoxin acting directly on the excitable membranes and disrupting ion conduction. It primarily affects the sodium channel, delaying the disappearance of increased sodium conduction caused by stimulation, prolonging the transmembranous sodium flux, and consequently causing repeated firing of the sensory and the motor neurons, brief depolarization of neurons, and sustained muscular contraction. High concentrations, on the other hand, inhibited the neuronal membrane ion conduction and blocked excitation (1).

No significant correlation between the neurotoxic action and the insecticidal activity has been observed so far. Some pyrethrin derivatives were found to have a strong action on nerves but a weak insecticidal action, or vice versa (1).

2. Toxicity

The pyrethrins are marginally toxic to mammals and are much safer than most organic insecticides. The oral dose was rapidly metabolized in the body with no substantial residues (1). On the other hand, intravenous injection of pyrethrin I was very toxic to mammals (4). There is no evidence for the presumed action of these compounds on insects and invertebrates, but widely different actions were observed in various vertebrates. The symptoms of intoxication in vertebrates resembled those seen in insects; overexcitation and tremors appeared a few minutes after medication (1). Mammals were less sensitive to the oral doses of pyrethrin; this could be partly due to rapid metabolism and poor gastrointestinal absorption of the drug. The insecticidal activity of the pyrethrins on mammals whether given intravenously or intragastrically did not vary with their toxicity (4).

Pyrethrosin was shown to be toxic to warm-blooded animals; injection of 52 mg/kg SC to rabbits caused death within 48 hours (2).

CLINICAL STUDIES

1. As Insect Repellent

<Chuchongju> is often used to make mosquito-repellent incense. The 1% oil preparation of <Chuchongju> applied to the skin repelled mosquitoes for approximately three hours. A good antimalarial effect was achieved by a similar preparation used by the Indian army (5).

2. Eradication of the Mosquito, Fly, Louse, etc.

The kerosene preparation of the herb is commonly used. Maggots in manure jars may be eradicated by sprinkling the inside of the jars with the powdered <Chuchongju> (6).

3. Scabies

The available preparations are the <Chuchongju> powder and the 5% ointment, but they are not as efficacious as sulfur.

ADVERSE EFFECTS

In sensitive person, skin rash, rhinitis, or asthma may develop upon contact with <Chuchongju> preparations. Poisoning due to the orally ingested herb triggers nausea, vomiting, gastrointestinal colic, diarrhea, headache, tinnitus, nightmares and syncope. Convulsions may occur in children (6).

REFERENCE

1. Wouters W et al. (reviewer). General Pharmacology 1978 9(6):387.

2. Zhao CG et al. Chinese Journal of Physiology 1934 8(2):167.

3. Huang RL. Ziran Kexue (Natural Sciences) 1952 2(2):135.

4. Elliott M et al. Nature 1973 244:456.

5. Zhang BH et al. Chinese Journal of Health 1958 (2):101.

6. Editorial Group. National Collection of Chinese Materia Medica. Vol. 2. People's Medical Publishing House. 1975. p. 449.

(Xue Chunsheng)

QINJIAO 秦艽

<Qinjiao> refers to the root of *Gentiana macrophylla* Pall., *G. straminea* Maxim., *G. crassicaulis* Duthie, or *G. dahurica* Fisch. (Gentianaceae). Bitter and pungent to the taste and with a "mild" property, the herb is antirheumatic, channel-deobstruent, muscle-relaxant, antipyretic, and analgesic. It is prescribed in rheumatism, pain of joints and extremities, muscle spasm, hectic fever in pulmonary tuberculosis, fever in children due to nutritional disorders, and jaundice.

CHEMICAL COMPOSITION

<Qinjiao> contains alkaloids gentianine, gentianine and gentianol, gentiopicroside, carbohydrates, and volatile oil.

PHARMACOLOGY

1. Anti-inflammatory Effect

Gentianine was shown to mitigate formaldehyde-induced paw swelling in rats and accelerate its subsidence. Swelling was basically relieved by injection of 90 mg/kg IP daily for 10 days; the anti-inflammatory efficacy was equivalent to that of sodium salicylate 200 mg/kg (1). Likewise, pretreatment with gentianine injection 90 mg/kg also reduced egg white-induced paw swelling in rats and accelerated its subsidence. However, gentianine was ineffective in bilaterally adrenalectomized rats and in normal rats anesthetized with pentobarbital sodium (2). Another experiment proved that gentianine markedly and dose-dependently decreased the vitamin C content in the rat adrenal glands. No such action, however, was achieved in hypophysectomized animals and in animals under pentobarbital sodium anesthesia (1). Hence, it is postulated that the anti-inflammatory effect of <Qinjiao> was realized through activation of the pituitary-adrenocortical function via the nervous system. The dye diffusion method, moreover, showed that injection of gentianine 90 mg/kg IP to rats markedly decreased capillary permeability boosted by injection of egg white (3).

2. Effect on the Central Nerous System

<Qinjiao> was shown to have sedative, analgesic, and antipyretic actions, and an inhibitory effect on the reflex intestinal secretion. Intragastric or intraperitoneal administration of gentianine to mice produced sedation; it also potentiated the hypnotic action of pentobarbital sodium in mice and rats.

However, central stimulation leading to paralysis and death occurred with increased dosages (>364 mg/kg IP) (3,4).

The hot plate method proved that the analgesic action of <Qinjiao> in mice could be reinforced and prolonged when the seeds of *Hyoscyamus niger*, the rhizome of *Corydalis turtschaninovii* f. *yanhusuo*, and the root tuber of *Aconitum chinense* were used concomitantly. However, no synergism was observed between <Qinjiao> and morphine (5). It was proved that injection of gentianine at 90 mg/kg IP to rats exposed to heat radiation elevated the pain threshold by 47% after 20 minutes, but the effect disappeared after 40 minutes (3).

Gentianine at 20–40 mg/kg SC, IP or IV dose-dependently inhibited the reflex intestinal secretion in dogs due to perfusion of mercurous chloride into the intestinal fistulae (4).

3. Antianaphylactic Shock and Antihistaminic Effect

Injection of gentianine 90 mg/kg IP to rabbits markedly decreased the symptoms of egg white-induced anaphylactic shock (3). The same dosage administered intraperitoneally to guinea pigs also markedly abated asthma and convulsion induced by histamine aerosol (3).

4. Hyperglycemic Effect

Injection of gentianine 180–250 mg/kg IP to rats elevated the blood glucose level 30 minutes after medication; the duration of action was approximately 3 hours. The dosages of 150–250 mg/kg IP also produced hyperglycemia in mice; the higher the dosage, the stronger the action. The hyperglycemic effect of gentianine injection did not appear in adrenalectomized animals however. Also, a significant reduction of liver glycogen was observed concurrent with hyperglycemia. Adrenergic blocking agents partially or completely blocked the hyperglycemic action of gentianine, indicating that it was mediated primarily by the release of epinephrine (6).

5. Effect on the Cardiovascular System

Gentianine had prominent but brief hypotensive and bradycardic effects on anesthetized dogs and rabbits. Blood pressure was lowered promptly and dose-dependently after injection of 5–20 mg/kg IV. However, the original blood pressure was usually recovered in 2–10 minutes and no tachyphylaxis developed. Neither intravenous injection of atropine nor bilateral vagotomy blocked the hypotensive effect, indicating that it was not related to the vagus nerve. Gentianine also depressed the isolated frog heart: At the concentration of 1:2,000 the gentianine infusion progressively reduced the heart rate, while increasing the concentration to >1:1000 caused insufficient diastole and decreased cardiac output apart from bradycardia. The hypotensive effect is probably secondary to direct cardiac depression (3).

6. *Effect on Smooth Muscles*

Injection of gentianine 5–20 mg/kg IV to anesthetized dogs did not modify the ileal movement. Likewise, concentrations of 1:10,000–1:2500 had no effect on the movement of the isolated guinea pig ileum, but antagonized histamine- and acetylcholine-induced intestinal contractions. The 1:5000 concentration virtually antagonized the action of histamine but not quite that of acetylcholine (3).

7. *Bacteriostatic Effect*

In vitro, the ethanol extract of <Qinjiao> inhibited *Shigella dysenteriae*, *Salmonella typhi*, *Vibrio cholerae*, and *Staphylococcus aureus* (7). The aqueous extract (1:3) also exhibited various degrees of inhibitory effect on some common skin fungi *in vitro* (8).

8. *Toxicity*

The LD_{50} of gentianine in mice were determined to be 486 mg/kg PO and 300 mg/kg IP (3). No significant ill effects were observed after a single dose of 420–520 mg/kg PO in rats, a single dose of 240 mg/kg PO or 80 mg/kg IV in dogs, or 100 mg/kg PO once daily for 3 days in monkeys and cats. In subacute toxicity tests, injection of gentianine to rats at doses of 50, 90 and 120 mg/kg IP once daily for 14 days did not produce changes in the physical appearance of the animals, but pathological examination revealed the presence of protein in the glomeruli and renal tubules as well as pulmonary edema in some animals (3).

CLINICAL STUDIES

1. *Rheumatic or Rheumatoid Arthritis*

<Qinjiao> is one of the important ingredients in many antirheumatic compound prescriptions such as Decoction of Angelica pubescens-Loranthus parasiticus, and Major Gentiana macrophylla Decoction. The herb is mainly used in rheumatic arthritis. G. macrophylla Injection, 2 ml/ampoule, is a sterilized solution of the total alkaloids of <Qinjiao>; each ampoule contains total alkaloids equivalent to 10 mg of gentianine. It is administered intramuscularly to treat rheumatic and rheumatoid arthritis. Excellent analgesic, detumescent, and antipyretic effects, as well as a restorative effect on articular function were achieved with this agent (9). However, an early report suggested that orally administered gentianine was not altogether effective in rheumatic arthritis (3).

2. *Epidemic Cerebrospinal Meningitis*

In twenty-one cases cured in 3–7 days by injection of G. macrophylla Injection, 0.625 g(crude drug)/ml, 2–5 ml IM every 6 hours, not a single case developed sequelae or side effects during treatment (10).

ADVERSE EFFECTS

Four cases of rheumatic arthritis given gentianine 100 mg PO thrice daily for 4–13 days experienced severe nausea and vomiting, successively. Palpitation and bradycardia occurred in one case after receiving the 100-mg dose, but the patient recovered rapidly (3).

REFERENCE

1. Song ZY et al. Acta Physiologica Sinica 1958 22(3):201.

2. Ji XJ et al. Acta Physiologica Sinica 1959 23(2):151.

3. Liu GT et al. Acta Physiologica Sinica 1959 23(3):203.

4. Chen XY. Acta Physiologica Sinica 1959 23(4):311.

5. 47–12 Class of Shenyang Medical College. Medical Research of Shenyang Medical College 1958 (2):8.

6. Xu LN et al. Acta Pharmaceutica Sinica 1965 12(6):357.

7. Wang Y et al. Acta Botanica Sinica 1954 3(2):121.

8. Cao RL et al. Chinese Journal of Dermatology 1957 (4):286.

9. Editorial Department. National Medical Journal of China 1978 (7):444.

10. Yiyang County Institute of Medical Sciences. Harbin Zhongyi (Harbin Journal of Traditional Chinese Medicine) 1960 3(5):27.

(Zeng Zhaoxian)

QINPI 秦皮

<Qinpi> is the dried bark or branch of *Fraxinus rhynchophylla* Hance. (*F. chinensis* Roxb. var. *rhyncophylla* (Hance) Hemsl.), *F. chinensis* Roxb., *F. bungeana* DC., *F. paxiana* Lingelsh., or *F. stylosa* Lingelsh. (Oleaceae). Also called <Huaquliu>, the herb is bitter, puckery, and "cold". It has "damp-heat" clearing, antiasthmatic, antitussive, and vision-improving effects and is reputed to purge the liver of intense heat. It is useful in dysentery, leukorrhea, swollen eyes, conjunctivitis, corneal opacity, and arthralgia.

CHEMICAL COMPOSITION

<Qinpi> contains coumarins fraxetin, fraxin, aesculin and its aglycone aescuktin, and tannin. The bark of *F. rhynchophylla* additionally contains alkaloids.

PHARMACOLOGY

1. Antibacterial Effect

In vitro, the <Qinpi> decoction was inhibitory but not lethal to *Staphylococcus aureus, Escherichia coli, Shigella flexneri*, and *Shigella sonnei* (1,2). The MIC of aescuktin against *Neisseria catarrhalis, Staphylococcus aureus, Escherichia coli*, and *Shigella flexneri* were 1:2500, 1:2000, 1:1000, and 1:2000, respectively. Aesculin, at concentrations of 10–20 mg/100 ml, inhibited *Staphylococcus aureus, Neisseria catarrhalis*, alpha streptococcus, and *Neisseria gonorrhoeae* (3).

2. Anti-inflammatory Effect

Aesculin and fraxin markedly inhibited the increase of capillary permeability induced by histamine but were inactive against bradykinin (4,5). Aescuktin and aesculin inhibited the erythematous reaction of the back of guinea pigs to ultraviolet irradiation: the former agent was found to be more potent (4). A significant anti-inflammatory effect on egg white- and dextran-induced paw swelling in rats was achieved with aescuktin 100 or 200 mg/kg IP, manifested by the amelioration and rapid subsidence of ankle-joint swelling. The dosage used in this experiment for both aescuktin and sodium salicylate was the same — 200 mg/kg; but that of the former was only one-half of the LD_{50} in mice, and that of the latter was one-third of the LD_{50}. Obviously, the effect of aeskutin on these two pathological models was more potent than sodium salicylate (6). Aesculin at 10 mg/kg IP inhibited rat paw swelling induced by carrageenin, dextran, and serotonin. Its inhibitory effect was weaker on paw swelling due to formaldehyde than on that elicited by carrageenin. In addition, aesculin inhibited cotton pledget-induced granulation in rats. Fraxin at 10 mg/kg IP inhibited paw swelling in rats induced by carrageenin, dextran, formaldehyde, and histamine. It was found to be more potent than aesculin, with effective rates of 49, 53, 64, and 27%, respectively. It was less potent than aesculin in inhibiting serotonin- and bradykinin-induced paw swelling (7).

Another report claimed that six hours after injection of aescuktin 200 mg/kg IP to rats, the vitamin C content of the adrenal glands was calculated to be 258 mg/100 g (glandular weight) which was much lower than in the control group (308 mg/100 g glandular weight). The anti-inflammatory action of aescuktin, therefore, probably relates to the stimulation of the adrenocortical function (6).

3. Effect on the Cardiovascular System

Aescuktin (1:2000) was shown to inhibit the isolated toad heart, whereas aesculin (1:1000) slightly stimulated it. These agents had no significant action on the toad heart *in situ*. Experiments showed that both aescuktin (1:2000) and aesculin (1:1000) perfused into the isolated rabbits auricular vessels were not significantly active, whereas aescuktin (1:2000) perfused into the blood vessels of the toad hind limb caused vasoconstriction. Aescuktin or aesculin 3–10 mg/kg administered intravenously to anesthetized cats or rabbits caused mild hypertension lasting for 30 minutes; this effect was not accompanied by any significant change in the respiration (6).

4. Antitussive, Expectorant, and Antiasthmatic Effects

A significant antitussive action was demonstrated by intraperitoneal injection of the aescuktin suspension or aesculin aqueous solution 320 mg/kg in mice with cough induced by ammonia solution aerosol. The phenol red excretion method proved that these two agents have significant expectorant actions. Aescuktin 12.5 g/kg produced a significant antiasthmatic effect in histamine-dosed guinea pigs. In addition, the 0.25% aescuktin also had smooth-muscle relaxant and antihistaminic effects on isolated guinea pig bronchi (3).

5. Sedative, Anticonvulsant and Analgesic Effects

Administration of aescuktin or aesculin 100 mg/kg IP or PO to mice markedly prolonged cyclobarbital-induced sleep; the former agent was more potent than the latter. Injection of aescuktin 100 mg/kg IP mice antagonized electroshock and also delayed the onset of convulsion induced by strychnine and pentylenetetrazole. The herb was also shown to have an analgesic action: Using the Nilser method, it was demonstrated that injection of aescuktin 100 mg/kg IP to mice resulted in an analgesic rate of 70% against 75% obtained with codeine 25 mg/kg and 80% from aspirin 500 mg/kg. Although their analgesic rates are quite close, these is a great disparity in the dosage administered.

Thus, the analgesic effect of aescuktin was deemed to be stronger than that of aspirin but weaker than that of codeine (6). As proved in the hot plate method, the analgesic efficacy of aesculin 10 mg/kg PO in mice was 14.8% of that produced by morphine 5 mg/kg SC (8).

6. Effect on Smooth Muscles

Aescuktin, at a concentration of 1:2500 inhibited the isolated rabbits intestinal muscle and the isolated rat uterus, as manifested by the decrease in contraction amplitude, prolongation of the relaxed phase, and reduction in contraction frequency; the effect of aesculin on smooth muscles was inconspicuous (6,9).

7. Effects on Urine Output and Uric Acid Excretion

Early studies reported that fraxin exerted diuretic and uricosuric actions in rheumatic patients (10,11). Aesculin administered to rabbits via different routes increased the excretion of uric acid; injection of the drug into the ear vein triggered an initial increase followed by a decrease in the urine output, and augmented uric acid excretion (12,13). Uricosuria is attributed to the stimulation of the sympathetic nervous system and also to a direct action on the kidneys, thereby suppressing the reabsorption of uric acid (12).

8. Pharmacokinetics

The orally administered aesculin was absorbed from the upper small intestine, but not from the stomach and large intestine (12). After intravenous injection of ^{3}H-aesculin to guinea pigs, high drug levels were found in the adrenal glands, testicles, and especially in the kidneys. Four hours after the intravenous injection in rats, the highest concentration was detected in the mitochondria of the renal medulla, next in the cell nucleus and then in the microsome. The drug also appeared in the gallbladder and brain. In rats, the oral or intravenous dose was disposed of primarily unchanged in the urine and feces (13,14). But it was largely metabolized in guinea pigs (14,15).

9. Toxicity

Aescuktin and aesculin have low toxic profiles. The LD_{50} of aesculin in mice was 11.5 g/kg PO, whereas that of aescuktin was 39 g/kg (6). The MLD of the latter compound was 250 mg/kg IV. Sedation, convulsion, coma, and death from respiratory paralysis were associated with poisoning from aescuktin and aesculin. No toxic reactions were observed after administration of aescuktin 1 g/kg PO daily to mice for 2 weeks (9). Fraxetin and fraxin could paralyze the CNS in mice and rabbits, causing respiratory arrest and death (10).

CLINICAL STUDIES

1. Bacillary Dysentery

1.1 The <Qinpi> decoction (18 g of crude drug/40 ml) was used to treat 50 children with bacillary dysentery; 21 of them had positive stool culture. The daily dosage for patients under 1 year (11 cases) was 8–10 ml; for 1–3 years (16 cases), 10 ml; and for over 3 years (24 cases), 15 ml; divided into four doses by mouth. Each course lasted 7–14 days. Treatment was discontinued during midcourse in 2 cases because of severe vomiting. Body temperature and bowel movement were normalized in an average of 1.9 and 8.1 days, respectively. There days after medication all 21 cases registered negative in the stool culture; the average cure rate was 80%.

1.2 Fraxetin 50–100 mg/kg/day divided into 2–3 doses for 5–6 days was used to treat 77 children with acute bacillary dysentery; the effective rate was over 70%; the antibacterial rate was higher in cases receiving high dosages (16). Aescuktin 5 mg/kg daily was employed in 67 cases; a cure was achieved in 4 cases, improvement in 11, and no response in 15 (17).

2. Chronic Bronchitis

The 1:1 <Qinpi> aerosol, 2 ml each time for a course of 10 applications, was used to treat 422 cases. Two courses were generally required. The extract tablet (0.3 g of the extract/tablet), 2 tablets thrice daily for 3 courses (each lasting 10 days), was employed in 50 cases. These medications were very effective for the short-term control of dyspnea (18).

3. Miscellaneous

The eye wash prepared from the decoction of 5–15 g <Qinpi>, the seed of *Cassia tora* and whole *Equisetum hiemale*, or the oral decoction of <Qinpi>, the rhizome of *Coptis chinensis*, and the stem and leaf of *Lophatherum gracile* was efficacious in conjunctivitis.

ADVERSE EFFECTS
The <Qinpi> decoction has low toxicity; vomiting was its sole side effect (19).

REFERENCE

1. Zhejiang People's Academy of Health. Preliminary Studies on the in vitro Antibacterial Action of 200 Kinds of Chinese Traditional Drugs. 1970.

2. Changzhou First People's Hospital. Health Information (Changzhou Health Bureau) 1975 (9):40.

3. General Hospital of Shenyang Military Region of the Chinese PLA. Chinese Traditional and Herbal Drugs Communications 1973 (6):13.

4. Yamagmi I et al. Chemical Abstracts 1970 72:53570d.

5. Japan Centra Revuo Medicina 1972 285(5):570, Vide Jiangsu College of New Medicine. Encyclopedia of Chinese Materia Medica. Vol. 2. Shanghai People' s Publishing House. 1977. p. 1768.

6. Hu YH et al. Xinyiyaoxue Zazhi (Journal of Traditional Chinese Medicine) 1975 (8):41.

7. Nakaya S. Folia Pharmacologica Japonica 1970 66(2):18.

8. Folia Pharmacologica Japonica 1972 68(1):25p.

9. Li J et al. Journal of Peking Medical College 1943 (5):180.

10. Watanabe C. Folia Pharmacologica Japonica 1947 43(2):35.

11. Japan Centra Revuo Medicina 1937 54:273, Vide Jiangsu College of New Medicine. Encyclopedia of Chinese Materia Medica.

12. Nakaya S et al. Folia Pharmacologica Japonica 1969 65(2):113.

13. Nakaya S et al. Folia Pharmacologica Japonica 1968 64(1):45.

14. Folia Pharmacologica Japonica 1970 66(4):139.

15. Folia Pharmacologica Japonica 1971 67(2):199.

16. Zhang XZ et al. Shanghai Zhongyiyao Zazhi (Shanghai Journal of Traditional Chinese Medicine) 1962 (9):30.

17. Yu DX et al. Chinese Journal of Paediatrics 1962 11(5):353.

18. 211th Hospital of Shenyang PLA Units et al. Chinese Traditional and Herbal Drugs Communications 1973 (1):21.

19. First Teaching Hospital of Xi' an Medical College. Chinese Journal of Paediatrics 1959 10(3):237.

(Chen Jiayu)

GUIZHI 桂枝

<Guizhi> is the tender twig of *Cinnamomum cassia* Presel. (Lauraceae). It is sweet, pungent and "warm". It has diaphoretic, muscle-relaxant, channel-warming and -deobstruent effects. It is used to treat common cold, myalgia, arthralgia, and amenorrhea with abdominal cramp.

CHEMICAL COMPOSITION

See under <Rougui> or bark of *Cinnamomum cassia* Presl.

PHARMACOLOGY

1. Effect on the CNS

1.1 *Sedative effect. Cinnamic aldehyde* isolated from <Guizhi> produced a significant sedative effect in mice. The oral doses 250–500 mg/kg diminished the spontaneous activity, and antagonized methamphetamine-induced euphoria as well as rod rotation-induced ataxia in the animals. It also prolonged cyclobarbital sodium-induced sleep (1). EEG determination further proved its sedative action. It was found that in rabbits with subcortically implanted electrodes, the dose of 50 mg/kg IP tended to increase the low amplitude fast wave and slightly prolong the arousal wave (response to sound) (1).

1.2 *Anticonvulsant effect.* Injection of cinnamic aldehyde 500 mg/kg IP to mice delayed the death of the animals from tonic convulsions induced by strychnine, but did not antagonize the effect of pentylenetetrazole. Administration of Radix Bupleuri-Ramulus Cinnamomi Decoction 4 g/kg PO daily to mice for 11 days markedly antagonized audiogenic seizures (2). The decoction was also shown to have an anticonvulsant effect on experimental convulsions of the nerve ganglions of snail gastropodia. The 2% powdered extract of Radix Bupleuri-Ramulus Cinnamomi Decoction inhibited changes in the action potentials of the ganglionic cells of snail gastropodia; these changes resembled those induced by pentylenetetrazole in the cat cortical cells during convulsion. The individual drugs of this prescription — Radix Bupleuri, Ramulus Cinnamomi, Radix Paeoniae, and Rhizoma Zingiberis Recens — also exerted similar inhibitory actions, indicating that all of them had an anticonvulsant effect (3).

1.3 *Analgesic effect. Cinnamic aldehyde* had no significant analgesic effect on mice as proved in the tail pressure method, but it weakly inhibited writhing induced by intraperitoneal injection of acetic acid (1).

1.4 *Antipyretic effect.* A hypothermic action was exhibited in mice with normal body temperature, and an antipyretic action in rabbits with typhoid or paratyphoid vaccine-induced fever, by the <Guizhi> decoction, cinnamic aldehyde, and sodium cinnamate (1,4). Due to their central and peripheral actions, these drugs caused cutaneous vasodilation (5), regulated blood circulation, and directed blood flow towards the body surface, thus promoting heat dissipation and diaphoresis.

2. Blood-Stimulant and Emmenagogic Effects

The oil of <Guizhi> bark has been shown to have a specific hyperemic effect on the uterus and has been used since ancient times to induce abortion. Because of its specific hyperemic effect, and dilative effect on rabbits capillaries, it is postulated that <Guizhi> potentiates the blood-stimulant and stasis-eliminative actions of other drugs, such as Ramulus Cinnamomi-Poria Pill (6).

3. Antitussive Effect

The pulmonary excretion of the absorbed <Guizhi> bark oil thinned bronchial secretions, thus producing expectorant and antitussive effects (7).

4. Diuretic Effect

Injection of the <Guizhi>-containing "Wuling San" (Five-Drug Powder of Poria) to the ureteral fistulae of unanesthetized dogs at 0.25 g/kg IV markedly increased the urine output; among the ingredients in this powder, <Guizhi> had the most potent diuretic action. It is therefore inferred to be the chief diuretic principle of this prescription (8).

5. Effect on the Immunologic Function

In the study on nephritis, it was found that the <Guizhi> extract inhibited the activation of complements in the heterophil antibody reaction, and it is thought to have a strong antiallergic effect. Thus, "Wuling San" is efficacious in allergic nephritis. It was also discovered that Radix Bupleuri-Ramulus Cinnamomi Decoction was also effective in allergic dermatitis or urticaria, and its chief antiallergic agent is believed to be <Guizhi> (9,10).

6. Antibacterial Effect

The <Guizhi> decoction was a potent inhibitor of *Staphylococcus aureus* and *S. albus, Salmonella typhi* and common pathogenic skin fungi (11,12): The cinnamic oil and cinnamic aldehyde inhibited *Mycobacterium tuberculosis* (13,14). Likewise, the <Guizhi> decoction (1:20) inhibited type A Asian influenza virus Jingke 68–1 strain and $ECHO_{11}$ virus (15).

7. Toxicity

Refer to the monograph on <Rougui>.

CLINICAL STUDIES

1. Epilepsy

Satisfactory results can be achieved with Radix Bupleuri-Ramulus Cinnamomi Decoction Plus Radix Paeoniae in the treatment of epilepsy. Out of 433 treated cases (mostly with poor response to other anticonvulsants), 115 were cured and 79 markedly improved; the markedly effective rate was 44.8%. Many cases achieved stable and long-term therapeutic effects, while the EEG patterns were improved and epileptic attacks controlled in some. Comparative analysis of the clinical symptoms and EEG in 123 cases revealed disappearance of epileptic waves along with cessation of the seizures in 46% of the cases and residual epileptic waves in 38% of asymptomatic cases (16).

2. Common Cold of the "Wind-Cold Type", Rheumatism, Cough, Dyspnea, "Retention of Phlegm and Fluid", Amenorrhea and Abdominal Cramp

The usual dosage is 3–9 g given as decoction by mouth (17).

2.1 *Prophylaxis of influenza.* The Compound Ramulus Cinnamomi Aerosol (Ramulus Cinnamomi and Herba Elsholtziae, each 12.5 g, enough for as many as 150 applications), is sprayed into the pharynx twice daily to prevent influenza. This drug is reported to have reduced the incidence of influenza and cold and also markedly decreased their symptoms, in the general population (18).

3. Cardiac and Renal Edema

<Guizhi> is usually used with the sclerotium of *Poria cocos*. "Wuling San" can be used for allergic nephritis (10,17)

4. Miscellaneous

Prescriptions composed of <Guizhi> and the root of *Angelica sinensis* etc. have therapeutic value in the management of frostbite (19). One case of hysteromyoma was reportedly cured after taking 60 doses of the modifed Ramulus Cinnamomi-Poria Pill (20).

REFERENCE

1. Harada M et al. Journal of the Pharmaceutical Society of Japan (Tokyo) 1972 92(2):135.

2. Takato M et al. The Japanese Journal of Pharmacognosy 1976 30(2):109.

3. Sugaya A. The Japanese Journal of Pharmacognosy 1975 29(2):160.

4. Noguchi E. The Japanese Journal of Pharmacognosy 1967 21(1):17.

5. Zhang LS. Nihon Yakubutsugaku Zasshi 1942 35(2):176.

6. Takase T. Chemical Structure and Physiological Effect. 1941. p. 204.

7. Akamatsu K. Wakanyaku. 1970. p. 420.

8. Wang LW et al. Abstracts of the Symposium of the Chinese Society of Physiology (Pharmacology). 1964. p. 133.

9. Zhang XM. Developments in Chinese Traditional Drugs (Hunan Institute of Medical and Pharmaceutical Industry) 1975 (1):10.

10. Hosono. Practical Kampo 1976 (9):3.

11. Wang Y et al. Acta Botanica Sinica 1954 3(2):121.

12. Maruzzella JC. Journal of Pharmacy and Pharmacology 1959 (11):188.

13. Okazaki K. Journal of the Pharmaceutical Society of Japan (Tokyo) 1952 72(9):1131.

14. Ito H. Folia Pharmacologica Japonica 1970 66(4):366.

15. Virus Section, Academy of Traditional Chinese Medicine. Xinyiyaoxue Zazhi (Journal of Traditional Chinese Medicine) 1973 (1):26.

16. Aimi S et al. The Journal of the Society for Oriental Medicine in Japan 1968 19(1):33.

17. Zhongshan Medical College (editor). Clinical Applications of Chinese Traditional Drugs. 1st edition. Guangdong People' s Publishing House. 1975. p. 8.

18. You YZ. The References of Traditional Chinese Medicine (Information Department of the Academy of Traditional Chinese Medinice) 1974 (8):21.

19. Xia ZF. Journal of Traditional Chinese Medicine 1956 (10):978.

20. Anxiang County Hospital of Traditional Chinese Medicine. Hunan Yiyao Zazhi (Hunan Medical Journal) 1974 (1):42.

(Chen Quansheng)

JIEGENG 桔梗

<Jiegeng> refers to the root of *Platycodon grandiflorum* A. DC. (Campanulaceae). It has a sweet, bitterish and pungent taste with a slightly "warm" property. It is credited with expectorant, throat-demulcent, and pus-discharging effects. Thus, it is usually used in cough with excessive sputum, pharyngolaryngitis, pulmonary abscess, and vomiting of blood with pus. Traditionally, the peeled root is used. However, it has been shown that the unpeeled root is similar to the peeled root in expectorant effect, toxicity and saponin content (1).

CHEMICAL COMPOSITION

<Jiegeng> contains platycodin, α-spinasterol, α-spinasterol-β-D-glucoside, Δ^7-stigmasterol, betulin, inulin, platycodonin, and platycogenic acids A, B and C.

PHARMACOLOGY

1. Expectorant and Antitussive Effects

Administration of the <Jiegeng> decoction 1 g/kg PO to anesthetized dogs markedly increased mucous secretion in the respiratory tract; its potency resembled that of ammonium chloride (2). Likewise, a marked expectorant effect was demonstrated in anesthetized cats (3).

It was reported that platycodin was a more potent expectorant than the root of *Polygala tenuifolia* but weaker than that of *Polygala senega* L. However, the result of the phenol red test in mice showed that platycodin was weaker than the root of *Polygala tenuifolia* (4). The oral doses of platycodin irritated the pharyngeal and gastric mucosae, reflexedly increasing mucous secretion in the respiratory tract and diluting the sputum for easy expectoration (5). The crude preparation of platycodin had an antitussive effect (6–8), its ED_{50} in guinea pigs was determined to be 6.4 mg/kg IP (7).

2. Hypoglycemic Effect

The aqueous or ethanol extract of <Jiegeng> at 200 mg/kg PO lowered the blood glucose level of rabbits; the hypoglycemic curve of the aqueous extract was similar to that of tolbutamide 25–50 mg/kg PO. In rabbits with alloxan-induced diabetes, the aqueous or ethanol extract given at 500 mg/kg PO for 4 days also produced a hypoglycemic effect, simultaneous with restoration of the decreased liver glycogen level. The extracts also inhibited dietary hyperglycemia. In this respect, the ethanol extract was more potent than the aqueous extract (9).

3. Inhibition of Gastric Secretion and Anti-peptic Ulcer Effect

The crude preparation of platycodin at a dose lower than one-fifth of the LD_{50} inhibited gastric secretion and prevented peptic ulcer in rats (8). The dose 100 mg/kg virtually inhibited gastric secretion induced by ligation of the pylorus. Intraduodenal administration of the crude preparation of platycodin 25 mg/kg to rats prevented the formation of peptic ulcer; the strength of its action was equivalent to that of atropine 10 mg/kg SC. However, the prophylactic effect of the dose 100 mg/kg PO against the formation of stress ulcer was two times weaker than that of atropine 10 mg/kg SC. The crude preparation of platycodin markedly decreased the ulcer index in rats induced by acetic acid. The therapeutic effect achieved in the group receiving platycodin 25 mg/kg per day was higher than that in the group given the licorice extract FM_{100} 200 mg/kg per day (6,10).

4. Anti-inflammatory Effect

The crude preparation of platycodin was shown to have an anti-inflammatory effect (6). The intragastric doses equivalent to one-tenth to one-fifth the LD_{50} antagonized carrageenin- and acetic acid-induced swelling of rat hind limbs. Oral administration of doses less than one-tenth of the LD_{50} once daily also markedly inhibited cotton pledget-induced granulation in rats. The drug was effective against adjuvant-induced arthritis in rats (8,11). It decreased the capillary permeability of mice with allergic reaction (11). Writhing and peritoneal exudation induced by intraperitoneal injection of platycodin in mice was inhibited by oral administration of the same agent (8).

<Jiegeng> had no direct antibacterial effect, but its aqueous extract was shown to enhance the phagocytic function of macrophages, the bactericidal power of neutrophiles, and the lysozymal activity (12).

5. Effect on the Circulatory System

Intravenous injection of the crude preparation of platycodin to rats resulted in a transient fall in the blood pressure, bradycardia, and respiratory depression. High concentrations produced a negative inotropic effect on the isolated guinea pig auricle (7). Intra-arterial injection of 200–800 µg of the crude platycodin to anesthetized dogs reduced the vascular resistance of the coronary artery and hind limb vessels, thereby increasing the blood flow in these vasculatures, with a potency equal to that of papaverine. Likewise, injection of 4 mg/kg IV increased the blood flow in these vessels and simultaneously produced transient hypotension. Vasodilation was believed to be due to a direct action on the peripheral blood vessels (7,13).

6. Miscellaneous Actions

The crude preparation of platycodin had sedative, analgesic, and antipyretic actions (6,8,14); it inhibited the spontaneous activity in mice and prolonged cyclobarbital sodium-induced sleep but did not prevent the development of convulsion caused by electric shock and pentylenetetrazole (14). This agent reduced hepatic cholesterol and increased the fecal excretion of sterols and cholic acid in rats (15). It also exhibited anticholinergic and antihistaminic actions by inhibiting ileal contraction in guinea pigs due to acetylcholine and histamine (11). <Jiegeng> 2 g/kg PO produced anti-edema diuretic effects in rats with congestive edema following bilateral ligation of the jugular vein (16). *In vitro*, the 1:10 herb decoction inhibited *Epidermophyton floccosum* (17).

7. Toxicity

The LD_{50} of the <Jiegeng> decoction in mice was determined to be 24 g/kg PO. All 5 rabbits given the decoction at 40 g/kg PO died within 24 hours, whereas the other 5 rabbits dosed with 20 g/kg survived (1). Platycodin had a very pronounced hemolytic effect (18); it had a hemolytic index of 1:10,000. Thus it cannot be administered by injection. The orally administered drug loses its hemolytic effect after being decomposed in the alimentary tract. Its MLD in mice was determined to be 770 mg/kg SC (19). The LD_{50} of the crude preparation of platycodin in mice and rats were 420 and >800 mg/kg Po, or 22.3 and 14.1 mg/kg IP, respectively (8). At large intragastric doses platycodin reflexedly stimulated the vomiting center, causing nausea and vomiting (19).

CLINICAL STUDIES

1. Respiratory Tract Inflammation

Two cases of lung abscess were reported to have been effectively treated with Radix Platycodi White Powder (composed of Radix Platycodi, Fructus Crotonis, and Bulbus Fritillariae Cirrhosae) (20). Radix Platycodi Decoction (composed of Radix Platycodi and Radix Glycyrrhizae) was also useful in lung abscess and lobar pneumonia. <Jiegeng> is often combined with other antitussives and expectorants in compound formulae (e.g. Anti-Cough, Cough-Stop, Rhizoma Pinelliae Liquid) widely used in the treatment of common cold, cough, upper respiratory tract infection, bronchitis, and pneumonia.

2. Pharyngitis, Carbuncle and Furuncle

The <Jiegeng> decoction can be administered orally to treat pharyngitis. The powder prepared from <Jiegeng> and the kernel of *Coix lachryma-jobi* may be used to treat dental caries and gingivitis. Suppurant Decoction (composed of Radix Platycodi, Radix Glycyrrhizae and Rhizoma Zingiberis Recens) and Suppurant Powder (composed of Fructus Aurantii, Radix Paeoniae and Radix Platycodi) are useful in treating furuncle and carbuncle (19).

3. To Promote Gastric Function

Radix Platycodi-Rhizoma Pinelliae Decoction (composed of Radix Platycodi, Pericarpium Citri Reticulatae, Rhizoma Pinelliae and Rhizoma Zingiberis Recens) is used to treat postpartum gastric dysfunction. Radix Platycodi-Fructus Aurantii Decoction (composed of Radix Platycodi and Fructus Aurantii) is useful in chest or upper abdominal fullness caused by exogenous "cold" pathogenic factor (19).

REFERENCE

1. Zhou WZ et al. Chinese Pharmaceutical Bulletin 1979 14(5):202.

2. Tang RY et al. Chinese Medical Journal 1952 38(1):4.

3. Gao YD. Chinese Medical Journal 1954 46(5):331.

4. Zhu XL. Japan Centra Revou Medicina 1943 80:179.

5. Zhu Y. Pharmacology and Applications of Chinese Medicinal Materials. People's Medical Publishing House. 1958. p. 146.

6. Takagi K et al. Chemical Abstracts 1975 82:261d.

7. Takagi K et al. Journal of the Pharmaceutical Society of Japan (Tokyo) 1972 92(8):969.

8. Takagi K. Metabolism and Disease 1973 10 (5):474; Hunan Institute of Medical and Pharmaceutical Industry (translator). Foreign References on Chinese Materia Medica. 1st edition. 1975. p. 13.

9. Eda et al. Folia Pharmacologica Japonica 1971 67(6):223p.

10. Kawashima K et al. Chemical and Pharmaceutical Bulletin 1972 20(4):755.

11. Takagi K et al. Journal of the Pharmaceutical Society of Japan (Tokyo) 1972 92(8):961.

12. Nihon Yakugakkai Dai 98 Nen Tekisai. Kampo Kenkyu 1978 5:168.

13. Takagi K et al. The Japanese Journal of Pharmacology 1974 23(5):709.

14. Takagi K et al. Journal of the Pharmaceutical Society of Japan (Tokyo) 1972 92(8):951.

15. Mashcherskaya KA et al. Chemical Abstracts 1968 68:20785s.

16. Yamabara et al. Chemical and Pharmaceutical Bulletin 1979 27(6):1464.

17. Zheng WF et al. Chinese Medical Journal 1952 38(4):315.

18. Zhao SX et al. Journal of East China College of Pharmacy 1956 (1):37.

19. Sheng ZN. Xinzhongyiyao (Modernized Traditional Chinese Medicine) 1957 8(4):17.

20. Wang HT. Journal of Traditional Chinese Medicine 1955 (4):25.

(Wu Chongrong)

EZHU 莪术

<Ezhu> is the rhizome obtained from *Curcuma zedoaria* Rosc., *C. aromatica* Salisb., or *C. kwangsiensis* S. Lee et C.F. Liang (Zingiberaceae) (1). Pungent, bitter and "warm", the herb is credited with vital-energy-stimulant, stasis-deobstruent, digestant and analgesic activities. It is mainly used in the treatment of distention and pain of the abdomen associated with dyspepsia, abdominal pain due to blood stasis, hepatomegaly, splenomegaly, amenorrhea due to blood stasis, and wounds and injuries.

CHEMICAL COMPOSITION

<Ezhu> contains 1–2.5% of volatile oil which is mainly composed of sesquiterpenes. The volatile oil contains more than 20 components: curzerenone (zedoarone), the major component; curdione; epicurcumenol; curzerene; pyrocurcuzerenone; curcumol (curcumenol); isocurcumenol; procurcumenol; dehydrocurdione; furanodienone; isofuranodienone; furanodiene; zederone; curcumin; etc.

Curdione and curcumol are antineoplastic agents recently isolated in China, identical to constituents isolated from the rhizome of the same species in other countries. Antineoplastic agents isolated from the volatile oil of *C. wenchowensis* were also identical to curdione or curcumol.

PHARMACOLOGY

1. Antineoplastic Effect

The 100% *C. wenchowensis* injection at 0.3–0.5 ml IP to mice afforded a mean inhibition rate of over 50% against sarcoma 180, but was inactive against Ehrlich ascites carcinoma in mice. Crystal I (curcumol) and crystal II (curdione) (2), obtained from the volatile oil of *C. wenchowensis* rhizome, injected to mice at 75 mg/kg SC had high inhibition rates against sarcoma 37, cervical cancer U_{14}, and Ehrlich ascites carcinoma but was weak against sarcoma 180. A series of immune reactions were observed in markedly shrunken tumors including: marked increase in fibroblasts surrounding the tumor tissue, presence of a layer of lymphocytes within the tumor mass, and phagocytic engulfment of tumor cells. Under the electron microscope, the treatment group showed more pronounced changes in the neoplastic cellular nucleus mainly manifested in the reduction of the nucleus/cytoplasm ratio, tendency of nuclear configuration to normalize, and diminution of chromatins, nucleoli and interchromatin granules. These phenomena indicate that curcumol has an inhibitory effect on the nuclear metabolism of the sarcoma cells in mice. Results of *in vitro* studies revealed that curcumol and curdione destroyed Ehrlich ascites carcinoma cells, causing degeneration and necrosis of the latter (3).

In vitro inhibition tests showed that various concentrations of the injection preparation of the <Ezhu> oil directly destroyed the tumor cells with characteristic strength and swiftness. Higher concentrations were needed to destroy 90% of the tumor cells (4). *In vivo* studies on the 615 purebred mice models with transplanted tumors of TM_{755} and R_{615} strains revealed that the <Ezhu> oil 50 mg/animal IP was significantly efficacious, affording a tumor inhibition rate of 35–60%. After active immunization of 615 purebred mice with L_{615} leukemic cells treated with <Ezhu>-oil, one-third of the surviving animals could withstand an attack by 100,000 L_{615} cells, and survived for a long period. The <Ezhu> oil also afforded protection to mice inoculated with L_{615} tumor vaccine that was exposed to 10,000 rads of X-ray; 40% of the animals survived the challenge. On the other hand, 100% of the mice inoculated with heat-deactivated tumor vaccines died after the challenge; These results suggest that the <Ezhu>-tumor vaccine not only has a good immunoprotective effect but is also specific. When the splenocyte suspension of the surviving animals was transferred to mice of the same strain, the animals were protected against an attack of 10^5 L_{615} cells. Thus, the long-term survival rate after challenge was 10%, but after inoculation with the <Ezhu>-tumor vaccine, the long-term survival rate of the mice after challenge was up to 40%. These findings indicate that a significant immunoprotective effect is achieved with the drug through enhancement of the specific immunity of the host (4). The mode of the antineoplastic action of <Ezhu> involves a direct action and the participation of the host immune reaction (3,4).

Clinical observation after intratumor injection of the <Ezhu> oil revealed partial necrosis and sloughing of cancerous tissues, smooth uterine cervix, and the attainment of a clinical cure. These morphological changes indicate a direct cytocidal effect of the drug on cancer. Pathological examinations showed engulfment of the malignant cells by proliferating small lymphocytes, extensive hyperplasia of the cellular tissue of the lymph sinuses, and marked lymphocytosis following administration of <Ezhu>. All these findings indicate the presence of a significant host immune reaction in the responsive patients (5). Cytopathological studies proved that the blood of cancer patients was highly coagulable, and that large amounts of fibrin precipitated around and inside the tumor masses to form a fibrinous reticulum impeding deep penetration of antineoplastic drugs and immunoactive cells, thus interfering with the antineoplastic effect. Traditional drugs, which stimulate blood circulation and eliminate stasis, directly or indirectly benefit the treatment of tumor as they are capable of altering this pathological state (6).

2. Antibacterial Effect

In vitro, the volatile oil of *C. wenchowensis* inhibited the growth of *Staphylococcus aureus*, beta *Streptococcus hemolyticus, Escherichia coli, Salmonella typhi*, and *Vibrio cholerae* (7).

3. Prevention of Leukopenia

Intraperitoneal injection of either the <Ezhu> oil, fresh <Ezhu> oil 10 ml/kg, or curcumol (0.3%) 10 ml/kg to mice for 8 days markedly offset leucopenia induced by intraperitoneal injection of cyclophosphamide 150 mg/kg, and also promoted the rise of WBC count. These results indicate that <Ezhu> can increase the leukocyte count (8).

4. Antithrombotic Effect

The <Ezhu> oil affected some stages of thrombus formation. It antagonized the delay in platelet aggregation due to ADP and epinephrine; this effect was believed to be induced by curcumin (9,10).

5. Effect on the Gastrointestinal Smooth Muscle

In the digestive tract, <Ezhu> has a similar action to fresh ginger; it directly stimulated the smooth muscle and was useful in the treatment of colic due to flatulence (11). Low concentrations of <Ezhu> increased the tonicity of the isolated rabbit intestine, whereas high concentrations related the intestinal tract (12).

6. Effect on the Ovary, Endometrium, and Embryo

The ethanol extract of <Ezhu> and its sesquiterpenes showed a very marked abortifacient effect in rats and mice during the early gestational period, and also an anti-implantation effect in dogs; toxic effects were minimal (13). Four daily intragastric administrations of the herb suspension (equivalent to 15 g(crude drug)/kg) to separate groups of mice for contraception, or to induce abortion of early pregnancy did not trigger a decidual reaction in the endometrium, but resulted in the suppression of the secretory phase, and degeneration and detachment of the embryos (14).

7. Pharmacokinetics

The absorption of the orally administered ^{3}H-curcumol was rapid and complete. Radioactivity appeared in rats 5 minutes after the intragastric dose and peaked in 15 minutes, maintaining high levels for one hour. The ratio of area under the drug-time curve after the intragastric dose to that of the intravenous dose in rats was 4.35:1, and the intragastric dose was four times that of the intravenous dose. Hence, absorption of the orally administered ^{3}H-curcumol was relatively complete. The 72-h fecal excretion of the intragastrically administered ^{3}H-curcumol in rats represented only 6.77% of the administered dose, indicating that most of the drug was absorbed form the gastrointestinal tract. Therefore, the oral route is considered to be a relatively good route of administration. High drug concentrations following the intravenous or oral dose were detected in the liver and kidneys, calculated to be 2–2.5 times those found in other tissues. The radioactivity in other organs varied with the biphasic plasma radioactivity. During the first phase, plasma radioactivity sharply fell; $t\frac{1}{2}(\alpha)$ of the drug was determined to be 33 minutes, indicating rapid distribution in the body. On the other hand, during the second phase, plasma radioactivity slowly dropped, and the $t\frac{1}{2}(\beta)$ was 12.5 hours, indicating slow elimination. The radioactivity showed a high affinity of the drug for adipose tissue where high levels could still be detected 4 hours after medication. However, the distribution of curcumol in tumor tissues did not significantly differ from that in other tissues. ^{3}H-Curcumol by intravenous or oral administration crossed the blood-brain barrier as shown by the presence of radioactivity in the brain tissue. The amount excreted in the urine and feces 72 hours after the intragastric dose in rats represented 48.63 and 6.77% of the oral dose, respectively, in contrast to 54.75 and 14.35% after the intravenous injection. These results indicate that the drug is excreted in the urine and feces, and the main route of excretion is through the kidney. Though biliary excretion accounted for about 50%, only 6.77% of the oral dose was excreted in feces in a period of 72 hours. These facts indicate extensive enterohepatic circulation (15).

8. Toxicity

The LD_{50} of the <Ezhu> oil injection for clinical use, containing 1% <Ezhu> oil and 10% Tween 80, were 819.8 mg/kg IP and 789.1 mg/kg IM in mice. However, the high amount of Tween 80 in the injection increased the toxicity of the <Ezhu> oil (16).

Subacute toxicity studies revealed that the <Ezhu> oil at 1 mg/kg IM in the dog, or 5 ml/kg in the mouse, for 8 weeks did not produce significant toxic effects or abnormalities in the histology of various tissues (16). No significant difference was noted between the oil extracted from the fresh <Ezhu> and that from the dried one, as far as the TD and LD_{50} of their intraperitoneal dose in mice were concerned (17).

The acute LD_{50} of curcumol and curdione in mice were 250 and 414 mg/kg IP, respectively, and the subacute LD_{50} were 163.4 and 215.3 mg/kg IP daily for 7 days, respectively (3). The acute LD_{50} of the highly soluble curcumol o-phthalate was 136 mg/kg IP in mice (18). Hemolysis was induced by the injection prepared from the dried and fresh <Ezhu>, as well as by the slower-acting vehicle, Tween 80. Thus *in vivo* hemolytic studies with rabbits revealed that the volatile oil of <Ezhu> at 2.0, 1.0, and 0.5 ml IM all induced hemolysis. This finding suggests that the volatile oil itself is a hemolytic factor (19). Administration of the <Ezhu> extract at 15 mg/kg PO for 4 or 7 days resulted in marked hepatic and renal damages seen under the microscope, leading to progressive hepatic necrosis, most marked 3 weeks after cessation of medication. The kidneys generally appeared congested, with marked swelling of the tubular epithelial cells (19).

CLINICAL STUDIES

<Ezhu> is chiefly used to treat cervical cancer. The mixture of 1% <Ezhu> oil or 1% <Ezhu> injection with 0.5% curcumol or curzerenone is injected into the tumor mass; the same agent is concomitantly used for local application and intravenous or intra-arterial injection. Out of 165 early

cases so treated, 52 cases achieved a short-term cure, 25, marked effects, 41 some improvement, and 47 unresponsive; the aggregate effective rate was 71.4% (20). A comprehensive review of 343 cases of early cervical cancer undertaken by The 4th Conference of the National Coordinating Group for <Ezhu> Therapy of Malignant Tumor showed that a short-term cure was attained in 102 cases, marked effects in 63, some improvement in 75, and no effect in 103, the aggregate effective rate being 70% (21). The herb is generally believed to be more efficacious for the early stage of cervical cancer, thereby obviating the need for surgery and radiotherapy, and is reported to have few toxic and side effects (20,21).

ADVERSE EFFECTS

In comparison with the pretreatment readings, no abnormality was found in the routine blood tests of 165 cases treated with <Ezhu>, as well as in the hepatic and renal functions of some patients (20). Neither were there changes in the bleeding and coagulation times, platelet count, and hemoglobin (21). However, severe pain may occur during intratumor and local injection. Rapid injection may cause chest discomfort, flushing, and dyspnea (20,21). A sour and peppery taste in the mouth is also experienced by patients during injection.

REFERENCE

1. Editorial Committee. China's Pharmacopoeia. Part 1. 1997. p. 460.

2. Xu HX et al. Journal of Shenyang College of Pharmacy 1978 (10):20.

3. Tumor Section, Faculty of Medicine Liaoning College of Traditional Chinese Medicine. Xinyiyaoxue Zazhi (Journal of Traditional Chinese Medicine) 1976 (12):28.

4. Tumor Research Unit, Zunyi Medical College. Acta Academiae Medicinae Zunyi 1978 (1):10.

5. Zhu JC. Acta Academiae Medicinae Wenzhou 1979 (1):30.

6. Li YK et al. Chinese Traditional and Herbal Drugs Communications 1979 (10):31.

7. Nigam SS et al. Chemical Abstracts 1970 73:63548n.

8. Pu TC et al. Acta Academiae Medicinae Wenzhou 1979 (1):51.

9. Cardiovascular Section, Institute of Materia Medica of Beijing Academy of Traditional Chinese Medicine. Combined Western and Traditional Chinese Therapy of Cardiovascular Diseases (Academy of Traditional Chinese Medicine) 1977 (3):47, 50, 52.

10. Wang MC et al. Compiled Information on Combined Western and Traditional Chinese Medicine. Lanzhou Medical College. 1978. p. 57.

11. U.S. Dispensatory. 24th edition. 1947. p. 1652.

12. Zunyi Medical College. Xinyiyaoxue Zazhi (Journal of Traditional Chinese Medicine) 1976 (12):39.

13. Chen ZZ et al. Proceedings of the Northeastern Sichuan Symposium on Family Planning Techniques. Sichuan Health Bureau. 1979.

14. Chen ZZ et al. Proceedings of the Sichuan Symposium on Family Planning Techniques (Sichuan Health Bureau) 1980 (2):191.

15. Su CY et al. Acta Pharmaceutica Sinica 1980 15(5):257.

16. Wang LW. Acta Academiae Medicinae Zunyi 1979 (2):7.

17. Pharmacology Section, Wenzhou Medical College. Acta Academiae Medicine Wenzhou 1979 (1):55.

18. Yu RH et al. Journal of Shenyang College of Pharmacy 1978 (10):25.

19. Pathology Department, Chongqing Health School. Sichuan Selected Information on Tumor Prevention and Treatment. Sichuan Office of Tumor Prevention and Treatment. 1975. p. 114.

20. Curcuma Rhizome Research Group, Luda Hospital of Obstetrics and Gynecology. Xinyiyaoxue Zazhi (Journal of Traditional Chinese Medicine) 1977 (3):13.

21. Wu XH et al. Acta Academiae Medicinae Wenzhou 1979 (1):43.

(Chu Yan)

LAIFUZI AND LUOBO 萊菔子與蘿蔔

<Laifuzi> is the ripe seed of *Raphanus sativus* L. (Cruciferae); the fresh root tuber <Luobo>, withered old root <Digulou> and leaf <Luoboye> are also used as medicine.

<Laifuzi> has a pungent and sweetish taste as well as a "mild" property; when roasted it has a "warm" property. It is digestant, antiflatulent, antitussive and mucolytic. It is, therefore, a known remedy for dyspepsia, tightness of the chest with abdominal distention, cough, and asthma with expectoration.

<Luobo>, which is a common edible vegetable, has a pungent and sweetish taste and a slightly "cold" property. When cooked, it tastes sweet and has a "mild" property. <Luobo> is known for its digestant, mucolytic, detoxicant and anti-inflammatory actions and is considered to relieve gastrointestinal distress. It is used in dyspepsia with abdominal distention, aphonia due to cough, hematemesis, epistaxis, thirst, dysentery, and migraine.

<Digulou> is sweet and "mild". It is diuretic and detumescent. It is prescribed in edema and dysuria.

<Luoboye> is indicated for appetite-prohibiting dysentery.

CHEMICAL COMPOSITION

<Laifuzi> contains small amounts of volatile oil and large amounts of fixed oil. The volatile oil contains methyl mercaptan, α-hexanal, and β-hexanal; the fixed oil contains large quantities of erucic acid, linoleic acid, linolenic acid, and glycerol sinapate. The fixed oil also contains sinapine and raphanin. Recent chemical assay showed that <Laifuzi> contains phenolic compounds, alkaloids, and flavones (1).

<Luobo> contains carbohydrates, lignin, methyl mercaptan (trace amount), trigonelline, choline, adenine, and glycosides such as glucoraphenin.

PHARMACOLOGY

1. Antimicrobial Effect

The aqueous extract of <Laifuzi> markedly inhibited staphylococcus and *Escherichia coli* (2), and also inhibited in different extents *Trichophyton concentricum*, Schlemm' s *Dermatomyces favosa, Microsporum audouini, Dermatomyces ferrugineum, Microsporum lanosum* and *Nocardia asteroides* (3). Raphanin was shown to be the antibacterial principle. Experiments proved that at 1 mg/ml, raphanin markedly inhibited many kinds of bacteria *in vitro* (2); the MIC against staphylococus, *Shigella dysenteriae, Salmonella typhi,* and *Escherichia coli* were 40, 125, 125, and 200 μg/ml, respectively. At concentrations exceeding 250 μg/ml, it inhibited the growth of some fungi. Serum weakened the antibacterial activity of raphanin; the sulfur compounds such as hydrogen sulfide, mercaptoacetic acid, cystine, and glutathione abolished it. Raphanin also inhibited viruses; the DNA viruses were more susceptible than the RNA viruses. It interfered with the synthesis of interferon, that is, 10 μg/ml achieved significant inhibition and 35 μg/ml complete inhibition (4). Sulforaphen, a kind of erucic oil isolated from <Laifuzi>, at 1% concentration inhibited the growth of streptococcus, *Pseudomonas aeruginosa*, pneumococcus and *Escherichia coli*, but the 0.1% solution was devoid of significant action (5). Recently, raphanin and sulforaphen were considered to be the same substance (6).

All the acidic, neutral, and alkaline substances isolated from the ether extract of the root tuber of the black radish exhibited antibacterial activity; of these the acidic substance was the most potent. Gram-positive bacteria were more sensitive to these agents than the gram-negative organisms. These substances also inhibited mycobacteria and pathogenic fungi. However, the presence of serum reduced their antibacterial potency by one-half (7). An acidic complex, raphin, obtained by further isolation, had a wide-spectrum antibacterial activity; at 4–20 μg/ml, it inhibited the growth of *Staphylococcus aureus*, *Streptococcus pyogenes*, *Corynebacterium diphtheriae*, *Mycobacterium*, *Bordetella pertussis* and also some pathogenic fungi. Raphin was also shown to have a therapeutic effect on experimental local staphylococcal infection in mice (8). In addition, the <Luobo> juice was reported to be lethal to *Trichomonas vaginalis* (9,10); however, another paper reported that it was inactive (11).

2. Detoxicant Effect

In vitro, mixing of raphanin with bacterial exotoxin detoxified the latter. At a concentration of 1:200, it neutralized five times the lethal dose of tetanin and at 1:500, four times the lethal dose of diphtherial toxin. Cutaneous necrosis caused by diphterial toxin was reduced by raphanin diluted to 1:1600 (8).

3. Hypotensive Effect

The aqueous extract of <Laifuzi> had a significant hypotensive effect. The intravenous injection caused a fall in the blood pressure of anesthetized rabbits, cats, and dogs; its action was characterized by a slow onset and prolonged effect. It reflexedly elicited deep and rapid respiration but did not significantly alter the ECG (12).

4. Anti-inflammatory and Analgesic Effects, and Influence on the Adrenocortical Function

A compound formula, Osteohyperplasia Pill, (Radix Rehmanniae Conquitae, Herba Cistanches, Caulis Spatholobi, Herba Pyrolae, Herba Epimedii, Rhizoma Drynariae, and Semen Raphani) produced a significant anti-inflammatory action and inhibited tissue hyperplasia and inflammatory exudation of croton oil-induced granulocyst in rats. Analysis of the individual drugs in this formula revealed that the anti-inflammatory effect was provided by Radix Rehmanniae Conquitae, Herba Cistanches, and Semen Raphani. Intraperitoneal injection of the 250% <Laifuzi> aqueous extract markedly inhibited inflammatory hyperplasia in croton oil-induced granulocyst in rats, but its anti-exudative effect was weak (13). Osteohyperplasia Pill also significantly inhibited carrageenin-induced paw swelling and hyperplasia of cotton pledget-induced granulation in rats; however, the inhibitory effect on tissue hyperplasia disappeared after adrenalectomy, indicating that this action was accomplished via the adrenal glands. The pill also caused thymic atrophy in mice and reduced the vitamin C content of rat adrenal glands; but the latter effect disappeared with hypophysectomy. These results indicate that the basic anti-inflammatory mechanism of Osteohyperplasia Pill involves the activation of the pituitary-adrenocortical function (14). Another report claimed that "Tan Yin Wan" (Pill for Phlegm and Fluid Retention) could activate the pituitary-adrenocortical function; study of the individual drugs of this formula revealed that <Laifuzi> itself was without such action (15). In addition, Osteohyperplasia Pill was proved to have an analgesic effect in mice by the hot plate method, electrical stimulation of the tail, and acetic acid-induced writhing (16).

5. Miscellaneous Actions

Long-term feeding of a variant of this herb, *Raphanus sativus* var. *major* to albino rats reduced the iodotyrosine (* literal translation would be iodotyramine) content of the thyroid gland after injection of ^{131}I, suggesting disruption of thyroxin synthesis (17). Experiments indicated that "Tan Yin Wan" markedly inhibited the ^{131}I uptake of the thyroid gland in rats and mice. The drug also significantly synergized with methylthiouracil in causing thyroid hyperplasia. "Tan Yin Wan" therefore can markedly inhibit the thyroid function. Studies of the ingredients of this pill, however, revealed that <Laifuzi> was not the main bioactive constituent (18). <Luobo> stimulated the digestive glandular secretion and produced cholagogic, choleretic and diuretic actions (19). It increased the tonicity and decreased the contraction amplitude of the isolated rabbit intestine (20). Raphanin, at concentrations of 1:1000–1:10,000, inhibited the germination of seeds and the growth of rabbit testicular cells *in vitro* (2,21). It was reported that the radish lignin had a marked anitneoplastic action. In addition, the 1:800 raphanin decreased the heart rate and tension of the isolated frog heart (2).

6. Toxicity

The LD_{50} of the <Laifuzi> aqueous extract in mice was determined to be 127.4(123.8–131.1)g/kg IP. Most of the treated animals died of seizures within one hour. Administration of 100, 200, and 400 g/kg PO daily to rats for 3 weeks did not produce significant changes in the blood picture, liver and kidney functions, or important organs (12).

The acidic substance of the root tuber of black radish at 3 g/kg SC or 2 g/kg IP produced no toxic reactions in mice. The dose of 1 g/kg SC resulted in only transient and mild toxic effects in rabbits (7). Injection of raphanin at 10 mg IV killed mice but the 5-mg dose was not lethal (2).

CLINICAL STUDIES

1. As Stomachic and Digestant

Good therapeutic effects were achieved with the stir-fried <Laifuzi>, the fruits of *Crataegus pinnatifida* and *Hordeum vulgare*, and <Shenqu> (a kind of fermented herb mixture) in cases of "gastrointestinal stasis" with symptoms of abdominal distention, borborygmus, eructation, acid regurgitation, and tenesmus.

2. Chronic Bronchitis

<Laifuzi> is an expectorant and antiasthmatic commonly used in treating bronchitis. "Sanzi Yangqin Decoction" (Semen Raphani, Semen Sinapis Albae, and Fructus Perillae) is effective in treating cough, dyspnea, and chest tightness due to excessive sputum. As reported in recent literature, "Boshi Pill" or "Bozao Pill" containing the stir-fried <Laifuzi> and other herbs was reported to be effective against chronic bronchitis of the "heat-phlegm" and "damp-phlegm" types, respectively (22,23). Optimal prophylactic and therapeutic effects in chronic bronchitis were obtained with "Tan Yin Wan" containing the "Sanzi Yangqin Decoction" plus Rhizoma Atractylodis, Rhizome Zingiberis, Radix Aconiti Praeparata, Cortex Cinnamomi, Rhizome Atractylodis Macrocephalae, and Radix Glycyrrhizae. It was particularly effective against phlegm and fluid retention in patients with hypofunction of the "spleen" and "kidney" (24,25).

3. Constipation and Intestinal Obstruction

<Laifuzi> was found to be effective in intractable constipation, and constipation in children (26,27). In combination with other drugs, <Laifuzi> was also effective in treating intestinal obstruction such as that due to ascarides (28) and adhesions (29). Radix et Rhizoma Rhei-Semen Raphani Decoction (Semen Raphani, Radix et Rhizoma Rhei, and Radix Aucklandiae) was used to treat 124 cases of intestinal obstruction due to adhesion; 98 cases were cured and 9 improved. Generally 3–5 doses (in mild cases one dose) were sufficient to ensure a cure (29). <Laifuzi> with mirabilite was also effective in intestinal obstruction due to adhesions (30).

4. Trichomonas Vaginitis

Trichomonas vaginitis was effectively treated by intravaginal application of a cotton ball impregnated with radish juice or of ground radish (10,31). Sixty-two out of 68 cases so treated were cured (31).

5. Hypertension

Semen Raphani Tablet was clinically tried in the management of 70 cases of essential hypertension. Marked effects were obtained in 31 cases and some improvement in 29. The systolic pressure was lowered by a mean of 25.6 mmHg and the diastolic pressure by a mean of 13.0 mmHg. In most patients, the optimal antihypertensive effect appeared in 2–5 weeks of medication. Different degrees of amelioration were achieved in respect of dizziness, headache, insomnia, palpitation, numbness of the extremities and lassitude, and ECG. The action of the tablet was similar to that of reserpine. *Dosage and preparation*: Each tablet 0.4 g is equivalent to 5 g of the crude drug; 4–6 tablets twice daily, and in individual patients, thrice daily, are recommended (32,33).

6. *Miscellaneous*

Osteohyperplasia Pill was shown to be effective in hypertrophic spondylitis (34,35) or Kaschin Beck disease (36). The radish leaf is an effective folk remedy for dysentery and diarrhea (37). In addition, radish paste was used locally to treat ulcerations in tuberculosis of cervical lymph nodes (38). Fresh radish juice has been used as the major therapeutic agent in treating silicosis (39). Radish juice was also used effectively in pulmonary tuberculosis with hemoptysis (40), as a retention enema in allergic colitis, diarrhea after colon operations, diarrhea due to indigestion, and chronic ulcerative colitis (41). The powder of <Laifuzi> mixed with vinegar was also effective in treating painful swellings (42).

REFERENCE

1. Liu DY. Jilin Zhongyiyao (Jilin Journal of Traditional Chinese Medicine) 1979 (1–2):119.

2. Ivanovics G et al. Nature 1974 160:297.

3. Cao RL et al. Chinese Journal of Dermatology 1957 (4):286.

4. Zelepukha SI. Antimikrobiye Svoistva Rastenii Upotrebliaemykh v Pischchu. Izd 'Uradzhai'. 1973. p. 93.

5. Schmid H et al. Chemical Abstracts 1984 42:7249f.

6. Koczka I et al. Chemical Abstracts 1950 44:5538c.

7. Negrash AK. Chemical Abstracts 1965 62:3105b.

8. Zelepukha SI. Antimikrobiye Svoistva Rastenii Upotrebliaemykh v Pischchu. Izd 'Uradzhai'. 1973. p. 141.

9. Pshchemichnikova AS. Akushcherstvo I Ginekolokiia 1953 (1):71.

10. Wang TG et al. Chinese Journal of Obstetrics and Gynecology 1956 (4):316.

11. Chen XY. Chinese Journal of Obstetrics and Gynecology 1956 (4):395.

12. Basic Sciences Research Unit, Fourth Hospital. Acta Academiae Medicinae Jilin 1978 (1):37.

13. Basic Sciences Research Unit, Fourth Hospital. Acta Academiae Medicinae Jilin 1976 (4):29.

14. Pharmacological Research Group for Osteohyperplasia Pill, Changchun College of Traditional Chinese Medicine. Journal of Bethune University of Medical Sciences 1978 (4):34.

15. Bronchitis Coordinating Research Unit, Xi'an Medical College. Xinyiyaoxue Zazhi (Journal of Traditional Chinese Medicine) 1974 (1):35.

16. Pharmacological Research Group for Osteohyperplasia Pill, Changchun College of Traditional Chinese Medicine. Journal of Bethune University of Medical Sciences 1978 (4):28.

17. Makhkamov GM et al. Chemical Abstracts 1966 64:14532b.

18. Pharmacology Group, Bronchitis Coordinating Research Unit Xi' an Medical College. Shaanxi Medical Journal 1975 (3):51.

19. Borisov MI. Lekarstevennye Sboistva Sel' skokhoziaistveiiykh Rastenii. Izd ' Uradzhai' . 1974. p. 40.

20. Acute Abdomen Research Unit, Zunyi Medical College. Information on Medical Sciences and Technology (Zunyi Medical College) 1974 (5):71.

21. Klosa J. Chemical Abstracts 1951 45:1650h.

22. Chronic Bronchitis Group, Xiangfan College of Traditional Chinese Medicine. Xiangfan Science and Technology 1973 (3):7.

23. Chronic Bronchitis Group, Xiangfan College of Traditional Chinese Medicine. Xiangfan Science and Technology 1973 (3):1.

24. Institute of Traditional Chinese Medicine, Chinese Academy of Medical Sciences (Shaanxi Branch). Journal of Traditional Chinese Medicine 1961 (3):88.

25. Chronic Bronchitis Research Unit, Shaanxi College of Traditional Chinese Medicine. Shaanxi Medical Journal 1972 (1):6.

26. Guo YZ. Xinzhongyi (Journal of New Chinese Medicine) 1976 (2):57.

27. Yang CB. Xinzhongyi (Journal of New Chinese Medicine) 1975 (1):25.

28. Xi ZR. Acta Academiae Medicinae Anhui 1976 (3) :43.

29. Chang JY. Zhongji Yikan (Intermediate Medical Journal) 1980 (6):45.

30. Surgery Department, Yingkou County Hospital. Liaoning Yiyao (Liaoning Medical Journal) 1975 (1):56.

31. Fan XH. Chinese Journal of Obstetrics and Gynecology 1956 (3):213.

32. Chen QD. Journal of Bethune University of Medical Sciences 1978 (4):71.

33. Chen QD. Journal of Traditional Chinese Medicine 1980 (4):12.

34. Liu BL. Xinzhongyi (Journal of New Chinese Medicine) 1973 (2):11.

35. Liu BL. Journal of Barefoot Doctor 1977 (1):31.

36. Osteoarthritis Deformans Group. Compiled Information on Traditional Chinese Medicine. Fourth Teaching Hospital of Jilin Medical College. 1975. p. 97.

37. Guan ZF. Fujian Zhongyiyao (Fujian Journal of Traditional Chinese Medicine) 1957 (4):29.

38. Zhuang MQ. Barefoot Doctor (Changwei District Health Bureau) 1976 (6):16.

39. Zeng LK et al. Xinzhongyiyao (Modernized Traditional Chinese Medicine) 1958 9(7):10.

40. Niu XC. Chinese Journal of Prevention of Tuberculosis 1960 (2):90.

41. Wang XZ et al. Shaanxi Zhongyi (Shaanxi Journal of Chinese Traditional Medicine) 1980 1(3):45.

42. Wu WY. Fujian Medical Journal 1981 (1):26.

(Deng Wenlong)

XIAKUCAO 夏枯草

<Xiakucao> refers to the plant *Prunella vulgaris* L. (Labiatae) Itself, or its fruitspike, or inflorescence. It is bitter, pungent, and "cold". The herb is noted for its heat-clearing effect on the liver and for its discutient action. It is a remedy for headache with vertigo, acute conjunctivitis, lymph node tuberculosis, goiter, mastitis, and hypertension.

CHEMICAL COMPOSITION

The whole plant contains triterpenoid saponins, of which the aglycones are oleanolic acid. It also contains free oleanolic acid, ursolic acid, rutin, hyperoside, cis-caffeic acid, trans-caffeic acid, alkaloids, and soluble salts (3.5%, of which 68% is potassium chloride).

The fruitspike contains anthocyanins of delphinidin and cyanidin, d-camphor, d-fenchone, and ursolic acid.

PHARMACOLOGY

1. Effect on the Circulatory System

The aqueous extract, ethanol-water extract, and 30% ethanol extract of <Xiakucao> produced hypotension in anesthetized animals (1). The <Xiakucao> decoction administered to dogs at 100 mg/kg IV produced a marked hypotensive effect and also tachyphylaxis (2). Intravenous injection of the decoction 1–1.5 g to dogs lowered blood pressure by 40–60 mmHg, which was readily restored to the original levels in 2–5 minutes. Intraperitoneal injection of 3–4 g decreased the blood pressure by 30–40 mmHg in 15–30 minutes; the hypotensive effect lasted 1–2 hours. Intragastric administration of 2–5 g to dogs resulted 30–60 minutes later in mild hypotension lasting two hours. A similar result was demonstrated in sheep given an intravenous injection of 1–1.5 g (3). Antihypertenisve effect was also produced by chronic oral administration of 2 g/kg twice daily in dogs with ' chronic skin bridge in the neck'. Two weeks of oral administration to dogs with renal hypertension decreased the blood pressure; this was subsequently restored to the original level after cessation of medication (2).

Experiments proved that the stem, leaf, fruitspike and the whole of *P. vulgaris* had hypotensive activity; of these the fruitspike was the least potent. The hypotensive action was attenuated by vagotomy (3). Intravenous injection of the total inorganic salts of <Xiakucao> to dogs at doses equivalent to 1.5–3 g of the crude drug had no significant effect on the blood pressure. However, increasing the dosage by more than onefold reduced the blood pressure by 10 mmHg. Therefore, it is believed that the hypotensive action of this herb does not primarily originate from the inorganic salts (3). A paper reported that the 30% tincture of the stem and leaf was rich in potassium salt. Intragastric administration of the fruitspike preparation which has low potassium content to anesthetized dogs did not result in hypotension, and removal of the inorganic salts abolished the hypotensive effect of <Xiakucao>. It is therefore postulated that the hypotensive effect obtained by intravenous injection of <Xiakucao> preparation is closely related to the presence of inorganic salts (4).

Low concentrations of the <Xiakucao> decoction perfused into isolated toad and rabbit hearts had an exciting effect, increasing the amplitude of cardiac contraction, whereas high concentrations significantly decreased the contraction amplitude and caused incomplete contraction and dilation. Intravenous injection of the 10% <Xiakucao> decoction 0.2 ml to rabbits promptly and markedly increased the amplitude of cardiac contraction and slightly decreased the blood pressure. It is considered that the hypotensive dosage did not product cardiac depression (5).

The 50% <Xiakucao> decoction perfused into the blood vessels of toad hind limbs initiated vasodilation which became weak when the concentration was increased to 100%; mild contractions were observed in some individual experiments. Apparently, <Xiakucao> has a biphasic effect on the blood vessels. Only vasodilation was achieved in acute experiments on animals, because small doses were used (6).

2. Antibacterial Effect

In vitro the <Xiakucao> decoction inhibited to different extents *Shigella dysenteriae, Salmonella typhi, Vibrio cholerae, Escherichia coli, Proteus vulgaris*, staphylococcus and *Mycobacterium tuberculosis* var. hominis (7,11). The ethanol extract inhibited *Pseudomonas aeruginosa* in the agar culture medium (12). *In vitro* the aqueous extract (1:4) was shown to inhibit some common pathogenic skin fungi to different extents (13). The pulmonary tuberculosis index and pulmonary lesions in mice with experimental tuberculosis were slightly reduced by daily feeding of the herb powder 5–7.5 g/kg following the infection. The mortality rate, however, approximated that of the control (14).

3. Antineoplastic Effect

Daily injection of the 100% <Xiakucao> decoction to mice 0.4–0.6 ml/animal SC for 2 weeks inhibited Ehrlich ascites carcinoma and sarcoma 180. However, during the treatment period, reduced food intake, significant weigh loss, and increase in the mortality rate were observed. Hence, the drug has no clinical value (15,16).

4. Effect on Smooth Muscles

The 50% <Xiakucao> decoction caused prominent and prolonged tonic contraction of the isolated uterus of nonpregnant rabbits. In contrast, its effect on the pregnant uterus was weak. The decoction increased rhythmic peristalsis of the isolated rabbit intestine; the duodenum was especially sensitive to it while the ileal response was weaker (17).

CLINICAL STUDIES

1. Hypertension with "Hyperactivity of the Liver"

The presenting symptoms included headache, tinnitus, blurred vision, fever accompanied by restlessness, sweating, anxiety, and insomnia. <Xiakucao> 30 g or used with the seed of *Cassia tora* 30 g may be given in the form of a decoction (18). Twenty cases of essential hypertension were reported to have been treated with Compound Spica Prunellae Mixture; better responses were acheived in the first- or second-stage cases (19).

2. Tuberculosis

Radix Pulsatillae-Spica Prunellae Decoction was reported to be effective in the treatment of tuberculosis of cervical lymph nodes. About 0.5–1 month after medication, the enlarged lymph nodes gradually subsided or had shrunk markedly, and the purulent ulcerations were healed (20). Sixty cases of infiltrative pulmonary tuberculosis were treated with a decoction composed of <Xiakucao>, *Artemisia apiacea*, and turtle shell. As a results, lesions were virtually absorbed in 24 cases and partially absorbed in 12 cases, and cavities healed or shrunk in 1 case (21). Out of 21 cases of pulmonary tuberculosis treated with Prunella-Humulus Mixture (Spica Prunellae and Herba Humuli, each 30 g), 17 cases benefitted. The medication was markedly effective in cough and poor appetite, and secondarily in fever, chest pain, and hemoptysis. It was quite effective in the exudative and mixed types and to a lesser extent in the cavernous type (22).

3. Acute Icteric Hepatitis

Symptomatic remission was obtained by 75 patients treated with <Xiakucao> (23).

4. Miscellaneous

Two cases of thyroid adenoma confirmed by scintillation scanning were given <Xiakucao> and golden carp cooked in a bain-marie. Cold nodules disappeared along with other symptoms after two months of medication (24).

REFERENCE

1. Li GC et al. Abstracts of the 1956 Academic Conference of the Chinese Academy of Medical Science. 1956. p. 70.

2. Zhang BH. Abstracts of the 1963 Symposium of the Society of Physiology (Beijing Branch). 1963. p. 78.

3. Kexue Yu Jishu (Science and Technology) — Medicine 1957 2(1):13.

4. Pharmacology Department, Jiangsu College of New Medicine. Internal information. 1972.

5. Pharmacology Department, Xi' an Medical College. Acta Academiae Medicinae Xi' an 1958 (5):18.

6. Student Scientific Research Group of Xi' an Medical College. Acta Academiae Medicinae Xi' an 1958 (5):28.

7. Liu GS. Chinese Journal of New Medicine 1950 1(2):95.

8. Microbiology Department, Shandong Medical College. Acta Academiae Medicinae Shandong 1959 (8)42.

9. Jiangsu Sanitation and Anti-epidemic Station. Chinese Traditional Drugs for Tuberculosis. Jiangsu Sanitation and Anti-epidemic Station. 1977. p. 44.

10. Medical Laboratory, 254th Hospital of the Chinese PLA. Tuberculosis (Beijing Institute of Tuberculosis) 1972 (1):31.

11. Bacteriology-Immunology Department, Beijing Institute of Tuberculosis. Journal of Beijing Institute of Tuberculosis 1960 2:53.

12. Wang WS et al. Chinese Pharmaceutical Bulletin 1959 7 (10):522.

13. Cao RL et al. Chinese Journal of Dermatology 1957 (4):286.

14. Feng YQ et al. Acta Academiae Medicinae Primae Shanghai 1964 (2):241.

15. Guangxi Medical College. Compiled Information on Medical Sciences and Technology. Guangxi Medical College. 1960. p. 49.

16. Guangxi Medical College. Compiled Information on Medical Sciences and Technology. Guangxi Medical College. 1960. p. 48.

17. Ma GD et al. Acta Academiae Medicinae Xi' an 1958 (5):16.

18. Zhongshan Medical College (editor). Clinical Applications of Chinese Traditional Drugs. 1975. p. 70.

19. Pan MJ. Fujian Zhongyiyao (Fujian Journal of Traditional Chinese Medicine) 1963 8(3):17.

20. Chen LG. Medical and Health Information 1976 (1):21.

21. First Staff Hospital of Huanggang Convalescent Hospital of the General Logistics Department of the Chinese PLA. Tuberculosis (Beijing Institute of Tuberculosis) 1972 (1):60.

22. Preventive Medicine Department, Jiangxi Institute of Tuberculosis. Antituberculosis Information (Jiangxi Institute of Tuberculosis) 1972 (1):16.

23. Yantai Hospital of Infectious Diseases. Shandong Medical Journal 1964 (11):39.

24. Cheng XW. Fujian Medical Journal 1980 (2):55.

(Yuan Wei)

CHAIHU 柴胡

<Chaihu> refers to the root obtained from *Bupleurum chinense* DC. (*B. falcatum* auct. Sin. non L.), *B. scorzonerifolium* Willd. (*B. falcatum* L. var. *scorzonerifolium* (Willd.) Ledeb.), or from *B. falcatum* L. (*B. scorzonerifolium* Willd. var. *stenophyllum* Nakai) widely used and studied in Japan (Umbelliferae). Another species which is also used as medicine is *B. rotundifolium* L.

<Chaihu> is bitter to the taste with a slightly "cold" property. It is considered to be diaphoretic, gastrointestine-regulative, liver-function restorative, and "spleen"-invigorative (by encouraging the upward flow of vital energy and nutrients). It is used to treat fever in common cold, alternating chills and fever, distention and pain of the chest and costa, malaria, prolapse of the uterus and rectum, and irregular menstruation.

The toxic species *B. longiradiatum* Turcz. should not be used as a source of <Chaihu>.

CHEMICAL COMPOSITION

The root of *B. chinense* mainly contains saponins and the corresponding sapogenins. *B. chinense* also contains rutin, volatile oil (bupleurmol), fixed oil (glycerides of oleic acid, linolenic acid, palmitic acid and stearic acid), spinasterol, adonistal, and triterpenoid glucosaponins (1).

The root of *B. falcatum* contains about 2.8% of saikosides (mixture of crude saponins), from which saikosaponins a, b, c, and d, and saikogenins A, B, C, D, E, F and G were isolated. Saikogenins A, B, C, D and E were not considered as true sapogenins but as the reaction products between saikogenins E, F and G and reagents.

The whole plant of *B. scorzonerifolium* contains quercetin, isoquercetin, isorhamnetin, rutin, and narcissin (2).

Two crystals, kaempferitin and kaempferitin-7-rhamnoside, were recently isolated from the flavonoids of the stem and leaf of *B. chinense* and *B. scorzonerifolium* (3,4).

PHARMACOLOGY

1. Effect on the CNS

<Chaihu> has marked sedative, analgesic, antipyretic, hypothermic, and antitussive effects (5–11).

1.1 *Antipyretic effect.* Oral administration of the <Chaihu> decoction 5 g/kg to rabbits with fever induced by heat resulted 1.5 hours later in normal, or initially subnormal body temperature which normalized later (12). The *Bupleurum* stem decoction had no antipyretic effect in rabbits with triple-vaccine-induced fever, whereas the injections prepared from the root, or the steam distillate of the stem and leaf produced a satisfactory antipyretic effect. The saponins of the former and the volatile oil of the latter appear to be the active antipyretic components (13). In rabbits with fever induced by intravenous or subcutaneous injection of *Escherichia coli*, subcutaneous injection of the 5% aqueous solution of the ethanol extract of <Chaihu> (1.1 g of the crude drug/ml) 0.5 ml/kg did not produce any antipyretic effect; the dose 2.0 ml/kg lowered the body temperature slightly, but did not restore it to normal. Increasing the dose to 2.2 ml/kg, however, produced a significant antipyretic action (14). <Chaihu> also had an antipyretic effect in rabbits with fever induced by expired mixed typhoid vaccine, or by the refined lipopolysaccharides obtained from the cell wall of *Escherichia coli* (5). Oral administration of the saikosides of <Chaihu> to rats at doses less than one-fifth of the LD_{50} also produced hypothermic and antipyretic effects (7). In mice with fever induced by subcutaneous injection of the beer yeast suspension, either *B. chinense* volatile oil 300 mg/kg or the saponins 380 and 635 mg/kg (corresponding to one-fifth and one-third of the LD_{50}) injected intraperitoneally 5–8 hours after the yeast injection produced a marked antipyretic effect (15).

1.2 *Sedative effect.* Numerous experiments proved that various kinds of *Bupleurum* preparations, the saikosides of the root and fruit, and saikogenin A had significant sedative effects. Sedation was achieved in mice after oral administration of the saikosides 200-800 mg/kg (5–7). The rod climbing test revealed that the sedative effect of the saikosides in mice resembled that of meprobamate; the ED_{50} for inhibiting the spontaneous activity was determined to be 347 mg/kg PO (9,16). The saikosides also markedly inhibited the conditioned escape and avoidance in rats, suggesting the possible presence of a tranquilizing effect (9). Oral administration of the saikosides extracted from *B. longiradiatum* or *B. chinense* 500 mg, or of saikogenin A to mice prolonged cyclobarbital sodium-induced sleep (9,17). Injection of saikogenin A 100 mg/kg IP produced inhibition in the rod climbing test of mice. It also antagonized the stimulant effect of methamphetamine, deoxyephedrine, and caffeine in mice (9,17).

1.3 *Analgesic Effect.* The tail pressure test showed that the saikosides administered orally had an analgesic effect on mice (7). Injection of the crude sapogenin A and the syrupy residue, S-R, at doses 50 and 100 mg/kg IP, respectively, inhibited writhing induced by intraperitoneal injection of acetic acid in mice. One to five doses of S-R at 2 g/kg PO produced a stronger inhibitory effect than a single dose of 0.5 g/kg of aspirin. A significant analgesic effect was also demonstrated by S-R on pain caused by tail compression (9).

Injection of the total saponins of *B. chinense* 478 mg/kg IP (one-fourth of the LD_{50} to mice produced a marked analgesic effect on pain caused by introduction of electrical current into the animals' tails. In contrast, the volatile oil from the same species was inactive (15).

1.4 *Antitussive Effect.* The saikosides had a potent antitussive effect (6–9,18); the ED_{50} in guinea pigs as proved in the mechanical stimulation test was 9.1 mg/kg IP, which was equipotent to codeine phosphate 7.6 mg/kg IP (6,9).

2. Anti-inflammatory Effect

Carrageenin-induced paw swelling in rats was markedly inhibited by injection of *B. chinense* saponins and the volatile oil at doses 478 and 190 mg/kg IP (one-fourth of the LD_{50}) (15) respectively, and also by saikogenin A (S-A) and the syrupy residue (S-R) (9). Oral administration of the saikosides 400 mg also inhibited paw swelling induced by dextran, serotonin, and croton oil (9,17,19). The saikosides were shown to inhibit the increase in vascular permeability induced by acetic acid, histamine and serotonin (9,17). Kaempferitin and in particular kaempferitin-7-rhamnoside also reduced capillary permeability (20). Another report stated that kaempferitin injection intraperitoneally had an anti-inflammatory effect on croton oil-induced ear swelling of mice, whereas the oral dose had no significant effect (21).

Intramuscular injection of 1 mg, or administration of 10 mg of saikosaponins a and d, or daily administration of the saikosides 100 mg/kg PO for 7 days antagonized exudation of granulocyst and granulation due to implanted cotton pledgets (9,17). Experiments proved that the anti-inflammatory potency of the saikosaponins was similar to that of prednisolone (22). The anti-inflammatory effect achieved with <Chaihu> alone was similar to that of its compound formulae. The anti-granulocyst action of <Chaihu> was more potent than its anti-exudative action. A more efficacious anti-exudative action was achieved with Radix Bupleuri-Ramulus Cinnamomi Decoction than with the single drug <Chaihu> (5,22).

Intraperitoneal injection of saikosaponins a and d to rats did not alter body and adrenal weights, as well as the hematocrit, but significantly decreased plasma 17-hydroxycortisone (23). Later work revealed that 30 minutes after intraperitoneal injection of saikosaponins a and d, plasma corticosterone was greatly increased along with the development of transient hyperglycemia, whereas saikosaponin c had no such effect (24). It was also observed in animal experiments that the weight of the adrenal glands increased in proportion to the dosage of the saikosaponins, whereas the reverse was observed of the thymic weight. Transection of the adrenal glands revealed that the diameters of the medulla and cortex in the treatment group were slightly increased by 4 and 14%, respectively, relative to the control. Microscopic examination disclosed a significant thinning of the glomerular zone of the adrenal glands, and markedly reduced cortical lymphocytes in the thymus gland with inconspicuous corticomedullary demarcation (25). To sum up, the saikosaponins apparently produce an anti-inflammatory effect by stimulating and enhancing the adrenocortical function.

3. Effect on the Digestive System

3.1 *Liver*. Both the aqueous extract and decoction of <Chaihu> (1:20) increased the total bile output and bile salt content in dogs (26). Another experiment indicated that *B. chinense* also had cholagogic and choleretic actions, with the fruit exhibiting the most potent effect, and the flower a weak activity. The flavones are probably the choleretic component (5). The <Chaihu> preparations significantly checked experimental liver damage induced in animals by bacteria (typhoid vaccine), carbon tetrachloride and *Penicillium* mold (27,28). <Chaihu>, licorice, and Radix Bupleuri-Glycyrrhizae Mixture, all markedly mitigated hepatic damage (e.g. hepatocellular degeneration, necrosis, etc.), induced by carbon tetrachloride in rats. They caused the almost complete restoration of intracellular glycogen and RNA content in hepatocytes, marked decrease in serum transaminase activity, reduction of liver cirrhosis, inhibition of fibrous hyperplasia, and acceleration of fibrous tissue resorption; Radix Bupleuri-Glycyrrhizae Mixture gave the best effect (5,27,29). It was also reported in literature that oral administration of the liquid preparation of *B. rotundifolium* (Pekvokrin) 0.5 mg/kg to dogs with carbon tetrachloride-induced hepatitis quickly restored to normal the deranged hepatobiliary secretory function and the chemical composition of the bile (e.g. bilirubin, bile salt, and cholesterol) (28). Administration of the saikosides 500 mg/kg PO daily for 3 days caused the recovery of the liver function in rats with carbon tetrachloride-damaged liver (30). The saikosaponins also caused the recovery of the impaired liver function and tissue damage induced by galactosamine (31). In contrast, the total flavones given orally offered no protection to mice against carbon tetrachloride-induced hepatitis; this might be due to its poor absorption from the gastrointestinal tract (32).

3.2 *Gastrointestinal tract.* The saikosaponins, at concentrations of $1–2 \times 10^{-4}$, were capable of stimulating the isolated intestinal smooth muscle without being antagonized by atropine (10). The saikosides, at 3×10^{-6}, enhanced acetylcholine-induced contraction of the isolated small intestine of guinea pigs but had no effect on contraction induced by histamine, suggesting that the saikosides had anticholinesterase activity (9). However the flavone extract of <Chaihu>, which contained kaempferitin, exerted a spasmolytic action on the isolated intestinal muscles (3).

Perfusion of the saikosaponins into the intestine increased the gastric pH and inhibited gastric secretion (18). In rats with ligated pylorus, the saikosides markedly inhibited gastric secretion, decreased pepsin activity, and tended to decrease the ulcer index. Like saikosides, the S-R portion administered into the duodenum also decreased the ulcer index, but had no significant effect on gastric secretion (9,30). In rats with experimental ulcers induced by acetic acid, oral dosing of saikosides 10 mg/kg daily for 15 days also decreased the gastric ulcer index, but large doses, 150 or 100 mg/kg tended to aggravate the ulcers. This finding is attributed to a direct stimulation of the gastric mucosa by the saikosides (9,33). Similar results were also observed in histamine-induced ulcers in guinea pigs (9,34). In prophylactic studies, oral administration of the saikosides 500 mg/kg resulted in striking inhibition of stress ulcer precipitated by ' fixed drowning stress' (35); this effect the probably a central origin. On the other hand, the S-R portion failed to prevent stress ulcer but slightly improved aspirin-induced gastric ulcer (9).

4. Effect on the Circulatory System

Studies on the isolated frog heart and the isolated guinea pig auricle showed that the saikosaponins at $1–2 \times 10^{-4}$ had myocardiodepressant effect (10). The flavone extract, which contained kaempferitin, increased the amplitude of cardiac contraction without altering the heart rate (36). The saikosides at doses less than one-fifth of the LD_{50} also lowered the blood pressure and decreased the heart rate in rats (7). Intravenous injection of the aqueous solution of the flavones to rabbits produced marked hypotension and bradycardia; about 48.6% reduction in the blood pressure was achieved 5 minutes after medication and the action persisted for 20 minutes (32). A trandsient fall in the blood pressure and decreased heart rate occurred in dogs after injection of the saikosides 5 mg/kg IV. In addition, the saikosides had a significant hemolytic action (9). The structurally different saikosaponins exhibited different types of hemolytic activity; their hemolytic potency was as follows: $d>a>b_1>b_2>c$. Within a certain range of concentration, the hemolytic effect of the saikosaponins was inhibited by adenine and creatinine (37).

5. *Effect on Blood Lipids*

Experiments proved that <Chaihu> did not modify the serum cholesterol and phospholipid levels in normal rabbits but increased the cholesterol/phospholipid ratio in rabbits fed with cholesterol (38). The saikosaponins also lowered the cholesterol and triglyceride levels in rats given feeds containing cholesterol 1% and cholic acid 0.5%; their effect on triglycerides was more pronounced (39). Saikosaponins a and d as well as the saikogenins A and D had anticholesterolemic effects, increasing the excretion of cholesterol and its metabolites in the bile and stool (8,9,40).

6. *Effect on Metabolism*

6.1 *Protein synthesis.* Daily injection of the mixture of the saikosides a, c, and d (3:2:2) at 2 mg/100 g IM for 4 days significantly enchanced protein synthesis in rat liver slices as reflected by a marked increase in the incorporation of ^{14}C-leucine into protein (39,40).

6.2 *Blood glucose.* The oral doses of *B. falcatum* rapidly increased the blood glucose level which peaked in 0.5–1 hour and then gradually returned to the original level 5 to 6 hours later (14). The saikosaponins elevated the blood glucose level in rats which had fasted for 18 hours. Thus, 4 hours after intraperitoneal injection of glucose 300 mg, a marked increase in the liver glycogen was observed which paralleled the dosage of the saikosides. The effectiveness of <Chaihu> on liver diseases may relate to its role in the promotion of protein synthesis and increase of liver glycogen (9).

6.3 *Normobaric hypoxia.* As shown in experiments on mice, intraperitoneal injection of 100 or 150 mg/kg of the total flavones extracted from the stem and leaf of *B. chinense* increased their tolerance to normobaric hypoxia; the mechanism of its action awaits further study (32).

7. Effect on the Immunologic Function

The 300% *B. chinense* injection markedly enhanced formation of anti-sheep erythrocyte antibody in twice-immunized mice. It had no significant effect on the production of antitoxin in rabbits immunized four times with tetanin, but markedly strengthened the inhibition of leukocyte transformation. Thus, it is preliminarily held that *B. chinense* reinforces both humoral and cellular immunities (41).

8. Effect on Urine Excretion

Oral administration of <Chaihu> at 400 mg/kg to water-loaded rats inhibited urine excretions; large doses, i.e., 800 mg/kg, produced the opposite effect, probably due to the stimulation of the renal tubules by substantial amounts of the saikosides absorbed from the alimentary tract (9). Clinical observation revealed that a marked diuretic effect was achieved with small doses of the <Chaihu> granules given orally to subjects with poor water excretion; no such effect was obtained with large doses which paradoxically caused edema of the extremities, face, shoulder and neck, and tenderness of the lower chest (42).

9. Effect on Pathogens

In vitro studies revealed that <Chaihu> inhibited the growth of *Mycobacterium tuberculosis*, leptospirae, and cowpox virus (5,43,44). The <Chaihu> injection had a therapeutic effect on warts in man (45). Optimal effects were often obtained with the <Chaihu> decoction in the treatment of malaria and hemoglobinuric fever (hemolytic malaria). Hence, it is postulated that <Chaihu> has an antiplasmodial action (13).

10. Structure-Activity Relationship of Saikosaponins

Studies on the anti-inflammatory (anti-granulocyst) and antilipemic activities of saikosaponins a, c and d proved that saikosaponins a and d possessed significant activities, whereas saikosaponin c was inactive. The decisive factors were the saikogenins, of which A and D were found to be active while C was not. The structure mainly responsible for the effects might be 4-α-hydroxymethyl or the sugar moiety (39,40). The cross-linking $13\beta_1$, 28-epoxyoleanene system was found to play an important role in the hemolytic activity of the saikosaponins, and the number of the vertical C-16β-OH, the C_{25}-OH radicals, and the sugar moiety also had a significant influence (37).

11. Pharmacokinetics

Stool and urine analyses after intramuscular injection of the ^{14}C-saikosaponins a and d to animals showed that the fecal excretion of the two saikosaponins in 2 and 7 days accounted for 50 and 85%, respectively, of the administered dose; only a small percentage was excreted in the urine on Day 1. The oral doses were poorly absorbed. Hence, to attain an anti-inflammatory effect similar to that achieved with the intramuscular dose, the oral dose had to be ten times as large (39).

12. Toxicity

<Chaihu> has a low toxicity. The MLD of the 10% <Chaihu> extract solution administered in moles was 100 mg/kg SC (12). The saikosides may cause hemolysis in rats; the LD_{50} in mice was 4.7 g/kg PO and the LD_{50} in guinea pigs was 53.8 mg/kg IP (6). The saikosides of *B. longiradiatum* and *B. falcatum* at doses 1.0–2.0 g/kg were reportedly nontoxic (17). However, studies in China revealed that the total saponins of *B. longiradiatum* was more toxic than *B. chinense*, and that they had poor therapeutic effects; the powder of the <Chaihu> derived from this plant was not recommended for oral use or for making pills or injections.

CLINICAL STUDIES

1. Fever

Optimal antipyretic effect was achieved with *B. chinense* in fever due to common cold, influenza, malaria, and pneumonia. According to a clinical study of 143 cases treated with the herb, fever subsided within 24 hours in 98.1% of the influenza cases and 87.9% of the common cold cases (46). In another series of 40 cases of pathological fever, <Chaihu> also produced an antipyretic effect in 97.5%, and achieved a reduction of 1–2°C in the body temperture in 77.5%. However, only a transient antipyretic effect may be achieved in cases of infection as body temperature could go up again after some time unless antibiotics are given concomitantly (47).

In traditional Chinese medicine, Minor Bupleurum Decoction is often used to treat alternate spells of fever and chills as well as in fever due to exogenous pathogenic factors.

2. Infectious Hepatitis

Satisfactory therapeutic effects were obtained in 100 cases of infectious hepatitis treated with B. chinese Injection. *Dosage and administration*: B. chinense (1:2) Injection 10–20 ml in 50% glucose for intravenous injection 1–2 times a day or, 20–30 ml in 250–500 ml of 10% glucose for intravenous infusion once a day. Children, 5–10 ml per day. In cases of chronic hepatitis with hepatomegaly, add Radix Salviae Miltiorrhizae Injection to the solution; vitamins C and B complex were given as adjuvants by mouth. Each course lasted 10 days with 4–5 days interval allowed between courses. After treatment, patients usually showed marked improvement in mental state, appetite, and subjective symptoms; amelioration or disappearance of pain over the liver area was achieved in 4–5 days in most patients. For patients with hepatosplenomegaly, shrinkage to the costal margin position occurred in children after one therapeutic course, whereas the recovery in adults was slower. Of the liver functions, the transaminase activity and icterus index recovered faster than the thymol turbidity and flocculation tests. Sixteen cases of hepatitis B registered negative for HBAg after 1–7 therapeutic courses. According to clinical experience, rapid reduction in the transaminase level in active hepatitis could be achieved in most patients by a daily dose of 40–50 ml for a period of about 10 days. Upon recovery, the dosage had to be appropriately reduced to preclude the development of poor appetite and increased thymol turbidity which would further prolong the treatment course. This rebound phenomenon is probably due to the accumulation of <Chaihu> in the body. A few patients developed xerostomia after receiving the <Chaihu> liquid (48). Another author also reported that <Chaihu> may decrease the transaminase level in hepatitis patients (49).

Clinically, <Chaihu> prescriptions are perceived to be effective against chronic hepatitis (50). There is also a report on the therapeutic effect of the herb on dyspeptic syndrome in hepatobiliary diseases (51).

3. Warts

A 60% effective rate was achieved in 25 cases of warts intramuscularly given <Chaihu> distillate 2 ml (equivalent to 1 g of the crude drug) for a course of 20 days. Of 6 cases of verruca vulgaris, 3 were cured, 1 improved, 2 unresponsive; of 12 cases of verruca plana, 3 were improved, 1 was unresponsive; one case of verruca accuminata was cured (45). Local acupoint injection with B. chinense Injection was applied to 5 cases of warts. Skin lesions rapidly sloughed off or disappeared in 4 cases after 2–6 injections.

Dosage and administration: Verruca vulgaris: 0.5–1.0 ml injected at sites 2.4 mm from the base of the wart once every 2–3 days; verruca plana: 4 ml each time to 2–4 acupoints around the skin lesion, i.e. 1 ml to each of the acupoints "Waiguan", "Quchi", etc. Once a day or on alternate days. A cure was generally obtained after 10 treatments (52).

4. Acute Pancreatitis and Acute Biliary Tract Infection

Based on the principles: "to soothe the liver and regulate the flow of vital energy", "to remove toxic heat", and "to purge intense heat", Major Bupleurum Decoction, modified according to patient's needs, was used with good effects in the treatment of acute pancreatitis and acute biliary tract infection (53,55).

5. Uremia

It was reported that Tincture of Lespedeza, which contains the bioactive component kaempferitin, was effective in mild uremia and azotemia of various origins (56).

6. Oral Candidiasis

A report from abroad claimed that 7 cases of oral candidiasis refractory to nystatin, trichomycin or amphotericin had been effectively with "Chaihu Qinggan Tang" (Liver-Clearing Decoction of Bupleurum chinensis (57).

ADVERSE EFFECTS

Mild lassitude, sedation and drowsiness occurred in 30% of subjects who took small doses of the <Chaihu> granules (equivalent to 0.6 g of the crude drug). These reactions did not affect daytime activities. On the other hand, 80% of subjects given large doses were deeply sedated, with 17% complaining of poor sleep, drowsiness during the day time, and decreased work efficiency (9). Large doses of the <Chaihu> granules caused impairment of appetite in most individuals, while the reverse was experienced by persons with strong constitutions. Volunteers had 1–2 bowel movements daily with pronounced flatulence and abdominal distention. These symptoms could be relieved by concomitant oral administration of licorice (42). Three incidences of allergic reaction were recently reported in patients given intramuscular injection of the <Chaihu> preparation (58).

REFERENCE

1. Takeda K. Metabolism and Disease (Wakan Yaku Supplement) 1973 10(5):676.

2. Minaeva VG et al. Rasti Resyrs 1965 1(2):233.

3. Shi YN. Chinese Traditional and Herbal Drugs 1980 11(6):241.

4. Zhang WX et al. Bulletin of Chinese Materia Medica Research (Beijing Institute of Chinese Materia Medica) 1980 (1):1.

5. Shanxi Medical College. Shanxi Medical and Pharmaceutical Journal 1974 (1):481.

6. Takagi K et al. Chemical Abstracts 1969 71:69253t.

7. Takagi K et al. (Liu YQ translator). References on Medicine Abroad — Pharmacy 1975 (1):34.

8. Wang JM et al. Guowai Yixue (Medicine Abroad) — Traditional Chinese Medicine and Materia Medica 1979 (4):1.

9. Shibata M. Metabolism and Disease (Wakan Yaku Supplement) 1973 10(5):687.

10. Takagi K. Metabolism and Disease (Wakan Yaku Supplement) 1973 10(5):474.

11. Takagi K. Chemical Abstracts 1975 82:261d.

12. Kariyone T. Wakan Yakuyo Shokubutsu 1940. p. 130.

13. Phytochemistry Department, Beijing Institute of Chinese Materia Medica et al. Bulletin of Chinese Materia Medica Research (Beijing Institute of Chinese Materia Madica) 1979 (2):1.

14. Zhu Y. Pharmacology and Applications of Chinese Medicinal Materials. People's Medical Publishing House. 1958. p. 34.

15. Zhou ZC et al. Chinese Pharmaceutical Bulletin 1979 14(6):252.

16. Sandberg F. Arzneimettel Forschung 1959 (9):203.

17. Imaoka I. Chemical Abstracts 1970 73:43769g.

18. Shibata M. Chemical Abstracts 1974 80:116158p.

19. Takagi K et al. Chemical Abstracts 1970 72:30185t.

20. Makarov VA et al. Farmakologiia I Toksikologiia 1969 32(4):438.

21. Pharmacology Department Beijing Institute of Chinese Materia Medica. Bulletin of Chinese Materia Medica Research 1980 (1):13.

22. Arichi S. The Journal of the Society for Oriental Medicine in Japan 1971 22(3):28.

23. Yamamoto M et al. Arzneimettel Forschung 1975 25(7):1021.

24. Oura et al. (Li GQ translator). Guowai Yixue (Medicine Abroad) — Traditional Chinese Medicine and Materia Medica 1980 (3):38.

25. Arichi S et al. Japan Centra Revuo Medicina 1980 (1):133.

26. Petorovskii GA. Farmakologiia I Toksikologiia 1957 20(1):75.

27. Liver Diseases Research Unit, Shanxi Medica College. Madical and Health Communications (Shanxi Medical College) 1973 (2):6.

28. Peseinik Ikh. Farmakologiia I Toksikologiia 1973 36(1):103.

29. Liver Diseases Research Unit, Shanxi Medical College. Medical and Health Communications (Shanxi Medical College) 1973 (3):17.

30. Shibata S et al. Chemical Abstracts 1977 87:62641g.

31. Ariehi S et al. Chemical Abstracts 1978 89:20944z.

32. Pharmacology Department, Beijing Institute of Chinese Materia Medica. Bulletin of Chinese Materia Medica Research 1980 (1):18.

33. Takagi K. The Japanese Journal of Pharmacology 1969 19:418.

34. Journal of the Pharmaceutical Society of Japan (Tokyo) 1967 87:889.

35. Takagi K et al. The Japanese Journal of Pharmacology 1968 18(1):9.

36. Markarov VA et al. Chemical Abstracts 1972 76:138196u.

37. Hiroko A et al. Planta Medica 1978 34(1):160.

38. Aonuma S. Chemical Abstracts 1958 52:4016b.

39. Yamamoto M. Metabolism and Disease (Wakan Yaku Supplement) 1973 10(5):695.

40. Zhang YM (translator). Chinese Traditional and Herbal Drugs Communications 1976 (8):47.

41. Wu HS et al. Hubei Journal of Traditional Chinese Medicine 1980 (1):37.

42. Hosono et al. The Journal of Society for Oriental Medicine in Japan 1970 21(1):8.

43. Wang SY. Kexue Tongbao (Science Bulletin) 1958 (12):379.

44. Zhejiang People's Academy of Health. Medical Research Information (Zhejiang Medical College) 1971 (3):35.

45. Wang HZ et al. Xinyiyaoxue Zazhi (Journal of Traditional Chinese Medicine) 1975 (3):48.

46. Nanjing Medical College. Encyclopedia of Chinese Materia Medica. Vol. 2. Shanghai People's Publishing House. 1978 p. 3763.

47. Wuxi First People's Hospital. Wuxi Yiyao (Wuxi Medical Journal) 1973 (1):42.

48. Pingliang District First People's Hospital. Technical Information on Combined Western and Traditional Chinese Medicine 1976 (1):1.

49. Sun ZY. Shanghai Journal of Traditional Chinese Medicine 1965 (3):1.

50. Metabolism and Disease (Wakan Yaku Supplement) 1973 10(5):702.

51. Helio C. Chemical Abstracts 1970 72:30225f.

52. Xu JG. Dermatological Research Communications 1978 (1):59.

53. Wu XZ et al. Journal of Traditional Chinese Medicine 1965 (7):12.

54. Liu CR. Hunan Yiyao Zazhi (Hunan Medical Journal) 1974 (5):24.

55. Jiang JM et al. Journal of Traditional Chinese Medicine 1980 (1):23.

56. Stecher PG. The Merck Index. 8th edition. Merck and Co. 1969. p. 597.

57. Awata (Chen PY translator). Guowai Yixue (Medicine Abroad) — Traditional Chinese Medicine and Materia Medica 1980 (3):37.

58. Li JX. Journal of Traditional Chinese Medicine 1980 (6):31.

(Wang Yusheng)

DANGSHEN 黨參

<Dangshen> refers to the root of *Codonopsis pilosula* (Franch.) Nannf. (Campanulaceae). The plants *C. tangshen* Oliver, *C. nervosa* (Chipp.) Nannf. and *C. clematidea* (Schrenk) Clarke are also sources of <Dangshen>. The herb is sweet and "mild". It tonifies the vital-energy and the "spleen" and is chiefly used in shortness of breath with palpitation, lassitude and physical weakness, and watery stool with poor appetite.

CHEMICAL COMPOSITION

<Dangshen> contains saponins, trace amounts of alkaloids, carbohydrates, mucilage, and resin.

The root of *C. tangshen* contains volatile oil, scutellarein glucoside, trace amounts of alkaloids, polysaccharides, inulin, and saponins.

The root of *C. clematidea* contains two alkaloids, codonopsine and codonopsinine.

PHARMACOLOGY

1. Effect on Animal Motoricity

A paper reported that the intragastric dose of the <Dangshen> decoction 0.25 g markedly enhanced the swimming ability of weight-loaded mice (1). However, another paper reported that intragastric administration of the <Dangshen> injection (ethanol extract of the <Dangshen> decoction) 0.5 g daily for 5 days did not enhance the swimming ability of weight-loaded mice (2).

2. Effect on Organismic Responses

In experiments, mice were placed inside an oven at 45–47°C after receiving a subcutaneous dose of 0.2 g of the <Dangshen> injection. It was found that the survival time of the treatment group was significantly longer than that of the control. This finding indicates that <Dangshen> increases the tolerance of animals to high temperature (2).

3. Promotion of Phagocytosis

Daily intragastric administration of the <Dangshen> decoction, 0.25 g of 1–2 weeks, accelerated the clearance of the intravenously injected ^{131}I-plasma protein colloidal particles from the blood, suggesting an enhancement of reticuloendothelial phagocytosis. The sporophore of *Ganoderma lucidum* and the root of *Astragalus membranaceus* were also reported to have this effect. Thus, a more striking effect was obtained when <Dangshen> was combined with the sporophore of *Ganoderma lucidum* as in the G. lucidum Mixture (3). Both *in vitro* an *in vivo* studies proved that Linctus of Radix Codonopsis Pilosulae and Fructus Lycii markedly promoted the phagocytic function of the peritoneal macrophages in mice (4).

4. Effect on the Blood and Hematopoietic System

Subcutaneous injection of the aqueous or ethanol extract of <Dangshen> and, especially, oral administration of the <Dangshen> powder to rabbits caused an increase of erythrocytes, decrease of leukocytes, and relative increase of neutrophils and decrease of lymphocytes. After splenectomy, the extracts still increased erythocytes; but their effect was weak, and the leukocyte count was decreased while the change in differential count was unchanged. <Dangshen> also increased the amount of hemoglobin, and this effect was likewise greatly attenuated after splenectomy. Feeding splenectomized animals with <Dangshen> plus the fresh spleen heightened these effects, suggesting association of the herb' s action with the spleen. However, the effects of <Dangshen> were short-lived, i.e., the pretreatment blood picture was restored 20 days after cessation of the <Dangshen> diet (5–7).

The <Dangshen> decoction 5 g/kg injected subcutaneously to rabbits also markedly increased erythrocytes and hemoglobin, and markedly decreased leukocytes (1). Another article showed that daily intragastric administration of the decoction 2 g/kg for 3 days decreased, though statistically insignificantly, both red and white blood cell counts. Increasing the dose to 5 g/kg caused a marked increase in leukocytes but no significant decrease in erythrocytes (8). Subcutaneous administration of the <Dangshen> injection at 0.3 g/day to mice for 5 days markedly increased the leukocyte and reticulocyt counts and slightly reduced the erythrocytes and hemoglobin. Yet, when the drug was given intragastrically for the same period of time, the erythrocytes, leukocytes and hemoglobin were significantly increased, while there were no significant effects on the reticulocytes and lymphocytes. In studies employing similar methods, no significant effects were observed in rats after the oral doses of the docoction, or in rabbits after the intraperitoneal doses of the injection liquid (9). Given these inconsistent results, it is imperative to carry out further studies in order to ascertain the effects of <Dangshen>.

The 1:40 aqueous extract of <Dangshen> had no hemolytic action; but it reacted with erythrocytes to produce discoloration and turbid precipitation (10). The 100% injection was also devoid of hemolytic action but it promoted blood coagulation an markedly shortened the plasma recalcification time (9,11).

5. Effect on Blood Glucose

The decoction 6 g/kg PO markedly elevated the blood glucose level in rabbits (8). The herb injection at 0.5 g/mouse IP and 1 g/kg IV in rabbits also caused pronounced hyperglycemia. On the other hand, <Dangshen> injection, 1 g administered subcutaneously to rats for 13 days, did not modify the blood glucose level. Experiments on mice indicated that the injection antagonized insulin-induced hypoglycemia, but was ineffective against that induced by epinephrine (9). The extract evoked a hyperglycemic effect in rabbits at 0.8 kg/kg SC, but had no effect when given orally. Removal of the sugars from the extract by enzymolysis prior to subcutaneous administration abolished the hyperglycemic effect, suggesting that the hyperglycemic effect was related to the sugars contained therein (6,7).

6. Effect on the Cardiovascular System

Transient hypotension was produced by the aqueous and ethanol extracts of <Dangshen> injected intravenously to anesthetized dogs and rabbits (1,7,8,12). The intravenous doses of <Dangshen> injection, i.e., 0.5 g/kg in anesthetized rabbits and 0.25 g/kg in anesthetized dogs, promptly decreased the blood pressure, which was also rapidly reversed. Tachyphylaxis from repeated dosings was absent. The hypotensive effect of <Dangshen> was not modified by bilateral vagotomy, intravenous injection of atropine, diphenhydramine, or procaine, suggesting that the effect was not attributed to by stimulation of parasympathetic receptors and interoceptors, or to histamine release (12). Some authors claimed that the herb extract markedly antagonized the pressor effect of epinephrine (1,13); another paper, however, reported that it had no such effect (12). Codonopsine injected intravenously to anesthetized cats, at doses exceeding 20 mg/kg, decreased the blood pressure (14). Low concentrations of the herb injection or the ethanol extract inhibited isolated toad heart, whereas high concentrations caused cardiac arrest (9,12). No hypotensive effect was observed in chronic hypertensive dogs given the aqueous extract 4 g/kg/day PO (15).

7. Miscellaneous Actions

<Dangshen> injection administered intraperitoneally produced no hypothermic effect in normal rabbits, nor any antipyretic effect on febrile response by bacterial vaccine (2). The decoction increased the tonicity and slightly decreased the contraction amplitude of the isolated small intestine of rabbits (16). The injection produced stimulant effects on isolated rat uteri (9). *In vitro*, meningococcus was moderately sensitive to the injection, whereas *Corynebacterium diphtheriae, Neisseria catarrhalis, Escherichia coli, E. paracolon* (17), and *Mycobacterium tuberculosis* var. *hominis* were slightly sensitive (18). There was report to the effect that the decoction markedly promoted the growth of halophilic bacteria, *Salmonella enteritidis*, and *Shigella shigae* (19).

8. Toxicity

The LD_{50} of <Dangshen> injection in mice was determined to be 79.21 ± 3.60 g/kg IP. Subcutaneous injection of the herb 0.5 g to rats for 13 days did not produce toxic reactions. Intraperitoneal injection of 1 g to rabbits for 15 days caused no toxic symptoms or changes in the SGPT level (6). The LD$_{50}$ of codonopsine in mice was 666–778 mg/kg IP (14).

CLINICAL STUDIES

1. Neurosis

Compound <Dangshen> Injection, which contains 1 g of <Dangshen> and 50 mg of vitamin B per ml, clinically tried in 144 cases, at a daily dose of 2 ml/person IM, for two weeks as a therapeutic course, with certain effectiveness (20).

2. Hematopoietic Diseases

Either used alone or with other drugs, <Dangshen> showed therapeutic value in the management of anemia, chlorosis, leukemia and thrombocytopenia (5,6).

3. "Asthenia of Spleen and Stomach" (Poor Gastrointestinal Function)

<Dangshen> may be used to treat "asthenia of the spleen and stomach", poor appetite with loose bowel, scanty saliva and polydipsia. Instant teas prepared from two parts of <Dangshen> and one part of the fruit of *Lycium barbarum* were said to offer better results (4).

4. Postgastrectomy Therapy

The modified "Sijunzi Tang" (Decoction of Four Noble Herbs) (Radix Codonopsis Pilosulae, Rhizoma Atractylodis Macrocephalae, Poria, Radix Glycyrrhizae, Radix Polygoni Multiflori, and Radix Paeoniae Albae) was given as a "postoperative decoction" in 154 cases of gastric operations. It was reported that the amount of fluid replenishment could be reduced by the oral decoction given 16–24 hours after the operation (21).

5. Gastric Ulcer

"Liuwei Tang" (Decoction of Six Drugs) (Radix Codonopsis Pilosulae, Rhizoma Atractylodis Macrocephalae, Poria, Radix Aucklandiae, Fructus Amomi, and roasted Radix Glycyrrhizae) was used to treat 20 cases of gastric ulcer. Eighteen cases benefitted, of which 10% achieved a short-term cure (21).

6. Hyperemesis Gravidarum (Vomiting of Pregnancy)

"Liujunzi Tang" (Six Major Herbs Decoction) (Radix Codonopsis Pilosulae, Rhizoma Atractylodis Macrocephalae, Poria, Pericarpium Citri Reticulatae, Rhizoma Pinelliae, and roasted Radix Glycyrrhizae) was given to 93 cases with satisfactory therapeutic results. Vomiting stopped after 2 doses in 50 cases, after 4 doses in 24 cases, and after 5–8 doses in 16 cases, while in the remaining 3 cases an antiemetic effect was obtained after 10–14 doses (24).

7. Nephritis

Nephritis and albuminuria were reported to have been effectively treated with <Dangshen> and the root of *Astragalus membranaceus* (6). Others reported the use of "Dangshen Guilu Pill" (Radix Codonopsis Pilosulae, Colla Plastri Testudinis, Colla Cornus Cervi, Colla Corii Asini, Radix Rehmanniae Conquitae, and Radix Angelicae Sinensis) in the treatment of 11 cases of chronic nephritis, of which 6 cases benefitted (22,23).

ADVERSE EFFECTS

<Dangshen> has a low toxicity; it has no ill effects in general clinical application. Overdosage (exceeding 60 g per dose) might cause precordial discomfort and arrhythmia; but these reactions disappeared spontaneously upon discontinuation of the medication (5).

REFERENCE

1. Zhou LJ et al. Jiangxi Yiyao (Jiangxi Medical Journal) 1961 (12–13):29.
2. Wang SM et al. Shanxi Yiyao (Shanxi Medical Journal) 1973 (9):22.
3. Isotopes Laboratory, Beijing Institute of Tuberculosis. Xinyiyaoxue Zazhi (Journal of Traditional Chinese Medicine) 1974 (8):13.
4. Zhu CW et al. Studies on Chinese Proprietary Medicine 1979 (5):46.
5. Jiang TL. The References of Traditional Chinese Medicine 1976 (4):33.
6. Zhu Y. Pharmacology and Applications of Chinese Medicinal Materials. People's Medical Publishing House. 1958. p. 247.
7. Jing LB et al. Contr Inst Physiol Nat Acad Peiping 1935 2:61, 145.
8. Zhang ZW et al. Harbin Zhongyi (Harbin Journal of Traditional Chinese Medicine) 1963 (3):43.
9. Wang SM et al. Shanxi Yiyao (Shanxi Medical Journal) 1973 (9):28, 35, 56.
10. Zhao SX et al. Journal of East China College of Pharmacy 1956 (1):37.
11. Wang SM et al. Shanxi Yiyao (Shanxi Medical Journal) 1973 (9):58.

12. Wang JM. Shanghai Zhongyiyao Zazhi (Shanghai Journal of Traditional Chinese Medicine) 1956 (1):36.

13. Jing LB et al. Chinese Reports of the Institute of Physiology (National Peiping Research Institute) 1935 1:63.

14. Khanov MT et al. Chemical Abstracts 1972 77:135091r.

15. Zhang BH. Abstracts of the 1963 Symposium of the Society of Physiology (Beijing Branch). 1963. p. 78.

16. Acute Abdomen Research Unit, Zunyi Medical College. Xinyiyaoxue Zazhi (Journal of Traditional Chinese Medicine) 1974 (12):39.

17. Wuhan Sanitation and Anti-epidemic Station. Hubei Science and Technology — Medicine 1972 (6):37.

18. Chen YY et al. Jiangxi Yiyao (Jiangxi Medical Journal) 1961 (12–13):31.

19. Hygiene Department, Institute of Industrial Health of the Chinese Academy of Medical Sciences. Hygiene Research 1972 (1):13.

20. Pharmaceutics Department, Xiaogan County People's Hospital. Hubei Science and Technology — Medicine 1976 (3):25.

21. Guangdong College of Traditional Chinese Medicine et al. Chinese Traditional Prescriptions. Shanghai People's Publishing House. 1974. p. 157.

22. Mei GW et al. Guangdong Yixue (Guangdong Medical Journal) — Traditional Medicine Edition 1964 (1):32.

23. Sha CG et al. Journal of Traditional Chinese Medicine 1961 (2):23.

(Liu Wenqing)

XUCHANGQING 徐長卿

<Xuchangqing> refer to the whole plant of *Cynanchum paniculatum* (Bunge) Kitag. (*Pycnostelma paniculatum* (Bunge) K. Schum.) (Asclepiadaceae). Also called <Liaodiaozhu>, the herb tastes pungent and has a "warm" property. It is credited with detoxicant, anti-inflammatory, detumescent, emmenagogic, channel-deobstruent and analgesic activities. It is mainly used in the treatment of flatulence, stomachache, toothache, menstrual disorder, pruritic eczema, snake bite, and wounds and injuries.

CHEMICAL COMPOSITION

The whole herb contains paeonol 1%, flavone and small amounts of alkaloids (1,2).

PHARMACOLOGY

1. Effect on the CNS

1.1 *Analgesic effect.* Injection of <Xuchangqing> 5 or 10 g/kg IP to mice was shown to produce an analgesic effect in the hot plate method; this effect appeared 10 minutes after medication and lasted over one our (3). Paeonol also increased the pain threshold in mice. However, it was demonstrated by other workers that C. paniculatum Fluid Extract which was devoid of paeonol still delayed the reaction to pain, and increased the pain threshold as well as analgesic rate (4), suggesting the presence of analgesic constituents other than paeonol in <Xuchangqing>.

1.2 *Sedative Effect.* Paeonol has a sedative effect (refer to the monograph on <Moudanpi>. In the radiant heat and the tremble cage methods, the dose 5 g/kg IP of C. paniculatum Injection devoid of paeonol markedly reduced the spontaneous activity but did not prolong the barbiturate-induced sleep in mice (3). However, transient episodes of convulsion appeared in rabbits give the intravenous injection. Whether or not this result was due to the differences in routes of administration or species used requires further study (4).

2. Effect on the Cardiovascular System

Injection of <Xuchangqing> 3 g/kg IP daily for 7 days to rabbits failed to eliminate T wave elevation on the ECG due to acute myocardial ischemia elicited by intravenous infusion of pituitrin (3). However, injection of the <Xuchangqing> decoction 10 –15 g/kg IP to mice caused a marked increase in the ^{86}Rb uptake of the myocardium; therefore, the herb is believed to be capable of increasing the coronary flow, improving myocardial metabolism, and consequently relieving myocardial ischemia (3,5).

Paeonol decreased the blood pressure of animals (5). The paeonol free <Xuchangqing> preparations also lowered the blood pressure and decreased the heart rate in dogs, rabbits, and rats. Hence, apart from paeonol, there could be other antihypertensive constituents in the herb (3,5).

3. Effect on Experimental Hyperlipidemia and Atherosclerosis

Daily administration of the herb 3 g/kg PO to rabbits with hyperlipidemia induced by cholesterol diet caused a marked reduction in the serum total cholesterol and β-lipoprotein in the 5th and 9th weeks, relative to the control. The incidence of atherosclerotic changes was also comparatively low, i.e., 3/10 in the treatment group, against 7/9 in the control. In the treatment group, large lipid plaques in the arterioles were dispersed and minimal, and damage to the adrenal glands, reticuloendothelial system and the liver was relatively mild. In addition, from studies of changes in the basophilic leukocytes in rabbits with experimental hyperlipidemia, it was found that after nine weeks of medication the basophilic leukocytes increased with the decrease in cholesterol level. This event shows the antilipemic action of <Xuchangqing> (3,6).

4. Effect on Smooth Muscles

C. paniculatum Injection caused a decrease in the tension of the isolated ileum of guinea pigs and antagonized strong ileal contractions induced by barium chloride, but not those produced by acetylcholine or histamine. However, the same methods showed that paeonol markedly antagonized strong contractions of the isolated ileum of guinea pigs induced by acetylcholine, histamine, and barium chloride (7).

5. Antibacterial Effect

The agar well diffusion method showed that *Staphylococcus aureus* was moderately sensitive to <Xuchangqing>, while *Escherichia coli, Shigella sonnei, Pseudomonas aeruginosa*, and *Salmonella typhi* were insensitive to it. <Xuchangqing> also inhibited alpha streptococcus (8). *In vitro* dilution method demonstrated that the 1:4 decoction of <Xuchangqing> inhibited *Shigella flexneri* and *Salmonella typhi*, whereas the 1:2 decoction inhibited *Pseudomonas aeruginosa, Escherichia coli*, and *Staphylococcus aureus* (9). Paeonol at the concentration 1:15,000 inhibited *Escherichia coli* and *Bacillus subtilis* and at 1:2000 inhibited *Staphylococcus aureus, in vitro* (10).

6. Toxicity

The LD_{50} of the paeonol free <Xuchangqing> preparation in mice was 32.9±1.0 g/kg IP (3,5).

Injection of this agent at 5 g/kg IV to rabbits produced convulsion lasting 30–60 seconds, but the animals were able to get up after 1–2 minutes and recover gradually; they appeared to be well within 48 hours (3).

CLINICAL STUDIES

1. Analgesia

The effect of <Xuchangqing> on rheumatic pain and toothache was excellent. It was also effective in lumbar muscular strain, stomachache, abdominal pain, cancer pain, and postoperative pain. *Dosage and administration*: 0.5% aqueous or oil solution of paeonol 50 mg or 100 mg can be given by intramuscular or acupoint injection 1–2 times daily (1,11).

2. Skin Diseases

Clinically, the herb may be used to treat skin diseases such as eczema, urticaria, psoriasis, contact dermatitis, and neurodermatitis. *Dosage and administration*: Dry herb powder 6–12 g decocted in water can be taken by mouth, or used as an external wash; C. paniculatum Injection can be administered intramuscularly (12, 13).

3. Chronic Bronchitis and Asthma

The decoction of the dried herb 6–12 g can be given by mouth (12,14).

4. Malaria

A single oral dose of the decoction of the dried herb 9–12 g was tried in 122 cases. In 88.5% of the treated cases, the blood smear was found to be negative for the plasmodium 2–3 days after medication; clinical symptoms disappeared, and there were no relapses during a period of one month. In 4.9% of the cases, the malarial symptoms were controlled during three weeks with no incidence of relapse, but positive blood smear persisted, and in 6.6% of the cases the symptoms and blood examination were unchanged (15).

5. Miscellaneous

Oral administration of the dried <Xuchangqing> 6–12 g decocted, and local application of the crushed fresh herb can be used to treat viper bites (11). The compound preparations of this herb were found to reduce patients' blood cholesterol and blood pressure (16).

REFERENCE

1. Pharmaceutics Department, Nanjing Hospital of Traditional Chinese Medicine. Chinese Traditional and Herbal Drugs Communications 1973 (2):38.

2. Lin YX et al. Acta Pharmaceutica Sinica 1963 10(9):576.

3. Hebei College of New Medicine. Research of New Traditional Chinese Medicine 1975 (1):36.

4. Editorial Group. National Collection of Chinese Materia Medica. People' s Medical Publishing House. 1975. p. 699.

5. Drug Therapy Section, Hebei College of New Medicine. Xinyiyaoxue Zazhi (Journal of Traditional Chinese Medicine) 1973 (10):30.

6. Antihypertensive Agents Section of the Pharmacology Department, Institute of Materia Medica of the Chinese Academy of Medical Sciences. Acta Pharmaceutica Sinica 1960 7(8):250.

7. Reference materials of the pharmacology section of Nanjing College of Pharmacy. 1972.

8. Editorial Group. South Zhejiang Herbal. New edition. 1975. p. 269.

9. Hubei Science and Technology — Medicine 1971 (2):211.

10. Ota T et al. Japan Centra Revuo Medicina 1963 184:125.

11. Shanghai No. 1 Pharmaceutical Factory. Pharmaceutical Industry 1973 (7):7.

12. 'May 7th' Health School of Rongcheng Country (Shandong). Chinese Traditional and Herbal Drugs Communications 1970 (4):25.

13. Minjia Production Brigade Health Post (Mia Commune of Yidu County, Shandong). Chinese Traditional and Herbal Drugs Communications 1974 (3):45.

14. Information o the prevention and treatment of chronic bronchitis. Shangqiu District (Henan):1974. p. 52.

15. Chinese Traditional Drugs Research Group, Liji Commune Health Centre (Gushi County, Henan). Xinyiyaoxue Zazhi (Journal of Traditional Chinese Medicine) 1975 (6):36.

16. 197th Hospital of the Chinese PLA. New Chinese Medicine 1973 (1):14.

(Bao Dingyuan)

CHOUWUTONG 臭梧桐

<Chouwutong> is the leaf of *Clerodendron trichotomum* Thunb. (Verbenaceae). The root and stem may also be used medicinally. Also known as <Bajiaowutong>, the herb has a bitter and sweetish taste, and a "mild" property. It is antirheumatic, analgesic, and hypotensive. It is chiefly use in treatment of rheumatism, hemiplegia, migraine, and severe intermittent headache. It has been used recently as a folk remedy for hypertension.

CHEMICAL COMPOSITION

<Chouwutong> contains clerodendrin, acacetin-7-glucurono-(1→2)-glucuronide (1), bitter substances (2), inositol, and alkaloids. Two crystals were recently isolated and named clerodendronins A and B (3). The former has a marked sedative effect, and the latter a marked analgesic effect. Both substances have a very weak hypotensive effect.

The hypotensive components of <Chouwutong> easily dissolve in water, but do not readily dissolve or are insoluble in ethyl ether, ethanol, and chloroform (4,5). They were thought to be alkaloids (6) or high molecular weight organic acids (7).

The root of *C. trichotomum* contains clerosterol, clerodolone, and clerodone.

PHARMACOLOGY

1. Hypotensive Action

Both chronic and acute studies on laboratory animals consistently confirmed the hypotensive effect of <Chouwutong> (3–11).

The effect of the <Chouwutong> decoction intragastrically administered to dogs with renal hypertension was found to be superior to that of the back of *Eucommia ulmoides* but inferior to that of the total alkaloids of *Rauvolfia* (12). The <Chouwutong> infusion or extract given orally to rats with renal hypertension reduced the blood pressure by 16–57.4% 3–10 days after medication. The blood pressure was restored within two weeks of discontinuation of medication. On the other hand, the intravenous injection of these extracts initiated a biphasic hypotensive action in anesthetized dogs and rats. The first phase was characterized by the prompt appearance of a pronounced but brief action lasting not longer than 45 minutes. The second phase featured a weak but prolonged action usually appearing 30–50 minutes after medication. Only the second phase was produced by the intramuscular or oral doses of the extracts, and only the first phase was achieved by the intravenous dose of the decoction; the oral dose was inactive (*presumably referred to the first phase action). Consequently, the first phase of the hypotensive action is thought to be nonspecific with no therapeutic value (4).

The herb harvested prior to the flowering stage was found to be more potent than that collected later. Prolonged storage decreased its potency (4,5,7). Disputes abound regarding the hypotensive mechanism of <Chouwutong>. Some workers believed that the hypotensive effect was mediated by the CNS and baroreceptors of the cardiac blood vessels (13), while others attributed it to direct vasodilation (6), or related it to the brain, ganglions, and peripheral blood vessels (11).

The hypotensive action of <Chouwutong> was markedly weakened in decerebrated cats (14). Hexamethonium or spinal section at the level of the second cervical vertebra virtually abolished the second phase of the hypotensive action (15). Moreover, the pressor reflex due to electrical stimulation of the peroneal nerve and compression of the carotid artery was inhibited for a long time by <Chouwutong>. The herb also markedly weakened and even reversed the pressor response to electrical stimulation of the afferent vagus nerve (13, 15). <Chouwutong> acted on the baroreceptors of pulmonary vessels causing reflex hypotension (13), but this effect was completely or virtually abolished by blockade of the baroreceptors by intravenous injection of procaine (13,15). Vagotomy, atropinization, or bilateral occlusion of the carotid sinuses did not modify the hypotensive effect. In experiments with the cat nictitating membrane, it was shown that the infusion of <Chouwutong> (15) and clerodendronin A (16) had a weak ganglionic blocking action and that they synergized with hexamethonium. The herb did not antagonize the effects of epinephrine on blood pressure and nictitating membrane, nor did it enhance the hypotensive effect of acetylcholine (10,15,16).

<Chouwutong> perfused into the blood vessels of toad hind limbs produced a direct vasodilatory effect (9,10,15). In denervated rabbit ears, pronounced vasodilation was initiated by <Chouwutong> but it was brief; this does not, however, quite conform with it prolonged hypotensive action. In an experiment with dogs, the first hypotensive phase was characterized by a significant reduction in the splenic volume. In contrast, the second phase brought a slight increase in the splenic volume but produced no changes in the volume of the hind limb. The herb directly initiated vasoconstriction in rabbit ears and rat hind limbs (15). Therefore, the hypotensive mechanism involves primarily the inhibition of the vasomotor center, and the reflex mechanism of vascular baroreceptors. The slight inhibition of ganglions plays a secondary role, whilst there is no connection between the direct vasodilatory and specific hypotensive actions of the herb.

2. Sedative Effect

<Chouwutong> had a sedative effect; it prolonged the anesthesia produced by pentobarbital sodium but was itself devoid of a hypnotic effect. It failed to antagonize strychnine- and caffeine-induced convulsions (10,17). <Chouwutong> synergized with earthworms in antagonizing caffeine-induced convulsions (18). The sedative index and potency of clerodendronin A were greater than those of reserpine (19).

3. Analgesic Effect

<Chouwutong> was proved to have an analgesic effect in mice by stimulating electrically the tail

(20). Clerodendronin B at doses of 4 and 8 mg/10 g IP in mice produced a more striking and prolonged analgesic effect than morphine at 10 and 20 mg/kg, respectively. Clerodendronin B at 60 mg/kg IV (equivalent to 10 g/kg of the crude drug) produced a transient hypotensive effect only. Hence, it is inferred that the analgesic and the hypotensive principles of the herb are not identical substances (3).

4. Anti-inflammatory Effect

<Chouwutong>, *Bidens bipinnata*, or *Siegesbeckia orientalis* used on its own did not inhibit formaldehyde- or egg white-induced paw swelling in rats. But a significant anti-inflammatory action was obtained by combining <Chouwutong> with *Bidens bipinnata* as in "Guanjie Ling" (Arthritis Drug), or with *Siegesbeckia orientalis* as in Herba Siegesbeckiae-Folium Clerodendri Trichotomi Pill. The decoction or ethanol extract of <Chouwutong> at 20 g/kg PO once daily for 5 days was as effective as sodium salicylate at 300 mg/kg IP. The efficacy of the combined preparations seemed to have resulted from the synergism of the drugs and not to be due to a newly formed substance in the mixture (21). Both the steroids and total alkaloids isolated from Guanjie Ling were effective against experimental paw swelling in rats. But the total alkaloids produced a significant effect only at doses exceeding 520 g(crude drug)/kg. For the steroids, even larger doses were required. It is evident that these two constituents were not the chief anti-inflammatory principles (22).

Guanjie Ling by mouth caused a marked decrease in the vitamin C content of rat adrenal glands; it appeared to stimulate the secretion of the adrenal cortex. It did not, however, effect the urinary excretion of 17-ketosteroids in guinea pigs and in patients with rheumatoid arthritis. Additionally, Guanjie Ling significantly inhibited egg white-induced paw swelling in adrenalectomized rats, suggesting that its anti-inflammatory effect was not entirely dependent upon its action on the pituitary-adrenal system (23).

5. Miscellaneous Actions

Long-term intragastric administration of <Chouwutong> preparations to rats increased the gelatinoid substance of the thyroid gland, which is not considered as a toxic reaction but is attributed to inhibition of the sympathetic nerves responsible for regulating thyroid secretion into the blood stream (24). <Chouwutong> was also found to have an anthelmintic activity (25).

6. Toxicity

In mice, the LD_{50} of <Chouwutong> infusion was 19.4 g/kg IV. The dose 150 g/kg PO caused no deaths within 72 hours. The doses 0.25 and 2.5 g/kg given to rats via the same route daily for 60 days did not produce any abnormalities in the urine, blood, body weight, and pathological examination. Only a few of the animals had an increased water intake and appeared sedated, less active, and diarrheic (4). Likewise, the herb decoction administered to dogs at 10 g/kg PO had no effect on the liver, blood, and ECG, but the dose 20 g/kg induced vomiting (12).

The toxic effects of clerodendronins A and B were minimal; the LD_{50} of clerodendronin A in mice was 1.84 g/kg IP (equivalent to 370 g/kg of the crude drug). Oral doses as high as 10 times this dose did not cause death in rats. On the other hand, the LD_{50} of clerodendronin B in mice was 3.21 g/kg IP (equivalent to 550 g/kg of the crude drug) (3).

CLINICAL STUDIES

1. Hypertension

Tablets prepared from <Chouwutong> powder can be given by mouth at a daily dosage of 10–16 g in 3–4 doses. Out of 171 cases of hypertension treated with this preparation, 78 cases (45.16%) showed decreases in the diastolic pressure of over 20 mmHg and 62 cases (36.26%) had over 10 mmHg reduction. Marked therapeutic effects generally appeared in 5 weeks, and the efficacy increased with the duration of therapy. Concurrent improvement in symptoms including headache and dizziness was also obtained. A rebound elevation of the blood pressure occurred 1–2 weeks after discontinuation of medication unless a dosage of 2–4 g daily was maintained (26). In another report of 430 cases, the therapeutic effect of <Chouwutong> was said to be slightly better than that of the *Rauvolfia* preparations (27). The combination of <Chouwutong> with earthworms was found to be more efficacious than the herb used alone (28).

2. Rheumatic Arthritis

Excellent therapeutic effects were achieved by combining this herb with *Siegesbeckia orientalis* (Herba Siegesbeckia-Folium Clerodendri Trichotomi Pill) (29), or with *Bidens bipinnata* (Herba Bidensis Bipinnatae-Folim Clerodendri Trichotomi Pill) (30) against rheumatic arthritis (refer to the monograph on <Xixiancao> for the therapeutic effect of Herba Siegesbeckiae-Folium Clerodendri Trichotomi Pill).

3. Chronic Bronchitis

The fresh stem and lead of *C. trichotomum* 200 g made into a decoction can be administered by mouth in 3 doses daily, 10 days as a therapeutic course. In 88 cases which received 3 therapeutic courses, the decoction was found to be effective in cough, expectoration and asthma, but marked effects were slow to appear and unstable (31).

4. Malaria

Two hundred and twenty-six cases of different types of malaria were treated with Clerodendron trichotomum Tablet (0.25 g/table) initially at doses of 10 tablets every 6 hours for 2 days, and then, 5 tablets thrice daily for 5 days, a total of 7 days. All symptoms were controlled within 4 days. The blood smear revealed that 82.3% became negative for the plasmodium in 2 days, 97.3% in 4 days and 98.6% in 7 days. No relapse occurred in 3 months (32).

ADVERSE EFFECTS

Generally, <Chouwutong> does not produce adverse effects. The high dosages employed to treat bronchitis caused arrhythmia, nausea, and vomiting in a few patients, and systemic edema of lower extremities, as well urticaria in individual patients, but these were mostly not serious (31).

REFERENCE

1. Okigawa M et al. Tetrahedron Letters 1970 (33):2935.

2. Journal of the Pharmaceutical Society of Japan (Tokyo) 1964 84(5):472.

3. Xu SY et al. Acta Academiae Medicinae Anhui 1960 3(2–3):8, 12.

4. Xu SY et al. Acta Pharmaceutica Sinica 1962 9(12):734.

5. Yan YJ et al. Acta Academiae Medicinae Qingdao 1957 (1):5.

6. Shanghai Institute of Hypertension. Compiled Information on Hypertension Research. 1st edition. 1959. p. 107.

7. Li CH et al. Academic Papers of the Second Military Medical College. Vol. 1. 1959.

8. Institute of Materia Medica, Chinese Academy of Sciences. Kexue Tongbao (Science Bulletin) 1956 (7):93.

9. Zou TF et al. Acta Academiae Medicinae Qingdao 1957 (1):14.

10. Shen JQ et al. Shanghai Zhongyiyao Zazhi (Shanghai Journal of Traditional Chinese Medicine) 1957 (4):5.

11. Shanghai College of Traditional Chinese Medicine et al. Abstracts of the Scientific Papers of Shanghai College of Traditional Chinese Medicine. 1st edition. 1959. p. 59.

12. Wang XL et al. Acta Pharmaceutica Sinica 1960 8(2):88.

13. Li CJ et al. Acta Academiae Medicinae Jilin — Special Issue on Traditional Chinese Medicine and Materia Medica 1959 (4):107, 115.

14. Pharmaceutics Department, Shanghai Institute of Pharmaceutical Industry. Journal of the Shanghai Institute of Pharmaceutical Industry 1958 (4):65.

15. Xu SY. Acta Physiologica Sinica 1962 25(4):272.

16. Li CC et al. Abstracts of the 1959 Symposium of Shanghai First Medical College. 1959. p. 35.

17. Xu SY. Scientific Papers of Anhui Medical College. Vol. 2. 1959. p. 1.

18. Xu SY. Scientific Papers of Anhui Medical College. Vol. 2. 1959. 51.

19. Xu SY. Information Exchanges of Anhui Medical College. 1960. p. 8.

20. Wang YR et al. Shanghai Zhongyiyao Zazhi (Shanghai Journal of Traditional Chinese Medicine) 1957 (4):11.

21. Liu GT et al. Acta Pharmaceutica Sinica 1964 11(10):708.

22. Zhu XY et al. Acta Pharmaceutica Sinica 1965 12(2):129.

23. Zhu XY et al. Abstracts of the 1962 Symposium of the Chinese Pharmaceutical Association. 1962. p. 330.

24. Morphology Group, Hypertension Research Unit of Anhui Medical College. Scientific Papers of Anhui Medical College. Vol. 2. 1959. p. 74.

25. Breitwieser K. Chemical Abstracts 1944 38:4754 (8).

26. Ding JM et al. Shanghai Zhongyiyao Zazhi (Shanghai Journal of Traditional Chinese Medicine) 1957 (3):6.

27. Shanghai Eleventh People's Hospital. Compiled Information on Traditional Chinese Medicine Research. 1st edition. Shanghai Health Bureau. 1959. p. 1.

28. Hypertension Group. Acta Academiae Medicinae Anhui 1960 3(2–3):20.

29. Tao WG. Journal of Traditional Chinese Medicine 1957 (11):608.

30. Chinese Academy of Medical Sciences. Medical and Health Express 1959 (45):15.

31. Kaijiang County Coordinating Research Group on Chronic Bronchitis. Sichuan Communication on Chinese Traditional and Herbal Drugs 1972 (4):28.

32. Li ZR et al. Journal of Traditional Chinese Medicine 1961 (5):31.

(Xue Chunsheng)

ZHEBEIMU 浙貝母

<Zhebeimu> refer to the bulb of *Fritillaria verticillata* Willd. var. *thunbergii* Bak. (Liliaceae). It is bitter and slightly "cold". Its actions are reputed to be antitussive, mucolytic, discutient and detumescent. It is, therefore, useful in cough (*due to common cold; characterized by thick sputum, etc.), pulmonary abscess, laryngitis, lymph node tuberculosis, pyogenic infection and ulcers of the skin.

CHEMICAL COMPOSITION

<Zhebeimu> contains alkaloids peimine, peiminine, peimidine, peimiphine, peimisine, and peimitidine. The last four are in trace quantities. It also contains propeimine, a steroid. A glycoalkaloid, named peiminoside, was recently isolated. Hydrolysis of peiminoside yields peimine and a molecule of glucose. The hypotensive effect of peiminoside is stronger than that of peimine.

PHARMACOLOGY

1. Antitussive Effect

Injection of peimine or peiminine 4 mg/kg SC to guinea pigs with cough induced by sulfur dioxide produced no antitussive effect (1). Likewise, administration of <Zhebeimu> 0.4 g/kg PO to cats with cough induced by injection of iodine solution into the costal pleural cavity did not produce an antitussive effect (2). On the other hand, "Bei Xin Powder" (the commercial product of its young buds) and the ethanol extract of <Zhebeimu>, separately given to mice at 2 and 4 g/kg PO before cough induction with sulfur dioxide, resulted in a conspicuous antitussive effect lasting for as long as 2 hours. A significant antitussive effect was also produced by injection of the <Zhebeimu> alkaloids 3 mg/kg IP in mice (3).

2. Effect of the Circulatory System

Both peimine and peiminine perfused into isolated frog hearts at concentrations of 1:5000–1:1000 caused bradycardia and atrioventricular block (4). Peimine and peiminoside administered by intravenous injection to anesthetized dogs (10 mg/kg), cats (1–3 mg/kg), and rabbits (5–10 mg/kg) decreased the blood pressure. Injection of peiminoside 2 mg to the left coronary vessel of open-chest dogs did not modify the blood pressure but increased the heart rate and coronary flow (5).

3. Effect on Smooth Muscles

Perfusion of low concentration (1:5,000,000) of peimine into isolated cats and rabbit lungs dilated the bronchial smooth muscle, whereas high concentrations (1:10,000–1:1000) constricted it (6). These effects resembled those of atropine (7).

Peimine at 10^{-5}–2.5×10^{-4} increased the tension and contraction amplitude of the isolated rabbits uterus even to the extent of uterine spasm. The pregnant uterus was found to be more sensitive to the drug than the nonpregnant one. The same dosage mainly increased the amplitude and frequency of uterine contraction in albino rats. Peimine 0.5 mg was equipotent to pituitrin 1 unit, or ergometrine 0.04 mg, in causing uterine contraction in rabbits. Peimine could still stimulate the uterus after atropine blockade of the contractile effect of acetylcholine, but this effect was diminished or absent if it was administered after dibenzylamine blockade of epinephrine (8). Therefore, the action of peimine is probably due to the stimulation of adrenergic receptors. Peimine at a concentration of 2×10^{-5} was capable of increasing the contraction amplitude and frequency of peristalsis of the isolated rabbit small intestine (4).

4. Miscellaneous Actions

Peiminine briefly inhibited salivation in dogs; the action was 20–30 times weaker than that of atropine. Hence, oral doses of <Zhebeimu> do not cause xerostomia (9). In addition, the 1% peiminine hydrochloride solution caused mydriasis and loss of the light reflex in cats, pigeons, rabbits, and dogs. The mydriatic action was found to be stronger and more prolonged than that of homatropine in rabbits and pigeons (10).

5. Toxicity

Peiminine is more toxic to cats and rabbits. The MLD of the drug in rabbits was 10–12 mg/kg IV and that in cats, 8–10 mg/kg. All the animals died in 1–2 hours. Toxic symptoms included respiratory depression, mydriasis, tremor, convulsion, incontinence of urine and feces, and finally respiratory failure leading to death (11).

CLINICAL STUDIES

1. Common Cold, Acute Upper Respiratory Tract Infections, Bronchitis, and Pneumonia

In cases of cough with dry mouth, itchy throat, and thick yellowish sputum, <Chuanbeimu> may be administered in combination with the fruits of *Forsythia suspensa* and *Arctium lappa* as in the formula Morus-Prunus Decoction (12). F. verticillata Flower Extract Tablet was used to treat 245 cases; it was 76.5% effective for cough due to upper respiratory tract infections and 68.2% for that due to chronic bronchitis. *Dosage and administration*: F. verticillata Flower Extract Tablet (each 0.35 g, equivalent to 1 g of the crude drug) 3 tablets thrice daily (13).

2. Scrofula and Chronic Lymphadenitis Colli

<Chuanbeimu> can be used with the root of *Scrophularia ningpoensis*, oyster shell, fruit-spike of *Prunella vulgaris*, and the root of *Rehmannia glutinosa* such as in Prescription for Lymphadenitis Colli (12).

3. Gastric and Duodenal Ulcers

In order to prevent constipation caused by the calcium carbonate-rich cuttlefish bones used to treat ulcers, <Chuanbeimu> is often prescribed as an adjuvant such as in the Os Sepiae-Bulbus Fritillariae Powder (12).

4. Infected Lumps

Especially in mastitis, <Chuanbeimu> may be used as an adjuvant remedy in concert with the flower bud of *Lonicera japonica*, the flower of *Chrysanthemum morifolium*, and the whole of *Taraxacum mongolicum* (12). *Dosage*: generally 9–15 g, or a maximum of 18–30 g in treating scrofula (tuberculosis of cervical lymph nodes) (12).

REFERENCE

1. Wo SZ. Chinese Medical Journal 1954 40(11):853.

2. Huang QZ. Chinese Medical Journal 1954 40(5):325.

3. Institute of Materia Medica, Zhejiang People's Academy of Health. Progress in Scientific Research. Vol. 2 Zhejiang People's Academy of Health. 1966.

4. Chen KH et al. Journal of the American Pharmaceutical Association 1933 22(7):638.

5. Kikushi K et al. Folia Pharmacologica Japonica 1961 57:49.

6. Zhang YD et al. Reports on Pharmacological Studies (Institute of Physiology, National Peiping Research Institute) 1935 1(1):89.

7. Liu SG et al. Reports on Pharmacological Studies (Institute of Physiology, National Peiping Research Institute) 1935 1(1):169.

8. Wang JG et al. Abstracts of the Symposium of the Chinese Society of Physiology (Pharmacology). 1964 p. 43.

9. Zhang YD et al. Reports on Pharmacological Studies (Institute of Physiology, National Peiping Research Institute) 1935 1(2):199.

10. Zhang FC et al. Reports on Pharmacological Studies (Institute of Physiology, National Peiping Research Institute) 1935 1(2):181.

11. Liu SG et al. The National Medical Journal of China 1936 22(2):107.

12. Zhongshan Medical College (editor). Clinical Applications of Chinese Traditional Drugs. 1975. p. 483.

13. Shaoxing Chinese Medicine Factory. Chinese Traditional and Herbal Drugs Communications 1972 (3):59.

(Yuan Wei)

YIMUCAO 益母草
(APPENDIX: CHONGWEIZI 附: 茺蔚子)

<Yimucao>, also called <Chongwei>, is the whole plant of *Leonurus heterophyllus* Sweet (Labiatae). Other plants which may be used as <Yimucao> are *L. heterophyllus* Sweet f. *leucanthus* C. Y. Wu et H.W. Li, *L. sibiricus* L., and *L. turkestanicus* V. Krecz. et Kuprian.

The herb has a bitter and pungent taste, and a slightly "cold" property; it is nontoxic. It is menstruation-regulative, blood-stimulant, stasis-eliminative, regenerative, diuretic, and detumescent. It is, therefore, used to treat irregular menstruation, amenorrhea, dysmenorrhea, incessant lochial discharge, and adema in acute nephritis.

CHEMICAL COMPOSITION

<Yimucao> contains about 0.01–0.04% of leonurine, a derivative of guanidine. It also contains stachydrine, leonuridine, benzoic acid, potassium chloride (large amounts), lauric acid, linolenic acid, β-linolenic acid, oleic acid, and a phytosterol with mp 124–125°C. It was reported that five crystalline substances were isolated from the herb, two were alkaloids leonurines A and B, and three were non-alkaloids.

PHARMACOLOGY

1. Effect on the Uterus

The decoction, ethanol extract of <Yimucao> and leonurine, all, had a stimulant effect on the uteri of many animals including the rabbits, cat, dog, and guinea pig (1–3). The <Yimucao> decoction stimulated the isolated uteri of nonpregnant rabbits, also those of early and late pregnancy, and postpartum period. Stimulation of the uteri *in situ* was induced 30 minutes after a quick intravenous injection of the decoction; the potency and duration of action increased with the dosage. In rabbit uterine fistulae, intragastric administration of the <Yimucao> decoction produced marked excitation after 15–20 minutes, with or without intrauterine distention (4). The stimulant effect of the total alkaloids on the isolated guinea pig uteri resembled that of ergometrine (5). Both of the aqueous and the ethanol extracts of <Yimucao> produced conspicuous excitation of the isolated and *in situ* uteri, but in the case of the latter a brief inhibitory effect appeared prior to stimulation. This inhibitory action was absent with the aqueous solution after ether extraction. Therefore, <Yimucao> probably contained two bioactive principles, one inhibitory and the other excitatory (6).

Leonurine increased the contraction amplitude of the uterus isolated at proestrus or from ovariectomized rats premedicated with 50 μg of estradiol intramuscularly. A correlation was observed between the action and dosage of leonurine. At concentrations of 0.2–1.0 μg/ml, the dosage and uterine tension showed a linear relationship; maximum tension was attained at concentrations of 2 μg/ml or higher. At times, leonurine produced a biphasic effect on the spontaneously contracting specimens. The minimal effective dose or abruptly increased concentration (exceeding fivefold the original concentration) elicited a brief inhibition of 10–20 minutes' duration prior to the appearance of excitation in specimens with spontaneous contraction. High concentrations of the drug (> 20 μg/ml) produced an inhibitory effect on account of its local anesthetic effect on the myometrium. The contracting effect of leonurine on the uterus lasted a few hours but was stopped by washing away the drug. Atropine 2 μg/ml did not modify this effect (7).

Leonurine A also produced significant stimulation on the isolated uteri of rabbits and cats but on rabbit uteri *in situ* (8). However, the <Yimucao> injection prepared by distillation was devoid of uterine contracting effect (9). The active uterine stimulant principle mainly resided in the leaf; the root had a very weak action and the stem was inactive (4).

2. Effect on Intestinal Smooth Muscles

Low dosage of leonurine decreased the tonicity of the isolated rabbit intestinal tract and increased its contraction amplitude, whereas high dosage decreased the amplitude of contraction but increased its frequency (1,3).

3. Effect on the Circulatory System

Small doses of leonurine enhanced contraction of the isolated frog heart, but large doses caused inhibition which might be due to stimulation of the vagus nerve endings. Perfusion of frog blood vessels with leonurine caused vasoconstriction directly proportional to the concentration of the test solution. Leonurine 2 mg/kg injected intravenously to anesthetized cats promptly caused hypotension which was quickly reversed in a few minutes. Such brief hypotensive effect was observed even after bilateral vagotomy but it became less conspicuous in animals premedicated with atropine. The hypotensive effect of leonurine is therefore attributed to stimulation of the vagus nerve endings and not of the vagal nuclei. In warm-blooded animals, leonurine produced marked vasodilation and antiadrenergic effects (10). Another report claimed that in dogs the <Yimucao> injection decreased the extent of lesions due to experimental myocardial infarction, reduced the infarction area and protected the subcellular structures of the myocardium (11). In rats with isoproterenol-induced myocardial ischemia, <Yimucao> improved or normalized the ischemic ECG, increased the coronary flow, improved the microcirculation, decreased the heart rate, and antagonized platelet aggregation (12).

4. Effect on the Respiratory Center

Intravenous injection of leonurine to anesthetized cats markedly increased the respiratory rate and amplitude, but high dosage reversed the stimulant effect to inhibition, eliciting weak and irregular breathing. Bilateral vagotomy did not modify the stimulant effect, suggesting direct stimulation of the respiratory center by the drug (1,3,10).

5. Miscellaneous Actions

A pronounced increase in urine output was seen in rabbits injected with leonurine 1 mg/kg IV, and curariform effect was exerted by the drug on frog neuromuscular specimens (1). High concentrations caused hemolysis of the rabbit blood suspension (1,3).

6. Toxicity

<Yimucao> has a low toxicity. Animal feed, containing 50% of the dried <Yimucao> powder, given to adult male rats for 80 days did not produce toxic effects or modify fertility (7). The LD_{50} of the <Yimucao> injection in mice was 30–60 g/kg IV (13). Intraperitoneal injection of leonurine to rats at 2 mg daily for 4 days produced no significant adverse effects (7). The MLD of leonurine was 0.4–0.6 g/kg SC in frogs (1). Subcutaneous injection of the total alkaloids of the herb 30 mg/kg daily to rabbits for 2 weeks did not affect the food intake, fecal and urinary excretions, and body weight. The LD_{50} of the total alkaloids in mice was 572.2 ± 37.2 mg/kg IV (5).

CLINICAL STUDIES

1. Irregular Menstruation, Postpartum Uterine Hemorrhage, Incomplete Involution of Uterus, and Menorrhagia.

The <Yimucao> decoction, fluidextract, or compound prescriptions may be given orally (3,5, 14–17). The effect of the <Yimucao> extract on the involution of the uterus resembled that of the ergot extract (3,15). It was superior to the latter agent in treating lochiorrhea (15). Nevertheless, the onset of its uterine contracting effect was slow; only 16.4% of the uteri showed increase in contractility after one hour of medication and 25% within two hours; the effect was not dose-dependent (16). *Dosage and administration*: Decoction 15–20 g daily; fluidextract 2–3 ml thrice daily.

2. Nephritis

The simple decoction of <Yimucao> was satisfactorily used in 80 cases of acute glomerulonephritis, except in 9 cases where antibiotics were additionally required to combat complications such as pneumonia. The therapeutic course lasted 5–36 days. Not a single case relapsed during the follow-up period of from 6 months to 5 years. *Dosage and administration*: 90–120 g daily of the dried herb, or 180–250 g daily of the fresh herb (18). When <Yimucao> was used in 13 cases of edema due to acute or chronic nephritis, edema rapidly subsided, urinary and fecal outputs increased, and appetite improved (19). It was found in the course of clinical practice that through its blood-stimulant and stasis-eliminative actions, <Yimucao> improve and increases renal blood flow, thereby enhancing the repair and regeneration of glomeruli and renal tubules, reversing fibrosis and eliminating inflammatory lesions and albuminuria, and consequently restoring renal function (20).

3. Hypertension

The decoction, tincture, or aqueous extract of <Yimucao> may be used to treat essential hypertension (21). In 56 cases of hypertension treated with Compound Clerodendron trichotomum Tablet (Herbal Leonuri, Folium Clerodendri Trichotomi, Spica Prunellae, Herba Siegesbeckiae), the patients' blood pressure was lowered after one day of medication, and the effect was maximal on the tenth day (22).

4. Coronary Disease

Intramuscular injection of Yimucao Injection, or intravenous infusion of this injection in glucose solution, to 11 cases of coronary disease produced the following results: 9 cases showed marked symptomatic improvement, and 2 improvement; on the ECG, 6 cases showed significant improvement and 4 slight amelioration, while one case was unresponsive (13).

5. Miscellaneous

"Xiaoyan Zhidai Wan" (Anti-inflammatory and Antileukorrheal Pill) (Herba Leonuri, Radix Sanguisorbae (fried), etc.) was used in treating chronic cervicitis, vaginitis of various causes, endometritis, and salpingitis. After 10 days' treatment, the leucorrhea became clear and scanty, and there was concurrent amelioration of lower abdominal distention and pain, as well as low-back pain (23). It was reported that satisfactory results were achieved in the treatment of urticaria with the <Yimucao> extract 30 g twice daily (24) and in the treatment of 3 cases of postpartum urinary retention with <Yimucao> plus acupuncture (25); marked and rapid antilipemic effect of Antilipemic Prescription (Herba Leonuri, pulp of Fructus Crataegi, etc.) was achieved in 35 cases of hyperlipidemia (26).

ADVERSE EFFECTS

<Yimucao> has low toxicity; multiple and long-term oral doses produced no adverse reaction (14,19). The intramuscular dose did not cause toxic side effects other than xerostomia and shortened sleep (13). No ill effects were known from the clinical use of the sterilized injection of the total alkaloids 15 mg/ml (5).

(APPENDIX: CHONGWEIZI 附: 茺蔚子)

<Chongweizi>, also called <Xiaohuma> (*error in Chinese edition as Xiaomahu), is the fruit of *Leonurus heterophyllus*. It is sweet to the taste and slightly "cold". It contains leonurinine (27), alkaloids I, II, and III (28), oil (mainly oleic acid and linolenic acid) (29), and vitamin A-like substances (30).

The aqueous extract, the ethanol-water extract, and the 30%-ethanol extract of <Chongweizi> were shown to decrease the blood pressure of anethetized animals (31). Alkaloids A, though producing an insignificant action on the uterus *in situ*, showed a pronounced stimulant effect on the isolated uteri of cats and guinea pigs, increasing not only the tension but also the force and frequency of contraction (8).

The lotion, syrup, and injection preparations prepared from <Chongweizi> and the branches and leaves of *Morus alba* had therapeutic value in 214 cases of hypertension (32).

A single oral dose of about 30 g of <Chongweizi> may cause poisoning in 4–6 hours. Toxic manifestations mostly appear from 12 to 48 hours after a cumulative dose of 60 to 140 g. The symptoms include general weakness, immobility of the lower extremities, generalized soreness, chest tightness, and in severe cases, perspiration and prostration; the mental state, speech, pulse, and tongue usually remain normal (33).

REFERENCE

1. Kubota H et al. Journal of the Pharmaceutical Society of Japan (Tokyo) 1930 11(2):159.

2. Zhang FC et al. Reports on Pharmacological Studies 1935 1(1):103.

3. Zhang JR. Xinzhongyiyao (Modernized Traditional Chinese Medicine) 1952 3(6):111.

4. Lu FH et al. Chinese Medical Journal 1954 40(9):699.

5. Chengdu Institute for Drug Control. Chengdu Medical and Health Information (Revolutionary Committee of Chengdu Health Bureau) 1971 (1):88.

6. Yuan W et al. Chinese Medical Journal 1954 40(9):692.

7. Kong YC et al. The American Journal of Chinese Medicine 1976 4(4):373.

8. Pharmacology Section, Shanghai First Medical College. Collected Information of Scientific Research and Technological Innovation. Shanghai Medical College. 1959. p. 9.

9. Chinese Materia Medica Department, Beijing Institute for Drug Control. Chinese Traditional and Herbal Drugs Communications 1972 (6):49.

10. Zhu Y. Pharmacology and Applications of Chinese Medicinal Materials. Vol. 1. People's Medical Publishing House. 1958. p. 217.

11. Xiyuan Hospital of the Academy of Traditional Chinese Medicine. Xinyiyaoxue Zazhi (Journal of Traditional Chinese Medicine) 1978 (7):57.

12. Coronary Disease Coordinating Research Group, Shanghai College of Traditional Chinese Medicine. Xinyiyaoxue Zazhi (Journal of Traditional Chinese Medicine) 1980 (10):68.

13. Zou QJ et al. Shanxi Medical and Pharmaceutical Industry 1978 (4):21.

14. Western Sichuan Institute of Health. Xi' nan Yaokan (Southwestern Journal of Pharmacy) 1952 2(1):233.

15. Fu XS et al. Chinese Journal of Obstetrics and Gynecology 1956 (3):202.

16. Liao XG et al. Chinese Journal of Obstetrics and Gynecology 1958 (1):1.

17. Qin JZ. Xinzhongyiyao (Modernized Traditional Chinese Medicine) 1958 9(6):16.

18. Yao YC et al. Journal of Traditional Chinese Medicine 1966 (4):26.

19. Lin PS. Journal of Traditional Chinese Medicine 1959 (6):18.

20. Guo ZY. New Medical Information (Jiangxi College of Traditional Chinese Medicine) 1979 (1):62.

21. Shass EIU. Fel' dsh I Akusher 1950 15(12):49.

22. Cooperative Medical Clinic of Linxi Production Brigade (Fangyang Commune, Changtai Country). Medical Research Information (Fujian Institute of Medical Sciences) 1977 (3):23.

23. Huaqiao Commune Health Centre (Changyang County, Hubei). Xinyiyaoxue Zazhi (Journal of Traditional Chinese Medicine) 1973 (5):30.

24. Shanghai College of Traditional Chinese Medicine. Studies on Chinese Proprietary Medicine 1980 (4):47.

25. Shan JM. Journal of Traditional Chinese Medicine 1964 (5):3.

26. New Chinese Medicine Department, Yuanchun Worker's Hospital (Guangzhou). New Medical Communications (Guangzhou Health Bureau) 1977 (5):26.

27. Xu ZF. Journal of the Chinese Chemical Society 1934 2(3):337.

28. Wang X et al. Abstracts of the Chinese Pharmaceutical Association (Beijing Branch). 1957. p. 57.

29. Xu ZF. Journal of the Institute of Chemistry (National Research Academy) 1932:(8):1.

30. Peter GM et al. Chinese Journal of Physiology 1936 10(2):273.

31. Li GC et al. Abstracts of the 1956 Academic Conference of the Chinese Academy of Medical Sciences 1956 (2):70.

32. Zhang TK et al. Liaoning Zhongji Yikan (Liaoning Journal of Paramedics) 1979 (11):34.

33. Jiang YP et al. Journal of Traditional Chinese Medicine 1964 (3):15.

(Yang Yasi)

SANGYE 桑葉

<Sangye> is the leaf of *Morus alba* L. (Moraceae). It is bitter, sweet and "cold" and is reputed for its diaphoretic as well as vision-improving effects. It is mainly used in common cold due to pathogenic "wind-heat", cough, pharyngalgia, dizziness, headache, and acute conjunctivitis.

CHEMICAL COMPOSITION

<Sangye> contains ecdysterone, inokosterone, lupeol, traces of β-sitosterol, rutin, moracetin, isoquercetin, scopoletin, scopolin, α-hexenal, β-hexenal, cis-β-hexenol, cis-γ-hexenol, benzaldehyde, eugenol; linalool, benzyl alcohol, butylamine, acetone, trigonelline, choline, adenine, amino acids, vitamins, chlorogenic acid, fumaric acid, folic acid, formyltetrahydrofolic acid, myoinositol, copper, and zinc. It also contains phytoestrogens.

PHARMACOLOGY

1. Antibacterial Effect

In vitro, the fresh <Sangye> showed a strong action against *Staphylococcus aureus*, beta *Streptococcus hemolyticus, Corynebacterium diphtheriae*, and *Bacillus anthracis*, and also some effectiveness against *Escherichia coli, Salmonella typhi, Shigella dysenteriae*, and *Pseudomonas aeruginosa* (1). The <Sangye> decoction had a leptospiricidal action (2).

2. Hypoglycemic Effect

Both <Sangye> and ecdysterone were found to be hypoglycemic in rats with alloxan-induced diabetes mellitus, and in mice with hyperglycemia elicited by epinephrine, glucagon or insulin antiserum (3,4). Ecdysterone promoted glycogenesis from glucose without altering the blood glucose level in normal animals (4). Some investigators considered that the fall in blood glucose level was precipitated by stimulation of insulin secretion by some amino acids in <Sangye> (5,6).

3. Miscellaneous Actions

<Sangye> caused inhibition of rodent intestinal muscles and stimulation of uteri at estrus. Intravenous injection of the dilute extract of the herb caused a transient fall in the blood pressure (5). Ecdysterone promoted cellular growth, stimulated the mitosis of dermal cells to form new epithelium, and enhanced

exuviation of insects. In man, it promoted protein anabolism, eliminated cholesterol, and reduced blood lipids (7). Feeding mice with phytoestrogens obtained from the ethanol extract of <Sangye> retarded the growth (8). The 10% <Sangye> injection administered into the quadricep or instilled into the conjunctival sac of rabbits did not produce local irritation. No allergic "Sang Ju Yin" (Morus-Chrysanthemum Decoction) increased the phagocytic index of macrophages and eosinophilic leukocytes (10).

4. Toxicity

The safety does of the 10% <Sangye> injection in 20-g mice by single intraperitoneal injection was equivalent to 250 times the human dose. Intraperitoneal injection of this agent to mice at a dose 60 times the human dose for 21 days did not cause damage on the liver, kidneys, and lungs, but much higher doses caused degeneration and hemorrhage of these organs (9).

CLINICAL STUDIES

1. Common Cold

"Sang Ju Ganmao Wan" (Morus-Chrysanthemum Cold Pill) (Folium Mori, Flos Chrysanthemi, Radix Platycodi, Semen Armeniacae Amarum, Rhizoma Phragmatis, Fructus Forsythiae, Herba Menthae, Radix Glycyrrhizae) is useful in the early stage of the common cold with symptoms of cough, mild fever, headache, and nasal congestion, and also useful in the early stage of measles (11).

2. Upper Respiratory Tract Infections

The concentrate of "Qing Wen Tang Yihao" (Antipyretic Decoction No. I) (Folium Mori, Rhizoma Phragmatis, Gypsum Fibrosum Crudae, Folium Isatidis, Rhizoma Imperatae, Radix Glycyrrhizae) was use with good effects in 40 children suffering from upper respiratory tract infections with symptoms of acute fever and cough; 22 of these cases were given the decoction alone (12).

3. Whooping Cough

"Sang Xing Tang" (Morus-Prunus Decoction) (Folium Mori, Semen Armeniacae Amarum, Radix Adenophorae, Bulbus Fritillaria, Semen Soyae Praeparatum, Cortex Gardeniae, and Pericarpium Pyri) was used to treat 72 cases of whooping cough. Improvement of different extents was achieved in 69 cases after one dose; the cough was completely relieved in 24 cases after 3 doses (13).

4. Elephantiasis of Lower Limbs

The 10% <Sangye> injection 5 ml was given once or twice daily for 15–21 days as a therapeutic course, or the 25–50% injection 4 ml once daily. Three days after medication, the diseased limb was bound, resulting in softening of the skin and tissue, and reducing the limb circumference (9).

5. Miscellaneous

"Mingmu Xiaoyan Wan" (Vision-Improving and Anti-Inflammation Pill, composed of 18 herbs including Folium Mori) was effectively used to treat deep keratitis. The drug shortened the duration of the ailment, facilitated resorption of corneal opacity, reduced vascularization, and variably improved vision (14). Some effectiveness was achieved with compound formulae of <Sangye> in corneal ulcer (15), esophagitis, atrophic gastritis, chronic cholecystitis, aphonia, and bronchiectasis complicated with hemoptysis (16). "Sang Ma Wan" (Morus-Sesame Pill) (Folium Mori, Semen Sesami) was reported to be effective against vertigo, blurred vision, chronic cough, constipation due to depletion of "body fluid", and rough dry skin (17).

ADVERSE EFFECTS

The <Sangye> injection may cause local pain. Some patients may develop chills, fever and dizziness, possibly induced by the precipitates of the injection. They are usually mild and do not interfere with the treatment. More severe reactions such as general malaise, lumbar, back and lower-limb pains, and immobility were observed in individual patients. These disappeared progressively after 1–2 days of bed rest (9).

REFERENCE

1. Lingling District Sanitation and Anti-epidemic Station. Hunan Yiyao Zazhi (Hunan Medical Journal) 1974 (4):50.
2. Xuzhou Medical College. Information on New Chinese Medicine 1971 (1):27.
3. Sharaf AA et al. Chemical Abstracts 1963 60:4650g.
4. Yoshida T et al. Biochemical Pharmacology 1971 20(12):3263.
5. Sharat A et al. Planta Medica 12 Jg, Heft 1, 1964 71–76.
6. Liu YG. Xinzhongyi (Journal of New Chinese Medicine) 1979 (1):50.
7. Beijing Medical College et al. Chemical Studies of Chinese Traditional Drugs. People's Medical Publishing House. 1980. p. 420.
8. Saxena SK. Chemical Abstracts 1979 91:69467d.

9. Linyi County (Shandong) Sanitation and Anti-epidemic Station et al. Chinese Traditional and Herbal Drugs Communications 1972 (6):32.

10. Qian RS. Journal of Traditional Chinese Medicine 1980 (3):75.

11. Tianjin Institute for Drug Control and Research. Chinese Traditional and Herbal Drugs Communications 1977 (10):27.

12. Pediatics Department, OPD of the First Hospital. Scientific and Technical Information (Fourth Military Medical College of the Chinese PLA) 1977 (10):7.

13. Xue JX. Xinzhongyi (Journal of New Chinese Medicine) 1979 (3):43.

14. Li YZ et al. Xinyiyaoxue Zazhi (Journal of Traditional Chinese Medicine) 1977 (11):22.

15. Chen YL. New Chinese Medicine 1977 (8):406.

16. Li XP. Zhejiang Zhongyiyao (Zhejiang Journal of Traditional Chinese Medicine) 1978 (2):17.

17. Institute of Chinese Materia Medica, Chinese Academy of Medical Sciences et al. Handbook of Chinese Medicinal Preparations. People's Medical Publishing House. 1973. p. 325.

(Gong Xuling)

SANGZHI 桑枝

<Sangzhi> comes from the tender branches of *Morus alba* L. (Moraceae). It has a slightly bitter flavor and a "mild" property. It is antirheumatic and improves limited joint movement. It is, therefore, used to treat rheumatism and contracture of limbs.

CHEMICAL COMPOSITION

The bark of *M. alba* contains mulberrin, mulberrochromene, cyclomulberrin, cyclomulberrochromene, and betulinic acid. The wood contains morin, dihydromorin, dihydrokaempferol, 2,4,4',6-tetrahydroxybenzophenone and 2,3',4,4',6-pentahydroxybenzophenone.

PHARMACOLOGY AND CLINICAL STUDIES

1. Increase in Lymphocyte Transformation Rate

<Sangzhi> benefits patients with low lymphocyte transformation rate. Twenty cases with low lymphocyte transformation rate (portal cirrhosis of the liver, chronic nephritis, chronic hepatitis, hepatitis B carrier, *Staphylococcus aureus* carrier, allergic subsepticemia, chronic bronchitis) were evenly divided into two groups. One group was given an oral decoction of 30 g <Sangzhi> daily in addition to other conventional treatment, whereas the control group was given conventional treatment only. After one month of treatment, the lymphocyte transformation rate in the control group was found to be not significantly different, but that in the <Sangzhi> group was markedly increased compared with the pretreatment level (1).

2. Chronic Brucellosis

"Sang Liu Tang/Wan" (Morus-Salix Decoction/Pill) (Ramulus Mori, Ramulus Salix Babylonicae, Herba Erodii seu Geranii, Cortex Acanthopanacis, Radix Angelicae Sinensis, Myrrha, Fructus Chaenomelis, Flos Carthami, Radix Ledebouriellae) was of therapeutic value in 54 cases unresponsive to antibiotics (2).

3. As Hair Tonic

Hair growth in rabbits and sheep were promoted by the specially prepared "Yangmao Sangzhi Jinchuye" (Ramulus Mori Hair Tonic Extract) (3).

REFERENCE

1. Yan QH et al. Xinyiyaoxue Zazhi (Journal of Traditional Chinese Medicine) 1979 (10):36.

2. Changyi County Sanitation and Anti-epidemic Station. Barefoot Doctor (Changwei District, Shandong) 1978 (4):18.

3. Sasaki. Japan Centra Revuo Medicina 1943 81:432.

(Gong Xuling)

SANGSHEN 桑椹

\<Sangshen\> refers to the fruit-spike of *Morus alba* L. (Moraceae). Sweet and sour to the taste and of "warm" property, it tones up the liver and "kidney" and is credited with hematinic and secretory effects. It is mainly used to treat dizziness, vertigo, tinnitus, palpitation, premature greying of the hair, and constipation in anemia.

CHEMICAL COMPOSITION

\<Sangshen\> contains vitamins B_1, B_2 and C, and carotene. The fatty acids of its oil are mainly composed of linoleic acid and small amounts of stearic acid and oleic acid.

PHARMACOLOGY AND CLINICAL STUDIES

The 100% \<Sangshen\> decoction moderately induced lymphocyte transformation (1). Fructus Mori Ointment (Fructus Mori, crystal sugar or honey) is useful in syndromes due to anemia and "wind pathogenic factor", arthralgia due to blood stasis, constipation in elderly persons, insomnia and restlessness, soreness and weakness of the low-back and legs, and premature greying of the hair (2).

REFERENCE

1. Microbiology Section of Clinical Medicine Research Department, General Hospital of Nanjing PLA Units. Jiangsu Yiyao (Jiangsu Medical Journal) 1978 (10):45.
2. Institute of Materia Medica, Academy of Traditional Chinese Medicine. Handbook of Chinese Medicinal Preparations. People's Medical Publishing House. 1973. p. 498.

(Gong Xuling)

SANGBAIPI 桑白皮

<Sangbaipi> refers to the root bark of *Morus alba* L. (Moraceae). It is sweet and has a "cold" property. It has antiasthmatic, diuretic and detumescent effects and is mainly used to treat cough and asthma due to pathogenic "heat" in the lungs, facial edema, and dysuria.

CHEMICAL COMPOSITION

<Sangbaipi> contains flavone derivatives mulberrin, mulberrochromene, cyclomulberrin, cyclomulberrochromene, and morusin. It also contains betulinic acid, scopoletin, α-amyrin, β-amyrin, undecaprenol, and dodecaprenol. Mulberrofuran A was recently isolated (1).

PHARMACOLOGY

1. Diuretic and Cathartic Effects

Diuresis was produced in rabbits by <Sangbaipi> decoction at 2 g/kg PO (4%, 50 ml/kg) (2), and in rats by the aqueous or n-butanol extract at doses of 300–500 mg/kg PO or IP (3). This action was not accompanied by increases in urine output and in excretion of sodium, potassium, and chloride. Administration of the aqueous extract 3 g/kg PO to mice caused watery stool, suggesting that the drug has a purgative effect (3).

2. Effect on the Cardiovascular System

Different degrees of hypotension were produced with the decoction, the aqueous, ethanol, n-butanol, and other extracts of <Sangbaipi>, administered intravenously, intraduodenally, or orally to normal or hypertensive dogs, rabbits, or rats; the duration of the effect was prolonged and it was accompanied by bradycardia (3–8). The hypotensive effect was inhibited by atropine or bilateral vagotomy but unaltered by chlorpheniramine (3–5). It was, however, reported that bilateral vagotomy or spinal section between the fifth and sixth cervical vertebrae did not abolish the hypotensive action, indicating the possible existence of a cholinergic substance in the extracts (4,5).

The <Sangbaipi> produced in China had a stronger hypotensive action but was more toxic than the Japanese produce (9).

The <Sangbaipi> extract inhibited the isolated frog heart but its action was blocked by atropine (4,5). The n-butanol extract 1 mg/ml initially caused a significant increase succeeded by weak inhibition of the contraction rate and contractility of the isolated rat atrium, whereas the aqueous extract only produced weak inhibition (3). The <Sangbaipi> extract initiated vasoconstriction in the frog hind limb and vasodilation in the isolated rabbit ear; it also increased brachial blood flow, which was blocked by atropine (3–5).

3. Effect on Smooth Muscles

Experiments on dogs showed that injection of the n-butanol extract at 50 mg/kg IV markedly enhanced gastrointestinal motility, whereas the aqueous extract was ineffective. The n-butanol extract 0.1 mg/ml relaxed the isolated ileum of guinea pigs, inhibiting its spontaneous motility; it also weakly stimulated the antrum cardiacum strip of rats (3). Stimulation of the isolated rabbit intestine and uterus was also effected by the <Sangbaipi> extract (4,5).

4. Effect on the Nervous System

4.1 *Sedative and tranquilizing effects.* The aqueous or n-butanol extract of <Sangbaipi> at doses exceeding 50 mg/kg IP exhibited sedative and tranquilizing effects in mice, decreasing the spontaneous activity and the sensitivity to pain and touch, as well as causing mydriasis (3).

4.2 *Anticonvulsant effect.* Both the n-butanol and aqueous extracts of the herb slightly inhibited electroshock in mice but the animals' extensor muscle remained tense. The mortality rate in the experimental group was significantly lower than that in the control (3).

4.3 *Analgesic effect.* The aqueous extract demonstrated a prominent analgesic effect on acetic acid-induced writing and in tail-squeeze experiments on mice; it elevated the pain threshold. On the other hand, the dose 2 g/kg PO was as potent as 0.5 g/kg of aspirin (3).

4.4 *Hypothermic effect.* A hypothermic action was demonstrated in mice by the intraperitoneally administered n-butanol extract; the oral dose was inactive in rats (3).

5. Antibacterial Effect

Staphylococcus aureus, Salmonella typhi and *Shigella flexneri* (1,10), as well as to some extent trichomyces, (11) were inhibited by the 100% <Sangbaipi> decoction, whereas *Mycobacterium tuberculosis* was not sensitive (12).

6. Miscellaneous Actions

<Sangbaipi> suppressed paw swelling induced in rats by carrageenin and dextran. It also has a weak antitussive action (3). The <Sangbaipi> extract used alone had no effect on the leech musculi dorsa

but increased the tonicity of the frog musculi rectus abdominis. Pretreatment of these specimens with physostigmine markedly potentiated the effect of the extract. This preparation also slightly increased the secretion of the parotid glands of rabbits (4). An inhibition rate of around 70% of human cervical carcinoma JTC-26 strain was produced *in vitro* by infusion of the herb (13).

7. Toxicity

The LD_{50} of a yellow powder (obtained from <Sangbaipi> after repeated treatment with petroleum ether, ethanol, ether, acetic anhydride, water, and ethyl acetate) in mice was determined to be 32.7 mg/kg IV (4). No deaths were observed in mice after administration of 10 g/kg PO or IP, or 5 g/kg IV of the n-butanol or aqueous extract (3). The ethanol extract was considered to be low in toxicity because no ill effects were observed in experimental animals receiving a single large dose or multiple small doses (7).

CLINICAL STUDIES

1. Edema

Edema of pregnancy was effectively treated with the "Wupi Yin" (Cortex Mori, Cortex Poria, Pericarpium Arecae, Pericarpium Citri Reticulatae, Cortex Zingiberis Rescens) plus the style of *Zea mays*. In severe cases the sclerotium of *Polyporus umbellatus*, and the rhizome of *Alisma plantago-aquatica*, etc. were added to this basic prescription (14).

2. Bronchitis

Acute bronchitis may be treated with the decoction of <Sangbaipi>, the kernel of *Prunus armeniaca*, the root of *Scutellaria baicalensis*, the bulb of *Fritillaria cirrhosa*, the leaf of *Eriobotrya japonica*, the root of *Platycodon grandiflorum* and the root bark of *Lycium chinense*, each 9 g (15). Asthmatic bronchitis may be treated with "Dingchuan" Tang" (Antiasthmatic Decoction) (16).

3. Miscellaneous

Some patients suffering from esophageal or gastric cancer obtained symptomatic remission after treatment with "Sangpi Kujiu/Cu Tang" (Cortex Mori Bitter Wine/Vinegar Decoction) (17). Suture thread prepared from <Sangbaipi> was used to suture wounds in dogs; since the thread was usually absorbed by the tissue, stitch removal was precluded (18).

REFERENCE

1. Normura T et al. Chemical Abstracts 1979 90:55116f.

2. Rao MR. Chinese Medical Journal 1959 45:67.

3. Yamatake Y et al. The Japanese Journal of Pharmacology 1976 26(4):461.

4. Tanemura I. Folia Pharmacologica Japonica 1960 56:704.

5. Tanemura I. Folia Pharmacologica Japonica 1960 56:44.

6. Suzuki B et al. Japan Centra Revuo Medicina 1944 86:14.

7. Feng KY et al. Xinyiyaoxue Zazhi (Journal of Traditional Chinese Medicine) 1974 (3):43.

8. Watanabe K. Japan Centra Revuo Medicina 1942 77:17.

9. Xu CS. Japan Centra Revuo Medicina 1966 219:498.

10. Microbiology Section. Journal of Nanjing College of Pharmacy 1960 (5):10.

11. Lee HK et al. Chemical Abstracts 1966 65:11009e.

12. Wang SY. Kexue Tongbao (Science Bulletin) 1958 (12):379.

13. Sato A. Kampo Kenkyu 1979 (2):51.

14. Mu DG. Journal of Barefoot Doctor 1978 (5):3.

15. Editorial Group. National Collection of Chinese Materia Medica. People's Medical Publishing House. 1975. p. 677.

16. Hudong Hospital of Yangpu District (Shanghai). New Chinese Medicine 1972 (9):14.

17. Huang YR. Fujian Zhongyiyao (Fujian Journal of Traditional Chinese Medicine) 1965 10(3):23.

18. Chen JM et al. Wuhan Zhongyi (Wuhan Journal of Traditional Chinese Medicine) 1958 (Inaugural Issue):68.

(Gong Xuling)

SANGJISHENG 桑寄生

<Sangjisheng> refers to the leaf and branch of *Loranthus parasiticus* (L.) Merr. or *L. yadoriki* Sieb. (Loranthaceae). (*The plants should be more correctly identified as *Taxillus chinensis* (DC) Danser and *T. sutchuenensis* (Lecomte) Danser, respectively). It is sweet with a bitter aftertaste and a "mild" property. It tones up the liver and "kidney", prevents abnormal fetal movements, fortifies bones, muscles and tendons, and initiates antirheumatic and channel-deobstruent effects. It is therefore used in the treatment of rheumatism, soreness and weakness of the low-back and kness, numbness of the lower extremities, abnormal fetal movements, threatened abortion, and hypertension.

CHEMICAL COMPOSITION

<Sangjisheng> contains avicularin (quercetin-3-arabinoside) and small amounts of quercetin.

PHARMACOLOGY

1. Action on the Cardiovascular System

The aqueous extract, the ethanol-water extract, and the 30%-ethanol extract of <Sangjisheng> precipitated hypotension in anesthetized animals (1). The <Sangjisheng> injection dilated the coronary vessels of the isolated normal and fibrillating hearts of guinea pigs, and greatly increased the coronary flow; it also antagonized coronary constriction due to pituitrin, decreased the heart rate and strengthened cardiac contractility after inhibiting it (2).

Brief episode of hypotension of different degrees and tachyphylaxis developed in anesthetized dogs following injection of avicularin at 0.05–2 mg/kg IV (3). The *L. yadoriki* tincture 0.1–0.25 g (crude drug)/kg injected intravenously to anesthetized dogs and cats also produced a conspicuous hypotensive effect, but no tachyphylaxis occurred. Significant hypotension was also observed when the drug was intragastrically administered. Vagotomy or atropinization only slightly delayed or weakened its hypotensive effect but did not abolish it. The drug diminisned the pressor reflex to compression of the common carotid artery and stimulation of the afferent sciatic nerve. The hypotensive action was still apparent despite sinus nerve blockade. The drug did not reinforce or antagonize the action of epinephrine, and had no direct vasodilatory effect on the normal rabbit ears. *L. yadoriki* has central inhibitory activity; its hypotensive effect was postulated to be central or reflexize (4).

2. Central Depressant Effect

L. yadoriki markedly inhibited excitation produced by caffeine in mice and delayed the death of pentylenetetrazole-treated mice. These results indicate the presence of a significant central depressant activity (4).

3. Diuretic Effect

Avicularin injected to anesthetized dogs at 0.5–2 mg/kg IV produced diuresis of different degrees. In a chronic experiment with rat, both oral and parenteral dosages of 34 mg/kg resulted in a marked diuretic effect directly proportional to the dosage employed (3).

4. Antimicrobial Effect

In vitro, the 10% decoction or extract of <Sangjisheng> inhibited poliomyelitis virus and some enteroviruses ($ECHO_6$, $ECHO_9$, Coxsackie A_9, B_4, B_5, etc.). This effect was not due to metabolic modifications that trigger the inhibition of intracellular synthesis of virus; instead, it was attributed to a direct deactivating effect (5). *In vitro* studies showed that the herb inhibited the growth of *Salmonella typhi* and staphylococcus (6).

5. Miscellaneous Actions

The *L. yadoriki* tincture reduced the tension of the isolated rabbit intestine but did not modify the contraction rhythm. High concentrations caused transient contraction of the nonpregnant rabbit uterus (4).

6. Toxicity

The LD_{50} of *L. yadoriki* tincture in mice was determined to be 11.24 g(crude drug)/kg IP, and that of avicularin was 1.17 g/kg. The cause of death was attributed to paroxysmal seizure-induced respiratory arrest (1,4).

CLINICAL STUDIES

1. Angina Pectoris

The granule infusion of <Sangjisheng> was administered by mouth to 54 cases of angina pectoris for a course of from 4 weeks to 5 months. The effects usually appeared after 1–2 weeks of medication along with the subjective improvement of symptoms; ECG was improved in 44% of the treated cases (2).

2. Arrhythmia

Thirty-seven cases of arrhythmia were treated with the <Sangjisheng> injection intramuscularly 2–4 ml twice daily, or intravenously 12 ml daily, or by intravenous infusion of 18–20 ml daily, for a course of 14 days. The drug was effective in 76.9% of the cases with ventricular premature beats, in 75% with paroxysmal atrial fibrillation and in 55.5% with atrial premature beats. It was ineffective against chronic atrial fibrillation. Its clinical effects resembled those of verapamil or lidocaine; however, these drugs were not used as controls (7).

3. Frostbite

According to a report (8), first-degree frostbite was treated locally with an ointment prepared from the <Sangjisheng> decoction dried over low heat and reconstituted with distilled water, alcohol and white clay, while second-degree frostbite was responsive to a mixture of the <Sangjisheng> extract, glycerin, ointment base and zinc oxide powder.

ADVERSE EFFECTS

The granule infusion of <Sangjisheng> my cause dizziness, blurred vision, general malaise, loss of appetite, abdominal distention, mild diarrhea, and xerostomia in individual patients (2).

REFERENCE

1. Li GC. Abstracts of the 1956 Academic Conference of the Chinese Academy of Medical Sciences. 1956. p. 70.
2. Huaihai Pharmaceutical Factory (Shanghai) et al. Xinyiyaoxue Zazhi (Journal of Traditional Chinese Medicine) 1973 (3):16.
3. Li WS et al. Acta Pharmaceutica Sinica 1959 7(1):1.
4. Wang YS et al. Acta Academiae Medicinae Sichuan 1959 (2):88.
5. Zeng Y et al. Chinese Medical Journal 1964 50(8):521.
6. Li SS (editor-in-chief). Abstracts of Research Literature on Chinese Traditional Drugs (1820–1961). Science Press. 1971. p. 502.
7. Xu JM. Tianjin Pharmaceutical Industry 1978 (1,2):46.
8. Chen JJ. Chinese Journal of Surgery 1961 (11):784.

(Huang Heng)

ZHIZI 栀子

<Zhizi> refers to the fruit of *Gardenia jasminoides* Ellis. (Rubiaceae). The leaf, flower, and root may also be used as medicine. <Zhizi> is also know as <Huangzhizi> and <Shanzhizi>. It has a bitter flavor and a "cold" property. It has tranquilizing, "damp-heat"-clearing, and stasis-discutient actions, and is known to remove pathogenic "heat" from the blood. It is, therefore, used to treat irritability in febrile diseases, jaundice, acute conjunctivitis, epistaxis, hematemesis, hematuria, pyogenic infections and ulcers of the skin, and externally for sprains as well as painful swellings due to blood-stasis.

CHEMICAL COMPOSITION

The fruit of *G. jasminoides* contains gardenoside, geniposide (genipin-1-glucoside), genipin-1-β-D-gentiobioside, gardoside (8,10-dehydrologanin), scandoside methyl ester, α-mannitol, β-sitosterol, nonacosane, crocin and crocetin. The peel also contains ursolic acid.

PHARMACOLOGY

1. Effect on the Digestive System

1.1 *Liver function.* The extract of <Zhizi> produced no significant effect on the contents of y and z proteins and GOT in liver of normal rats, but increased the activity of hepatic uridine diphosphate-glucose dehydrogenase. In the case of animals with ligated common bile duct, however, the extract lowered the abnormally elevated GOT, decreased the y protein and z protein contents and increased the activity of uridine diphosphate-glucose dehydrogenase in the liver. The extract of <Zhizi> blocked bromsulphalein (BSP) excretion from the liver (1). Another paper reported that genipin administered to rats slightly increased GOT and GPT levels (2). <Zhizi> also reduced liver damage due to carbon tetrachloride (3).

1.2 *Secretion, excretion and metabolism of bile.* Experiments on rats and rabbits indicated that <Zhizi> had cholagogic and choleretic actions. Bile secretion was enhanced by the ethanol extract, crocin, crocetin, and genipin (4,5). Genipin, given to rats whether orally, intravenously, or intraduodenally at a dose of 25 mg/kg, increased bile secretion. The most prominent effect was achieved via duodenum, whereby the efficacy obtained was close to that of sodium dehydrocholate (6). In anesthetized dogs, intraintestinal or intravenous administration of drugs, which "regulate vital energy and relieve stasis", increased bile secretion to different extents; the strongest choleretic action was exhibited by prescriptions composed of the shoot of *Artemisia capillaris*, the fruit of

Gardenia jasminoides and the root and rhizome of *Rheum palmatum* (7). Cholecystography performed in man after administration of the <Zhizi> decoction revealed significant gallbladder contraction (8), indicating a cholagogic effect. However, early reports claimed that the aqueous or ethanol extract of <Zhizi> orally administrered to rabbits had no effect on bile secretion (9) and gallbladder contraction (10). In animal experiments, the solutions of sodium crocin and sodium crocetin, as well as the aqueous and ethanol extracts of <Zhizi>, were shown to decrease the serum bilirubin in rabbits with ligated common bile duct (5,9). The extent of the decrease directly correlated with the drug dosage, i.e. the higher the dosage, the greater the decrease. The ethanol extracts had a weaker action than aqueous extracts (9). Apparently, the herb enhanced the metabolism of bilirubin. At present, the decremental effect of <Zhizi> on serum bilirubin is thought to be rather complicated, because the herb neither increased the activity of bilirubin uridine diphosphate glucuronyl transferase (UDP-GT) nor increased the contents of y and z proteins (1).

1.3 *Gastric secretion and motility.* Intraduodenal administration of genipin 25 mg/kg to rats with ligated pylorus decreased the gastric secretion and total acidity and increased the pH value; its strenght was one-tenth to one-fifth that of atropine sulfate (6). Injection of geniposide and genipin to rats at 100 and 25 mg/kg IV respectively inhibited spontaneous gastric peristalsis and pilocarpine-induced gastric contraction; but the effects were short-lived (6). At low concentration (1:25,000), the ethanol extract stimulated the motility of the small intestine of rats and rabbits, while at high concentration (1:1000) it produced inhibition (11). Genipin was also shown in experiments on the isolated mouse and guinea pig ilea to have relatively weak anticholinergic and antihistaminic actions (6). Geniposide was reported to have a cathartic action (12). Drugs which are reputed to regulate the vital energy and relieve stasis, such as Artemisia capillaris Decoction, could relieve gastrointestinal spasm and enhance the propulsive movement of the gastrointestinal tract of mice (7).

2. Effect on the CNS

Injection of the ethanol extract of <Zhizi> 5.69 g/kg IP to mice decreased the spontaneous activity of the animals, indicating a sedative effect. It also synergized with cyclobarbital sodium in prolonging sleep by almost twelve times. However, the extract could not antagonize amphetamine-induced activity and convulsions induced by pentylenetetrazole, strychnine nitrate and electric shock. It also had no analgesic action.

Body temperature of mice dropped by a mean of 3°C one hour after intraperitoneal injection of the ethanol extract; in rats after the 200-mg/kg dose, the effect was sustained for more than 7 hours (13). Ursolic acid was considered by some authors to be the active principle responsible for sedation and antipyrexia. This compound was shown to increase the half-convulsive dose of pentylenetetrazole in mice and to have a significant anticonvulsant action (14,15). Although the aqueous extract, geniposide, and genipin had no sedative and antipyretic actions, they were shown to produce analgesia as they were able to inhibit acetic acid-induced writing in mice (6).

3. Effect on the Cardiovascular System

A hypotensive effect was exhibited by the <Zhizi> decoction and ethanol extract in anesthetized and non-anesthetized cats, rabbits, and rats whether administered orally, intraperitoneally or intravenously. The intravenous route produced a rapid but transient effect. <Zhizi> was devoid of any influence on the pressor effect of epinephrine and the pressor reflex of blocked carotid arterial blood flow, and had no potentiating effect on the hypotensive action of acetylcholine. The hypotensive action of <Zhizi> was not affected by administration of antihistaminic drugs such as diphenhydramine; hence, it was not related to histamine release. Likewise, intravenous injection of procaine failed to alter the hypotensive effect of this herb, indicating no involvement of the afferent nerves. <Zhizi> had no blocking action on the nerve ganglions. However, its hypotensive action was greatly attenuated or completely abolished by bilateral vagotomy. Atropine also cancelled its effect. Thus, the site of action is inferred to be in the CNS and the hypotensive effect is attributed to increased excitability of the medullary parasympathetic centers (11). Another report stated that <Zhizi> had no significant effect on the peripheral resistance. In perfusion experiments, the extract decreased the myocardial contractility of isolated rat hearts. Hypotension in anesthetized dogs and rats elicited by injection of the <Zhizi> extract 500 mg/kg IV was a consequence of the reduction in stroke volume and cardiac output (16). The incidence of arteriosclerosis in cholesterol-fed rabbits was reduced by injection of crocetin 0.01 mg/kg IM (17). High dosage (1 g/kg IV) of the methanol extract of <Zhizi> produced ECG aberrations of myocardial damage and atrioventricular block in rats (16), but injection of genipin 30 mg/kg IV to anesthetized rabbits had no significant effect on the blood pressure, heart rate, and ECG (6).

4. Antibacterial Action

In the well diffusion method, *Staphylococcus aureus*, *Diplococcus meningitidis*, and *Micrococcus catarrhalis* were shown to be inhibited by <Zhizi> (3). *In vitro*, the aqueous extract of the herb inhibited many types of skin fungi (18,19). The decoction was also lethal to leptospirae (20) and adult schistosomes (21).

5. Toxicity

The acute LD_{50} of the fluidextract of <Zhizi> was determined to be 31.79 g/kg SC in mice (22). Another report claimed that geniposide and the aqueous extract of the herb had a very low toxicity; no death occurred in animals after administration of geniposide 3 g/kg PO. IP or IV, and after injection of the aqueous extract 5 g/kg IP. The 72-h LD_{50} of a single dose of genipin were 237 mg/kg PO, 190 mg/kg IP, and 158 mg/kg IV (6). The lethal dose of crocin and sodium crocetin in mice was found to be 15 and 5 g/kg SC, respectively (23).

CLINICAL STUDIES

1. Infectious Diseases

Out of 19 cases of acute icteric hepatitis treated with the <Zhizi> decoction, 7 were completely cured and 10 nearly cured; the average duration of hospitalization was 30.3 days (24). In addition, <Zhizi> had therapeutic value in acute bacterial cystitis, and infections of the skin and mucous membrane (3).

2. Sprain and Contusion

A dressing of the <Zhizi> powder and alcohol employed in 407 cases of sprain of the extremities improved local blood stasis, swelling and pain. These symptoms disappeared in 30 hours and limb functions recovered in an average of 5.1 days (3,25).

3. Hemostasis

The sterilized <Zhizi> powder can be used as a hemostatic agent for upper gastrointestinal tract bleeding and also in local bleeding. Dosage: 3–6 g, orally, thrice a day (26).

REFERENCE

1. Kong YC et al. Comparative Medicine East-West 1977 513–47:241; Zou ZC (abstracter). Guowai Yixue (Medicine Abroad) — Traditional Chinese Medicine and Materia Medica 1980 (2):42.

2. Yuda M et al. Kampo Kenkyu 1975 (5):5.

3. Wenzhou District Health Bureau. South Zhejiang Herbal. New edition. 1975. p. 336.

4. Harada M et al. Kampo Kenkyu 1975 (1):28.

5. Miwa T. Folia Pharmacologica Japonica 1954 50(1):25.

6. Harada M et al. Journal of the Pharmaceutical Society of Japan (Tokyo) 1974 94(2):157.

7. Nankai (Tianjin) Medical College. Chinese Medical Journal 1973 (1):33.

8. Jiang WX et al. Shanxi Medical Journal 1963 7(3):1.

9. Li XX. Chinese Journal of New Medicine 1951 2(9):660.

10. 243 Logistics Unit of the Chinese PLA. Xinyiyaoxue Zazhi (Journal of Traditional Chinese Medicine) 1974 (4):44.

11. Zhang SF. Acta Pharmaceutical Sinica 1965 12(10):636.

12. Lin QS. Chemical Studies of Chinese Traditional Drugs. Science Press. 1977. p. 603.

13. Chinese Traditional Anesthesia Group, Pharmacology Section of Nanjing College of Pharmacy. Jiangsu Yiyao (Jiangsu Medical Journal) 1976 (1):27.

14. Bian XM et al. Chinese Traditional and Herbal Drugs Communications 1976 (9):15.

15. Liu GQ et al. Chinese Traditional and Herbal Drugs Communications 1979 (5):33.

16. Chow HY et al. The American Journal of Chinese Medicine 1976 4(1):47.

17. Gainer JL. Chemical Abstracts 1974 81:45530m.

18. Zheng WF. Chinese Medical Journal 1952 38(4):315.

19. Cao RL et al. Chinese Journal of Dermatology 1974 (4):286.

20. Information on New Chinese Medicine (Xuzhou Medical College) 1971 (1):27.

21. Zhang CS. Chinese Medical Journal 1956 42(5):409.

22. Tu GR et al. Abstracts of the 1964 Symposium of the Society of Physiology (Beijing Branch). June 1964.

23. Miwa T. Japan Centra Revuo Medicina 1955 117:702.

24. Lou FL et al. Academic Information. Vol. 14. Second Military Medical College of the Chinese PLA. 1962. p. 14.

25. Lin SH. Journal of Traditional Chinese Medicine 1964 (12):450.

26. Notes on Science and Technology (236 Logistics Unit of the Chinese PLA) 1971 (2):4.

(Zhang Zunyi)

LUOFUMU 蘿芙木

<Luofumu> refers to the root of *Rauvolfia verticillata* (Lour.) Baill, *R. yunnanensis* Tsiang, *R. yunnanensis* Tsiang var. *angustifolia* Wu, and *R. latifrons* Tsiang (Apocynaceae).

In other countries the plant, *R. serpentina* Benth is used as medicine (1,2). This species has also been introduced into China.

<Luofumu> has a bitter flavor and a "cold" property. It is latent-heat-clearing, antipyretic, and detumescent and is reputed to reduce pathogenic intense "heat" in the liver. It is, therefore, used as a remedy for fever in common cold, pharyngolaryngitis, headache and vertigo in hypertension, abdominal pain of acute diseases (such as cholera), vomiting, urticaria, scabies, mania, and for snake and scorpion bites.

CHEMICAL COMPOSITION

<Luofumu> contains three groups of alkaloids (13). The first group includes strongly-alkaline quaternary ammonium compounds serpentine, serpentinine, sarpagine, and samatine. The second group includes tertiary amine derivatives yohimbine, ajmaline, ajmalicine, tetraphylline, and tetraphyllicine. The third group includes weakly-alkaline secondary amines reserpine, rescinnamine, deserpidine, raunesine, and canescine.

The kinds and quantity of alkaloids vary with the growing location or source. The total alkaloid content of Indian *R. serpentina* of 0.8–1% was regarded as meeting the standard. The root of *R. verticillata* grown in Guangxi, China, contains 1–2% of alkaloids (3), and that grown in Yunnan, China, contains 1–3% (4). The whole root, root bark, peeled root, stem bark and leaf of *R. verticillata* grown in Guangdong, China, contains 0.8, 1.4–1.5, 0.5, 0.88 and 0.6% of alkaloids, respectively (5). Reserpine is the major alkaloid of the *Rauvolfia* species, in the root of which the reserpine content varies from 0.002% to 0.16% (1).

"Jiangyaling" (Verticil) is the trade name of an extract of the alkaloids of *R. verticillata*. It is a mixture of more than 20 alkaloids (6).

PHARMACOLOGY

Among the three groups of alkaloids in <Luofumu>, the quaternary ammonium alkaloids such as sarpagine had significant ganglionic blocking and antiadrenergic actions (6), whereas samatine of the same group displayed only ganglionic blocking action (7). The quaternary ammonium compounds are poorly absorbed when administered orally. The tertiary ammonium alkaloids such as ajmaline posessed an antiarrhythmia action. The weak secondary ammonium alkaloids such as reserpine, rescinnamine, and deserpidine exhibited a strong central tranquilizing and a prolonged hypotensive action. The crude preparation and the total alkaloids of <Luofumu> manifested all the above mentioned actions, but their actions could be characterized primarily as hypotensive and sedative.

1. Hypotensive Effect

1.1 China-produced < Luofumu> crude preparations.

1.1.1 Decoction of the root bark of Guangdong-produced <Luofumu> 22.5 mg(crude drug)/kg injected intravenously to anesthetized dogs sharply decreased the blood pressure, the effect lasting from 40 minutes to 3 hours. The dose of 30 mg(crude drug)/kg IM decreased the blood pressure; the lowest reading, which was 38% lower than the control, was recorded in 0.5–1 hour; the hypotensive effect lasted 2–6 hours. With the oral dose 750 mg(crude drug)/ kg, the blood pressure started to fall within 0.5 hour and the action sustained for 6 hours; the lowest level attained was about 50% of the original level (5,8,9).

1.1.2 The crude preparation of Guizhou-produced <Luofumu> 100–200 mg(crude drug)/kg injected intravenously to anesthetized animals sharply decreased the blood pressure by 40–110 mmHg; injection of 400 mg(crude drug)/kg IM produced a gradual but significant effect. An antihypertensive effect similar to that of serpina from the total alkaloids of the Indian *R. serpentina* in rabbits with renal hypertension was exhibited by the crude preparation at 1–2 g/kg/day for a course of 15 days (10).

1.1.3 The acidified-alcohol extract of Guangdong-produced <Luofumu> also had a significant hypotensive action. Intravenous injection of 100–150 mg(crude drug)/kg of the extract produced a hypotensive effect similar to 1 mg/kg of the total alkaloids obtained from the leaves. Blood pressure of hypertensive dogs was lowered by the leaf extract 1–2 g/kg PO, with attendant side effects such as bradycardia, sedation, and diarrhea. The oral doses 20, 40, or 80 mg/kg of the total alkaloids of the leaves also lowered the blood pressure of hypertensive rats (11,12).

1.2 The total alkaloids of the Chinese-produced <Luofumu> (Trade name: Verticil) has a faster, stronger, and longer lasting action than serpina (9). When used intravenously, the antihypertensive action of Verticil was mainly contributed by the quaternary and tertiary alkaloids which had rapid ganglionic and adrenergic blocking actions. But, when used orally, the antihypertensive effect was produced by the secondary alkaloids (6). This is because the secondary alkaloids reserpine, rescinnamine etc. are more easily absorbed from the intestinal tract and have a very slow onset.

Intravenous injection of 0.5–1 mg/kg of the total alkaloids from <Luofumu> produced in Guangdong, Guangxi, Yunnan or Hainan Island caused a marked and prolonged hypotension in anesthetized dogs. Treatment of hypertensive dogs with doses of 2–10 mg/kg decreased their blood pressure and produced sedation. Some animals developed tremor and diarrhea; the most conspicuous side effects were seen with <Luofumu> from Guangdong followed by that from Yunnan and the least from Guangxi. However, based on their LD_{50} in mice by the oral route, the toxicity of the <Luofumu> produced from Guangxi and Hainan was highest, next, that from Yunnan and, lowest, that from Guangdong mainland (13).

The soluble alkaloids of <Luofumu> given to anesthetized dogs at 1 mg/kg IV or to anesthetized cats at 2–3 mg/kg IV lowered the blood pressure by 50% for 2–3 hours; it also exerted a ganglionic blocking action, antagonized the pressor effect of epinephrine and inhibited the pressor reflex caused by unilateral blockade of the carotid arterial blood flow, electrical stimulation of the afferent vagus or sciatic nerve. Blood pressure in most dogs with experimental hypertension was reduced by oral administration of 10 mg/kg/day of the total alkaloids for 4 weeks (14).

Hemodynamic studies on anesthetized dogs showed that the total alkaloids of <Luofumu> decreased the arterial pressure and the total peripheral resistance as well as dilated the coronary arteries. In rats with renal hypertension, the total alkaloids improved ischemia of the myocardium, kidney, and liver. Intravenous injection of a large dose (5 mg/kg) to rabbits decreased the cerebral blood flow which, proportionately, was more marked than that of the blood pressure; hence, the cerebral vascular resistance was substantially increased, compared with the pretreatment value. Intra-arterial injection of a small dose (0.2 mg) into the carotid artery neither altered the systemic blood pressure nor caused cerebral vasodilation (14–18). The reduction of blood pressure paralleled the depletion of catecholamines in the tissues (19).

A strong, quick, and prolonged hypotensive action in anesthetized cats was achieved by intravenous injection of 0.5–3 mg/kg of the total alkaloids of the root of *R. yunnanensis*. After the medication, the pressor reflex caused by stimulation of the afferent vagus nerve or by blockade of the right common carotid artery was weakened, suggesting inhibition of the central or peripheral sympathetic function. There was also an attenuation or even reversal of the pressor action of epinephrine, indicating blockade of the peripheral α-adrenergic receptors but not β-receptors. The bradycardia caused by this drug in cats could not be completely abolished by vagotomy. However, pronounced tachyphylaxis developed. The reduction in blood pressure following the second medication was only around 50% of the first treatment. In isolated rabbit ears, hind limbs, and hind limbs with intact sciatic or femoral nerve, the total alkaloids of *R. yunnanensis* were shown to have no direct vasodilatory action (20).

After intravenous injection of 1 mg/kg of the total alkaloids of <Luofumu> (*R. yannanensis* var. *angustifolia*), the area under the curve (the magnitude of blood pressure drop against time of the hypotensive action) was 32% which was slightly smaller than the 45% obtained with the total alkaloids of <Luofumu> from *R. verticillata* at an equivalent dosage. The former agent was shown to have an antiadrenergic action, and to weaken the pressor reflex; in spinal cats, however, the hypotensive effect was weaker, indicating inhibition of the vasomotor center. Systemic use of the total alkaloids from the root of *R. yunnanensis* var. *angustifolia* caused vasodilation in the isolated rabbit ear with intact nerves. This effect was mediated by the sympathetic nervous system (21).

Injection of the alkaloids of the root of *R. verticillata* minus reserpine to anesthetized dogs at 1 mg/kg IV still produced a prominent hypotensive effect; this was also true of daily oral administration of 10–30 mg in hypertensive dogs; however, sedation, tremor, miosis, and relaxation of the nictitating membrane developed concurrently. These findings indicate that apart from reserpine, there are other alkaloids in the herb that also possess hypotensive and sedative actions.

1.3 *Reserpine ("Xueanping", serpentine).* Reserpine possesses most actions of the <Luofumu> alkaloids; it lowered the blood pressure and decreased the heart rate; its hypotensive actions is characteristically mild, long-lasting and with a long latent period. Even at high dosage the action of reserpine appeared as late as one hour after medication and peaked in 2–4 hours. Increasing the dosage prolonged the duration of action but did not proportionately increase the magnitude of effect (1,2). Hence, excessively low blood pressure does not usually occur. Low oral doses of reserpine usually decreased the blood pressure after a few days; the peak effect occurred 2–3 weeks later; the effect lasted up to a few weeks after discontinuation of the medication.

The hypotensive action of reserpine was assessed in the past as being due to inhibition of the sympathetic nervous center (1,2,23,24). However, electrophysiologic studies revealed that the impulses of preganglionic sympathetic fibers were not decreased but increased by reserpine, indicating that reserpine did not diminish the excitability of the sympathetic nervous system.

In 1957, it was found that reserpine depletes the sympathetic neurotransmitter norepinephrine. Thus, when the sympathetic nervous system is stimulated, although the impulse reaches the nerve terminal, there are not enough neurotransmitters released from the sympathetic terminal, resulting in a marked weakening of cardiovascular stimulation, and thus precipitating bradycardia, vasodilation, and hypotension (25,26). In either normotensive (27) or hypertensive animals (28), the hypotensive effect of reserpine paralleled the depletion of catecholamines in the tissue. Restoration of catecholamine levels in the tissue after cessation of reserpine treatment usually takes 2–4 weeks (25–28). Since depletion and replenishment of catecholamines in the tissue take some time, reserpine, therefore, has a slow onset and a long duration of action. The mechanism of catecholamine depletion by reserpine (29) is attributed to the interference of the function of synaptic vesicles which store the neurotransmitters, making the active uptake and storage of norepinephrine and its precursor, dopamine, impossible, allowing the inactivation of the catecholamines by monoamine oxidase (MAO).

Concomitant with catecholamine depletion, reserpine also increased the levels of acetylcholine in the tissue. Apart from the weakening of the sympathetic nervous function, reserpine was shown in China to increase the tone of the parasympathetic nerves (30).

2. Tranquilizing Effect

2.1 *Crude preparations of <Luofumu> (R. verticillata) from China.* The decoction of the root bark of Guangdong-produced <Luofumu> given to mice intragastrically at 10 g/kg resulted one hour later in sedation lasting more than 24 hours; though sedated, the animals were easily aroused by touch. There was no evidence of respiratory depression, and the sedative effect was completely reversible (9).

2.2 *Total alkaloids of <Luofumu> (R. verticillata) from China.* Tranquilization was achieved with the total alkaloids 10 mg/kg/day in dogs with experimental hypertension (14). However, the agent did not display antagonism to and even synergized with central stimulants (32).

2.3 *Reserpine.* Like chlorpromazine, reserpine has been shown to have a central tranquilizing action causing sedation, loss of concentration, sommnolence and light sleep. It also produced tameness in fierce and aggressive animals and sedation of manic patients. Small doses of reserpine, which do not alter the blood pressure, decreased the positive conditioned response (31) and inhibited the conditioned avoidance in dogs (2).

The central actions of reserpine, including the tranquilizing and the extrapyramidal actions, were closely associated with the depletion of norepinephrine, dopamine and serotonin in the brain (33,34).

3. Miscellaneous Actions

The alkaloids such as reserpine and rescinnamine also inhibited the thermotaxic centers and lowered the body temperature; they also produced parasympathetic hyperactivity such as increased intestinal peristalsis, gastrointestinal secretions, appetite, and body weight. Intra-amniotic injection of reserpine was reported to be effective in terminating mid-term pregnancy (35).

4. Toxicity

The decoction of <Luofumu> from China at 60 g/kg PO was not lethal to mice; the LD_{50} was determined to be 4 g/kg SC (32). In acute toxicity experiments on mice, the LD_{50} of a single intragastric dose of the total alkaloids of various <Luofumu> produced in China was determined to be as follows: Guangxi *R. verticillata* root 690 mg/kg (13), Hainan *R. verticillata* root 820 mg/kg (13), Yunnan *R. verticillata* root 870, 1150 mg/kg (4,13), Guangdong *R. verticillata* root 1320 mg/kg (13), Hainan *R. verticillata* leaf 2350 mg/kg (8), *R. yunnanensis* var. *angustifolia* root > 2000 mg/kg (20).

The acute LD_{50} of the pure alkaloid, reserpine, was 500 mg/kg PO in mice (1), whereas the absolute lethal dose was 16 mg/kg IP. A difference of thirtyfold in these values suggested incomplete absorption of the oral dose. The acute LD_{50} of a single intravenous injection of reserpine in rabbits was 15 mg/kg (36). Chronic toxicity studies revealed that administration of reserpine to rats at 2 mg/kg PO daily for 6 months caused sedation but did not significantly change the food intake and body weight. Rabbits could tolerate daily injection of 0.1 mg/kg IV for 12 days very well; no pathological changes were found in dissection of internal organs (36). Thus, reserpine has relatively low toxicity which is functional rather than organic.

CLINICAL STUDIES

1. Hypertension

More than 200 cases of hypertension were treated with 6–15 mg of the total alkaloids of the root of *R. verticillata* produced in Yunnan (37) daily, orally, for a course of 3 weeks to 2 months; the first- and second-stage cases definitely benefitted, whereas in the third-stage cases with organic changes in heart, kidneys, or brain vessels, the treatment was virtually ineffective. Unlike reserpine, the total alkaloids had milder side effects but produced tachyphylaxis (20). Fifty cases were treated with the Guizhou-produced *R. verticillata* (38); a short-term effective rate of 92% was attained, in which 54% had marked decrease in the blood pressure, 12% moderate decrease and 26% had low reduction. Again, it was more effective in the first- and second-stage cases. The symptoms — dizziness, headache and palpitation — were improved, and side effects such as somnolence and lassitude were infrequently reported.

Hypertension is frequently treated with reserpine at 0.125–0.5 mg PO; this treatment is more effective in early cases (39–45). Hypertensive crisis treated with high dosage of reserpine (2 mg IM) showed steady and satisfactory lowering of blood pressure in 3–4 hours. However, the medication caused marked drowsiness which is difficult to differentiate from hypertensive encephalopathy (46,47). Precautions should be taken in this regard.

2. Psychosis

Calmness and patient compliance were reportedly achieved with reserpine in treating manic psychosis such as paranoid and catatonic schizophrenia, mania, and paranoia (48,49). Initially, reserpine in large doses (2–4 mg) may be given intramuscularly 1–2 times daily; when patients appear sedated this is replaced by oral administration of 2–6 mg/day in 1–2 doses. Overdosage can cause depression and parkinsonian syndrome. Hence, the lowest possible dose should be used for maintenance therapy. Reserpine is contraindicated in depressive psychosis because of possible aggravation, and in some cases, suicidal attempts (50,54).

3. Pruritic Dermatosis

Two hundred and one cases of psychologically related pruritic skin diseases, 52 of which with complete medical records, were treated with the tablet of the total alkaloids of the root of *R. verticillata* at 4–8 mg thrice daily for an average of 2 weeks. The medication was effective for neurodermatitis, chronic eczema, chronic urticaria, contact dermatitis, and seborrheic dermatitis; the best result was achieved in urticaria. The aggregate effective rate was 89% and the marked effect cases represented 44%, improved cases 32%, abated cases 13%, and unresponsive cases 11% (51). Another paper reported the treatment of 102 cases of pruritic skin diseases (80 with complete medical records) with reserpine at 0.5–1 mg/day PO (in 2–4 doses); the aggregate effective rate was 74%. There were 10% cured, 44% markedly improved, 20% significantly improved and 26% unchanged (52). The total alkaloids were shown to have milder and fewer side effects than reserpine (51). The weakly alkaline secondary ammonium alkaloids of <Luofumu> (including reserpine), due to their central sedative action, were effective for psychologically-related skin diseases in proportion to the degree of psychological involvement (52). Additionally, as pruritus is related to histamine, the efficacy of reserpine may be attributed to its ability to deplete tissue histamine.

4. Secondary Malnutrition

Malnourished, thin and weak patients refractory to therapy of a diet high in calories, protein and vitamins benefitted from small doses of reserpine which weakened the catabolic effects of the sympathetic nerves, strengthened the assimilative effects of the parasympathetic nerves, and increased the appetite; the body weight gradually increased (on average, 0.25 kg per week) and physical strength also improved (53).

5. Hyperthyroidism

Reserpine is useful in improving the hyperthyroidism symptoms of hyperactivity of the sympathetic nervous system, irritability, palpitation, and high blood pressure.

ADVERSE EFFECTS

The total alkaloids of <Luofumu> from China (Verticil) have milder side effects than reserpine. Severe ill effects are rarely seen. The main adverse effects are (1) central depressive symptoms such as dizziness, lassitude, somnolence, nightmares, short sleep, insomnia and, rarely, severe depression (43,50,54); (2) cardiovascular symptoms such as bradycardia, nasal congestion (may be relieved by naphazoline nose drops), and in isolated cases, cardiac failure (54); (3) digestive system symptoms including xerostomia, gastrointestinal hypermotility, watery or soft stool, and frequent bowel movement. This drug may increase acid secretion and may aggravate the symptoms or provoke bleeding of an existing peptic ulcer. Therefore, it is contraindicated or to be used with caution in patients with this condition (55–57).

REFERENCE

1. Bein HJ. Pharmacological Reviews 1956 8(3):435.
2. Liu TP. Shengli Kexue Jinzhan (Progress in Physiological Sciences) 1958 2(4):393.
3. Liu ZJ. Kexue Tongbao (Science Bulletin) 1957 (20):609.
4. Li XY et al. Scientia Sinica 1962 11:791.

5. Lou Q et al. People's Health Care 1959 1(1):67.

6. Zeng GY et al. Zhonghua Yixue Zazhi (National Medical Journal of China) 1977 57(1):56.

7. Jin GZ et al. Kexue Tongbao (Science Bulletin) 1959 (16):529.

8. Zeng GY et al. Acta Pharmaceutica Sinica 1959 7(9):361.

9. Luo Q et al. Kexue Tongbao (Science Bulletin) 1957 (12):376.

10. Xia BN et al. Acta Academiae Medicinae Guiyang 1960 (2):1.

11. Xia BN et al. Kexue Tongbao (Science Bulletin) 1957 (6):182.

12. Xia BN et al. Acta Pharmaceutica Sinica 1959 7(9):355.

13. Zeng GY et al. Acta Pharmaceutica Sinica 1959 7(9):370.

14. Pharmacology Section, Institute of Materia Medica of the Chinese Academy of Sciences. Acta Physiologica Sinica 1959 23(1):54.

15. Li XY et al. Acta Physiologica Sinica 1961 24(3−4):254.

16. Li XY et al. Acta Pharmaceutica Sinica 1959 7(9):336.

17. Li XY et al. Acta Pharmaceutica Sinica 1959 7(9):341.

18. Li XY et al. Acta Physiologica Sinica 1962 25(1):87.

19. Zhao GS et al. Acta Physiologica Sinica 1965 28(4):416.

20. Deng SX et al. Acta Pharmaceutica Sinica 1959 7(9):327.

21. Yue KL et al. Acta Pharmaceutica Sinica 1964 11(10):680.

22. Xu LN et al. Acta Pharmaceutica Sinica 1959 7(9):377.

23. Robson JB et al. Recent Advances in Pharmacology. 2nd edition. Churchill Ltd. 1956. p. 78.

24. Bein HJ. Psychotropic Drugs. Elsevier Publishing Co., Amsterdam. 1957. p. 325.

25. Bian CP. Shengli Kexue Jinzhan (Progress in Physiological Sciences) 1964 6(2):160.

26. Zheng MQ. Medical Information — Pharmacology. Medical Information Unit of Sichuan Health Bureau. 1964. p. 21.

27. Wu BJ et al. Shengli Kexue Jinzhan (Progress in Physiological Sciences) 1964 27(3):265.

28. Zhou EF et al. Acta Pharmaceutica Sinica 1965 12(8):496.

29. Weiner N. Annual Review of Pharmacology 1970 (10):273.

30. Zheng MQ et al. Acta Physiologica Sinica 1964 27(4):343.

31. Xu LN et al. Acta Physiologica Sinica 1961 24(3−4):151.

32. Luo Q et al. People's Health Care 1959 1(2):160.

33. Brodie BB et al. Journal of Pharmacology and Experimental Therapeutics 1960 129:250.

34. Garattini S et al. Journal of Pharmacy and Pharmacology 1961 31:548.

35. Zheng MQ et al. Chinese Journal of Obstetrics and Gynecology 1980 15(2):105.

36. Zhang CY. Psychotropic Drugs. Shanghai Sci-Tech Literature Publishing House. 1966. p. 127.

37. Chinese Academy of Medical Sciences. Reference Materials on Medical Sciences 1959 (11):2.

38. Zhang MX. Acta Academiae Medicinae Guiyang 1960 (2):7.

39. Dong CL. Chinese Journal of Internal Medicine 1956 4(4):251.

40. Cai XH et al. Chinese Journal of Internal Medicine 1957 5(6):458.

41. Shi XN et al. Chinese Journal of Internal Medicine 1957 5(6):463.

42. Shi XN. Chinese Journal of Internal Medicine 1958 6(12):1158.

43. Hu KN et al. Chinese Journal of Internal Medicine 1957 5(6):466.

44. Xu BY. Acta Academiae Medicinae Primae Shanghai 1957 (3):233.

45. Zhang ZJ. Chinese Journal of Obstetrics and Gynecology 1959 7(4):294.

46. Zhang MQ. Chinese Medical Journal 1963 49(9):612.

47. Wu WY. Chinese Journal of Paediatrics 1960 11(2):159.

48. Tan MX. Chinese Journal of Neurology and Psychiatry 1956 2(2):114.

49. Jia CY et al. Chinese Journal of Neurology and Psychiatry 1958 4(1):63.

50. Zhou YL et al. Chinese Journal of Internal Medicine 1958 6(12):1211.

51. Wang YF et al. Yunnan Medical Journal 1962 (2):43.

52. Yang TL et al. Chinese Journal of Dermatology 1959 7(6):387.

53. Zheng MQ. Chinese Medical Journal 1963 49(9):613.

54. Zhou YL et al. Chinese Journal of Internal Medicine 1958 6(12):1210.

55. He ZX et al. Chinese Journal of Internal Medicine 1958 6(12):153.

56. Fu RN et al. Chinese Journal of Internal Medicine 1958 6(12):1213.

57. Fang RX et al. Chinese Journal of Internal Medicine 1959 7(4):389.

(Zheng Mingqi)

Juhua 菊花

<Juhua> is the capitulum of *Dendranthema morifolium* (Ramat.) Tzvel. (*Chrysanthemum morifolium* Ramat.) (Compositae). The whole plant or its leaf may also be used as medicine.

<Juhua> tastes sweet and bitter with a slightly "cold" property. It is latent-heat-clearing, antipyretic, hepatic-depressant and vision-improving. It is a very popular remedy for common cold due to pathogenic "wind-heat", headache with vertigo, acute conjunctivitis, and hypertension.

CHEMICAL COMPOSITION

The flower, leaf and stem all contain volatile oils. The flower contains about 0.13% of volatile oil, chrysanthemin, adenine, choline, stachydrine, and traces of vitamin A analogues, vitamin B_1 and acacetin. It was reported that white chrysanthemum contains more flavonoid glycosides, and that it also contains adenosine, coumarins, and alkaloids (1).

PHARMACOLOGY

1. Effect on the Cardiovascular System

The alcohol-precipitated decoction of <Juhua> markedly dilated the coronary vessels and increased the coronary flow. Injection of 1 g(crude drug) into the constant-pressure perfusion fluid adjacent to the intubated heart increased the coronary flow by 62% within 2 minutes and at the same time slowed the heart rate by about 20%. The force of cardiac contraction was in many instances strengthened rather than weakened (chance proportion 3:2) (1). In larger doses, the decoction also increased the coronary flow of the *in situ* dog heart by about 40%, and increased the myocardial oxygen consumption by 27%, on average (2). It also reduced the ischemic ECG pattern, ST depression, induced by electrical stimulation of the CNS, but did not alter or decrease the heart rate. These results were essentially consistent with those from experiments with isolated rabbit hearts (3). It also increased the coronary flow and myocardial oxygen consumption of the isolated heart of rabbits with experimental atherosclerosis (4). The two extracts obtained by successive extraction of this <Juhua> preparation with ethyl acetate and chloroform, as well as the residual aqueous solution, increased the coronary flow of isolated hearts of normal rabbits and rabbits with ventricular fibrillation, but not as conspicuously as did the original preparation. On the other hand, the features of these extracts vary: the ethyl acetate extract had a slow onset but a prolonged effect, producing the highest increase in coronary flow; the chloroform extract was the weakest; the residual aqueous solution had a rapid but brief action and also caused asystole of normally pulsating isolated rabbit hearts and normalized ventricular fibrillation. It is therefore inferred that <Juhua> contains multiple cardioactive principles, and the pronounced effect of the alcohol-precipitated decoction is attributed to the synergism among these bioactive components (5).

Propranolol added to the perfusion fluid did not attenuate the effect of <Juhua> on coronary flow; on the contrary, it made it more marked. The modification in myocardial contractility was similar to that seen before addition of propranolol. It is preliminarily held that the incremental effect of the <Juhua> preparations on the coronary flow is not related to the myocardial metabolite-induced coronary dilation, nor does it involve the β-adrenergic receptors of the coronary vessels. Whether this effect is a result of a direct action on the coronary smooth muscles or of the lowered myocardial tension resulting in decreased coronary resistance, or involves other receptors, requires further study (6). In summary, the <Juhua> preparations could dilate coronary vessels, thereby reducing myocardial ischemia. Although the <Juhua> preparations increased the cardiac contractility and myocardial oxygen consumption, their dominant action is dilation of the coronary vessels (1).

Intraperitoneal injection of the fluidextract of <Juhua> to mice increased the tolerance of the animals to hypobaric hypoxia (7). This could be attributed not only to the factors mentioned above but also to its sedative effect (8). In addition, it was shown that chrysanthemin has a hypotensive action, and that the <Juhua> preparations inhibited the increased local capillary permeability due to intradermal injection of histamine; the efficacy of the 10-mg dose was equivalent to that of 2.5 mg of rutin (9).

2. Antimicrobial Effect

In vitro, the aqueous extract or decoction of <Juhua> was shown to inhibit many pathogenic bacteria, influenza virus PR_8, and leptospirae with an MIC of about 1:10–1:80 (10–15). The *in vivo* studies with mice revealed that the volatile oil distilled from the fresh aerial part of the plant had a strong antibacterial action against *Staphylococcus aureus, Escherichia coli,* and *Shigella flexneri*, but very weak action against *Pseudomonas aeruginosa*, and inactive against *Diplococcus pneumoniae* (16).

3. Miscellaneous Actions

Intragastric administration of the powder preparation of the herb shortened the coagulation time in rabbits. Compared with the crude drug, the powdered charred drug was more potent (17). In artificially induced fever of rabbits, the fluidextract of <Juhua> administered orally produced an antipyretic effect due to central depression (8). Another paper, however, claimed that significant antipyretic effect was achieved only with toxic dosage of the <Juhua> preparations (18).

4. Toxicity

<Juhua> has a very low toxicity. In acute toxicity studies on mice, most animals (8/10) survived

after administration of the decoction at 100 g/kg PO. Similarly, no deaths occurred after administration of the fluidextract at the same dosage. In subacute toxicity studies on rabbits, administration of the decoction or fluidextract 20 g(crude drug)/kg PO daily for 14 days did not produce significant changes in the ECG, BSP and phenol red excretion on the 7th day of medication. Some rabbits exhibited decreased appetite and body weight, diarrhea, and death ensued on about the 10th day of medication (7). The acute LD_{50} of the volatile oil of the aerial part in mice was determined to be 1.3475 ± 0.1311 g/kg IP; no abnormal reactions developed in mice after intraperitoneal injection of 4 mg per animal. Intramuscular dose of 4.8 mg in rabbits did not affect the body temperature or induce any local lesions. Injection of the volatile oil in mice at 0.4 mg/day IP daily for 10 days did not result in abnormalities of the blood picture and liver functions (19).

CLINICAL STUDIES

1. Coronary Disease, Hypertension, and Arteriosclerosis

In 61 cases of coronary disease treated with the concentrated <Juhua> decoction, the aggregate effective rate for angina pectoris was 80% of which 43.3% had marked effects; the aggregate effective rate for ECG was 45.9% of which 18.8% had marked effects. Remission or disappearance of angina pectoris was realized within 20 days in two-thirds of patients. The medication also markedly improved chest discomfort, palpitation, tachypnea, dizziness, headache, and numbness of the extremities. Nineteen out of 30 cases complicated with hypertension had decreases in blood pressure (2). In 164 cases of coronary disease treated with the <Juhua> fluidextract tablet for 2–4 months, the aggregate effective rate for symptomatic relief was 86.5% of which 35.6% were markedly improved, while the aggregate effective rate for ECG improvement was 45.3% of which 14.3% were markedly improved. However, no significant antihypertensive effect was achieved in those cases complicated with hypertension (20). These two kinds of <Juhua> preparation did not modify the heart rate. Determination of the serum cholesterol and triglyceride levels before and after treatment revealed no significant or consistent changes. Clinical use of formulae composed chiefly of the flower of *Dendranthema morifolium*, the flower bud of *Lonicera japonica*, the flower of *Sophora japonica*, and the fruit of *Crataegus pinnatifida* such as Lonicera-Dendranthema Decoction (21), Sophora-Dendranthema Decoction (22), Crataegus-Dendranthema Mixture (23), and Crataegus-Dendranthema Tea (24) were all effective in the treatment of hypertension with arteriosclerosis. Usually, symptoms including headache, vertigo and insomnia improved in 5–10 days in some patients, concurrently with reduction of the blood pressure and serum cholesterol. These medications were also effective in cerebral arteriosclerosis and coronary disease. Lonicera-Dendranthema Decoction produced the best antihypertensive effect; 35 out of 46 cases of hypertension so treated achieved normal blood pressure, while the remaining cases experienced different degrees of symptomatic improvement after 10–30 days' medication. The Crataegus-Dendranthema Tea had the best anticholesterolemic effect with an effective rate of 66.6%.

2. Upper Respiratory Tract Infection, Bronchitis, Tonsillitis, etc.

Intramuscular injection of an injection preparation of the distillate of the fresh *D. morifolium* plant from Hangzhou, which chiefly contains the volatile oil (with a blue substance called chamazulene) 4 or 8 mg/2 ml, had definite therapeutic and prophylactic value; the aggregate effective rate achieved in patients with upper respiratory tract infection, tonsillitis, acute bronchitis, and acute viral hepatitis was around 80% (19,25–27). Two well-known compound formulae are the Morus-Dendranthema Decoction and Morus-Dendranthema Cold Tablet. The Two Flowers Decoction (Flos Chrysanthemum, Flos Lonicerae, Radix Glycyrrhizae, and Semen Sterculiae Scaphigerae) was effective in the treatment of pharyngitis and sore throat (28).

3. Conjunctivitis, etc.

<Juhua> is often used with the fruit-spike of *Prunella vulgaris*, the ripe seed of *Cassia tora*, the fruit of *Tribulus terrestris*, and cicada slough; it may also be used with the fruit of *T. terrestris* and the whole plant of *Equisetum hiemale*, etc. for steam therapy of the affected eye (8). According to a report Lycium-Dendranthema-Rehmannia Decoction/Pill, modified as needed, was effective for optic neuritis and central retinitis (29).

4. Miscellaneous

The crushed fresh leaf of *D. morifolium* is often used locally to treat local infections (8,30). For example, the juice obtained from a few leaves of white chrysanthemum, and the flesh of a few live clams plus a small amount of borneol may be applied to mouth ulcers several times a day; a cure can be achieved in a few days (31). A mixture of equal amounts of the distillates of the frest plants *of D. morifolium* and *Ocimum basilicum* was effective when applied to burns of limited areas, ulcers, or infected wounds for prevention or treatment of infection (32).

ADVERSE EFFECTS

The concentrated decoction or fluidextract tablet of <Juhua> may cause upper abdominal pain or diarrhea in individual patients. Continuous use of the <Juhua> preparation in large doses may affect the gastrointestinal function but no other side effects have been reported (2,20). Very rarely, <Juhua> may cause allergic contact dermatitis (33).

REFERENCE

1. Physiology Section, Zhejiang Medical College et al. Communications of Zhejiang Medical College (Zhejiang Medical College) 1975 (2–3):70.

2. Coronary Disease Unit, First Teaching Hospital of Zhejiang Medical College. Medical Research Information (Zhejiang Medical College) 1975 (1):32.

3. Physiology Section, Zhejiang Medical College. Communications of Zhejiang Medical College (Zhejiang Medical College) 1975 (2–3):59.

4. Physiology Section, Zhejiang Medical College. Information on Coronary Disease Research. Zhejiang Medical College. 1975. p. 61.

5. Physiology Section, Zhejiang Medical College. Information on Coronary Disease Research. Zhejiang Medical College. 1975. p. 59.

6. Physiology Section, Zhejiang Medical College. Information on Coronary Disease Research. Zhejiang Medical College. 1975. p. 56.

7. Physiology Section. Acta Academiae Medicinae Zhejiang 1978 7(4):5.

8. Yuan F. Acta Academiae Medicinae Anhui 1977 (2):62.

9. Ohashina N et al. Japan Centra Revuo Medicina 1965 206:640.

10. Traditional Chinese Medicine and Materia Medica Research Unit of the Internal Medicine Department, First Teaching Hospital of Chongqing Medical College. Acta Microbiologica Sinica 1960 8(1):52.

11. Liu GS et al. Chinese Medical Journal 1950 68 (9–10):307.

12. Wang FL. Chinese Medical Journal 1950 68(5–6):169.

13. Zhang WX. Chinese Medical Journal 1949 67(11):648.

14. Microbiology Department, Xi' an Military Medical College et al. Shaanxi Journal of Medicine and Health 1959 1(1):14.

15. Xuzhou Medical College. Information on New Chinese Medicine (Xuzhou Medical College) 1971 (1):27.

16. Medical Laboratory and Pharmacy. Medical Techniques (Norman Bethune Hospital for International Peace of the Chinese PLA) 1974 (1–2):113.

17. Pharmacology Section, Shandong Institute of Traditional Chinese Medicine and Materia Medica. Chinese Pharmaceutical Bulletin 1965 11(12):562.

18. Nakamura. Tohoku Jikken Igaku 1925 (8):409; Qiu CB. New Compilation of Chinese Materia Medica. Shanghai Medical Publishing House. 1956. p. 274.

19. Pharmacy of Norman Bethune Hospital for International Peace of the Chinese PLA. Beijing Pharmaceutical Industry 1977 (3):8.

20. Zhejiang Coordinating Research Group for Clinical Trial of Dendranthema morifolium Tablet for Coronary Disease. Acta Academiae Medicinae Zhejiang 1978 7(4):9.

21. Shuangcheng County (Heilongjiang) People' s Hospital. Xinyiyaoxue Zazhi (Journal of Traditional Chinese Medicine) 1972 (2):32.

22. Liu LG. Hunan Information on Science and Technology 1973 (6):31.

23. Wuxiang County Hospital et al. Shanxi Medical and Pharmaceutical Journal 1977 (5):11.

24. Maoming Institute of Occupational Diseases. Guangdong Medical Information (Guangdong Institute of Medicine and Health) 1974 (11):30.

25. Pharmacy. Medical Techniques (Norman Bethune Hospital for International Peace of the Chinese PLA) 1976 (6):120.

26. Pediatrics Department. Medical Techniques (Norman Bethune Hospital for International Peace of the Chinese PLA) 1976 (6):39.

27. Wuyi County Hospital. Hengshui Science and Technology (Hengshui District Institute of Scientific and Technological Information, Hebei) 1979 (4):35.

28. EENT Department. Compiled Information on Combined Western and Tradtitional Chinese Medicine. 157th Hospital of the Chinese PLA. 1974. p. 350.

29. Cao SL. Teaching of Traditional Chinese Medicine (Guangxi College of Traditional Chinese Medicine) 1975 (1):59.

30. Chen XB. Guangxi Zhongyiyao (Guangxi Journal of Traditional Chinese Medicine) 1979 (2):26.

31. Wu YH. Guangdong Medical Information (Guangdong Institute of Medicine and Health) 1974 (9):40.

32. Surgery Department of the OPD. Medical Techniques (Normal Bethune Hospital for International Peace of the Chinese PLA) 1976 (6):108.

33. Schulz KH et al. Chemical Abstracts 1975 82:110222z.

(Dai Guangjun)

HUANGJING 黄荆

<Huangjing> comes from the fruit, root and leaf of *Vitex negundo* L. (Verbenaceae). It is bitter, "warm", and nontoxic. It is reputed to be antirheumatic, stomachic, antitussive, "cold-heat"-clearing, channel-deobstruent, expectorant, and sialogogic. It is mainly used to treat common cold, gastric diseases, carbuncle, furuncle, cough and asthma.

CHEMICAL COMPOSITION

The fruit and root of *V. negundo* contain flavonoid glycosides, cardiac glycosides, alkaloids, amino acids, and neutral resin. The fruit also contains small amounts of volatile oil, fixed oil and waxy substances. The bioactive components are flavonoid glycosides and cardiac glycosides. The leaf and fruit contain volatile oils which contain sabinen, small amounts of nishindine and resin. The leaf also contains p-hydroxybenzoic acid and protocatechuic acid.

PHARMACOLOGY

1. Expectorant, Antitussive, and Antiasthmatic Effects

The phenol red excretion test in mice showed that oral administration of the ether extract of the root of *V. negundo* produced an expectorant effect. On the other hand, in mice with cough induced by concentrated ammonia water aerosol, the decoction of the root given orally produced a pronounced antitussive effect (1–4). The decoctions of the root and seed produced bronchodilation in guinea pigs, and perfusion of these decoctions into isolated mouse lungs relieved spasm of the trachea and bronchi; the action of the seed was found to be stronger than that of the root (1,4). Significant spasmolytic and antiasthmatic actions were also shown in mouse lung perfusion studies by the lead salt-precipitated flavonoid glycosides of the root extract as well as by the cardiac glycosides isolated from the seeds; the latter was more potent (1).

2. Antibacterial Effect

In vitro, the decoctions of the seed and root inhibited *Staphylococcus aureus* and *Micrococcus catarrhalis*. The bacteriostatic action became stronger with prolonged decoction. It was also reported that the antibacterial action of <Huangjing> was not strong, and that its effectiveness agianst bronchitis was effected through the promotion of the absorption of the inflammatory exudates in the respiratory tract, not through any antibacterial action (3–5).

3. Miscellaneous Actions

The leaf of *V. negundo* had an anti-inflammatory action on formaldehyde-induced paw swelling of adrenalectomized male rats (4,6,7). Another paper reported that the leaf decoction could kill *Plasmodium flaciparum* (5).

CLINICAL STUDIES

1. Chronic Bronchitis

Seventeen of thirty-one cases benefitted from pills of the powdered seeds 6–9 g twice a day (morning and evening) for 4 therapeutic courses, each comprising 10 days (8). An effective rate of 84.2% was achieved in 335 cases of chronic bronchitis treated with the root decoction 50 ml twice daily for two courses of 10 days each (1,2). In 327 cases of chronic bronchitis treated with Compound Vitex negundo Fruit (Fructus Viticis (powder) 15 g, Placenta Hominis and Rhizoma Dioscoreae (powder) each 6 g, added to maltose to make into pills to be taken daily in three doses, for a course of 20 days), the effective rate was 94.8% (1–4). Fifty cases were treated with capsules of the volatile oil obtained from the branch and leaf; the effective rate was over 88.9% (9).

2. Malaria

The decoction of the fresh seed and root (15 g) may be administered by mouth 2 hours before malarial attack for 2 days. The leaf (or root) decoction (60 g) taken as tea for 7 days, or pills (the size of a mungbean) of the water-purified leaf powder at a daily dose of 9 g for several days, were reported to be effective for the prophylaxis of malaria (5).

3. Common Cold

The decoction of the fresh leaves of *V. negundo*, the whole plant of *Serissa serissoides* each 30 g, green onion, and ginger each 6 g may be taken by mouth (5).

REFERENCE

1. Shangrao District Office. New Medical Information (Jiangxi School of Pharmacy) 1973 (1):21.
2. Dexing Mobile Medical Team of the Academy of Traditional Chinese Medicine et al. Selected Information on Science and Technology of the Academy of Traditional Chinese Medicine. Information Department of the Academy of Traditional Chinese Medicine. 1972. p. 152.
3. Editorial Group. National Collection of Chinese Materia Medica. Vol. 1. People's Medical Publishing House. 1975. p. 767.

4. Shangrao District Health Bureau. Jiangxi Compiled Information of Prevention and Treatment of Chronic Bronchitis (Jiangxi Health Bureau) 1972 (3):73.

5. Guizhou Research Group on the Military Use of Chinese Traditional Drugs et al. Chinese Traditional Drugs Information (Guizhou Department of Scientific and Technological Information) 1972 (1):136.

6. Chaturved GN et al. Indian Journal of Medical Research 1965 53(1):71.

7. Singh RH et al. Indian Journal of Medical Research 1966 54(2):188.

8. Chishui County Coordinating Research Group on Chronic Bronchitis. Medical Information — Special Edition on Chronic Bronchitis. Guizhou Office for the Prevention and Treatment of Chronic Bronchitis. 1974. p. 63.

9. Shangrao District (Jiangxi) Health Bureau et al. Compiled Information. 1975. p. 127.

(Bao Dingyuan)

HUANGQIN 黄芩

<Huangqin> also known as <Kuqin>, is the root of *Scutellaria baicalensis* Georgi (Labiatae). Its other sources are *S. viscidula* Bge. <Huanghuahuangqin>, *S. amoena* C. H. Wright <Xi' nanhuangqin>, *S. rehderiana* Diels, *S. ikonnikovii* Juz., *S. likiangensis* Diels, and *S. hypericifolia* Lévl.

<Huangqin> is bitter and "cold". It is credited with "damp-heat"-clearing, "heat"-purgative, detoxicant and anti-inflammatory actions, and is known to prevent abnormal fetal movements. It is, therefore, useful for fever, cough (* with thick sputum), pneumonia, hemoptysis, jaundice, hepatitis, dysentery, acute conjunctivitis, abnormal fetal movements, hypertension, carbuncle and furuncle.

CHEMICAL COMPOSITION

The root contains 5 flavonoids: baicalein (scutellarein), baicalin (scutellarein-7-glucuronide), wogonin, wogonoside (wogonin-7-glucuronide), and neobaicalein. The root also contains β-sitosterol, benzoic acid, and enzyme of <Huangqin>. The stem and leaf contain scutellarin and baicalin.

PHARMACOLOGY

1. Antimicrobial Effect

<Huangqin> has a wide antibacterial spectrum. Different degrees of antibacterial activity were exhibited *in vitro* by the <Huangqin> decoction against *Staphylococcus aureus*, *Diplococcus pneumoniae*, *Streptococcus hemolyticus*, *Neisseria meningitidis*, *Shigella dysenteriae*, *Corynebacterium diphtheriae*, *Bacillus anthracis*, *Escherichia coli*, *Pseudomonas aeruginosa*, *Salmonella typhi*, *Salmonella paratyphi*, *Proteus vulgaris*, and *Vibrio cholerae* (1–8). The ethanol extract of the herb was also effective against *Neiserria meningitidis* and *Pseudomonas aeruginosa* (4,9). Antibacterial activity was also exhibited by the juice of the fresh leaf added to the *Staphylococcus* culture (10). One paper, however, claimed that the <Huangqin> decoction was inactive against 37 kinds of microbes including the above mentioned organisms (11). These divergent results may be due to the difference in the varieties of herb or to the experimental methods employed. <Huangqin> decoction inhibited *Mycobacterium tuberculosis* var. *hominis* and *M. tuberculosis* var. *bovis* (12–15); others claimed the opposite (16,17). The decoction had therapeutic value on experimental tuberculosis in mice but not in guinea pigs (15). The extract of <Huangqin> was shown *in vitro* to be active against 10 kinds of skin fungi including *Trichophyton violaceum* and *Microsporum audouini* (18), whereas the decoction was active against nine kinds of skin fungi including *Trichophyton violaceum* and *Microsporum canis* (19). *In vitro* studies revealed that the

decoction and the ethanol extract were inhibitory, and at high concentration, lethal to leptospirae (20). The extract and decoction also inhibited influenza virus PR_8 strain and type A Asian influenza virus (21–25). However, they were inactive against Xiantai virus, adenovirus type 7, and rhinovirus type 17.

Antimicrobial tests with baicalein and wogonin from the aqueous extract showed that only the former had a significant antibacterial activity (26). Another paper reported that *Vibrio cholerae* and *Staphylococcus aureus* were susceptible to wogonin *in vitro*, whereas *Salmonella typhi* and *Shigella dysenteriae* were not (27). In addition, baicalein at high concentrations was shown *in vivo* to inhibit the growth of amoeba (28).

2. Antiallergic and Anti-inflammatory Effects

Oral administration of baicalin 50 mg/kg/day to egg white-sensitized guinea pigs for 7 days protected the animals against allergic reaction due to re-inspiration of the antigen, significantly prolonging the latent period of convulsion. Both baicalin and baicalein markedly inhibited antigen-induced allergic contraction (Schultz-Dale reaction) of the isolated small intestine and trachea of sensitized guinea pigs; baicalein was shown to be more potent than baicalin (29,30). Similarly, baicalein had a stronger inhibitory action than baicalin on the passive systemic allergic reaction in guinea pigs and mice, as well as on the passive cutaneous allergy in guinea pigs (31). Experiments on isolated guinea pig intestines indicated that baicalein had antihistaminic and anticholinergic actions, whereas baicalin had none. These two compounds did not affect the binding of the antigen to the antibody but markedly decreased the release of chemical mediators from the lung slices of sensitized guinea pigs when exposed to antigens. Combined use of baicalin or baicalein with cysteine failed to decrease the amount of chemical mediators released, indicating that the suppression of allergic reaction was effected through inhibition of mercaptylase, which is responsible for the release of chemical mediators during antigen-antibody interaction (29).

Both baicalin and baicalein were shown to reduce the capillary permeability in the mouse ear (32). They also protected mice against experimental pulmonary hemorrhage induced by low atmospheric pressure (33).

3. Sedative Effect

Intraperitoneal injection of the <Huangqin> decoction 2 g/kg to mice inhibited the positive conditioned reflex, prolonging its latent period and increasing the frequency of reinforcement. If the positive conditioned reflex was established before the negative one, <Huangqin> could improve the negative conditioned reflex, thus intensifying the cortical inhibition (34). Intraperitoneal injection of baicalin 500 or 1000 mg/kg to mice resulted in a sedative effect lasting 2–3 hours (35). Mild sedation in rabbits was observed after intravenous injection of the <Huangqin> extract 1 g/kg. Central inhibition was increased and death could ensue by increasing the dosage (36).

4. Antipyretic Effect

The decoction at 0.24–0.48 g/kg IV (37) or 2 g/kg PO (38) or baicalin at 130 mg/kg IP for IV (35) subsided fever in rabbits given a mixed typhoid vaccine. An antipyretic effect was also achieved with the oral decoction on artificial fever induced by yeast in rabbits (39). However, it was also reported that no significant antipyretic effect was achieved with either the decoction or ethanol extract of the herb administered orally or intramuscularly in rabbits with fever induced by a mixed typhoid vaccine, whereas a transient and weak antipyretic action was produced by intravenous injection of the decoction. Since intravenous injection of normal saline also produced the same effect, it is considered that <Huangqin> is devoid of antipyretic action (40). Further studies are required as documented results are inconsistent. Baicalin administered either intravenously or intramuscularly to normal rabbits could not lower their body temperature (41).

5. Hypotensive Effect

The blood pressure of anesthetized dogs was markedly lowered by intravenous injection of the fluidextract 0.5 g/kg, oral administration of the extract 1 g/kg, intravenous injection of the decoction 60 mg/kg, and oral, intramuscular or intravenous administration of the ethanol extract 1 g(crude drug)/kg (36,39,42–44). Baicalin 10–20 mg/kg IV was also effective (35). Intravenous injection of the refined methanol extract produced hypotension in anesthetized rats (45). Oral or rectal administration of the tincture preparation lowered the blood pressure of dogs with neurogenic hypertension (46). A marked decrease of blood pressure was achieved in dogs with or without renal hypertension after giving the extract orally thrice daily for 4 weeks (47).

The mechanism of the hypotensive action was studies with the extract, the ethanol extract, and the refined methanol extract. Low concentrations produced stimulation and high concentrations inhibition of isolated frog and toad hearts (36,39). In anesthetized rats, the heart rate was decreased but the cardiac output was not significantly altered (45). The hypotensive effect in anesthetized dogs and rats was not modified by bilateral vagotomy or atropine injection (36,45). Vasodilation in the isolated rabbit ear, the isolated rabbit kidney and toad and rabbit hind limbs, as well as increased renal volume in anesthetized dogs, were noted. There was, however, neither antagonism to the pressor effect of epinephrine (36,42), nor weakening of the contraction of cat nictitating membrane caused by stimulation of the preganglionic carotid sympathetic nerves (36). In anesthetized rats, the total peripheral vascular resistance was decreased, the pressor response to blockade of the carotid artery was markedly inhibited, and the hypotensive reaction disappeared after spinal section at the 7th cervical vertebra (45). Intravenous injection of the herb solution in normal and arteriosclerotic rabbits caused vasodilation of the ears with intact nerves. When the herb solution was added to the perfusion fluid of the rabbit ear with intact nerves, it caused not only ear vasodilation but also a slight fall in the systemic blood pressure (48). To sum up, the fall in the blood pressure was chiefy effected by the inhibition of the vasomotor center, and secondarily through direct vasodilation. The herb may also stimulate the vascular baroreceptors, causing reflex hypotension (36,45,48).

6. Diuretic Effect

The aqueous extract, the ethanol extract, baicalin, baicalein, or wogonin given intravenously increased the urine output of anesthetized rabbits (49,50). Diuresis was also produced in normal rabbits by oral administration of the ethanol extract and in normal mice by intraperitoneal injection of baicalin or baicalein (32,50). Similarly, a diuretic effect was observed in anesthetized dogs after intravenous injection of the fluidextract or baicalin (35,42).

7. Cholagogic, Choleretic, and Spasmolytic Effects

Injection of the decoction 0.5 g/kg IV to anesthetized dogs increased bile secretion (51). In unanesthetized rabbits, intravenous injection of the aqueous extract, the ethanol extract, and baicalin produced a choleretic effect, whereas wogonin was inactive (52,53). Intravenous injection of baicalin reduced bilirubinemia in rabbits caused by ligation of the common bile duct (53). The decoction had an inhibitory effect on the motility of the isolated rabbit small intestine (54). Wogonin was shown to have spasmolytic effect against acetylcholine-induced spasm of the isolated mouse small intestine, whereas baicalein was inactive (55). Both the decoction and tincture inhibited the dog small intestine *in situ*, and only the tincture antagonized pilocarpine-induced excitation of the small intestine. Vagotomy did not modify the inhibitory effect on the intestine (39,56).

8. Detoxicant Effect

Intravenous injection of the tincture antagonized the toxic effects of strychnine in frogs, cats, and dogs, alleviated convulsion and lowered the mortality rate (57). Baicalin administered subcutaneously to mice reduced the toxic effects of strychnine and markedly increased the LD_{50} of strychnine by subcutaneous injection (58,59). Baicalein was shown to be devoid of detoxicant action in contrast to glucuronic acid. The glucuronic acid-treated group of carbon tetrachloride-poisoned mice showed high levels of liver glycogen compared with the baicalin-treated group; the baicalein-treated group had the lowest level. These results suggest that the detoxicant action of baicalin is probably due to the glucuronic acid contained (59).

9. Miscellaneous Actions

Intravenous or intramuscular injection of baicalin to rabbits caused a brief decrease followed by a marked increase in the total WBC count. Maximal effect was attained in 8 to 24 hours and normal values were re-established after 48 hours; however, the differential count was not significantly altered (41). The orally administered extract did not modify the serum cholesterol/total phospholipid ratio in normal rabbits, but lowered that of cholesterol-fed rabbits (60). The fluidextract increased the blood glucose level in rabbits (61).

10. Toxicity

Rabbits given the decoction at 10 g/kg PO or the ethanol extract at 2 g/kg IV appeared sedated; no death occurred in these animals (39). Injection of the aqueous extract at 2 g/kg IV to rabbits also produced sedative and hypnotic effects; but the animals died 8–12 hours later. However, when the dosage was reduced to 1 g/kg, sedation but no death occurred (36,41). A single oral dose of the aqueous extract 12 or 15 g/kg in dogs elicited no reactions during 48 hours of observation, except emesis in the high dosage group. Oral administration of this agent at 4 or 5 g/kg to dogs thrice daily for 8 weeks did not produce any significant abnormalities in the routine blood test and histology of internal organs. Loose bowel movement occurred only in the high dosage group but it disappeared upon discontinuation of the medication (47). The lethal doses of the various preparations in mice by subcutaneous injection were as follows: the ethanol extract 6 g/kg, baicalin 6 g/kg, and wogonin 4 g/kg (62). The LD_{50} of baicalin in mice was 3.081 g/kg IP (35). Another report claimed that after injection of baicalin 15 mg/kg IV to rabbits, restlessness and shortness of breath occurred, followed an hour later by significant sedation and hypnosis. All four experimental animals died within 48 hours (41). In conclusion, the various preparations of <Huangqin> have very low toxicity if given orally but high if given intravenously.

CLINICAL STUDIES

1. Respiratory Tract Infection in Children

Dosage of the 50% <Huangqin> decoction: below 1 year 6 ml, above 1 year 8–10 ml, and above 5 years adequately increased, to be given daily in three doses. In 63 cases (51 acute upper respiratory tract infection, 11 acute bronchitis, and 1 acute tonsillitis), 51 cases benefitted; body temperature was usually normalized in 3 days (63).

2. Chronic Bronchitis

Scutellaria-Lime Water Mixture (Radix Scutellariae and Radix Glycyrrhizae Decoction plus lime water) was used to treat 35 cases; relatively good responses were obtained in the simple type of the disease (63).

3. Scarlet Fever

The decoction of <Huangqin> given orally to 1577 persons markedly reduced the incidence rate of the disease (64).

4. Carriers of Epidemic Cerebrospinal Meningitis

Spraying of the aerosol of the 20% <Huangqin> decoction 2 ml (0.4 g crude drug) to the throat was effective in 209 cases (3).

5. Bacillary Dysentery

Equal amounts of <Huangqin> and the fruit of *Terminalia chebula* were made into powder by alum precipitation. The powder was used with symptomatic treatment in 100 cases. Clinical cure was attained in an average of 5.3 days (65). Likewise, an effective rate of 95.5% was obtained in 111 cases of acute bacillary dysentery treated with the sugar-coated tablet of *S. viscidula* powder, or the capsule of its aqueous fluidextract powder, or the decoction of the fresh or dried <Huangqin>. Symptoms disappeared rapidly with the decoction and fluidextract (66).

6. Leptospirosis

Tablets prepared from equal amounts of the fluidextracts of <Huangqin>, the flower bud of *Lonicera japonica*, and the fruit of *Forsythia suspensa* each 0.5 g (equivalent to 3.7 g of the crude drugs), were used to treat 65 cases at doses of 10–15 tablets every 6 hours, adequately reduced for children. Better results were achieved in moderate and mild cases (67).

7. Infectious Hepatitis

Baicalin was used to treat acute icteric and nonicteric hepatitis and active chronic hepatitis; it restored the liver functions and improved the clinical symptoms (68). Another author reported the therapeutic value of baicalin in patients with chronic hepatitis B, and in those with persistently positive HBsAg for more than one year (69).

8. Acute Biliary Tract Infections

Intravenous infusion of baicalin was employed in the treatment of 72 cases of acute biliary tract infections (30 biliary tract ascariasis complicated with cholecystitis and cholangitis, 25 acute cholecystitis, 10 acute retrograde pancreatitis, 5 cholecystitis complicated with cholelithiasis, one liver cirrhosis complicated with biliary tract infection, and one biliary tract infection with secondary liver abscess); 45 cases had marked improvement and 20 cases significant improvement (70).

9. Hypertension

An antihypertensive effect and symptomatic improvement were achieved by the <Huangqin> tincture tried in 51 cases of hypertension (71,72).

10. Miscellaneous

Salutary therapeutic effects were achieved in the treatment of 31 cases (36 eyes) of eye diseases with the alcohol-precipitated decoction of <Huangqin> and the flower bud of *Lonicera japonica*.

The preparation was given by subconjunctival injection for anterior eye diseases including corneal ulcer and scleritis and by postbulbar injection for posterior eye or retrobulbar diseases such as papillitis and postbulbar optic neuritis (73).

ADVERSE EFFECTS

According to clinical experience, <Huangqin> has a low toxicity. No ill effects, except rare gastric discomfort and diarrhea, were associated with either oral administration of the crude preparation of <Huangqin>, or injection of baicalin and baicalein (66–72). Intraocular injection of Scutellaria-Lonicera Injection (Radix Scutellariae, Flos Lonicerae) caused relatively severe local distending pain which could be alleviated by addition of an adequate amount of procaine to the injection liquid (73).

REFERENCE

1. Zhang CS. Modern Research on Chinese Materia Medica. Chinese Scientific Books and Instruments Company. 1954. p. 108.

2. Liu GS. Chinese Journal of New Medicine 1950 1(4):285.

3. Yan GH. Journal of Traditional Chinese Medicine 1960 (6):20.

4. Zhao ZY. Acta Microbiologica Sinica 1960 8(2):171.

5. Microbiology Section, Shandong Medical College. Acta Academiae Medicinae Shandong 1959 (8):42.

6. Lingling District (Hunan) Sanitation and Anti-epidemic Station. Hunan Yiyao Zazhi (Hunan Medical Journal) 1974 (4):50.

7. Li CL et al. Fujian Zhongyiyao (Fujian Journal of Traditional Chinese Medicine) 1960 (7):38.

8. Feng KY. Harbin Zhongyi (Harbin Journal of Traditional Chinese Medicine) 1965 (4–5):37.

9. Wang WS et al. Chinese Pharmaceutical Bulletin 1959 (10):522.

10. Yan GH et al. Chinese Pharmaceutical Bulletin 1960 (2):57.

11. Microbiology Section, Harbin Medical College. Heilongjiang Medical Journal 1959 (8):62.

12. Guiyang Institute of Tuberculosis. Chinese Journal of Prevention of Tuberculosis 1959 (6):37.

13. Chen YZ et al. Jiangxi Yiyao (Jiangxi Medical Journal) 1961 (12–13):31.

14. Guo J et al. Chinese Journal of Prevention of Tuberculosis 1964 5(3):481, 488.

15. Liu XK et al. Chinese Journal of Tuberculosis 1958 (3):204.

16. Laboratory of Liaoning Institute of Tuberculosis. Liaoning Medical Journal 1960 (7):29.

17. Microbiology Section, Harbin Medical University. Heilongjiang Medical Journal 1959 (8):63.

18. Cao RL et al. Chinese Journal of Dermatology 1957 (4):286.

19. Sun X. Chinese Medical Journal 1955 (6):536.

20. Xuzhou Medical College. Information on New Chinese Medicine (Xuzhou Medical College) 1971 (1):27.

21. Wang SY. Kexue Tongbao (Science Bulletin) 1958 (3):90.

22. Wang SY. Kexue Tongbao (Science Bulletin) 1958 (5):155.

23. Liu GS et al. Acta Microbiologica Sinica 1960 8(2):164.

24. Microbiology Department, Fourth Military Medical College. Shaanxi Journal of Medicine and Health 1959 (1):14.

25. Microbiology Section, Zhongshan Medical College. Information on Medical Sciences and Technology (Guangdong Institute of Medicine and Health) 1973 (8–9):33.

26. Wang XK et al. Acta Academiae Medicinae Sichuan 1959 (4):97.

27. Hsu HY. Journal of the Taiwan Pharmaceutical Association 1954 6:7; Chemical Abstracts 1956 50:1217c.

28. Zhang TM et al. Acta Academiae Medicinae Wuhan 1958 (1):11.

29. Eda et al. Folia Pharmacologica Japonica 1970 66:194.

30. Eda et al. Metabolism and Disease (Supplement) 1973 10(5):730; Li CG (translator). Foreign Research Information on Chinese Materia Medica — Rheum and Scutellaria. Hunan Institute of Pharmaceutical and Medical Industry. 1975. p. 24.

31. Eda et al. Folia Pharmacologica Japonica 1970 66:237.

32. Eda et al. Folia Pharmacologica Japonica 1966 62(1):39.

33. Okanishi T et al. Annual Report of Shionogi Research Laboratory 1952 (2):162; Chemical Abstracts 1957 51:9008c.

34. Pharmacology Department, Xi' an Medical College. Acta Academiae Medicinae Xi' an 1959 (8):102.

35. Pharmacology Department, Xi' an Medical College. Acta Academiae Medicinae Xi' an 1958 (5):30.

36. Tang RY et al. Acta Physiologica Sinica 1958 22:91.

37. Zhang FC et al. The National Medical Journal of China 1935 21:626.

38. Sun SX. Chinese Medical Journal 1956 42(10):964.

39. Pharmacology Department, Shanghai College of Traditional Chinese Medicine. Scientific Papers of Shanghai College of Traditional Chinese Medicine 1959 (2):3.

40. Chen MQ. Acta Pharmaceutica Sinica 1962 9:690.

41. Burns Research Group, Shenyang College of Pharmacy. New Pharmaceutical Communications (Shenyang College of Pharmacy) 1971 (2):16.

42. Jing LB et al. Chinese Reports of the Institute of Physiology (National Peiping Research Institute) 1936 3(3):259.

43. Wu J et al. Acta Academiae Medicinae Xi' an 1957 (4):38.

44. Wang JM. Shanghai Zhongyiyao Zazhi (Shanghai Journal of Traditional Chinese Medicine) 1956 (1): 36.

45. Huang N. The References of Traditional Chinese Medicine 1975 (1):45; The American Journal of Chinese Medicine 1974 2:375.

46. Usov LA. Farmakologiia I Toksikologiia 1958 21(2):31.

47. Lin JQ et al. Acta Physiologica Sinica 1958 22(3):249.

48. Wang RD et al. Abstracts of the First Congress of the Chinese Society of Physiology (Pharmacy). 1956. p. 55.

49. Kumazaki. Acta Scholae Medicinalis Universitatis in Gifu 1958 6:352.

50. Deng ZF et al. Chinese Medical Journal 1961 47(1):7.

51. Tong EY et al. Abstracts of the Symposium of the Chinese Society of Physiology (Pharmacology). 1964. p. 132.

52. Sato K. Journal of Kyoto Prefectural University of Medicine 1935 13(3):676.

53. Kumazaki. Folia Pharmacologica Japonica 1957 53(6):215.

54. Acute Abdomen Research Unit, Zunyi Medical College. Xinyiyaoxue Zazhi (Journal of Traditional Chinese Medicine) 1975 (10):36.

55. Shibata S et al. Journal of the Pharmaceutical Society of Japan (Tokyo) 1960 80:620.

56. Scientific Research Group of the Pharmacology Section, Xi' an Medical College. Acta Academiae Medicinae Xi' an 1957 (4):29.

57. Ibragimov FH. Osnovye Lekarstvennya Sredstva Kitaiskoi Meditsiny. Giml. 1960. p. 238.

58. Kuboki N et al. The Journal of Practical Pharmacy 1961 13(8):53.

59. Li XG. Chinese Pharmaceutical Bulletin 1964 10(4):160.

60. Aonuma S et al. Journal of the Pharmaceutical Society of Japan (Tokyo) 1957 77:1303.

61. Jing LB et al. Chinese Reports of the Institute of Physiology (National Peiping Research Institute) 1936 3(1):1.

62. Kumazaki. Japan Centra Revuo Medicina 1959 145:907.

63. Yue XS. Jiangxi Yiyao (Jiangxi Medical Journal) 1961 (11):16.

64. Jinzhou Suburbs Sanitation and Anti-epidemic Station. Chinese Traditional and Herbal Drugs Communications 1972 (3):35.

65. Zhongshan Medical College. New Chinese Medicine 1972 (8):31.

66. Sanitation and Anti-epidemic Department, Hospital of the 51084 Unit of the Chinese PLA et al. People' s Military Medicine 1977 (6):29.

67. Yuantong Commune (Chongqing County) Health Centre et al. Research Information on Chinese Traditional Drugs (Sichuan Institute of Chinese Materia Medica) 1971 (6):25.

68. Qi TP et al. Xinyiyaoxue Zazhi (Journal of Traditional Chinese Medicine) 1973 (8):24.

69. Huang MQ. Selected Information on Scientific Research (Jiangsu College of New Medicine) 1976 (2):42.

70. Shantou District People' s Hospital. Xinzhongyi (Journal of New Chinese Medicine 1976 (Supplement 1):24.

71. He YH. Shanghai Zhongyiyao Zazhi (Shanghai Journal of Traditional Chinese Medicine) 1955 (6):24.

72. He YH. Shanghai Zhongyiyao Zazhi (Shanghai Journal of Traditional Chinese Medicine) 1956 (1):24.

73. Ye LN. Xinyiyaoxue Zazhi (Journal of Traditional Chinese Medicine) 1973 (3):27.

(Liu Wenqing)

HUANGLIAN 黄連

<Huanglian> is the rhizome of *Coptis chinensis* Franch., *C. deltoideas* C. Y. Cheng et Hsiao, and *C. teetoides* C. Y. Cheng (*= *C. teeta* Wall.). (Ranunculaceae). These herbs are also known as <Weilian>, <Yalian>, and <Yunlian>, respectively.

The drug has a bitter flavor and a "cold" property. It is "heat" purgative, detoxicant, anti-inflammatory, latent-heat clearing, antipyretic, and "damp"-clearing. It is mainly used in the treatment of extreme irritability in fever, hematemesis, epistaxis, distention of the chest and abdomen due to "damp-heat", nausea, vomiting, dysentery, enteritis, acute conjunctivitis, furuncle, carbuncle, pyogenic infections or ulcers of the skin, and otitis media.

CHEMICAL COMPOSITION

<Huanglian> mainly contains berberine 5–8%, an isoquinoline alkaloid that has been synthesized. Other alkaloid constituents are coptisine, worenine, palmatine, and columbamine. In addition to alkaloids, <Huanglian> also contains obakunone and obakulactone.

The rhizome of *Coptis omeiensis* (Chen) C. Y. Cheng also contains jatrorrhizine. The whole plant of *C. chinensis* contains berberine, the yield of which peaks from July to October before the plant withers.

Reduction of berberine forms the colourless tetrahydroberberine with a change in pharmacological properties. Berberine for medicinal use is mainly isolated from *Berberis* species (refer to <Sankezhen> in volume). Methylation of berbamine in the residue of berberine extract yields a diquaternary ammonium iodide, named meberbamine iodide, a stereomer of tetrandrine dimethiodide.

PHARMACOLOGY

1. Antimicrobial and Antiprotozoal Effects

Reports on the antimicrobial effect of <Huanglian> in China and other countries are numerous (1–24). *In vitro*, the antibacterial spectra of <Huanglian> and berberine are essentially the same. They were very potent against staphylococcus, streptococcus, pneumococcus, *Vibrio cholerae*, *Bacillus anthracis*, and *Bacillus dysenteriae* (with the exception of *Shigella sonnei*), and to a lesser extent against *Bacillus subtilis, Klebsiella pneumoniae, Bordetella pertussis, Corynebacterium diphtheriae, Pasteurella pestis, Brucella* and *Mycobacterium tuberculosis*, but weak against *Escherichia coli, Proteus vulgaris*, and *Salmonella typhi*, and virtually inactive against *Salmonella paratyphi, Pseudomonas aeruginosa* and *Shigella sonnei*. Berberine was shown to be bacteriostatic at low concentrations and bactericidal at high concentrations (4). There is, however, a report on the absence of any bactericidal action from berberine *in vitro* (25). *In vivo*, <Huanglian> and berberine were proved to be effective against experimental cholera (26). However, intragastric administration of the herb failed to protect rabbits infected with *Corynebacterium diphtheriae* from ensuing death nor did it alleviate the local reaction (27). The herb exhibited no therapeutic effect on experimentally induced tuberculosis in rabbits and guinea pigs (28,29), except when large doses were given in mice (21).

Staphylococcus aureus, Streptococcus hemolyticus, and *Shigella flexneri* readily developed resistance to berberine used alone (4,30); they even utilized berberine (31,32). No cross resistance developed between berberine and penicillin, streptomycin, chlortetracycline, isoniazid, or p-aminosalicylic acid (33–34). Berberine and sulfonamides were shown to have similar antibacterial activity, but the former agent was not affected by serum (35). It appeared that berberine could eliminate the resistance (R) factor of the kanamycin- and chloramphenicol-resistant RS-2 strain of *Escherichia coli* and this phenomenon was thought to be due to selective inhibition of bacterial DNA replication following complexation of berberine with the bacterial attachment DNA (36). The compound formula of <Huanglian> displayed increased antibacterial activity with reduced resistance development (6).

In addition, <Huanglian> preparation or berberine was shown to inhibit various influenza viruses (37) and Newcastle disease virus (38) cultured in the chicken embryo, amoeba *in vitro* and in the rat (39,40), *Chlamydia trachomatis* (41), *Trichomonas* (42), *Leishmania tropica* (1,43), trypanosome (1,44), and 13 kinds of skin fungi including *Trichophyton violaceum, Epidermophyton floccosum, Microsporum canis* and *Nocardia asteroides* (45–47).

The antimicrobial mechanism of <Huanglian> has not yet been elucidated. However, it was reported that berberine strongly inhibited the intermediate process of carbohydrate metabolism of yeasts and bacteria, the oxidative decarboxylation of acetoacetic acid. Vitamin B_6, potassium permanganate (PP) and p-aminobenzoic acid antagonized the antibacterial effect of berberine (4, 48–50). In slightly alkaline medium, berberine inhibited the tryptophanase system of *Escherichia coli* and tyrosine decarboxylase of *Streptococcus faecalis*, and this inhibitory effect was antagonized by vitamin B_6 (51,52). Berberine decreased the RNA of *Vibrio cholerae*, thus inhibiting protein synthesis (24), and also markedly inhibited the incorporation of ^{14}C-thymidine, ^{14}C-uridine, or ^{14}C-phenylalanine into the pneumococcal polysomes and enlarged the *Escherichia coli* cell, making them polymorphic and filamentous (53). Gradient separation of berberine-treated *Vibrio cholerae* showed that 75% of the alkaloid was found in the adipose fraction. Furthermore, berberine treatment of *Vibrio cholerae* cultured in ^{14}C-glucose medium deactivated the bacterial toxin as well as permitting the escape of large amounts of radioactive substances into the culture medium (54). This may have resulted from autolysis of the already formed polysomes. Hence, berberine is considered to be damaging to the bacterial call membranes (53).

In dogs with experimental septicemi of *Staphylococcus aureus*, injection of berberine 19 mg/kg IV increased the leukocytic phagocytosis of *Staphylococcus aureus* and precluded the death of the animals (5). Berberine in low doses (2–5 mg/kg) enhanced the phagocytic function of the reticuloendothelial systems in rabbits (55).

2. Effect on the CNS

In conditioned reflex experiments with mice, low dosage of berberine (0.005 mg/20 g) enhanced the establishment of the positive conditioned reflex, whereas high dosage (0.05−0.1 mg/20 g) delayed the establishment. Both low and high dosages, particularly the latter, caused incomplete differentiation of the conditioned reflex. This might be related to its inhibitory effect on cholinesterase (56). Both Coptis Detoxicant Decoction and Coptis-Glycyrrhiza Mixture (equal amounts of Rhizoma Coptidis and Radix Glycyrrhizae) stimulated the central excitatory control mechanisms in mice but insignificantly depressed the inhibitory control mechanisms (57). In mice, berberine lowered the rectal temperature, decreased the spontaneous activity and prolonged the cyclobarbital- and pentobarbital-induced sleep (58,59). Significant antipyretic effect was exhibited by this agent against milk-induced fever in rabbits and that induced by yeast suspension in rats (60,61). Berberine at therapeutic doses stimulated respiration, probably through a direct action on the respiratory center, or via the chemoreceptors (62). However, it could have been a feedback phenomenon secondary to hypotension, or due to local stimulation produced by accumulation of the drug in the pulmonary tissue (63). Berberine in large doses caused paralysis of the respiratory center, ataxia, motor inhibition, and muscular flaccidity (64). Various behavioral studies using the revolving-rod, rod-climbing, pulling and avoidance methods showed that berberine at high dosage 15 mg/kg IP has a central depressive effect in mice (59). Nevertheless, at doses of less than 2 mg/kg IP or 300 mg/kg PO berberine did not produce any central effect (65,66).

Subcutaneous injection of 50–100 mg/kg of tetrahydroberberine to mice weakened the conditioned reflex and the orientation reaction, and concurrently produced analgesia, sedation, and muscle relaxation. The last effect was 3 times as potent as that of meprobamate. Tetrahydroberberine displayed mutual antagonism with amphetamine. The former potentiated the hypnotic action of barbital and chloral hydrate, but failed to antagonize convulsions induced by caffeine, pentylenetetrazole, strychnine, or nicotine (67,68).

Tetrahydroberberine converted the rapid waves of the frontal lobe of rabbit EEG to slow waves, and, like chlorpromazine, it caused persistent firing to the post-hippocampal region, and also caused muscle relaxation as well as the disappearance of the righting reflex. It did not produce hypothermia. It is suggested that tetrahydroberberine is a type of tranquilizer; the levorotatory isomer is more potent (69).

3. Effect on Peripheral Neurotransmitters

Berberine exerted a dose-dependent biphasic effect on acetylcholine in intact animals (70) and isolated organs (71–73). Generally, low dosage potentiated and high dosage antagonized it. At concentrations from 2×10^{-6} to 2×10^{-5}, berberine had no direct effect on the isolated frog musculi rectus abdominis, though it markedly enhanced the response to acetylcholine (70). As shown in the ECG, berberine antagonized acetylcholine-induced bradycardia and ST segment depression in rabbits

(74). The anticholinergic dose also antagonized pilocarpine but not potassium chloride (71). Berberine decreased the cholinesterase activity in dog and horse serum (70,72), and in rabbit brain homogenate (72,73), which was probably the mechanism of its cholinergic action. The anticholinergic activity of berberine may be explained by the fact that it is chemically similar to acetylcholine, both being quaternary ammonium compounds despite the great disparity in the structures of their other constituents (70–74).

Berberine significantly weakened the antagonistic effect of curare on the response of neuromuscular specimens of rats and frogs to acetycholine. The minimal effective doses of berberine, physostigmine and neostigmine are in the ratio of 10:20:1. Unlike that of physostigmine and neostigmine, the effect of berberine was slow to appear and repeated dosings or large doses did not weaken it (75). Meberbamine iodide had curariform muscle relaxant action (76). Berberine decreased the pressor effect of epinephrine (72,73,77). On the ECG, berberine was shown to counteract arrhythmia induced by epinephrine and norepinephrine in rabbits (74).

4. Effect on the Heart

Berberine at a low concentration (4×10^{-6}) excited the isolated cat heart and increased the coronary flow by 20–40%, whereas at 1×10^{-5}, it inhibited the heart. However, even at 1×10^{-4}, it did not stop the heart beat. This dose-dependent biphasic action was also observed in the *in situ* cat heart, isolated frog heart, cat and rabbit atria, and heart-lung preparation of dogs (60,71). Berberine exhibited a negative inotropic effect on the isolated rabbit heart. Perfusion of this agent at 1:1000 to frog hearts resulted in heart block (40). It also decreased the heart rate of toads (78), but caused tachycardia in the *in situ* dog heart (66). Study of the rabbit ECG revealed that apart from antagonizing autonomic neurotransmitters (74), berberine also inhibited the tachycardia induced by methamphetamine and dimethoxydeoxyephedrine and reversed the bradycardia elicited by neosynephrine, methoxamine, and the cholinesterase inhibitors DFP and neostigmine (79). Berberine also excited the isolated atria of rabbits, guinea pigs and rats, probably through selective stimulation of the β_1-adrenoceptors (61).

5. Effects on Blood Vessels and Blood Pressure

A clear hypotensive effect was observed after intravenous injection of berberine to anesthetized dogs, cats, rats and frogs as well as in unanesthetized rats; the extent and duration increased with the dosage. No tachyphylaxis developed from repeated dosing (58,61,78,80,81). The hypotensive dosage did not depress the heart (78,82). Concurrent with the hypotension, there were increases in the volume of the spleen, intestine, kidney, and extremities and in the perfusion volume of the systemic vasculature of frogs (63). Berberine was also shown to dilate the isolated renal blood vessels, prolong the hypotensive action of the vagus nerve and acetylcholine, and inhibit the pressor reflex of the carotid sinus (83). Another report, however, claimed that there was no connection between the action of berberine and the pressor reflex, and that the agent blocked the sympathetic ganglions (80). The hypotensive action of berberine was not modified by atropine, diphenhydramine, propranolol, phentolamine, and phenoxybenzamine, nor by decerebration and bilateral vagotomy, neither was it related to histamine release (58,73). The drug, however, inhibited cholinesterase, potentiated the hypotensive action of acetylcholine, and weakened the pressor reflex caused by stimulating the proximal sciatic nerve or by intravenous injection of epinephrine. It did not influence the contraction of the nictitating membrane caused by stimulation of the preganglionic fiber of the superior carotid sympathetic ganglions. The hypotensive mechanism of berberine is, therefore, appeared to be multiple and related to direct vasodilation, inhibition of cholinesterase, antagonism to epinephrine, and inhibition of the pressor reflex and the vasomotor center. The hypotensive action was reversed by ergotoxin (84). Pre-injection of large doses of atropine enabled berberine to reverse the pressor effect of acetylcholine (72,73). In addition, berberine acted on the chemoreceptors in the circulation-blocked marrow cavity, intestinal and carotid bodies, causing an increase in the blood pressure and respiration rate (62). A weak hypotensive action was also exhibited by tetrahydroberberine (68).

6. Effect on Smooth Muscles

Intravenous injection of berberine to dogs excitated the gastrointestinal smooth muscles, which was antagonized by large doses of atropine (60). Studies with isolated organs also showed that berberine excitated the smooth muscles of the stomach, intestine, bronchus, urinary bladder and uterus; this is consistent with its cholinergic effects (80,85). Low concentrations of the agent caused spasm of the isolated ileum of guinea pigs, whereas high concentrations produced a spasmolytic effect. The latter effect was probably due to antagonism of acetylcholine (40). Berberine also diminished contraction of the isolated ileum of guinea pigs caused by acetylcholine, carbachol, histamine, bradykinin, barium chloride, and potassium chloride, as well as contraction of the isolated rabbit uterus induced by serotonin (58). Low concentrations of berberine intensified prostaglandin-induced contraction of the isolated ileum of guinea pigs and high concentrations decreased it. The drug also reinforced calcium chloride-induced depolarization and contraction of the ileum of guinea pigs, and increasing the concentration of the drug did not diminish the ileal response to calcium chloride, indicating that berberine enhanced the action of calcium ions in excitation-contraction coupling (61).

7. Antineoplastic Effect

Early studies indicated that berberine was devoid of toxic effect on mitotic cells despite the presence of the stilbylamine group as in colchicine (86). Recent data, however, indicated that berberine and some of its derivatives have antineoplastic activity (77,87,88). Berberine inhibited respiration of ascites tumor cells by about 15% but had no influence on their glycolysis (48,89). Respiratory inhibition was attributed to inhibition of the yellow enzymes (86,90). Also, berberine inhibited the utilization of carboxamide by the cancer cells, thereby inhibiting the synthesis of purine and nucleic acids (91,92). Berberine and 9-berberolin were shown *in vitro* to inhibit Ehrlich ascites carcinoma and lymphoma NK/LY cells; but intraperitoneal injection of the drug in mice bearing these cancer cells produced unsatisfactory or no effects (87,93). In total packed cell volume studies, berberine and tetrahydroberberine derivatives were inactive against ascitic sarcoma 180, whereas 9-dimethylberberine and its acetate and benzoate salts and the thiophosphamine derivative of berberine displayed relatively strong antineoplastic activity (88,94).

8. Effect on Tissue Metabolism

Dose-dependently, berberine reduced the oxygen consumption of mouse liver and brain homogenates (95). In tissue culture the effects of berberine included metabolic inhibition, reduction of tissue oxygen consumption, fatty degeneration, and diminution of the oxygen consumption of frog skin, rat diaphragm and yeast. These effects are thought to be due to inhibition of intermediate metabolism (49,50). It was recently discovered that berberine and tetrahydropalmatine inhibited 90–100% of the NADH oxidase activity in the electron transfer granules prepared from calf heart, with a half-inhibitory concentration of 50 μM (96).

A single molecule of berberine had successfully been inserted into the DNA double helix of the calf thymus to form a complex (97). This agent also induced mutation of *Saccharomyces cereuisiae*, producing small colonies with impaired mitochondrial respiratory function, an event attributed to intercalation of berberine into the plasmid cyclic DNA, thereby inhibiting DNA synthesis, replication and transcription (53,98). A recent study revealed that the primary inhibitory effects of berberine on the DNA, RNA, protein, and lipid syntheses of sarcoma 180 cells *in vitro* were caused by inhibition of glucose utilization and its interaction with nucleic acids (98).

9. Effect on the Blood

Berberine was shown to cause shrinkage of red blood vessels, making them granular in shape, and to suppress the amebic movement of white blood cells (82). It decreased neutrophilic and eosinophilic cells on the one hand, and increased lymphocytes and monocytes on the other (99). A later report claimed that berberine had no effect on blood cells and coagulation time (63). In addition, <Huanglian> decoction had no significant effect on rabbit erythrocytes and leukocytes (100).

10. Miscellaneous Actions

Berberine was reported to have choleretic action (85), moderately increased bile output in anesthetized cats; its action lasted one hour, and normal output was restored after two hours. It increased the formation and storage of bile (101–103). It also caused an initial rise in the blood glucose level, followed by a progressive fall (85). The hypoglycemic action, however, was not confirmed in experiments on rabbits (104). As a fluorescent dye, berberine produced fluorescence of the mitochondria of *Saccharomyces ludwigii*, making these cells highly resistant to ^{60}Co irradiation as evidenced by their low mortality rate compared with the control. Berberine decreased the first and second death peaks of mice irradiated with ^{60}Co (105–107). It was also shown to have local anesthetic action, probably through interruption of the depolarization and repolarization of cell membranes (44,58).

The methanol extract of <Huanglian> suppressed various experimental paw swellings and granulation in rats. Local application of the herb suppressed granulation as effectively as butazone (108–110). An anti-inflammatory effect was also exhibited by the herb in rats following subcutaneous injection of cholera toxin into the neck (111). <Huanglian> and Sanguisorba Oil enhanced tissue healing of limited third-degree burns in rabbits and piglets caused by the napalm bomb (112). Berberine also reduced intraocular pressure (113). It had antidiuretic (99,114) and antidiarrheal effects; the latter was not due to an astringent action (115). A recent article reported that berberine counteracted stress gastric ulcer (66); but another paper claimed that this drug did not modify the secretion of gastric acid and juice and the formation of experimental gastric ulcer in rats (61). Since berberine could combine with the large molecular RNA and emit fluorescence, it may be used as a tool for quantitating RNA; this agent might also be useful in the determination of tissue herapin and mast cell count because it could stain heparin present in mast cells (116,117).

11. Pharmacokinetics

Small amounts of orally administered berberine were slowly absorbed, and the peak blood level was reached after 8 hours. The blood level following injection was also very low. Thirty minutes after oral administration of 0.4 g in man, drug concentration in blood was determined to be about 0.1 mg/%. This level was not raised despite administration of five doses, one every four hours.

On the other hand, after intravenous and subcutaneous injection, the blood level peaked in 10–20 minutes or one hour, respectively; drug levels declined sharply and were hard to maintain. Five minutes after an injection of berberine sulfate to the tail vein, dissection of the animals revealed that drug concentration in all tissues was higher than that in the blood. High concentrations were detected in the heart, kidneys, lungs, and intestine and lower in the muscle, stomach, liver, and spleen; low concentrations were found in the pancreas, eye ball, and brain. Drug concentration in all these organs, however, rapidly declined, leaving only traces after 24 hours, suggesting rapid distribution of berberine into all body tissues upon access to the circulation (10,118). Similar tissue distribution of berberine was also seen in mice killed 24 hours after subcutaneous injection of berberine (114). The drug was quickly metabolized in tissues into nonfluorescent substances and excreted (118). Berberine perfused into the isolated dog liver was metabolized into carbonates or compounds with a carboxyl group (119,120). The drug was recovered in the urine of subjects 30 minutes after an oral dose of 0.4 g; less than one-twentieth of that dose was, however, excreted in urine within 48 hours (14); fecal excretion of the drug was also low (121).

12. Toxicity

The MLD of berberine in rats, mice, guinea pigs and rabbits was determined to be 27.5–250 mg/kg IP; intraperitoneal or subcutaneous injection did not significantly lower the toxicity (53). The LD_{50} of berberine in mice was 24.3 mg/kg IP (58) and that in rats was 205 mg/kg IP. The LD_{50} of tetrahydroberberine in mice was 940 mg/kg PO, 790 mg/kg SC, and 100 mg/kg IV. Prolonged use did not result in accumulation or pathological changes (68).

CLINICAL STUDIES

1. Bacterial Infections

1.1 Infections of the alimentary tract

1.1.1 *Bacillary dysentery*. Over 1000 cases of bacillary dysentery were treated with various preparations of <Huanglian> (powder, dried fluidextract, syrup, decoction, berberine) by mouth and/or as an enema (aqueous extract or suspension), or with the various compound formulae chiefly containing <Huanglian> such as Radix Aucklandiae-Rhizoma Coptidis Pill, and Rhizoma Coptidis Pill by mouth. These preparations had the advantages of fast onset, short therapeutic course and few side effects. Their efficacy is comparable to those of chloramphenicol, synthomycin, and sulfathiazole-sulfaguanidine alternating treatment. Furthermore, <Huanglian> was safer than sulfonamides and had no side effects in severely dehydrated patients. Compared with patients receiving sulfonamide or chloramphenicol, those on <Huanglian> therapy had shorter hospitalization periods (48,122). When synthetic berberine and trimethoprim (TMP) were used to treat 257 cases of acute bacillary dysentery, a cure was achieved in 250 cases; this result was far better than that obtained with tetracycline plus furazolidone whereby only 47 out of 130 cases were cured. Moreover, there was less drug resistance in the former group (123).

1.1.2 *Acute gastroenteritis*. One hundred cases of acute gastroenteritis were all cured by oral administration of <Huanglian> powder, and around 70% of 57 cases of enteritis were effectively treated with berberine hydrochloride (122). Berberine was proven to be a good antidiarrheal agent in 50 children with gastroenteritis (124).

1.1.3 *Cholera*. Berberine was effective in controlling diarrhea in patients with mild and moderate cholera (125). Experimental treatment with berberine showed that it greatly prolonged the latent period of diarrhea induced by cholera toxin and suppressed the production of intestinal fluid. Hence, this agent is recommended as an adjunct for cholera therapy. In addition, berberine also antagonized experimental inflammation induced by local injection of cholera toxin (111,125–127). A paper reported that administration of <Huanglian> during the early stage of cholera produced excellent effects (128).

1.1.4   *Typhoid fever.* Capsules of the <Huanglian> powder 2 g every 4 hours by mouth until 3–5 days after complete recovery from fever were tried in 15 cases of typhoid fever. Thirteen cases had complete relief from fever in 56 days on average (129). The therapeutic effect of large doses of berberine on typhoid fever, 3.6–9 g/day in 4–6 doses, was confirmed by another report (130). Long-term treatment of 11 cases of typhoid carriers with Radix Aucklandiae-Rhizoma Coptidis Pill or berberine were reportedly ineffective (129).

1.1.5   *Chronic cholecystitis etc.* Two hundred and twenty-five patients obtained symptomatic relief 24–48 hours after oral administration of berberine 5–20 mg thrice daily before meals. The medication decreased the bilirubin content of the bile and increased the bile in gallbladder. The drug is probably also effective for toxic hepatitis caused by industrial toxic substances (131).

1.2   *Respiratory tract infections*

1.2.1   *Diphtheria.* Eleven cases of mild diphtheria were treated with <Huanglian> powder 0.6 g 4–6 times daily plus a gargle with 1% <Huanglian> solution. Fever subsided in 1–3 days; throat swab examination became negative in 2–8 days, and pseudomembrane disappeared in 2.6 days on average (122).

1.2.2   *Whooping cough.* In 57 cases of whooping cough treated with the 100% <Huanglian> decoction, a cure rate of 32.6% and a marked effective rate of 27% were achieved; marked effects were attained in 1.7 days of medication on average. The efficacy of the decoction was comparable to that of streptomycin or chloramphenicol (19).

1.2.3   *Pulmonary tuberculosis.* Oral doses of berberine 0.3 g thrice daily for 3 months as a therapeutic course had therapeutic value in 30 cases. Generally, early infiltrations were resorbed after one month, while progressive infiltrations were also improved (132). Different extents of resorption were also achieved after primary treatment with berberine, and in patients with unabsorbed infiltrations after long-term chemotherapy (122).

1.2.4   *Tuberculous pleurisy.* Very satisfactory results were achieved from berberine therapy of 58 cases of exudative tuberculous pleurisy. The patients were given berberine 0.2–0.3 g thrice daily by mouth; or 4–9 mg intramuscularly every 4–8 hours, or 4–6 mg by intrathoracic injection once or twice a week. Fever subsided in 8–15 days in 46.5% of the patients, and pleural fluid was absorbed in 11–20 days in 55.2%. The cure rate was 93.1%. In general, no side effects developed. <Huanglian> appeared to be suitable for patients allergic to streptomycin and isoniazid or for patients with drug-resistant bacteria (133).

1.2.5   *Bronchitis.* Berberine was effective in acute and chronic bronchitis, especially when also used as an aerosol (134).

1.2.6   *Pneumonia and lung abscess.* Satisfactory effects were reported of the oral use of the <Huanglian> powder or berberine in the treatment of lobar and other types of pneumonia (129,134). Oral administration plus intratracheal instillation of berberine in 32 cases of lung abscess was reported to be effective (135).

1.3 *Otorhinolaryngological infections*

1.3.1 *Otitis media and otitis externa.* The 10% <Huanglian> extract plus 3% boric acid had excellent effects in the treatment of 12 cases of chronic otitis media, 63 cases of acute suppurative otitis media, and 2 cases of diffuse otitis externa. Iontophoresis of the alcohol solution or 10% decoction of <Huanglian> was also effective for otitis media (122).

1.3.2 *Maxillary sinusitis.* Injection into the maxillary sinus with 2 ml of the 10% <Huanglian> decoction in 3% boric acid, or 2 ml of 0.2% berberine, was as effective as penicillin in treating suppurative maxillary sinusitis (122). The intrasinus injection of the 30% <Huanglian> solution 2 ml or local injection of the 0.1% berberine in glucose solution was also effective in treating chronic maxillary sinusitis (122,136).

1.3.3 *Chronic rhinitis.* Atrophic rhinitis was treated by bilateral inferior turbinal injection with 0.1% berberine in glucose solution, or with nasal inserts of gauze soaked with 10% <Huanglian> solution, once daily for a course of 7–10 days. The therapeutic effects included recovery of the olfactory sense, formation of eschars, and reduction of secretions (129,136).

1.3.4 *Acute and chronic tonsillitis.* An effective rate of 88.2% was achieved in 102 cases of chronic tonsillitis treated with 0.1% berberine in glucose solution injected into the tonsils, 3–5 ml once daily or on alternative days for a course of 7 injections (136). Therapeutic effects were obtained promptly with the oral dose or aerosol of berberine in 4 cases of acute tonsillitis (134).

1.3.5 *Extraocular inflammation, conjunctivitis, hordeolum, and blepharitis marginalis, etc.* Eye drops prepared from the <Huanglian> extract and borax, the <Huanglian> fluidextract, or the <Huanglian> ointment were found to be therapeutically effective in 68 cases of acute conjunctivitis (121,122). Washing the eyes with 5% <Huanglian> decoction several times cured more than 95% of the patients with acute simple conjunctivitis. No discomfort or irritation was reported (122). Bathing the eyes with 10% <Huanglian> decoction in 3% boric acid markedly improved hordeolum, various types of blepharitis marginalis, trachoma, keratitis, herpetic keratitis, superficial and deep corneal inflammation and ulcer, and acute and chronic conjunctivitis; iontophoresis of berberine solution plus application of silver nitrate solution onto the palpebral conjunctiva was also effective for the treatment of trachoma (122,137).

1.3.6 *Local inflammatory diseases of the mouth cavity and jaws.* The 10% <Huanglian> in boric acid solution used locally, or oral administration of crude <Huanglian> and gargle with <Huanglian> extract rapidly cured Vincent's angina; quick therapeutic results were also obtained with the compound Rhizoma Coptidis Powder (Rhizoma Coptidis, Indigo Naturalis, borax, Borneolum Syntheticum, Calomelas, Os Sepiae, Os Draconis, Radix Glycyrrhizae, Fructus Gardeniae, and Rhizoma Bletillae) applied on lesions of herpetic stomatitis, recurrent stomatitis, and traumatic oral mucosal ulcers (10,122,138). An aggregate effective rate of 81.1% was attained in over 100 cases of inflammation of the mouth cavity, maxilla and face treated with berberine orally (139).

1.4 *Gynecological inflammatory diseases.* <Huanglian> was reported to be efficacious in vaginitis, cervical erosion, and other gynecological inflammatory diseases (122,129).

1.5 *Local surgical infections.* Control of infection and satisfactory effects were achieved by external application of the 20% <Huanglian> vaseline dressing and the 3% <Huanglian> solution combined with oral administration of the <Huanglian> powder in 200 cases of various kinds of acute suppurative infections, furuncle and carbuncle, abscess, lymphadenitis, mastitis, paronychia, cellulitis, cholecystitis, and peritonitis; side effects were not known. Over 100 cases of multiple furunculosis and chronic folliculitis were chiefly treated locally with "Jinhuang San" (Golden Powder) and oral administration of the Detoxicant Decoction of Scutellaria and Coptis (Rhizoma Coptidis, Radix Scutellariae, Cortex Moutan, Radix Paeoniae Rubra, Flos Lonicerae, Fructus Forsythiae, Radix Glycyrrhizae, Fructus Gardeniae Nigra); the effective rate was 73% (122). Oral and external use of <Huanglian> was also very effective in treating various suppurative traumatic wounds (128).

1.6 *Systemic infections.* There were reports regarding the efficacy of <Huanglian> on scarlet fever, brucellosis, septicemia and pyemia due to *Staphylococcus aureus*, and on leprosy (122,127,140,149).

2. Other Infectious Diseases

The therapeutic effect of <Huanglian> used alone in the treatment of amebic dysentery was poor. Better results, however, were reported in a few cases of amebic dysentery treated with this herb plus the root of *Aucklandia lappa* and the fruit of *Prunus mume*, or with the compound formula consisting of this herb and the root of *Aucklandia lappa* (122). A recent study reported that berberine is an established chemotherapeutic agent for amebiasis (141). There were additional reports regarding its therapeutic effect on candidiasis of the lung, and on balantidiasis of the colon, as well as on its prophylactic and therapeutic values in measles (129,142,143).

3. Eczema

Satisfactory results were obtained from short courses of the <Huanglian>-castor oil preparation with or without vitamin C in the treatment of different types of eczema. These drugs were superior to zin oxide ointment (122).

4. Burns

Cure of burns may be achieved with Berberine-Radix Sanguisorbae Powder (2:100) in addition to conventional treatment (122). Rhizoma Coptitis Detoxicant Ointment (a compound formula) applied locally on all degrees of burns was not inferior to Western drugs, and possessed the added advantage of the requiring analgesics (144).

5. *Hypertension*

Daily administration of 0.74–4.0 g of berberine was shown to be effective and safe in 19 cases of primary, acute renal, and pre-eclamptic hypertension. The drug was more effective during the early and second stages than in the third stage of the disease. It was dually efficacious in hypertension complicated with acute nephritis, angina pectoris, coronary insufficiency, or bronchitis (145). Another paper claimed an effective rate of 70–93.3% in 88 cases of hypertension treated with berberine 0.6–1.8 g/day. A higher effective rate was obtained when reserpine was used concomitantly (146).

ADVERSE EFFECTS

According to ancient Chinese medical treatises, overdosage of <Huanglian> by mouth would cause nausea, vomiting, shortness of breath, and convulsion. The <Huanglian> ear drops or iontophoresis with the herb solution may cause dizziness and vomiting in some patients. <Huanglian> taken by mouth may produce transient diarrhea, abdominal distention, borborygmus, polyuria, loss of appetite, vomiting, nausea, and epigastric discomfort. No side effects were seen in adults given 12 g of the herb by mouth daily for 3 weeks, or a total dose of 100 g (115,122). It was reported that inadvertent administration of 4 days' doses of the herb within one day resulted in a dramatic improvement of cough, without any side effect (144). One case of allergic reaction due to intravenous injection of berberine had been reported, however (147). One case of drug rash caused by the <Huanglian> powder was also reported (148). Caution should be exercised as there are several recent cases of sudden circulatory and respiratory arrest after intravenous infusion of berberine; women with hypokalemia were particularly vulnerable (150).

REFERENCE

1. Zhang CS. Modern Research on Chinese Materia Medica. Chinese Scientific Books and Instruments Company. 1954. p. 120.

2. Xu ZL. Chinese Medical Journal 1947 33:71.

3. Zhan YQ. Chinese Medical Journal 1948 34:399.

4. Lin ZJ et al. Acta Physiologica Sinica 1957 21(3):213.

5. Chen MR. Acta Academiae Medicinae Sichuan (Special Edition on Comprehensive Studies of Coptis) 1959 (1):55.

6. Xu ZL et al. Acta Academiae Medicinae Sichuan (Special Edition on Comprehensive Studies of Coptis) 1959 (1):41.

7. Zhang NC. Proceedings of the Society for Experimental Biology and Medicine 1948 69:141.

8. Gao SY et al. Science 1949 110(1):11.

9. Zhang WX. Chinese Medical Journal 1949 67:648.

10. Liu GS. Chinese Journal of New Medicine 1950 1(2):95; 1(4):285.

11. Liu GS. Beijing Zhongyi (Beijing Journal of Traditional Chinese Medicine) 1953 2(1):20.

12. Liao YX. Acta Pharmaceutica Sinica 1954 2(1):5.

13. Gu QQ et al. Chinese Journal of Paediatrics 1956 7(2):93.

14. Xiang JM et al. Chinese Medical Journal 1957 43(4):276.

15. Sun K. Chinese Medical Journal 1955 41(5):449.

16. Lebedev DV. Medicine 1950 3:223.

17. Zhang YZ. Chinese Medical Journal 1958 44(6):592.

18. Wang SL. Shanghai Zhongyiyao Zazhi (Shanghai Journal of Traditional Chinese Medicine) 1956 12:30.

19. Zhao SQ et al. Chinese Medical Journal 1955 41(10):918.

20. Wang FL. Chinese Medical Journal 1950 68:169.

21. Yang ZC et al. Acta Academiae Medicinae Primae Shanghai 1957 (2):117.

22. Liu XK et al. Chinese Journal of Tuberculosis 1958 6(3):204.

23. Zhao CY et al. Acta Microbiologica Sinica 1960 (8):171.

24. Amin AH et al. Canadian Journal of Microbiology 1969 15:1067.

25. Brzezinska-Jazowa L et al. Chemical Abstracts 1964 61:3570a.

26. Dutta NK et al. Indian Journal of Medical Research 1962 50:732.

27. Cai FL et al. Acta Academiae Medicinae Henan 1959 (6):68.

28. Yu QT et al. Acta Academiae Medicinae Zhejiang 1959 (5):415.

29. Shao CY. Chinese Journal of Internal Medicine 1962 10(4):227.

30. Ni B et al. Acta Academiae Medicinae Primae Nanjing 1959 (1):19.

31. Gray PHH et al. Nature 1956 177:118z.

32. Gray PHH et al. Plant Soil 1957 8:354.

33. Du SC et al. Acta Academiae Medicinae Sichuan (Special Edition on Comprehensive Studies of Coptis) 1959 (1):49.

34. Zheng ZY et al. Chinese Medical Journal 1962 48(1):32.

35. Ukita T et al. Japanese Journal of Experimental Medicine 1949 20:103.

36. Hahn FE et al. Ann NY Acad Sci 1971 182:295.

37. Ye YL et al. Chinese Medical Journal 1958 44(9):888.

38. Gao SY. Science Record 1950 3(2−4):231.

39. Zhang TM et al. Chinese Medical Journal 1957 43(8):627.

40. Kulkarin SK et al. The Japanese Journal of Pharmacology 1972 22(1):11.

41. Sabit M et al. Indian Journal of Medical Research 1976 64(8):1160.

42. Ob-Gyn Section. Bulletin of Hunan Medical College 1958 (1):48.

43. Gupta D. Indian Medical Gazette 1929 64:67.

44. Seery TM et al. Journal of Pharmacology and Experimental Therapeutics 1940 69:64.

45. Zheng WF. Chinese Medical Journal 1952 38:315.

46. Sun X. Chinese Medical Journal 1955 41(6):536.

47. Jiangsu Institute of Dermatology. Dermatological Research Communications 1975 (2):203.

48. Traditional Chinese Medicine Research Department, Sichuan Medical College. Journal of Traditional Chinese Medicine 1958 (10):704.

49. Schmitz H et al. Chemical Abstracts 1952 46:4680i.

50. Hilwig I et al. Chemical Abstracts 1952 46:3166h.

51. Kuwano S et al. Chemical and Pharmaceutical Bulletin 1960 8:491.

52. Kuwano S et al. Chemical and Pharmaceutical Bulletin 1960 8:497.

53. Hahn FE et al. Antibiotics. Vol. III. JW Corcoran and FE Hahn. Springer-Verlag, Berlin. 1975. p. 577.

54. Modak S et al. Indian Journal of Medical Research 1970 58:1510.

55. Han ZW et al. Literature Compilation (Neimenggu Medical College) 1959 (1):46.

56. Feng DR et al. Scientific Papers of Sichuan Medical College (Abstracts of research papers in traditional Chinese medicine and materia medica). 1961. p. 16.

57. Feng DR et al. Scientific Papers of Sichuan Medical College (Abstracts of research papers in traditional Chinese medicine and materia medica). 1961. p. 17.

58. Sabit M et al. Indian Journal of Physiology and Pharmacology 1971 15(3):111.

59. Mardikar BR et al. Indian Journal of Medical Sciences 1973 27(6):540.

60. Pharmacology Section. Acta Academiae Medicinae Hubei 1959 Oct:39.

61. Sabit M et al. Indian Journal of Physiology and Pharmacology 1978 22(1):9.

62. Sun SH et al. Acta Academiae Medicinae Primae Shanghai 1956 (3):11.

63. Chopta RN et al. Indian Journal of Medical Research 1932 19:1193.

64. Turova AD. Shanghai Zhongyixue Zazhi (Shanghai Journal of Traditional Chinese Medicine) 1956 (1): 48.

65. Halder RK et al. Indian Journal of Pharmacology 1970 2:1.

66. Yamabara J. Folia Pharmacologica Japonica 1976 72:899.

67. Sadritdinov F. Chemical Abstracts 1966 65:14306e.

68. Sadritdinov F. Chemical Abstracts 1967 66:74714v.

69. Yamabara J. Folia Pharmacologica Japonica 1976 72(7):909.

70. Zhang CS. Acta Physiologica Sinica 1953 19(1):12.

71. Zhang CS. Journal of Pharmacology and Experimental Therapeutics 1941 71(2):178.

72. Folia Pharmacologica Japonica 1956 52(2):85.

73. Folia Pharmacologica Japonica 1957 53(1):63.

74. Furuya T. Folia Pharmacologica Japonica 1959 55:1152.

75. Shimamoto K et al. Folia Pharmacologica Japonica ©957 53(1):75.

76. Tan YZ et al. Special Edition on Anesthesia (Internal Information of Sichuan Medical College). 1978. p. 1.

77. Hano K. Acta Un Int Cancer 1959 15:122.

78. Fukuda H et al. Chemical and Pharmaceutical Bulletin 1970 18(7):1299.

79. Fukuda T. Folia Pharmacologica Japonica 1959 55:1162.

80. Wang JG et al. Acta Academiae Medicinae Lanzhou 1962 (1):65.

81. Chen SQ et al. Abstracts of the 4th Scientific Symposium of Sichuan Medical College. 1964. p. 86.

82. Ye SB et al. (reviewer). Acta Academiae Medicinae Sichuan (Special Edition on Comprehensive Studies of Coptis) 1959 (1):93.

83. Qu BL et al. Bulletin of Hunan Medical College 1962 (10):8.

84. Zhang HD et al. The National Medical Journal of China 1937 23:789.

85. Zhu Y. Pharmacology and Applications of Chinese Medicinal Materials. People's Medical Publishing House. 1958. p. 12.

86. Lettre H et al. Chemical Abstracts 1947 41:3218d.

87. Song CQ et al. (translator). References on Medicine Abroad — Pharmacy 1978 (2):95.

88. Petlychna LI et al. BA 1977 63(7):40192.

89. Schmitz H. Chemical Abstracts 1952 46:3159e.

90. Hirsch HH. Chemical Abstracts 1953 47:2888i.

91. Hano K et al. Gann 1957 48:443.

92. Hano K et al. Gann 1964 55(1):25.

93. Shvarev IF et al. Farmakologiia I Toksikologiia 1972 35(1):73.

94. Hoshi A et al. Gann 1976 67(2):321.

95. Pharmacology Section, Sichuan Medical College. Internal information.

96. Schewe T et al. Acta Biol Med Germ 1976 35:7.

97. Krey AK et al. Science 1969 166(3906):755.

98. Meisel MN et al. Doklady Akademii Nunk SSSR 1959 131:436.

99. Floriani L. Chemical Abstracts 1932 26:251(4).

100. Wang YS et al. Scientific Papers of Sichuan Medical College (Special edition on traditional Chinese medicine and materia medica). 1961. p. 14.

101. Turova AD et al. Chemical Abstracts 1963 58:2763b.

102. Velluda CC et al. Chemical Abstracts 1959 53:15345a.

103. Vartazaryan BA et al. Chemical Abstracts 1965 62:15304g.

104. Tang RY et al. Chinese Medical Journal 1958 44(2):150.

105. Meisel MN et al. Chemical Abstracts 1958 52:5535f.

106. Luchnik NV. Chemical Abstracts 1962 57:4985f.

107. Borodina VM. Iidr: Tsitologiia 1977 19(9):1067.

108. Fujimura H et al. Japan Centra Revuo Medicina 1971 276:344.

109. Fujimura H et al. Journal of the Pharmaceutical Society of Japan (Tokyo) 1970 90(6):782.

110. Wan MD et al. Abstracts of the Symposium of the Chinese Society of Physiology (Pharmacy). 1964. p. 77.

111. Akhter MH et al. Indian Journal of Medical Research 1977 65(1):133.

112. Seventh Military Medical College of the Chinese PLA. Research on Burns Prevention and Treatment. Jan 1960.

113. Leib WA et al. Chemical Abstracts 1960 54:11271g.

114. Furuya T. The Journal of Osaka Medical College 1957 17(1):19.

115. Akhter MH et al. Indian Journal of Medical Research 1979 90(2):233.

116. Yamagishi H. Journal of Cell Biology 1962 15(3):589.

117. Berlin G et al. Journal of Histochemistry and Cytochemistry 1978 26(1):14.

118. Xu ZL. Acta Academiae Medicinae Sichuan (Special Edition on Comprehensive Studies of Coptis) 1959 (1):36.

119. Ando J. Japan Centra Revuo Medicina 1958 136(5):745.

120. Furuya T. The Journal of Osaka Medical College 1956 16(3):18.

121. Furuya T. Chemical Abstracts 1959 53:1555a.

122. Jin DF (reviewer). Acta Academiae Medicinae Sichuan (Special Edition on Comprehensive Studies of Coptis) 1959 (1):102.

123. 302nd Hospital of the Chinese PLA. Chinese Journal of Internal Medicine 1976 New 1(4):219.

124. Sharda DC. Journal of Indian Medical Association 1970 54:22.

125. Patankar MR et al. Ind Pract 1972 25(10):454.

126. Sabit M et al. Indian Journal of Medical Research 1977 65(3):305.

127. Yang SF et al. Acta Academiae Medicinae Hubei 1959 (1):1.

128. Yao WH (reviewer). Wuhan Medical Journal 1966 3(2):144.

129. Jiangsu College of New Medicine. Encyclopedia of Chinese Materia Medica. Shanhai People's Publishing House. 1977. p. 4147.

130. Cheng SP et al. Chinese Journal of Internal Medicine 1959 7(8):744.

131. Turova AD et al. Chemical Abstracts 1964 61:15242f.

132. Hangzhou Second Medical College. Bulletin of Chinese Materia Medica 1958 4(11):384.

133. Zheng XW. Jilin Journal of Chemistry, Medicine and Health 1976 (2):22.

134. Zhang DF et al. Chinese Journal of Internal Medicine 1959 7(9):900.

135. Zheng Z et al. Chinese Journal of Internal Medicine 1963 11(7):567.

136. ENT Department, First Teaching Hospital of Shenyang Medical College. Medical Research 1976 (2):30, 32.

137. Pei CS et al. Zhongji Yikan (Intermediate Medical Journal) 1959 (8):14.

138. Wang SY. Acta Academiae Medicinae Primae Nanjing 1959 (1):141.

139. Ding ZL. Chinese Medical Journal 1962 48(5):310.

140. Zhang DF et al. Chinese Journal of Internal Medicine 1959 7(7):704.

141. Dutta NK et al. Journal of Indian Medical Association 1968 50:349.

142. Chen YP. Acta Academiae Medicinae Wuhan 1959 (9):71.

143. Liszka H et al. BA 1978 66(4):19660.

144. Anhui's People's Hospital. Special Issue on Burns 1973 (3):39, 46.

145. Cheng SP et al. Chinese Journal of Internal Medicine 1959 7(6):514.

146. Chen JL. Chinese Journal of Internal Medicine 1960 8(2):117.

147. Luo SR et al. Chinese Journal of Internal Medicine 1962 48(9):568.

148. Sun KC. People's Health Care 1959 (6):591.

149. Seda County (Sichuan) Sanitation and Anti-epidemic Station. Studies on Epidemic Prevention 1976 (4):340.

150. Editorial Committee. Chinese Journal of Internal Medicine 1981 20(1):44.

(Yang Zhengwan)

HUANGQI 黄耆

<Huangqi> is the root of *Astragalus membranaceus* (Fisch.) Bge., or *A. membranaceus* Bge. var. *mongholicus* (Bge.) Hsiao (Leguminosae). Sweet to taste and of slightly "warm" property, it is known for its vital-energy tonifying skin-reinforcing, diuretic, abscess-draining and tissue generative actions. It is, therefore, useful for palpitation with shortness of breath, spontaneous sweating, prostration, chronic diarrhea, prolapse of the uterus and rectum, chronic carbuncle and deep-rooted ulcer, and persistent sores.

CHEMICAL COMPOSITION

The root of *A. membranaceus* contains 2' 4' -dihydroxy-5,6-dimethoxyisoflavone, kumatakenin, choline, betaine, polysaccharides, glucuronic acid, and traces of folic acid.

PHARMACOLOGY

1. Enhancement of the Immunologic Function

The 32% <Huangqi> decoction given to mice orally at a dose of 0.5 ml daily or on alternate days for 1–2 weeks increased the phagocytic activity of the reticuloendothelial system (1). The phagocytic index was significantly increased even if the rehabilitation of the mouse reticuloendothelial system was disrupted by the injection of carbon particles prior to the administration of <Huangqi> (2). Concomitant use of rifampicine and G. lucidum Mixture (Radix Astragali, Radix Codonopsis Pilosulae, Ganoderma Lucidum) improved and regulated the suppressed immunologic function of mice. When used with antituberculous drugs, the mixture significantly decreased the mortality rate and prolonged the median survival time of tuberculous mice. These results are significantly better than that achieved with antituberculous drugs alone. G. lucidum Mixture also greatly enhanced the bactericidal function of the spleen (1). It was shown in antiviral studies that either the oral doses or nose drops of the <Huangqi> decoction protected mice from infection of parainfluenza virus type I (3,4). Results from 28 experiments using 1299 mice in total showed that the effect of <Huangqi> resembled, by and large, those of the interferon mediator, tilorone, and bronchitis vaccine. Oral administration or nasal spray of this herb offered protection against the common cold in an epidemiological study involving 1000 subjects (3). Though the herb was not itself an interferon inducer, it could promote the production of interferon by the mouse lung against parainfluenza virus type I and Newcastle disease virus (5). In patients susceptible to common cold, administration of this herb for two weeks or two months enhanced the induction of interferon by peripheral white blood cells as compared with the premedication stage. Similar results were demonstrated in studies with mice. The induction of leukocytes to produce interferon in patients could be one of the antiviral mechanisms of <Huangqi> (3). Addition of <Huangqi> to the culture of mouse renal cells increased their production of interferon in that the interferon titer was much higher in the <Huangqi> group than in the control group (5). Two months of oral treatment with this herb in subjects susceptible to common cold greatly increased the levels of SIgA and IgG in the nasal secretion. Moreover, quantitative changes in the SIgA were found correlated with the severity of the common cold (3). Tablets of the dried fluidextract of the whole plant given to 80 normal subjects by mouth greatly increased the IgM and IgE (6). These results indicate that <Huangqi> promotes humoral immunity. In comparison with the control, addition of the herb decoction to rat renal cell culture, whether before or after a challenge by follicular stomatitis virus, lowered the viral titer in the treated cells, indicating that <Huangqi> could inhibit the pathogenicity of virus on cell cultures. Further studies revealed that the inhibitory effect of <Huangqi> on viral multiplication is mediated by cells (5). In addition, <Huangqi> enhanced the specific rosette formation of mouse lymphocytes on sheep red blood cells (7). Atrophy of the immune tissues such as the spleen, thymus, and intestinal lymph nodes, as well as leukopenia, all caused by the immunosuppressant, prednisolone, were antagonized by the polysaccharides of the herb. Concomitant injection of the polysaccharides with the allergen via the same route produced a pronounced adjuvant effect wherein the number of plaque-forming cells was increased (8).

2. Effect on Cellular Metabolism

The addition of the 0.5% <Huangqi> to monolayer cultures of renal cells of the human embryo, hamster and mouse increased the number of living cells, caused vigorous cellular growth and doubled the life-span of these cells (3,9). <Huangqi> also delayed the natural ageing process of cultured human embryonic pulmonary diploid cells and markedly increased the maintenance time of the culture (3). Electron microscopic examination of the human embryonic renal cells cultured in the nutrient medium containing <Huangqi> (the final concentration being 0.3–0.5%), revealed an increase in the myelomembranous changes in the lysosomal membrane on the fourth and seventh days; histochemical studies showed a marked increased in glycogen granules, acid phosphatase and succinic dehydrogenase (9). These results suggested that <Huangqi> enhanced the physiological metabolism of cells. Daily intragastric administration of 0.5 ml of the decoction of *A. membranaceus* var. *mongholicus* (1:0.33 g) 0.5 ml to mice for 10 or 14 days markedly increased the plasma cAMP. A more prominent effect was achieved from daily intragastric administration of the <Huangqi> extract obtained by cation exchange resins 0.2 ml (equivalent to 6 g of crude drug) for 14 days (10). cAMP was also markedly increased in 80 normal subjects given tablets of the dried fluidextract of the herb (6).

In addition, the <Huangqi> injection (1:1) given subcutaneously at 0.3 ml/day for 5 days markedly increased the total WBC count and polynuclear leukocytes (11). One paper reported that <Huangqi> increased the hemoglobin in mice bearing U_{14} tumor (12).

3. Diuretic Effect

Studies on human subjects showed that <Huangqi> has a moderate diuretic action; it can increase the urine output and chloride excretion. The clinical dose of 0.2 g/kg increased urine output by 64% and sodium excretion by 14.5% (13–15). In rabbits, the orally administered decoction increased the urine output by 17.5%, while a 36% increase was obtained with the intraperitoneally administered ethanol extract (14). Diuresis was produced by injection of <Huangqi> at 0.5 g(crude drug)/mg SC (15,16) but not at 0.25 g/kg. In contrast, 1.0 g/kg of <Huangqi> decreased the urine output. The diuretic effect produced by a dose of 0.5 g/kg was equivalent to that obtained with 0.05 g/kg of aminophylline or 0.2 mg/kg of hydrochlorothiazide. No drug tolerance developed after 7 days of medication (15).

Approximately 15 minutes after injection of <Huangqi> 0.5 g/kg IV to anesthetized dogs, micturation was briefly inhibited but 1–1.5 hours later urine output was markedly increased (15,16). *A. ernestii* Comb. also had a diuretic action, but weaker (16).

4. Effect on Experimental Nephritis

Administration of <Huangqi> powder 4–5 g daily to rats for 3 days, prior to the production of nephrotoxic nephritis by injection of the rabbit anti-rat-kidney serum, markedly decreased proteinuria on the third day of the serum injection. Histological examination showed abatement of nephrosis. The antinephritis effect of the herb is thought to be related to the enhancement of metabolism and improvement of the systemic nutritional state (17). Prescriptions containing large amount of <Huangqi> used for the treatment of chronic nephritis in traditional Chinese medicine can also eliminate proteinuria (18).

5. Effect on the Cardiovascular System

The <Huangqi> decoction had no significant effect on the isolated frog heart, but the ethanol extract enhanced the contractility and increased the contraction amplitude of the isolated frog or toad heart. Large doses, however, produced cardiac depression (19–21). Intraperitoneal injection of the herb 0.5 g/kg to dogs had no significant effect on the heart rate but produced, 3–4 hours later, inverted and biphasic T waves and slightly prolonged ST intervals (16). Hypotension was elicited in rabbits, dogs or cats by the intravenous doses (19–27). Consecutive dosings resulted in tachyphylaxis. A longer hypotensive effect was produced by the intragastric doses (0.5–1.0 g/kg) (16). The hypotensive constituent was earlier thought to be an alkaline substance (22); however, recent studies found that the strength of the hypotensive action closely correlated with the amounts of γ-aminobutyric acid in the *Astragalus* root. This substance was therefore considered to be the active hypotensive principle (28). It is preliminarily held that the hypotensive mechanism is related to direct vasodilation, and that it has no significant connection with the vasomotor center, nerve ganglions, muscarinic receptors, and epinephrine and histamine release (25). Other authors also reported that <Huangqi> produced vasodilation including that of the coronary arteries (24,29). Significant vasodilation of hind limbs of anesthetized dogs and cats was elicited by the intravenous dose of the <Huangqi> injection; the same effect was achieved on the renal blood vessels. Large doses, however, caused reflex renal vasoconstriction due to hypotension (29). As with <Huangqi>, γ-aminobutyric acid at 10 mg/kg (equivalent to 30 times the γ-aminobutyric acid content in <Huangqi>) resulted in a similar vascular effect. Intra-arterial injection of small doses of <Huangqi>, however, markedly decreased the vascular resistance of the hind limb, whereas γ-aminobutyric acid was inactive. It is obvious from these facts that the vasoactivity of <Huangqi> could not be totally attributed to γ-aminobutyric acid (30).

6. Effect on Smooth Muscles

The 5% and 10% decoction of <Huangqi> markedly increased the tonicity, reduced the peristalsis, and increased the contraction amplitude of the rabbit intestinal tract *in vivo*, but they inhibited the isolated rabbit intestine and uterus (21). It was, however, also reported that the <Huangqi> decoction inhibited the motility of both the *in situ* and isolated rabbit intestines (20). The extract of *A. membranaceus* var. *mongholicus* was shown to increase the contraction amplitude of the isolated small intestine of guinea pigs (22). The <Huangqi> injection exerted a contracting action on the isolated rat uterus, with an efficacy equivalent to that of 0.0045 unit/ml of standard pituitrin (31).

7. Protection of Experimental Hepatitis

Histochemical examination of the liver of mice dosed with <Huangqi> revealed increase of glycogen, and activation of lysosomal and tissue dehydrogenases (29). In an experiment where the hepatic glycogen level was used as the criterion of therapeutic effect, oral administration of the 100% decoction 0.4 ml daily was found to protect the liver and to prevent the loss of hepatic glycogen in mice with acute toxic hepatitis induced by carbon tetrachloride given on the 8th experimental day (32).

8. Hormone-Like Effect

The extract, lactone, and sterol of this herb did not affect the body weight and the weight of the musculi levator ani or kidneys of rats and mice, indicating that they had no anabolic or androgen-like action (33). A paper reported that <Huangqi> produced estrogenic effects in mice by prolonging the estrous period (normally 1 day) to up to 10 days (34). The herb had no effect on the blood glucose level (35). The intravenous dose of the 1:1 <Huangqi> injection (1 g/kg) did not significantly affect the blood glucose level within 5 hours. Likewise, no significant hypoglycemic effect was achieved with the subcutaneous or intragastric dose (0.5 g/kg) of the injection in normal rats, or in rats with experimental hyperglycemia. However, the herb exhibited a tendency to increase the blood glucose level of animals with hypoglycemia induced by insulin (31).

9. Antibacterial Effect

In vitro, <Huangqi> was shown to be active against *Shigella shigae, Bacillus anthracis*, α-*Streptococcus hemolyticus*, β-*Streptococcus hemolyticus*, *Corynebacterium diphtheriae, Corynebacterium pseudodiphtheriae, Diplococcus pneumoniae, Staphylococcus aureus, Staphylococcus citreus, Staphylococcus albus*, and *Bacillus subtilis* (36,37).

10. Miscellaneous Actions

Subcutaneous injection of the <Huangqi> preparations to mice produced sedation for a few hours (22). Injection of the 100% <Huangqi> extract 1.0 mg/kg IV to dogs caused respiratory excitation (19). A report, however, claimed that the <Huangqi> decoction had no significant effect on the respiration of anesthetized rabbits (21). Since <Huangqi> contains many amino acids and carbohydrates, it is useful in the preparation of basic culture media, achieving results identical to beef extract-peptone (38).

11. Toxicity

No adverse effects were observed in mice within 48 hours of oral administration of <Huangqi> 75 g/kg (15) or 100 g/kg (16), which were several hundred times higher than the effective oral dose for diuresis (0.2 g/kg) in man. The LD_{50} of <Huangqi> in mice was determined to be 39.82 g/kg (16) or 40 g/kg IP (15). Another paper reported that injection of 50 g/kg IP to mice elicited no significant toxic reactions (25). Prostration, paralysis, dyspnea, and cyanosis, and in some animals, contracture of the extremities (15,16) were observed before the death of the animals. The LD_{50} of *A. ernestii* in mice was 38.25 g/kg IP (16). Daily injection of the herb 0.5 g/kg IP in rats for one month resulted in no derangement in the activity, food intake, micturation and defecation of the animals (15,16).

CLINICAL STUDIES

1. Common Cold

A satisfactory prophylactic effect against common cold was achieved in 1000 subjects given <Huangqi> orally or as a nasal spray, or Company Radix Astragali (Radix Astragali Crudae, Rhizoma Dioscoriae, Rhizoma Atractylodis Macrocephalae, Radix Rehmanniae Crudae, Pericarpium Citri Reticulatae, Poria), as evidenced by a decrease in the incidence of the disease and in the shortening of its course (3).

2. Chronic Persisting and Chronic Active Hepatitis

In 49 cases of chronic persisting hepatitis treated with the <Huangqi> injection, a marked effective rate of 61.2% and an aggregate effective rate of 85.7% were attained. Normalization of the GPT level was achieved in 80% of the responsive cases in 1–2 months (29).

3. Gastric and Duodenal Ulcers

An injection prepared from the alcohol-precipitated decoction of <Huangqi> (1.0 g/ml) administered intramuscularly at 2 ml twice daily for a course of one month was employed to treat 73 cases. Marked improvement in the subjective symptoms, particularly the vigor and appetite, was obtained. The barium test performed in 36 cases revealed healing of duodenal ulcer in 22.2%, improvement in 48.1%, and ineffective in 29.7%; the corresponding percentages for gastric ulcer were 64, 18, and 18% (39,40).

Out of 43 cases of peptic ulcer treated with the modified "Huangqi Jianzhong Tang" (Radix Astragali Decoction for Stomach Reinforcement) for a course of 25 days, 22 cases (51.2%) were cured, 17 (39.5%) had improvement and 4 cases (9.3%) were unchanged (41,42).

4. Malabsorption in Children

Eighty-nine children with impaired absorption of the small intestine (with "splenic deficiency", rickets, or susceptibility to respiratory tract diseases) were given the "Jianpi Fen" (Spleen-Invigorative Powder: Radix Codonopsis Pilosulae, Rhizoma Atractylodis Macrocephalae, Radix Glycyrrhizae) 3 g daily for one month. The following therapeutic effects were documented: increase of xylose clearance in 70 cases (78.8%), and reduction in 19 cases (21.2%), marked improvement of the clinical symptoms, and marked decrease in the incidence rate, particularly that of the respiratory tract (43).

5. Chronic Leukopenia

In 53 cases treated intramuscularly with <Huangqi> injection (1:1) 2 ml daily for a course of 1–2 weeks, the symptoms were improved and the WBC count increased to 4000–5000/mm^3 or higher; 31 cases were followed-up for 1–2 months and 80% were found to have WBC count maintained higher than 4000/mm^3 (44).

6. Miscellaneous

There are reports regarding the various therapeutic effects of compound prescriptions of <Huangqi> in chronic nephritis, chronic pyelonephritis (45), chronic bronchitis (46), sequelae of cerebrovascular accident (47), postpartum urinary retention (48), chyluria (49), and lepromatous leprosy (50).

REFERENCE

1. Isotopes Laboratory, Beijing Institute of Tuberculosis. Xinyiyaoxue Zazhi (Journal of Traditional Chinese Medicine) 1974 (8):12.

2. Hu YW et al. Studies on Epidemic Prevention 1977 (3):187.

3. Institute of Epidemic Prevention, Chinese Academy of Medical Sciences. Medical Research Communications 1978 (4):4.

4. Institute of Epidemic Prevention, Chinese Academy of Medical Sciences. Studies on Epidemic Prevention 1976 (2):124.

5. Institute of Epidemic Prevention, Chinese Academy of Medical Sciences. Studies on Epidemic Prevention 1976 (3):204.

6. Institute of Basic Medical Sciences, Chinese Academy of Medical Sciences et al. Zhonghua Yixue Zazhi (National Medical Journal of China) 1979 (1):23.

7. Microbiology Section, Department of Basic Sciences of Beijing Medical College. Journal of Beijing Medical College 1978 (3):156.

8. Shanghai Institute of Materia Medica, Chinese Academy of Sciences et al. Kexue Tongbao (Science Bulletin) 1979 (16):764.

9. Institute of Epidemic Prevention, Chinese Academy of Medical Sciences. Studies on Epidemic Prevention 1977 (3):180.

10. Isotopes Section of the Pharmacology Department, Basic Sciences Research Unit, Capital Hospital of the Chinese Academy of Medical Sciences et al. Medical Research Communications 1977 (10):27.

11. Shanxi Office of Drug Standard. Shanxi Medical and Pharmaceutical Journal 1974 (5–6):57.

12. Tumor Section, Institute of Chinese Materia Medica of the Academy of Traditional Chinese Medicine. The References of Traditional Chinese Medicine 1977 (3):21.

13. Xu SF et al. Acta Academiae Medicinae Primae Shanghai 1957 (1):38.

14. Deng ZF et al. Chinese Medical Journal 1961 (1):7.

15. Huang HP et al. Acta Pharmaceutica Sinica 1965 (5):319.

16. Chengdu Institute for Drug Control. Chengdu Medical and Health Information 1971 (1):90.

17. Jia JS et al. Abstracts of the 2nd National Symposium on Pathophysiology of the Chinese Society of Physiology. 1963. p. 63.

18. Zhang SJ et al. Chinese Journal of Internal Medicine 1960 (3):203.

19. Wang JM. Shanghai Zhongyiyao Zazhi (Shanghai Journal of Traditional Chinese Medicine) 1956 (1):16.

20. Pharmacology Section, Beijing College of Traditional Chinese Medicine. Beijing Zhongyi Xueyuan Xuebao (Journal of Beijing College of Traditional Chinese Medicine) 1960 (2):128.

21. Pan LS et al. Fujian Zhongyiyao (Fujian Journal of Traditional Chinese Medicine) 1963 (3):27.

22. Gao Q et al. Folia Pharmacologica Japonica 1959 55:51.

23. Terada et al. Folia Pharmacologica Japonica 1934 (2–3):40.

24. Fujita M et al. Folia Pharmacologica Japonica 1957 53:164.

25. Pharmacology Section, Shaanxi Institute of Traditional Chinese Medicine. Compiled Information on Combined Western and Traditional Chinese Medicine. 1971. p. 66.

26. Fujita M. Chemical Abstracts 1962 57:13887b.

27. Li GC et al. Abstracts of the 1956 Academic Conference of the Chinese Academy of Medical Sciences. Vol. 2. 1956. p. 70.

28. Hiroshi H et al. References on Medicine Abroad — Pharmacy 1977 (4):231.

29. Liu TP. Jiangsu Yiyao (Jiangsu Medical Journal) 1978 (2):32.

30. Shanxi Office of Drug Standard. Shanxi Medical and Pharmaceutical Journal 1974 (5–6):55.

31. Zhao LM. Shanxi Yiyao (Shanxi Medical Journal) 1973 (9):1.

32. Yan XW et al. Abstracts of the 1962 Symposium of the Chinese Pharmaceutical Association. 1963. p. 332.

33. Li JT et al. Abstracts of the 1964 Symposium of the Beijing Society of Physiology. 1964. p. 6.

34. Nagasawa M et al. Japan Centra Revuo Medicina 1941 73:589.

35. Jing LB et al. Chinese Reports of the Institute of Physiology (National Peiping Research Institute) 1936 (1):1.

36. Xu ZL. Chinese Medical Journal 1947 (3–4):71.

37. Zhang WX. Chinese Medical Journal 1949 (12):648.

38. Ajuvant Therapy Department, 60th Hospital of the Chinese PLA. Chinese Traditional and Herbal Drugs Communications 1976 (6):25.

39. Second Teaching Hospital, Jiangsu College of New Medicine. Selected Information on Scientific Research 1976 (2):47.

40. Digestion Unit of the Internal Medicine Department, Second Teaching Hospital, Jiangsu College of New Medicine. Jiangsu Yiyao (Jiangsu Medical Journal) 1977 (1):20.

41. Hui GX. Hunan Yiyao Zazhi (Hunan Medical Journal) 1977 (2):35.

42. Hui GX. Shanxi Medical Pharmaceutical Journal 1977 (2):39.

43. Pediatrics Department, Beijing College of Traditional Chinese Medicine. Zhonghua Yixue Zazhi (National Medical Journal of China) 1978 58(4):199.

44. Shanghai Medical Team of No. 32 Hospital of Qiannan. Guizhou Pharmaceutical Bulletin 1976 (2):34.

45. Wang DA. Jixi Science and Technology 1977 (3):1.

46. Chronic Bronchitis Group, Fifth Hospital of the Chinese PLA. Health Journal of Ningxia 1977 (3):25.

47. Luo K. Journal of Barefoot Doctor 1977 (7):21.

48. Second Obstetric Ward, Maternal and Child Health Centre Affiliated to Zhejiang Medical College. Notes on Science and Technology 1978 (1):19.

49. Cao MG et al. Journal of Traditional Chinese Medicine 1958 (6):397.

50. "Gulaodi" Research Group, Shaanxi College of Traditional Chinese Medicine. Shaanxi Medical Journal 1978 (1):20.

(Wu Tingkai)

HUANGBO 黃蘗

<Huangbo> is the bark obtained from *Phellodendron amurense* Rupr., and *P. chinense* Schneid. (Rutaceae) as well as from some varieties of these species. It has a bitter flavor and a "cold" property. It is credited with "damp-heat"-clearing, "heat"-purgative, detoxicant, anti-inflammatory, "asthenic heat"-clearing, as well as "kidney"- and vital-essence-tonifying actions. It is mainly used in dysentery caused by "damp-heat", jaundice, strangury, leukorrhea, eczema, pyogenic infections or ulcers of the skin, fever due to asthenia of the vital essence, nocturnal emission and spermatorrhea.

The book, "Benjing Fengyuan", describes the various actions of <Huangbo> as follows: "When raw it reduces sthenic 'heat', but wind-cured, it prevents the ascent of asthenic heat; when salted it relieves the lower abdominal cavity of intense heat, but gingered, it relieves 'phlegm' from the middle abdominal cavity; when charred with ginger juice, it eliminates "damp-heat", but charred with wine and salt, it cures heat of asthenia; and when processed with the juice of <Fuzi>, it treats asthenia of the vital essence, predominance of intense "heat" with flushing and 'yang' symptom-complex.

CHEMICAL COMPOSITION

<Huangbo> contains berberine, the amount of which varies with the variety and growing location (source), usually 1.6–4.0%. It also contains alkaloids phellodendrine, magnoflorine, palmatine and jatrorrhizine, and lactones obakulactone and obakunone.

PHARMACOLOGY

Refer to the monographs on <Huanglian> and <Sankezhen> for the pharmacological actions of berberine and palmatine, respectively.

1. Antimicrobial Effect

Various degrees of inhibitory action were exhibited by the decoction or ethanol extract of <Huangbo> *in vitro* against *Staphylococcus aureus, Staphylococcus albus, Staphylococcus citreus, Streptococcus hemolyticus, Diplococcus pneumoniae, Bacillus anthracis, Vibrio cholerae, Corynebacterium diphtheriae, Bacillus subtilis, Escherichia coli, Pseudomonas aeruginosa, Salmonella typhi, Salmonella paratyphi, Neisseria meningitidis*, and *Alcaligenes fecalis* (1–9). Many studies proved that the herb strongly inhibited *Shigella flexneri, Shigella sonnei, Shigella shigae*, and *Shigella schmitzii* (2,10–13). The antibacterial action of <Huangbo> was considered related to its strong inhibition of bacterial respiration and RNA synthesis (14). <Huangbo> also inhibited *Mycobacterium tuberculosis* (15,16), including strains resistant to streptomycin, p-aminosalicylic acid and isoniazid *in vitro* (4). The MIC "Sanhuang Powder" (Cortex Phellodendri, Rhizoma Coptidis, Radix Scutellariae) against *Mycobacterium tuberculosis* in deep culture was determined to be 1:12,800 (17). However, guinea pigs with experimental tuberculosis had an extremely poor response to the herb (18). The <Huangbo> decoction was also shown to have a strong leptospirocidal action (19,20).

The decoction and aqueous extract of <Huangbo> inhibited many kinds of pathogenic skin fungi to different extents, e.g., *Trichophyton violaceum, Epidermophyton floccosum, Microsporum canis, Trichophyton schoenleinii, Microsporum audouini* and *Epidermophyton inguinale* (21–24). The herb was also inhibitory to *Trichomona vaginalis* (25).

<Huangbo> had a significant selective inhibitory action against hepatitis B surface antigen (HBsAg); its action was not due to the tannins, berberine, phellodendrine, palmatine, or flavonoid glycosides (26–29).

2. Hypotensive Effect

Intraperitoneal injection of the alkaline substance of the ethanol extract of <Huangbo> to anesthetized cats produced a prolonged hypotensive effect (30); the average decrease in hypotension area within 90 minutes after injection of the fluidextract of <Huangbo> 2 g/kg IP was found to be 30% (31). "Erxian Mixture" (Cortex Phellodendri, Rhizoma Curculiginis, Herba Epimedii, Radix Morindae Officinalis, Rhizoma Anemarrhenae, Radix Angelicae Sinensis) given intraduodenally to anesthetized cats or to dogs with chronic renal hypertension also produced a hypotensive effect; <Huangbo> was the chief hypotensive component of this formula (32). Daily oral administration of 2 g/kg of <Huangbo> to rats with orchidectomy-induced hypertension also decreased the blood pressure (33). Berberine, phellodendrine, and palmatine have different potencies of hypotensive effect. Phellodendrine injected intravenously to rabbits, cats, or dogs decreased the blood pressure, augmented the pressor effect of epinephrine and norepinephrine, suppressed the pressor reaction to artificial asphyxia and stimulation of the afferent vagus nerve, and also suppressed the contraction of the nictitating membrane in cats due to stimulation of the preganglionic fibers (34). Xylopinin, a tertiary amine derivative synthesized from phellodendrine, also exhibited a significant hypotensive effect even at a dose as low as 0.05 mg/kg. The strength and duration of action increased with the dosage. The action was found to be of central origin, because it disappeared in cats with spinal section between the first and second cervical vertebrae. Atropinization, bilateral vagotomy, administration of diphenhydramine or hexamethonium, or bilateral extraction of the carotid arterial sinuses had no significant influence on the hypotensive action, but tolazoline, dibenzylamine and reserpine weakened it. Xylopinin also reversed the pressor effect of norepinephrine and epinephrine and inhibited contraction of the nictitating membrane in cats induced by electrical stimulation of the sympathetic superior cervical ganglion; it also antagonized the contraction of the nictitating membrane induced by epinephrine, etc. These findings suggest that xylopinin has significant antiadrenergic (sympatholytic) effect (35).

3. Effect on Smooth Muscles

<Huangbo> increased the force and amplitude of the contraction of isolated rabbit intestine. Similarly, berberine increased the intestinal contraction amplitude; obakunone increased the tension and contraction amplitude, whereas obakulactone relaxed the intestinal tract (36).

4. Miscellaneous Actions

Phellodendrine produced a muscle relaxant effect on the sciatic nerve-gastrocnemius specimen of rats. Although it did not modify the tonicity of the frog musculi rectus abdominis, it antagonized acetylcholine-induced contraction (34). <Huangbo> was reported to have a hypoglycemic action; intravenous injection of obakulactone at doses close to the lethal dose (0.05–0.1 g/kg) produced hypoglycemia in rabbits, whereas obakunone was inactive (37). <Huangbo> reportedly promoted the secretion of pancreatic juice in rabbits with pancreatic fistulae (8). Xylopinin was proved to have a central depressant effect (35). In addition, <Huangbo> killed sperms (38), wrigglers and house flies (39). The toxicity of the root of *Hemerocallis fulva* in mice could be reduced by concomitant administration of this herb (40). Recent data indicated that <Huangbo> markedly enhanced the production of antibodies in mice (41).

5. Toxicity

The LD_{50} of <Huangbo> in mice was determined to be 2.7 g/kg IP (32), and the MLD in mice by the same route was 0.52 g/kg (38). The LD_{50} of phellodendrine in mice was 69.5 mg/kg IP (34) and that of xylopinin, 71.5 mg/kg IP (35).

CLINICAL STUDIES

1. Bacillary Dysentery and Enteritis

<Huangbo> and its compound formulae are relatively effective in acute enteritis as well as in acute and chronic bacillary dysentery. For instance, a report claimed that all 31 cases of acute dysentery treated with the fluidextract of the herb were cured; fever subsided in a mean of 2.8 days; bowel movement normalized in 3.9 days, and stool culture became negative in 3.2 days (42). Another paper reported that 40 cases of chronic bacillary dysentery were all cured by <Huangbo>, evidenced by the disappearance of mucosal lesions as revealed by sigmoidoscopy. A cure was attained in 10 days on average. *Dosage and administration*: Pills were prepared with <Huangbo> powder and 10% alcohol and 4 g was given twice daily for a course of 7 days (43). The herb was also very effective in acute enteritis (44). It is usually prescribed as compound formulae, e.g., Pulsatilla Decoction (45–49).

2. Other Infectious Diseases

<Huangbo> and its compound formulae were considered effective against various infectious diseases. Twenty cases of epidemic cerebrospinal meningitis were cured with the fluidextract of the herb (50). The retention enema prepared from this herb and licorice was also efficacious (51). The prophylactic effect of a throat spray of the 50% <Huangbo> decoction against epidemic cerebrospinal meningitis was good; 92 out of 118 carriers became pathogen-free after a single spray (6). In the treatment of 27 cases of tuberculosis with the <Huangbo> powder, fever subsided, erythrocyte sedimentation rate reduced, appetite increased, and cough and expectoration abated (38). Another 12 cases responded to treatment with the dried fluidextract of <Huangbo> (52). In addition, <Huangbo> and its compound formulae showed different degrees of efficacy in acute conjunctivitis (53–55), chronic maxillary sinusitis (56), chronic suppurative otitis media (5), impetigo (57), various surgical infections (58,59), acute urinary tract infection (60), cervical erosion (61,62), candidial or trichomonal vaginitis (63–66), and chronic osteomyelitis complicated with fistulation (67). The <Huangbo> solution was reportedly used as an antiseptic agent in place of ethacridine in topical diseases (68).

3. Eczema

"Ermiao Powder" (Cortex Phellodendri, Rhizoma Atractylodis) was effective in various kinds of exudative eczema. A good response was obtained by <Huangbo> and its various compound formulae in eczema in infants and children, diaper rash, scrotal eczema, and other types of eczema (69–75).

4. Miscellaneous

There are reports on the treatment of edema of the prepuce in children (76,77), elephantiasis (78), sprain (79), and urinary tract bleeding (80), and on the fixation of fractures with the herb (81).

ADVERSE EFFECTS

One case of allergic skin reaction to the orally administered <Huangbo> was reported (82).

REFERENCE

1. Xu Z. News of Agriculture 1947 1(6):17.
2. Wang Y et al. Acta Botanica Sinica 1954 3(2):121.
3. Liu GS. Chinese Journal of New Medicine 1950 (1):95.
4. Osawa. Journal of the Society for Oriental Medicine in Japan 1959 (9):54.

5. Sun JL et al. Chinese Journal of Otorhinolaryngology 1960 (3):193.

6. Yan GH et al. Journal of Traditional Chinese Medicine 1960 (6):20.

7. Zhao ZY et al. Acta Microbiologica Sinica 1960 (2):171.

8. Japan Centra Revuo Medicina 1935 45:836; Jiangsu College of New Medicine. Encyclopedia of Chinese Materia Medica. Vol. 2 Shanghai People's Publishing House. 1977. p. 2032.

9. Yang HC et al. Chemical Abstracts 1953 47:8175c.

10. Xu ZL. Chinese Medical Journal 1947 33(3–4):71.

11. Medical Laboratory of the First Teaching Hospital. Acta Academiae Medicinae Xi'an 1958 (5):40.

12. Medical Laboratory. Papers of Beijing Railways Medical College. 1960. p. 47.

13. Li CL et al. Fujian Zhongyiyao (Fujian Journal of Traditional Chinese Medicine) 1960 5(7):38.

14. Coptis Research Unit, Sichuan Medical College. Acta Academiae Medicinae Sichuan 1960 2(1):1.

15. Jinzhou Hospital of Tuberculosis. Liaoning Medical Journal 1960 (7):26.

16. Guo J et al. Chinese Journal of Prevention of Tuberculosis 1959 (6):37.

17. Jinzhou Hospital of Tuberculosis. Liaoning Medical Journal 1960 (7):29.

18. Dai BD et al. Chinese Journal of Prevention of Tuberculosis 1964 (6):693.

19. Microbiology Section, Luda Health School. Medicine and Health (Luda Health Bureau) 1973 (2):63.

20. Hainan District Leptospirosis Research Group et al. Information on Medical Sciences and Technology (Guangdong Institute of Medicine and Health) 1973 (4):15.

21. Sun X. Chinese Medical Journal 1955 41(6):526.

22. Cao RL et al. Chinese Journal of Dermatology 1957 5(4):286.

23. Zheng WF. Chinese Medical Journal 1952 38(4):35.

24. Cao SN et al. Chinese Medical Journal 1962 (12):781.

25. Parasitology Section, Henan Medical College. Acta Academiae Medicinae Henan 1960 (7):23.

26. Hepatitis Group, Tianjin Sanitation and Anti-epidemic Section. Tianjin Medical Journal 1975 (7):343.

27. Infectious Diseases Unit of the Internal Medicine Department, Second Teaching Hospital of Chongqing Medical College. Chinese Journal of Internal Medicine 1976 (3):192.

28. Jing Q et al. Xinyiyaoxue Zazhi (Journal of Traditional Chinese Medicine) 1975 (9):38.

29. Jing Q et al. Tianjin Medical Journal 1976 (6):283.

30. Feng GH et al. Jiangxi Yiyao (Jiangxi Medical Journal) 1961 (7):29.

31. Zhu QZ et al. Acta Pharmaceutica Sinica 1962 9(5):281.

32. Chen WZ et al. Acta Pharmaceutica Sinica 1960 8(1):35.

33. Zhu QZ et al. Acta Pharmaceutica Sinica 1962 9(11):661.

34. Shimamoto K et al. Folia Pharmacologica Japonica 1962 58(2):138.

35. Shimamoto K et al. Folia Pharmacologica Japonica 1962 58(3):53.

36. Imamoto K. Japan Centra Revuo Medicina 1961 169:690.

37. Karai T et al. Journal of the Pharmaceutical Society of Japan (Tokyo) 1933 53(10):1057.

38. Furo N. Folia Pharmacologica Japonica 1958 54(3):33.

39. Sullivan WN et al. Chemical Abstracts 1944 38:3049b.

40. Xiao SH. Acta Pharmaceutica Sinica 1962 9(4):208.

41. Li P et al. Acta Academiae Medicinae Shangdong 1979 (4):31.

42. Luo LJ. Journal of Traditional Chinese Medicine 1957 (9):486.

43. Zhou YZ. Journal of Traditional Chinese Medicine 1959 (8):23.

44. Wu YS. Jiangxi Zhongyiyao (Jiangxi Journal of Traditional Chinese Medicine) 1957 (11):56.

45. Internal Medicine Department, Yaan District Hospital (Sichuan). Journal of Traditional Chinese Medicine 1959 (12):39.

46. Luo LJ et al. Chinese Journal of Parasitic and Infectious Diseases 1958 (4):214.

47. Luo LJ et al. Zhejiang Journal of Traditional Chinese Medicine 1957 (6):242.

48. Yu CP. Hunan Yiyao Zazhi (Hunan Medical Journal) 1977 (3):32.

49. Shi WY. Shanghai Zhongyixue Zazhi (Shanghai Journal of Traditional Chinese Medicine) 1959 (4):20.

50. Mao YJ. Chinese Journal of Internal Medicine 1960 8(1):70.

51. Hu JB. Zhejiang Journal of Traditional Chinese Medicine) 1960 (1):30.

52. Zijingshan (Jinzhou) Hospital of Tuberculosis. Zhongji Yikan (Intermediate Medical Journal) 1959 (11):52.

53. Chengguan People's Hospital of Enshi County. Xinzhongyi (Journal of New Chinese Medicine) 1975 (4):8.

54. Ji CY. Zhongji Yikan (Intermediate Medical Journal) 1960 (3):42.

55. Hefei Children's Health Centre. Chinese Medical Journal 1960 (4):292.

56. 204th Hospital of the Chinese PLA. Liaoning Medical Journal 1960 (4):7.

57. Scientific Research Unit, Miaoquan Commune Health Centre (Changshu County). Chinese Traditional and Herbal Drugs Communications 1970 (3):43.

58. Class 74 of Shangdong College of Traditional Chinese Medicine. Shaanxi Medical Journal 1976 (3):12.

59. Sun JH. Journal of Traditional Chinese Medicine 1965 (10):47.

60. Linfen People's Hospital. Xinyiyaoxue Zazhi (Journal of Traditional Chinese Medicine) 1977 (2):32.

61. Yuan WJ et al. Journal of Traditional Chinese Medicine 1979 (8):48.

62. Ye ZY. Health Journal of Hubei 1976 (5):46.

63. Liuda Production Brigade Health Post (Datong Commune of Qidong County, Jiangsu). New Chinese Medicine 1972 (2):53.

64. Gong ZF et al. Jiangxi Zhongyiyao (Jiangxi Journal of Traditional Chinese Medicine) 1958 (1):24.

65. Liu KT. Journal of Traditional Chinese Medicine 1965 (11):28.

66. Zhang XL. Journal of Traditional Chinese Medicine 1980 (8):77.

67. Zhang MJ. Chinese Journal of Surgery 1959 (2):131.

68. Ye NH. Zhejiang Journal of Traditional Chinese Medicine 1960 (3):140.

69. Chongqing Second Central Hospital. Journal of Traditional Chinese Medicine 1957 (5):247.

70. Xing RH. Barefoot Doctor (Changwei District Institute of Medical Sciences, Shangdong) 1974 (3):20.

71. Shenyang College of Pharmacy. Discovery and Popularization of Chinese Traditional Drugs 1970 (9):4.

72. Shen QX. Chinese Journal of Otorhinolaryngology 1959 (2):160.

73. Dang Q. Chinese Journal of Dermatology 1957 (2):153.

74. Yu DS. Dermatological Research Communications 1979 (1):54.

75. Weng XY. People's Military Medicine 1979 (9):76.

76. Song CG et al. Jiangsu Yiyao (Jiangsu Medical Journal) 1976 (4):40.

77. Zhong SL. Xinzhongyi (Journal of New Chinese Medicine) 1975 (1):47.

78. "626" Pharmaceutical Factory (Huaiyuan County, Anhui) et al. New Chinese Medicine 1973 (10):499.

79. Wang Q. Journal of Barefoot Doctor 1975 (2):14.

80. Urology Department, Third Teaching Hospital of Shanghai Second Medical College. Medical Exchanges 1975 (8):24.

81. Xiangtan People's Hospital. Chinese Journal of Surgery 1958 (11):1203.

82. Hu ZH. Shangdong Medical Journal 1963 (4):cover 4.

(Deng Wenlong)

HUANGJING 黄精

<Huangjing> is the rhizome of *Polygonatum sibiricum* Redoute, *P. cyrtonema* Hua, *P. macropodium* Turcz, *P. kingianum Coll. et Hemsl.*, and *P. cirrhifolium* (Wall.) Royle (Liliaceae). It is sweet and "mild" and is credited with "spleen"-tonifying, long-demulcent, vital-energy-tonifying and vital-essence-nourishing actions. It is useful for treating physical weakness, palpitation, shortness of breath, and dry cough.

CHEMICAL COMPOSITION

<Huangjing> contains mucilage. The rhizome of *P. cyrtonema* contains azetidine-2-carboxylic acid, aspartic acid, homoserine, digitalis glycoside, and anthraquinones.

PHARMACOLOGY

1. Effect on the Cardiovascular System

The aqueous extract, the ethanol-water extract, and the 30% ethanol extract of <Huangjing> were shown to have hypotensive effect in anesthetized animals (1). The 0.15% ethanol preparation of the herb increased the contractility of the isolated toad heart but did not alter the heart rate, whereas the 0.4% preparation or aqueous solution increased the rate of the isolated rabbit heart (2). The 1% "Rhizoma Polygonati-Radix Paeoniae Rubra Injection" markedly increased the coronary flow in the isolated guinea pig heart, slightly inhibited cardiac contractility and decreased the heart rate (3). The ethanol preparation of this herb, 0.2 g/kg, increased the coronary flow of the dog heart *in situ*, but had no significant effect on the femoral arterial pressure, heart rate, and central venous pressure. The ethanol preparation of <Huangjing> 0.2 g/kg was equipotent to aminophylline 0.75 mg/kg in increasing the coronary flow (2). Injection of 1.5 ml of Rhizoma Polygonati-Radix Paeoniae Rubra Injection through a coronary arterial tube at constant speed also markedly increased the coronary flow and, concurrently, transiently decreased the blood pressure (3).

2. Effects on blood lipids and atherosclerosis

In comparison with the control, intragastric administration of the 100% <Huangjing> decoction to rabbits with experimental hyperlipidemia 5 ml twice daily for 30 days resulted in marked decreases in blood triglycerides, β-lipoprotein, and cholesterol 10, 20 and 30 days after medication (4). Another report, however, claimed that no hypolipemic effect was achieved with the Rhizoma Polygonati Injection at 7.5 g IM (equivalent to 20 times the adult human oral dosage) injected to cholesterol-fed rabbits (5). Following daily intramuscular injection of 2 ml of Rhizoma Polygonati-Radix Paeoniae Rubra Injection for 14 weeks with one day off every 6 days, the aortic endothetial plaque formation and coronary atherosclerosis in the treatment group were milder than in the control group (6).

3. Antimicrobial Effect

In vitro studies showed that the aqueous extract of <Huangjing> (1:320) inhibited *Salmonella typhi, Staphylococcus aureus*, and acid-fast bacilli (7).

In guinea pigs with experimental tuberculosis, oral administration of 1 g/kg of <Huangjing> once daily for 60 days starting on the next day of infection and upon finding of lymph node enlargement produced a significant antitubercular effect. After medication, there was an increase in appetite, improvement in health, and 50% increase in the body weight of the animals; pathological examinations revealed mild lesions in the major organs and only a few tubercles in the lungs (8). The 2% <Huangjing> also inhibited to different extents common fungi in Sabouraud agar (9).

4. *Effect on Blood Glucose*

Oral administration of the <Huangjing> fluidextract to rabbits gradually increased the blood glucose level but decreased it later. The transient hyperglycemic effect was probably due to the carbohydrate content of the herb extract. The magnitude and duration of the hyperglycemic effect were directly proportional to the dosage employed. The fluidextract also markedly inhibited epinephrine-induced hyperglycemia (10).

CLINICAL STUDIES

1. *Coronary Disease*

A preparation of <Huangjing> and the root of wild *Paeonia lactiflora* was used to treat 100 cases of coronary disease. Various degrees of remission were obtained in 17 cases with angina pectoris; in 14 cases with ECG showing myocardial ischemia, 6 cases recovered, 5 improved, and 3 showed ineffective results. In 29 cases with chronic coronary insufficiency, 10 cases were recovered, 15 improved, and 14 unchanged. It was considered that the preparation could alleviate anginal pain, improve coronary blood flow, and could probably reduce blood lipids. This preparation was more effective in lowering the level of cholesterol than that of β-lipoprotein or triglycerides (1). the preparation was also shown to reduce blood glucose, platelet aggregation and prothrombin time (11).

2. *Pulmonary Tuberculosis*

Nineteen cases, of which 9 had positive sputum finding and 6 with cavities, were treated with the

<Huangjing> fluidextract for 2 months. Complete resorption of foci was achieved in 4 cases and improvement in 12; there was no response in 3 cases. Cavities in 2 cases healed and 4 were reduced in differing degrees. Six cases became negative in the sputum examination. Erythrocyte sedimentation rate was normalized in all cases except in two who had slightly higher readings than normal. Preliminarily, it is held that the herb has excellent therapeutic effects (12).

3. Tinea

With the exception of one patient, all 14 patients (19 tineal lesions) treated locally with the crude preparation of <Huangjing> were cured in a period of 2–30 days. The acute cases responded faster. This agent could also be used locally to treat tinea pedis and tinea cruris (13).

REFERENCE

1. Li GC et al. Abstracts of the Chinese Academy of Medical Sciences. 1956. p. 70.

2. Pharmacology Group, Coronary Disease Research Section of 244 Logistics Unit of the Chinese PLA. Sichuan Communications on Chinese Traditional and Herbal Drugs 1974 (2):20.

3. Pharmacology Section, Henan Institute of Traditional Chinese Medicine. References on Traditional Chinese Medicine Research — Special Edition on Coronary Disease. Henan College of Traditional Chinese Medicine and Henan Institute of Traditional Chinese Medicine. 1975. p. 15.

4. Pharmacology Section, Jinzhou Medical College. Science and Technology of Jinzhou Medical College 1977 (6):19.

5. General Hospital of Chengdu Military Region. Selected Information on Prevention and Treatment of Coronary Disease. Health Division of the Logistics Department of Chengdu Military Region of the Chinese PLA. 1975. p. 51.

6. Biochemistry Section, Henan Institute of Traditional Chinese Medicine. References on Traditional Chinese Medicine Research. Henan College of Traditional Chinese Medicine and Henan Institute of Traditional Chinese Medicine. 1975. p. 17.

7. Tang ZG. Chinese Medical Journal 1958 44(5):430.

8. Shao CY. Chinese Journal of Internal Medicine 1962 (4):227.

9. Li SC et al. Chinese Medical Journal 1958 44(5):434.

10. Min BQ. Yaowuxue Zazhi (Journal of Materia Medica) 1927 6(4):466.

11. Cardiovascular Unit of the Internal Medicine Department. First Teaching Hospital of Henan Medical College. Selected Information on Cardiovascular Diseases. Cardiovascular Unit of Henan Medical College. 1977. p. 50.

12. Feng YL. Zhejiang Yiyao (Zhejiang Medical Journal) 1960 (4):163.

13. Tang ZG. Chinese Medical Journal 1958 44(5):432.

(Yuan Wei)

HUANGDUJUAN AND BALIMA 黃杜鵑與八釐麻

<Huangdujuan>, also known as <Naoyanghua>, is the inflorescence of *Rhododendron molle* G. Don (Ericaceae) whose fruit is the drug <Balima> or <Liuzhouzi>.

 <Huangdujuan> tastes pungent and has a "warm" property; it is toxic. It has anesthetic, analgesic, and antirheumatic actions. It is chiefly used in the treatment of neuralgia, low-back ache, rheumatism, chronic bronchitis and also for wounds and injuries. The whole plant may be used as a remedy for scabies and tinea and as a pesticide against maggots.

CHEMICAL COMPOSITION

<Balima> contains andromedotoxin analogues, temporarily named rhomotoxin (1). <Huangdujuan> in addition contains rhododenkrin, rhodotoxin, andromedotoxin, sparassol, and flavonoids.

PHARMACOLOGY

1. Effect on the Cardiovascular System

Intravenous injection of rhomotoxin to anesthetized dogs reduced the blood pressure and heart rate. Its bradycardic effect was dose-dependent; 3.5 µg/kg IV decreased the heart rate by about 39%, while 20 µg/kg decreased it by about 70%. The hypotensive effect, however, was not dose-dependent; the duration of the hypotensive effect of 20 µg/kg was about 3 hours and was 10 times longer than that of 3.5 µg/kg. Compared with the hypotensive action, the bradycardic action was characterized by a faster onset and shorter duration. No interactions occurred between rhomotoxin and metaraminol, isoproterenol, propranolol, or phentolamine. Acetylcholine synergized with rhomotoxin in lowering the blood pressure, whereas atropine and vagotomy abolished the hypotensive and bradycardic effects. Procaine, on the other hand, weakened both effects of rhomotoxin. These findings suggest the involvement of the muscarinic and intravascular receptors. Sectioning of the carotid sinus nerve did not modify the hypotensive action, though it antagonized bradycardia. The contractility of the *in situ* heart was transiently and slightly weakened after intravenous injection of rhomotoxin, but the hypotensive effect remained prominent even after recovery of myocardial contractility, suggesting no connection between the hypotensive action and the effect in cardiac contractility. A brief decrease in the peripheral vascular resistance was induced by the herb. No direct vasodilatory response was elicited after administration of the herb through the femoral artery. However, evidence of cerebral vasodilation was seen clinically. In experiments with dogs, the herb markedly inhibited the pressor reflex of the carotid artery. Hence, it is postulated that the hypotensive action involved the inhibition of the vasomotor center and a direct action on peripheral blood vessels. In anesthetized open-chest dogs with intact or sectioned vagus nerves, intravenous injection of the herb caused a fall in the blood pressure, a decrease in the heart rate and concurrently, a reduction of the left ventricular pressure and ±dp/dt max. During inhibition of myocardial contraction the herb did not cause a significant rise in the LVEDP; on the contrary, LVEDP was occasionally decreased. Thus, rhomotoxin probably dilated the capacity vessels, decreased the venous return, and lowered the preventricular load. Within a certain dosage range, it caused sinus bradycardia but no ECG changes. Increasing the dosage, however, caused T wave changes, ST segment depression, and even arrhythmia (usually of the nodal rhythm, atrioventricular dissociation and premature beats) which recovered spontaneously if mild but converted to ventricular fibrillation in severe cases. Therefore, by stimulating the vagus nerve rhomotoxin inhibited the sinoatrial node, decreased the heart rate and, subsequently, allowed excitation of the ectopic pacemakers to initiate arrhythmia (1−3). Andromedotoxin also reduced the blood pressure and heart rate in cats and dogs (4). Yet another paper reported that andromedotoxin initially caused excitation, then paralysis, of the vagus nerve endings (5). Rhodotoxin caused dilation of the frog femoral and rabbit auricular blood vessels (6).

2. Analgesic Effect

As proved in the hot plate and electroshock experiments on mice, and in the central integration function test in rabbits, the orally administered <Huangdujuan> decoction produced analgesia (7). In experiments using electrical stimulation of the mouse tail to induce pain, the analgesic rates of the intragastrically administered <Huangdujuan> 0.5 g/kg and <Balima> suspension 0.2 g/kg were determined to be 35 and 37%, respectively. <Balima> suspension was more potent; the analgesic effect of 0.1 g/kg was equipotent to that of 0.05 g/kg of opium suspension. The analgesic indices of <Balima> and opium suspensions were very close: 28.9 and 30.0, respectively. However, increasing the dosage of <Balima> did not significantly increase the analgesic effect, but markedly increased the toxicity. The tinctures of <Huangdujuan> and <Balima> were less potent than their suspesions. Andromedotoxin prodiced a weaker analgesic effect and lower analgesic index than the crude preparations of <Huangdujuan> and <Balima> (8). The analgesic action of andromedotoxin was markedly reinforced by scopolamine but not by atropine (9).

3. Effect on Smooth Muscles

Rhodotoxin had a stimulant effect on the smooth muscles of the isolated rabbit intestine and uterus, but high doses produced inhibition (10). It weakly contracted the isolated rabbit bronchi (11). Andromedotoxin also excited the smooth muscles of the isolated rabbit bronchi and intestines (12).

4. Miscellaneous Actions

The response of the motor nerves inervating striated muscles to andromedotoxin was characterized by initial excitation and subsequent paralysis; the drug caused paralysis of higher nervous centres excluding the spinal cord (5,11). Both andromedotoxin and rhodotoxin have emetic action but the latter was 1.47 times stronger than the former (11). The emetic effect of andromedotoxin was of central origin, not due to stimulation of the gastric nerve endings (12).

5. Toxicity

The MLD of the <Huangdujuan> and <Balima> suspensions in mice was determined to be 3.4 and 2.89 g/kg PO, respectively. The LD_{50} of the extract and tincture of <Huangdujuan> was 5.85 and 5.13 g/kg, respectively. In contrast, the LD_{50} of the extract and tincture of <Balima> was 8.63 and 6.26 g/kg, respectively (8).

Both andromedotoxin and rhodotoxin depressed the respiration and heart. Overdosage resulted in death (3,5). The LD_{50} of these agents in mice was 3.437 and 0.143 µg/kg SC, respectively, whereas that in frogs by lymph-sac injection was 5.074 and 3.899 µg/kg, respectively. The MLD of both toxins in urethane-anesthetized cats and rabbits was comparable, about 400 µg/kg IV (13). The LD_{50} of rhomotoxin was 522 µg/kg IP in mice; death was preceded by dyspnea, hyperhidrosis, and convulsion (1).

CLINICAL STUDIES

1. Hypertension

Rhomotoxin was used in the treatment of 129 cases; 84 were given intravenous infusion of 2 mg in 200 ml of 10% glucose solution (an additional half-dose was given when necessary) at a rate of 30–40 µg (45–60 drog)/minute until the blood pressure was significantly decreased, or significant adverse reactions appeared. The other 45 cases were treated by intravenous push of 1 mg (1.5 mg in cases of severe hypertension) in 20–40 ml of 50% glucose solution; the injection was also stopped with the appearance of a "fall" in the blood pressure, or pronounced adverse reactions. Of the 129 cases so treated, only two were ineffective; 112 cases had marked improvement (i.e. lowering of diastolic pressure by more than 20 mmHg), and 15 cases some improvement. The duration of the hypotensive effect in the IV push group after one administration was 1.5–2 hours and 2–4 hours in the IV infusion group. It was cautioned that the blood pressure would further decrease 0.5–1 hour after discontinuation of medication. Hence, increasing the dosage hastily was discouraged as this could precipitate a series of dangerous symptoms such as shock (14). In addition, 34 cases of hypertension (stage I, 4 cases; stage II, 19 cases; stage III, 8 cases; and symptomatic hypertension, 3 cases) were given rhomotoxin by mouth. The hypotensive effect was most prominent 5–9 hours after a dose of 1 mg, and it lasted 1–4 hours. Blood pressure was essentially restored to the pretreatment level in 4–17 hours. For long-term oral treatment, rhomotoxin is recommended to be used in conjunction with other antihypertensive drugs. The intramuscular dosage is 0.5–1 mg; this route, however, is rarely employed because it causes pain at the site of injection (1).

2. Arrhythmia

Rhomotoxin was used in 19 cases of various supraventricular tachycardia. A significant reduction in the heart rate of 18 cases was achieved. The drug converted paroxysmal supraventricular tachycardia into sinus rhythm, prevented the attack of paroxysmal supraventricular tachycardia and paroxysmal atrial fibrillation; it was also effective for multiple premature beats (1). The 20% <Balima> decoction or tablet was given immediately at 3–15 ml (0.6–3.0 g) followed by 2–5 ml (0.4–0.6 g) 2–4 times daily; after onset of effects, the patients were put on maintenance dosage of 2–5 ml 1–2 times daily (2).

3. Anesthesia

A success rate of 94% was achieved in 154 operations using the 5–10% <Huangdujuan> for acupoint-injection anesthesia (0.1–0.2 ml for ear points and 0.2–1.0 ml for body points). The anesthetic effect obtained in operations on the head, neck, chest, and abdomen was better than in those on the spinal column, back, extremities, and perineum. The concomitant use of <Huangdujuan> with the flower of *Datura metel* for intravenous anesthesia potentiated the anesthetic effect of the latter, and abolished or reduced the attendant side effects — tachycardia, hypertension, and postoperative fever — of the latter agent. Operations could be carried out smoothly under anesthesia with intravenous infusion of alkaloids from the flower of *D. metel* 5–10 mg, intramuscular injection of 1.2 ml of 50% <Huangdujuan> and adequate doses of adjuvant anesthetics (15,16). Injection to ear acupoints with Compound R. molle Solution (Inflorescentia Rhododendri, Radix Aconiti Kusnezoffii, Rhizoma Ligustici, Radix Angelicae Sinensis) also produced anesthesia. However, muscle relaxation was unsatisfactory and there was visceral stretch reflex in abdominal operations (17).

4. Tinea Favus

Out of 565 cases of tinea favus treated locally with R. molle Ointment (Radix Rhododendri Mollis 120 g, sulfur 30 g, yellow vaseline 150 g) and low doses of griseofulvin (150 mg on alternate days in two doses for a course of 8–15 days) by mouth, 549 cases were cured (18).

5. Miscellaneous

<Huangdujuan> has therapeutic value in rheumatic and rheumatoid arthritis as well as in shock (19,20). In addition, a fumigant prepared from the dried leaves of *R. molle* was highly lethal to black *Apodemus* rats; with LD_{100} of 2.7 mg/l it was as potent as 1.0 mg/l of chloropicrin (21).

ADVERSE EFFECTS

Although satisfactory therapeutic effects were achieved by the herb in patients with arrhythmia and hypertension, some patients experienced transient adverse effects. The most common untoward effects were heartburn and generalized numbness, followed by dizziness, xerostomia, nausea, vomiting, and bradycardia. Overdosage could cause shock and even convulsion and unconsciousness, and flat or inverted T waves and various arrhythmia on the ECG. Severe reactions may necessitate the use of metaraminol and atropine. Hence, the herb should be used with caution in secondary hypertension and malignant hypertension, and contraindicated in critical cases. It does not cause orthostatic hypotension. No lesions of internal organs including the heart, liver, and kidneys were observed in its long-term use (1).

REFERENCE

1. First Teaching Hospital, Wuhan Medical College. Wuhan Journal of New Traditional Chinese Medicine 1973 (2):13.

2. Cardiovascular Research Group, First Teaching Hospital of Wuhan Medical College. Hubei Science and Technology 1972 (8):8.

3. Fang DC et al. Abstracts of the First National Symposium on Cardiovascular Pharmacology. 1980. p. 50.

4. Jiangsu College of New Medicine. Encyclopedia of Chinese Materia Medica. Vol. 1. Shanghai People's Publishing House. 1977. p. 1441.

5. Hardikar SW. Chemical Abstracts 1923 17:437(4).

6. Makino M et al. Chemical Abstracts 1929 23:3207.

7. Zhao Y. Journal of Military Medicine 1958 1(1):25.

8. Zhao GJ et al. Acta Pharmaceutica Sinica 1958 6(6):337.

9. Zhang TM et al. Acta Physiologica Sinica 1958 22(2):98.

10. Eda et al. Japan Centra Revuo Medicina 1951 117:703.

11. Zhu HB. Chinese Journal of Physiology 1931 5(2):115.

12. Yi. BE. Chinese Medical Journal 1939 25(1):45.

13. Makoto K. The Japanese Journal of Pharmacology 1956 (6):46.

14. Mao HY et al. Acta Academiae Medicinae Wuhan 1980 9(1):77.

15. Acupuncture Anesthesia Group, Teaching Hospital of Hubei College of Traditional Chinese Medicine. Health Journal of Hubei 1972 (5):49.

16. Hangzhou District People's Hospital. Jiangxi Medical Information 1972 (1):11.

17. Beijie People's Hospital (Jiangmen, Guangdong). New Chinese Medicine 1971 (10):29.

18. Douchang County Sanitation and Anti-epidemic Station. Jiangxi Medical Information 1976 (10):89.

19. Sun F et al. New Chinese Medicine 1977 (3):122.

20. Meixian District People's Hospital. Guangdong Medical Information 1975 (4):22.

21. Hemorrhagic Fever Research Group, Hubei Medical College. Scientific and Technical Information (Hubei Medical College) 1973 (5):18.

(Liang Yongyu)

HUANGHUAJIAZHUTAO 黄花夾竹桃

<Huanghuajiazhutao> comes from the leaf and seed of *Thevetia peruviana* (Pers.) K. Schum. (*T. neriifolia* Juss.) (Apocynaceae). Pungent, bitter and "warm", the herb is a known cardiotonic, diuretic, detumescent and anthelmintic. It is chiefly used as a remedy for cardiac failure, paroxysmal supraventricular tachycardia, and atrial fibrillation.

CHEMICAL COMPOSITION

The leaf, flower and seed of *T. peruviana* contain many cardiac glycosides. Seven cardiac glycosides were isolated from the kernel: thevetin A, thevetin B, peruvoside, neriifolin, ruvoside (theveneriine), perusitin and cerberin (1–3). The first two are weakly lipophilic primary glycosides, whereas the last five are lipophilic secondary glycosides. The efficacy of the secondary glycosides is several times higher than that of the primary glycosides. The early isolated thevetin is a mixture of thevetin A and thevetin B. A mixture of secondary glycosides (including mainly peruvoside, neriifolin and cerberin) was recently obtained in China from the defatted kernel of *T. peruviana*, also named thevetin (neriperside) (4). To avoid confusion, neriperside would be used hereafter.

PHARMACOLOGY

Pharmacological studies in early years demonstrated that <Huanghuajiazhutao> had digitalis-like cardiotonic action (5–8). The ethanol extracts of its leaf and flower (9–11), thevetin, and neriifolin (12–17) were shown to increase the contractility, decrease the rate, and inhibit the conduction of the *in situ* and isolated hearts of various animals. They also increased the cardiac output, improved the coronary circulation and accelerated the blood flow. Perfusion of the 1:10,000 thevetin solution into the isolated frog heart with weak contractions due to calcium deficiency quickly restored its strong and forceful pulsation. Overdosage, however, resulted in cardiac arrest at the systolic phase. In the case of barbiturates-induced heart failure in guinea pigs and cats, thevetin and neriifolin promptly restored cardiac contraction and increased cardiac contractility and tension. In cats, they even produced bradycardia, high blood pressure and typical ECG patterns of cardiac glycosides, e.g., prolonged P-R and R-R intervals, and depressed, flat or inverted T waves (13,18–20). Peruvoside greatly strengthened myocardial contraction in anesthetized cats and dogs with barbital- or butazolidine-induced myocardial damage and also in the heart lung preparation of guinea pigs. Its potency was approximately equal to that of ouabain but it had a greater safety range than the latter (21).

2. Sedative Effect

Neriperside produced a sedative effect in cats and monkeys, whereas K-strophanthin was inactive (19,20). Although neriifolin had no significant central depressant effects, its acetylated derivative, diacetylneriifolin, exerted a marked sedative effect. It was able to antagonize caffeine-induced hyperactivity and prolong cyclobarbital sodium-induced sleep in mice. These effects were attributable to the decreased molecular polarity and increased lipid solubility of the acetylated drug which can cross the blood-brain barrier with relative ease (16).

3. Effect on Smooth Muscles

The ethanol extracts of the leaf and flower had stimulant effects on isolated uteri and intestines of guinea pigs, rabbits, and cats; it increased the tone and even caused spastic contraction of uteri (7,10,11,22). Thevetin 0.5 cat unit induced abortion in cats during early pregnancy (22). No influence, however, was exhibited by these agents on the isolated uteri and intestinal musculatures of rats (10,11).

4. Diuretic Effect

Diuresis was promptly achieved with thevetin given intravenously to anethetized dogs and to dogs with ureteral fistula. Significant increase in urine output appeared in 1 to 1.5 hours after medication. The diuretic effect obtained in normal rats was most conspicuous on the fifth hour after the intraperitoneal administration (23).

5. Pharmacokinetics

Determination of the supplementary lethal doses of thevetin at 2, 4, and 6 hours after intraduodenal injection to cats with ligated pylorus showed the following absorption rates: 12.77, 37.79, and 8.14%, respectively (24). Using the same method, the absorption rates at 4, 6, and 8 hours after intraduodenal injection of 1 cat unit of neriifolin were 31.2, 33.8, and 37.1%, respectively (25). The 24-h accumulation of the 50% MLD of neriperside, ouabain, and digitoxin in pigeons were determined to be 0, 0, and 93%, respectively (16). Studies on the duration of action and accumulation of thevetin in guinea pigs revealed that after intravenous injection of 0.5 guinea pig unit, only 0.19 unit was retained in the body at Hour 2, and the LD determined at Hour 6 was closed to the normal lethal dose. On the other hand, after daily subcutaneous injection of 0.5 guinea pig unit (2.055 mg/kg) for 7 days, the LD determined on the 8th day still approximated the normal lethal dose. These results indicate that thevetin has no cumulative effect (26). Its hepatic elimination rate was 0% (24).

The absorption of neriifolin administered intragastrically was 14.51% at Hour 1, and 23.09% at Hour 2; complete absorption occurred at Hours 3, 4, and 6. Drug accumulation was low, and no drug was detectable after 72 hours (20). Its hepatic elimination rate was 27.12% (25).

6. Toxicity

<Huanghuajiazhutao> is extremely toxic. The MLD of thevetin and neriperside in pigeons were 1.574 ± 0.048 and 0.28 ± 0.0115 mg/kg, respectively (16,19). The MLD of thevetin, neriperside, and neriifolin in cats were 0.9752 ± 0.0239, 0.25 ± 0.0098, and 0.1508 ± 0.0059 mg/kg, respectively (19,24,25). In terms of frog units, neriifolin was also found to be the most toxic with the highest biological activity (refer to the following table) (1):

Cadiac glycoside	Frog unit/g
thevetin	12,500
thevetin A	19,500
thevetin B	5,500
peruvoside	32,000
neriifolin	41,000

The toxic manifestations of this herb were referrable to the digestive and nervous systems; they included nausea, vomiting, salivation, impairment of appetite and food refusal, drowsiness, lassitude, and shortness of breath, and, in a few animals, excitation and restlessness; most animals recovered within one week (9,10,23,27). Arrhythmia was a more serious toxic effect.

CLINICAL STUDIES

1. Heart Failure

Neriperside was effective to various extents in treating heart failure of different cause (4,28–30); it was more effective in heart failure due to hypertension and coronary disease than in that due to pulmonary heart disease. Its efficacy by intravenous injection was comparable to that of K-strophanthin. Hence, it is suitable as an emergency remedy in severe heart failure. Being a quick-acting oral cardiac glycoside, neriperside produced effects comparable to those of digoxin. Substitution of K-strophanthin with this agent and vice versa is feasible.

2. Pneumonia in Children Complicated with Cardiac Insufficiency

Out of 86 cases treated with neriperside, 26 achieved marked effects, 53 some improvement and 7 were unresponsive; the aggregate effective rate was 92.5%. Three cases showed toxic reactions during treatment (31).

3. *Paroxysmal Supraventricular Tachycardia and Paroxysmal Atrial Fibrillation*

Decrease in the heart rate was marked following injection or oral administration of neriperside. The negative chronotropic and the negative conduction action of this agent were stronger than those of K-strophanthin (4,30).

REFERENCE

1. Sun NJ. Acta Pharmaceutica Sinica 1962 9(6):359.

2. Lang HY et al. Acta Pharmaceutica Sinica 1964 11(11):464.

3. Voiglaender HW et al. Archiv der Pharmazie 1969 302(7):538.

4. Zhai SZ et al. Chinese Journal of Internal Medicine 1966 (14):414.

5. Chopra RN et al. Indian Journal of Medical Research 1933 20(1):903.

6. Chen KK et al. Archives of Pharmacodynamics 1950 84:81.

7. Chen KK et al. Journal of Pharmacology 1934 51:23.

8. Arnold HL et al. American Journal of Medical Sciences 1935 189:193.

9. Li CC et al. Acta Pharmaceutica Sinica 1960 8(6):235.

10. Li CC. Acta Pharmaceutica Sinica 1962 9(12):753.

11. Li CC. Acta Pharmaceutica Sinica 1962 9(4):199.

12. Modell W et al. Journal of Pharmacology 1948 (94):44.

13. Wang MD et al. Abstracts of the 1962 symposium of the Chinese Pharmaceutical Association. 1962. p. 305.

14. Pathophysiology and Pharmacology Sections, Kunming Medical College. Academic Bulletin (Kunming Medical College) 1960:130.

15. Yue KL et al. Yunnan Medical Journal 1965 7(2):40.

16. Yue KL et al. Abstracts of the Symposium of the Chinese Society of Physiology. 1964. p. 48.

17. Verma BB. Indian Journal of Physiology and Pharmacology 1964 8(1):8.

18. Wang DC et al. Abstracts of the Symposium of the Chinese Society of Physiology. 1964. p. 47.

19. Ke SL et al. Abstracts of the Symposium of the Chinese Society of Physiology. 1964. p. 49.

20. Revolutionary Committee of the Chinese Academy of Medical Sciences. Researches of the Chinese Academy of Medical Sciences 1970 (4):3.

21. Rao VE. The Indian Journal of Pharmacy 1973 35(4):107.

22. Li CC et al, Fuzhou Medical and Health Communications 1963 3(3):78.

23. Yue KL et al. Abstracts of the 1962 Symposium of the Chinese Pharmaceutical Association. 1962. p. 306.

24. Huang QZ et al. Acta Pharmaceutic Sinica 1965 12(12):824.

25. Huang QZ et al. Acta Pharmaceutica Sinica 1966 13(6):419.

26. Wang DC et al. Abstracts of the 1962 Symposium of the Chinese Pharmaceutical Association. 1962. p. 307.

27. Middleton WS et al. American Heart Journal 1936 (11):75.

28. Lung and Heart Diseases Unit of the Internal Medicine Department, Chaoyang Hospital of Beijing. Zhonghua Yixue Zazhi (National Medical Journal of China) 1976 56(1):36.

29. Xia DY. Zhonghua Yixue Zazhi (National Medical Journal of China) 1976 56(4):233.

30. Coordinating Group for Clinical Trial of Thevetin. Zhonghua Yixue Zazhi (National Medical Journal of China) 1976 56(1):32.

31. Pan YC et al. Zhonghua Yixue Zazhi (National Medical Journal of China) 1977 57(9):584.

(Huo Shaolan)

XUEDAN 雪膽

<Xuedan> is the root tuber of *Hemsleya amabilis Diels, H. macrosperma* C.Y. Wu, *H. chinensis* Cogn., *H. sphaerocarpa* Kuang et A.M Lu (Cucurbitaceae). It is also known as <Luoguodi>, <Qulian>, and <Jinguilian>.

<Xuedan> is bitter, "cold", and slightly toxic. It has latent-heat-clearing, antipyretic, detoxicant, anti-inflammatory, stomachic and analgesic actions. It is therefore a useful medication for dysentery, enteritis, bronchitis, acute tonsillitis, epigastric pain and stomachache.

CHEMICAL COMPOSITION

There are two principal kinds of constituents (1,2). The first kind includes tetracyclotriterpenoid bitter substances, called hemsleyadin, a mixture of dihydrocucurbitacin F-25-acetate and dihydrocucurbitacin F. The second kind includes saponins, called qingsidai, a mixture of 2 saponins with oleanolic acid as the aglycone. All *Hemsleya* species contain these two kinds of constituents but the quantity varies.

The root tuber of *H. amabilis* contains 1.5–2% of crude bitter principles and 5% of crude saponins, whereas those of *H. chinensis* have 0.2 and 10%, respectively (3).

PHARMACOLOGY

1. Antibacterial Effect

Hemsleyadin and the saponins of <Xuedan> were reported to have marked broad-spectrum antibacterial activity. Hemsleyadin 0.1 µg/ml inhibited *Shigella flexneri*. Its bacteriostatic concentration against *Salmonella typhi*, beta streptococcus, and *Escherichia coli* were 1000, 100, and 10 µg/kg, respectively (3). It was more potent than chloramphenicol in inhibiting *Salmonella typhi, Shigella dysenteriae*, and *Staphylococcus aureus* (4). The saponins at 0.1 µ g/ml strongly inhibited *Shigella flexneri* and beta streptococcus, and to different extents *Staphylococcus aureus, Escherichia coli, Salmonella typhi*, and *Salmonella cholerae suis* (4).

2. Antagonism on Coronary Disease

Intraperitoneal injection of the bitter fraction of this herb (including bitter principles) and bitter principles into mice and rats increased the myocardial blood flow, relieved the pituitrin-induced coronary vasoconstriction, decreased the myocardial oxygen consumption, antagonized the stimulant effect of epinephrine on myocardial oxygen consumption, and increased the tolerance of animals to hypoxia. The also protected rabbits against pituitrin-induced ST and T changes appeared on the ECG, but was inactive against arrhythmia (5,6).

Long-term or multiple administration of <Xuedan> tended to decrease the cholesterol in rabbits with experimental hypercolesterolemia and appeared to ameliorate arterial atheromatous plaques and fatty liver (5).

3. Hypotensive Effect

Intravenous injection of the total saponins of <Xuedan> to anesthetized dogs produced hypotension and tachyphylaxis. The intraduodenal route was ineffective (5). Intravenous injection of hemsleyadin A did not cause hypotension (7).

4. Antipyretic and Anti-inflammatory Effects

A weak antipyretic effect was achieved by intraperitoneal injection of hemsleyadin A against typhoid vaccine-induced fever in rabbits; it had no significant effect on the normal body temperature and nonvaccine-induced fever (7).

Intraperitoneal injection of the oleanolic acid obtained by acid hydrolysis of the saponins of the herb produced a marked anti-inflammatory effect on carrageenin- or formaldehyde-induced paw swelling in rats (8).

5. Miscellaneous Actions

Intraperitoneal injection of oleanolic acid offered effective protection against carbon tetrachloride-induced hepatic damage and SGPT elevation (9,10). Oleanolic acid inhibited the growth of sarcoma 180 in mice (11). Hemsleyadin A was shown to have no significant effect on the isolated guinea pig ileum and uterus (7).

6. Toxicity

The LD_{50} of a single intragastric dose of the bitter fraction of <Xuedan> (including hemsleyadin) was determined to be 1.52 g/kg (6). No death occurred with the intragastric dose of 10 g/kg of hemsleyadin A (3), suggesting substances other than hemsleyadin A had greater toxicity.

Dogs orally given 160 mg/kg of hemsleyadin A daily for 10 days showed no change in the hepatic and renal functions; in most animals erythrocytosis and leukocytosis of different degrees occurred (4). Injection of hemsleyadin or hemsleyadin A 20–40 mg/kg IV to rabbits caused slowing of the respiration and heart rates, decrease in the amplitude of cardiac contraction, conduction block and, finally, cardiac arrest. Thus, hemsleyadin has definite cardiotoxicity if given intravenously (6,7).

Intravenous injection of the saponins of the herb to cats at doses of 60, 120, and 200 mg/kg resulted in slight inhibition of the respiration, blood pressure, and heart rate. Note a single death occurred in mice given the oral dose of 10 g/kg. The LD_{50} of the saponins was 2.14 ± 0.11 g/kg IV and its hemolysis index was determined to be 1:600 (3).

No significant toxic manifestation developed in rats receiving oleanolic acid 180 mg/kg PO daily for 10 days, or a single dose of 1 g/kg SC or PO, nor in mice receiving a single dose of 1 g/kg SC or 2 g/kg PO (9,10).

CLINICAL STUDIES

1. Acute Bacillary Dysentery

In 444 cases of acute bacillary dysentery treated with the <Xuedan> tablet (0.5 g/tablet, 1–3 tablets thrice daily), <Xuedan> saponin tablet (30 mg/tablet, 2–3 tablets/dose) or hemsleyadin (5 mg/ tablet, 2–3 tablets/dose), a higher cure rate (around 84%) than that (62%) of the furazolidone group was attained. These medications were superior to the latter in controlling fever, abdominal pain, diarrhea, and tenesmus as well as in normalizing the stool (2).

2. Other Bacterial Infections

<Xuedan> was preliminarily found to be effective in acute tonsillitis, submaxillary lymphadenitis, periodontitis, and chronic bronchitis of the elderly (2). The treatment of pneumonia and septicemia in burns with <Xuedan> preparations was reported (12). The herb was also effective in pulmonary tuberculosis (3).

3. Cervicitis

Capsules or tablets, prepared from this herb plus the root of *Lithospermum erythrorhizon* and licorice, introduced deep into the vagina after a sitz bath every night for a course of 7 days, had been tried in 16,386 cases; an effective rate of 96% was attained (13).

4. Chronic Suppurative Maxillary Sinusitis

One hundred and fourteen inflamed sinuses were treated by intrasinus injection of a preparation of the <Xuedan> saponins (30 mg/2 ml) following irrigation once a week for 3 times. A short-term cure rate of 30.7% and an effective rate of 91.3% were achieved. The drug was found to be superior to penicillin and berberine (14).

5. Acute Icteric Hepatitis

Oleanolic acid 50–90 mg/day PO was tried in 153 cases, resulting in an aggregate effective rate of 93.5% and a cure rate of 70%. The cure rate achieved with oleanolic acid was higher than that (40%) of the control given Western medicines, whereas the time required for the biochemical parameters to improve was essentially not different (10).

6. Coronary Disease

A compound tablet prepared from the extracts of this herb plus the rhizome of *Dioscorea nipponica* and the flower bud of *Sophora japonica* was believed to be effective in resolving angina pectoris and lowering blood lipids in 276 cases treated for two months (5,6).

7. Pain

Excellent analgesia was achieved with the herb powder at doses of 0.3–0.5 g in over 60 cases of traumatic pain, toothache, sore throat, and abdominal pain. Drug effects usually appeared 2–5 minutes after medication and lasted from 40 minutes to 6 hours (15).

ADVERSE EFFECTS

The oral therapeutic dosages of <Xuedan>, its saponins, and bitter principles did not produce any significant side effects; higher dosages occasionally resulted in abdominal distention, sweating, and nausea. Intramuscular injection of hemsleyadin may cause local pain (4). The 1% <Xuedan> saponins 0.3 ml/kg administered by slow intravenous injection (1 ml/min) to man produced a hemolytic effect directly proportional to the administered dose. Leukocytosis and tachycardia developed concurrently. Normal WBC count was gradually restored after 5 hours. These reactions were absent in intramuscular administration (16). No aberrant ECG patterns were produced during intramuscular injection or intravenous infusion of the drug (2).

Daily doses of 50–120 mg of oleanolic acid by mouth did not cause significant toxic reactions nor any abnormalities in the blood, urine, and stool routine examinations and ECG, except some upper abdominal discomfort during the early stage of medication or upon administration on an empty stomach in some patients (10).

REFERENCE

1. Chemistry Department, Yunnan Institute of Materia Medica. Yaowu Yanjiu Tongxun (Drug Research Communications) 1973 (2):3, 15.

2. 69th Hospital of the Chinese PLA. Proceedings of the National Symposium on Combined Western and Traditional Chinese Medicine. 1974. p. 351.

3. 59th Hospital of the Chinese PLA. Xinyiyaoxue Zazhi (Journal of Traditional Chinese Medicine) 1973 (1):29.

4. Scientific Research Unit, Dexing (Jiangxi) Health Bureau et al. Xinyiyaoxue Zazhi (Journal of Traditional Chinese Medicine) 1975 (8):43.

5. Coronary Disease Unit, Sichuan Institute of Chinese Materia Medica. Sichuan Communications on Chinese Traditional and Herbal Drugs 1974 (1):17.

6. Coronary Disease Unit, Sichuan Institute of Chinese Materia Medica. Sichuan Communications on Chinese Traditional and Herbal Drugs 1976 (1):28.

7. Yunnan Institute of Materia Medica. Yaowu Yanjiu Tongxun (Drug Research Communications) 1973 (2):19.

8. Gupta MB et al. European Journal of Pharmacology 1969 6(1):67.

9. Hunan Institute of Medical and Pharmaceutical Industry. Chinese Traditional and Herbal Drugs Communications 1975 (3):47.

10. Hunan Institute of Medical and Pharmaceutical Industry. Chinese Traditional and Herbal Drugs Communications 1977 (4):33.

11. Deoliveira MM et al. Chemical Abstracts 1969 71:58886a.

12. 69th Hospital of the Chinese PLA. Chinese Traditional and Herbal Drugs Communications 1971 (2):51.

13. Pengxian (Sichuan) Institute of Chinese Materia Medica et al. Xinyiyaoxue Zazhi (Journal of Traditional Chinese Medicine) 1975 (2):34.

14. ENT Department, Sichuan Third People's Hospital et al. Chongqing Yiyao (Chongqing Medical Journal) 1976 (2):31.

15. Proceedings of the National Exhibition of Chinese Traditional Drugs and New Therapeutic Methods in Beijing (Surgical diseases). 1970. p. 8.

16. Pharmaceutical Factory, 58th Hospital of the Chinese PLA. Chinese Traditional and Herbal Drugs Communications 1972 (6):55.

(Xue Chunsheng)

XUELIAN 雪莲

<Xuelian> is the whole plant of *Saussurea laniceps* Hand.-Mazz., *S. medusa* Maxim., *S. involucrata* Kar. et Kir. ex Maxim., *S. tridactyla* Sch.-Bip., or *S. eriocephala* Franch. (Compositae). It is sweet with a slightly bitter aftertaste and a "warm" property. The herb is noted for its "kidney"-tonifying, yang-invigorative, menstruation-corrective, hemostatic, "cold"-discutient, and antirheumatic effects. It is mainly used in rheumatism, cough with thin sputum, lower abdominal pain in women, irregular menstruation, leukorrhea, metrorrhagia, retention of placenta, impotence, and snow blindness. Externally, it is used to treat wound hemorrhage.

CHEMICAL COMPOSITION

The drug contains alkaloids, flavonoids, lactones, sterols and volatile oil (1). The calcium salt of an acidic polysaccharide (2) and a substance (B2-1.0) (3) which caused uterine contraction were recently isolated from *S. medusa*.

PHARMACOLOGY

1. Abortifacient Effect

The abortifacient action of the <Xuelian> decoction given to pregnant mice at different gestational periods and also to rabbits during early pregnancy by intraperitoneal injection was confirmed to be excellent. Used during early pregnancy, the herb caused deformation and degeneration of the embryos and detachment of the endometrium, which may remain inside the uterine cavity or become expulsed through the vagina. In middle and late gestation, the drug usually expelled the whole embryo 5–6 hours after medication (4). The mode of action of the intrauterine dose was similar to, but more potent than, that of the intraperitoneal dose (4). In contrast, the oral dose was inactive. The bioactive component was probably the calcium salt of an acidic polysaccharide which is acid-labile and may be inactivated by gastric acid when given by mouth. The herb decoction lost its efficacy after two weeks of storage; the solution of this component was comparatively stable (2). The mechanism of the abortifacient action of <Xuelian> probably involved the inhibition of the decidual reaction, but not the degeneration of the corpora lutea (4). In *in vitro* human embryos, <Xuelian> did not significantly damage the trophoblastic cells or lower the activity of the enzymes involved in the synthesis of progestogens in the placental villi. In other words, this herb did not appear to inhibit the synthesis of progesterone (5). It appeared that the herb acted on the uterus to prevent the binding of hormones to the endometrial basal cells or the response of uterus to progestogens; hence, the herb suppressed the development of decidura, leading to abortion. Since the effect of <Xuelian> could be antagonized by increasing the dosage of progesterone, these two agents apparently competes with each other (4).

2. Effect on the Uterus

The <Xuelian> decoction at low concentrations caused strong and rhythmic contraction of the rat uterus isolated at estrus. This effect lasted more than one hour without increasing the tension. Higher concentrations caused stronger rhythmic contractions succeeded by progressive weakening and, finally, cessation of the contractions; spasm did not develop. Obviously, the features of the action of <Xuelian> differed from those of pituitrin. Intravenous injection of low doses of the <Xuelian> decoction to rabbits increased the amplitude and rate of uterine contraction; higher doses caused spastic contraction lasting 20 minutes (6). Other studies, however, could not confirm the uterotropic action of the herb decoction *in vitro*; the conclusion was that the herb was mainly inhibitory. But, B_2-1.0 and the calcium salt of the acidic polysaccharide obtained from *S. medusa* were found to exert prominent excitatory effect on muscle strips of mouse uterus at estrus and different stages of gestation. It was therefore considered that the decoction contained both inhibitory and excitatory components on the uterus. The actions of these two kinds of components can be separated from each other by injection on account of their different metabolic pathways. Furthermore, it was suggested that termination of pregnancy by <Xuelian> was attributed to uterine excitation (2,3). These effects may serve as the therapeutic basis for the use of <Xuelian> in the treatment of irregular menstruation, metrorrhagia, and retention of the placenta.

3. Effect on Other Smooth Muscless

The decoction and the total alkaloids of the herb were shown to inhibit the activity of isolated rabbit intestines. They markedly antagonized intestinal spasm caused by histamine, pilocarpine, acetylcholine, and pituitrin. A direct action was implied since the herb antagonized intestinal tonic contraction induced by barium chloride, and failed to antagonize salivation induced by pilocarpine. The total flavones of this herb caused intestinal tonic contraction, which could be antagonized by its total alkaloids (6,7). The total alkaloids also partially antagonized the histamine-induced contraction in isolated guinea pig bronchial rings (8).

4. Anti-inflammatory and Analgesic Effects

The decoction, ethanol extract, and total alkaloids of <Xuelian> markedly antagonized formaldehyde- or egg white-induced paw swelling in rats (6,8). The action of the ethanol extract resembled that of sodium salicylate. The total alkaloids also decreased the vascular permeability in rabbits (9). This herb was also proved by the hot plate method to have an analgesic effect in mice (10).

5. Effect on the Cardiovascular System

The <Xuelian> decoction was shown to antagonize the inhibitory effect of pentobarbital on the isolated toad heart. When given by intravenous injection, it enhanced the contractility of the rabbit heart *in situ* for 40–60 minutes. Yet it did not significantly affect the heart rate (6). On the other hand, the total alkaloids inhibited the isolated rabbit heart and even caused cardiac asystole (8).

The total alkaloids constricted the blood vessels of the isolated rabbit ear; this effect was blocked by phentolamine, suggesting mediation by α-receptors. The ethanol extract, in contrast, caused vasodilation which was not blocked by propranolol, indicating no involvement of β-receptors. This effect may be attributed to a direct action on the vascular smooth muscle (8).

Intravenous injection of the <Xuelian> decoction to anesthetized cats resulted in initially a transient fall, followed by elevation and, finally, by a secondary fall in the blood pressure. This effect lasted one hour. Repeated medication produced tachyphylaxis. A pressor effect was also achieved by the total alkaloids and total flavones in anesthetized rabbits and dogs, respectively; their actions were partially blocked by propranolol (7).

6. Toxicity

Pregnant mice injected with the abortifacient dose of the <Xuelian> decoction stored for two weeks all killed. This suggests not only a loss of the abortifacient effect but also an increase in the toxicity of the <Xuelian> decoction after long storage (2).

CLINICAL STUDIES

The traditional used of <Xuelian> have already been mentioned in the preceeding paragraphs. Recent studies showed that it may be effective in the induction of labor during the mid-term and early stages of gestation (5).

ADVERSE EFFECTS

Overdosage of <Xuelian> may cause profuse sweating. The herb is contraindicated in pregnant women.

REFERENCE

1. Li GH et al. Chinese Pharmaceutical Bulletin 1979 (2):86.

2. Lin QS et al. Pharmaceutical abstracts. In: Proceedings of the 1978 Shanghai Regional Symposium on Pharmacy. Chinese Pharmaceutical Association (Beijing Branch). 1978. p. 248.

3. Reproductive Physiology Research Unit, Beijing Medical College. Journal of Beijing Medical College 1978 (3):162.

4. Reproductive Physiology Research Unit, Beijing Medical College. Journal of Beijing Medical College 1976 (4):223, 227, 230.

5. Sun MZ et al. Journal of Beijing Medical College 1979 (2):79.

6. Pharmacology Department, Beijing Medical College. Journal of Beijing Medical College 1976 (1):43.

7. Li GH et al. Acta Academiae Medicinae Xinjiang 1978 (1):22.

8. Li GH et al. Acta Academiae Medicinae Xinjiang 1979 (2):63.

9. Li GH et al. Acta Pharmaceutica Sinica 1980 15(6):368.

10. Chen XY et al. Chinese Traditional and Herbal Drugs 1981 12(2):30.

(Xue Chunsheng)

XUESHANGYIZHIHAO 雪上一枝蒿

The root tuber of *Aconitum brachypodum* Diels (Ranunculaceae) is the drug <Xueshangyizhihao>. In some places, the drug is derived from other *Aconitum* plants such as *A. brachypodum* Diels var. *laxiflorum* Fletcher et Lauener, *A. brachypodum* Diels var. *crispulum* W.T. Wang, *A. bullatifolium* Lévl., *A. szechenyianum* Gay (*A. pendulum* Busch), and *A. flavum* Hand.-Mazz. It is also known as <Sanzhuanban> and <Tiebangchui>. The drug is bitter, tingling, "warm" and highly toxic. With detumescent, analgesic, and antirheumatic effects, it is used for the treatment of wounds and injuries, rheumatism, arthralgia, pyogenic infections or ulcers of the skin, and poisonous snake bites.

CHEMICAL COMPOSITION

<Xueshangyizhihao> contains aconitine, hypaconitine and atisine. Two slightly toxic alkaloids, anthorine and ψ-anthorine, were early reported as constituents of *A. szechenyianum*. Later, anthorines A and B were also isolated Bullatines B, E and F were isolated from *A. brachypodum* grown in Zhaotong, Yunnan. Bullatines A, B, C, D and G were isolated from *A. brachypodum* grown in Dongchuan, Yunnan.

PHARMACOLOGY

Refer to the monograph on <Fuzi> for the pharmacological actions of aconitine.

1. Analgesic Effect

As shown by electrical stimulation of the tail of mice, the 1 mg/kg-dose of bullatines A, B, C, or D, extracted from <Xueshangyizhihao> produced in Dongchuan, Yunnan, had an analgesic effect (1). Another paper, however, reported that significant analgesic effect in mice was achieved by subcutaneous injection of bullatine A 100 mg/kg, obtained from the same source, showing an analgesic index of only 7.5 which was one-eleventh that of morphine (2). The total alkaloids extracted from *A. flavum* also produced a strong analgesic action which was 43.7 times that of morphine, and was 300 times more toxic than the latter (3). <Xueshangyizhihao> of unknown species showed an analgesic index of only 4.07 in the hot plate method (4). All these results indicate that <Xueshangyizhihao>, despite its analgesic effect, has a low analgesic index and is not clinically safe.

2. Local Anesthetic Effect

The total alkaloid of *A. flavum* was to have a strong local anesthetic action. Its potency was proven experimentally to be 14 times that of dicaine hydrochloride and 159 times that of procaine hydrochloride; its toxicity, however, was 40 and 180 times those of the latter agents, respectively (3). On the other hand, bullatine A had no local anesthetic action (2).

3. Effect on the Cardiovascular System and Respiration

An early report stated that this herb had digitalis-like effect on the frog heart; the toxic symptoms were due to parasympathetic stimulation, and the ensuing cardiac insufficiency may be antagonized by atropine (5). Later studies showed that the aqueous extract of, and anthorines A and B isolated from, the herb produced in Yunnan exerted aconitine-like actions on isolated and *in situ* frog hearts (6). Experiments on anesthetized cats revealed that intravenous injection of the extract of *A. szechenyianum* caused arrhythmia, hypotension, and dyspnea. The arrhythmia induced by this extract mainly consisted of sinus bradycardia and ventricular tachycardia. In most cases, sinus bradycardia appeared first, but they often interchange. It is postulated that these effects are due to vagal stimulation and mainly to direct stimulation of the ectopic ventricular pacemakers. Hypotension caused by the extract was usually transient but at times irreversible. It often appeared before arrhythmia and therefore bore no causal relationship with alteration in the stroke volume but with reduced peripheral resistance. Moreover, stroke volume reduced by arrhythmia further lowered the blood pressure. Respiration was briefly stimulated only in individual animals, and was inhibited to different extents in most animals after the injection. The resulting symptoms included slow, weak, and irregular breathing and even brief respiratory arrest. Variation in the response to *A. szechenyianum* was considerable. The responses appeared following doses of 25 mg/kg in most animals, but, in some, after 50 mg/kg. Heat attenuated the drug effects; arrhythmia and hypotension, however, were still elicited by increasing the dosage. Experiments had shown that the decoction or extract (obtained by cold extraction) of *Podophyllum emodi* Wall. var. chinense Sprague strongly antagonized dyspnea and hypotension induced by *A. szechenyianum* but did not modify arrhythmia. Large doses of vitamin C antagonized arrhythmia induced by the herb, produced a prolonged pressor effect in case of hypotension, and stimulated the respiration (7).

4. Toxicity

A. szechenyianum produced in Yunnan was reported to be highly toxic to mice, and the 20% *A. szechenyianum* bait, which mice found indistinguishable from normal food, was useful as rat poison (8). The LD_{50} of the hydrochlorides of ballatines A, B, and D in mice were 21.96 ± 1.07, 2.99 ± 0.08, and 70.09 ± 2.78 mg/kg SC, respectively (1). In another report, the LD_{50} of bullatine A of similar melting point was determined to be 754 (694–814)mg/kg. Subcutaneous injection of large doses to mice caused an increase in activity, clonic convulsion, loss of the righting reflex, stimulation followed by depression of respiration, and finally, death due to respiratory paralysis. In contrast, no toxic manifestations resulted from an intravenous dose of 30 mg/kg in rabbits (2). The LD_{50} of the total alkaloids of *A. flavum* in mice was 1.09 ± 0.23 mg/kg IP (3). The LD_{50} of *A. szechenyianum* produced in Yunnan (ground with water) in mice was 2.512 mg/kg PO. Autopsy of the poisoned rabbits revealed myocardial swelling with punctate bleeding, disappearance of myocardial striation, and cerebral cellular swelling and degeneration (4). The toxicity of the herb may be reduced by autoclaving and heat processing (7,9).

CLINICAL STUDIES

<Xueshangyizhihao> is an analgesic commonly employed by folks and herbalists in the treatment of traumatic injuries and rheumatic pains. The usual oral dose of 25–50 mg is taken as powder or wine. The herb was shown to be efficacious in recent trials involving toothache, surgical would pain, and pain of advanced cancer. One hundred and fifty cases of low-back and leg pains, strain of lumbar and shoulder muscles, and sciatica were treated with local or acupoint injection of this herb at doses of 12.5–25 mg (maximum 50 mg) on alternate days for 3 days as a course. Excellent effects were obtained in 116 cases, improvement in 23 and no effect in 11. Drug effects usually appeared after 1–2 therapeutic courses (10). Other workers reported the effective use of the herb injection in treating rheumatism and traumatic pains. The peak analgesic effect appeared 30–60 minutes after the intramuscular dose and the action lasted 10–16 hours (9,11). In addition, good therapeutic effects also reported in the treatment of 98 cases of rheumatic arthritis, mild arthralgia, traumatic lumbago (without bone lesion) with injection containing 25 mg/ml of the crude herb at 1–2 ml/days IM, usually for 7–10 days (12).

ADVERSE EFFECTS

Although commonly prescribed by herbalists, <Xueshangyizhihao> is a very toxic drug. Its toxicity varies greatly with different species, and there are considerable differences in individual responses (13). Reports of poisoning and death due to the herb are numerous (4,14–26). The herb earned the sobriquet "Sanzhuanban" (meaning three-and-a-half turns) from the folk practice of grinding a piece of the herb with a small amount of water or wine in a porcelain bowl for 3.5 circles. Excessive grinding supposedly results in overdosage and poisoning. Thus, 10 cases of poisoning, including one dealth, due to ingestion of the solution obtained by grinding the herb for 4 to 11 circles, have been reported (4). The usual and maximum doses recommended in the Chinese pharmacopoeia are 25–50 and 70 mg, respectively. However, oral administration of 800–1000 mg of some species do not produce serious poisoning (13). Therefore, it is extremely important to distinguish the species from which the herb is derived and to be knowledgeable of its dosage. Extreme caution should be exercised when using this herb. Symptoms of poisoning may appear 10–30 minutes after oral administration, or instantly during injection, or as late as 6 hours after medication. The toxic symptoms involve multiple systems. Neurological symptoms include numbness of the lips, tongue tip, extremities and even of the whole body, immobility of extremities, slurred speech, salivation, hyperhidrosis, blurred vision, dizziness, spastic contractions, confusion and even coma; miosis is occasionally seen. Symptoms of the digestive system include nausea, vomiting, abdominal pain, and diarrhea. The circulatory symptoms include palpitation, nervousness, chest tightness, chest discomfort, slow pulse, arrhythmia and ECG signs of sinus bradycardia, dysrrhythmia, atrioventricular block or dissociation, frequent ventricular or supraventricular proiosystole, bigeminy, paroxysmal nodal tachycardia, and atrial fibrillation. In some instances, there may be hypotension, weak heart beat, cold extremities, pallor, and cyanosis — manifestations of shock, and death subsequent to circulatory and respiratory failure.

The emergency measures for <Xueshangyizhihao> poisoning are the same as for aconitine poisoning. Large doses of atropine will improve the ECG aberrations due to aconitine poisoning. Quinidine, propranolol, antihistamines, and procainamide will control aconitine-induced atrial fibrillation. Therefore, large doses of atropine (the earlier the better) as well as quinidine and procainamide are advocated in addition to general emergency measures (including gastric lavage) in order to treat cardiac toxicity. These maneuvers achieved good clinical results (13–17). Some practitioners hold the view that potassium chloride should be given, in addition to atropine, to relieve the excitatory effect of this herb on the myocardium; this method successfully rescued all 9 cases of poisoning (4). Oral administration of a decoction of 6 g of *P. emodi* var. *chinense* and large doses of vitamin C is also useful (7).

REFERENCE

1. Deng SX et al. Abstracts of the 1962 Symposium of the Chinese Pharmaceutical Association. Chinese Pharmaceutical Association. 1962. p. 259.

2. Tang XC et al. Acta Pharmaceutica Sinica 1966 13(3):227.

3. Pharmacology Section et al. Ningyi Tongxun (Communications of Ningxia Medical College) 1974 (9):19.

4. Internal Medicine Department, Hengyang Second Hospital. Hunan Yiyao Zazhi (Hunan Medical Journal) 1975 (2):27.

5. Li HM et al. The National Medical Journal of China 1943 29(5):457; Liu SS. Abstracts of Research Literature on Chinese Traditional Drugs (1820–1961). Science Press. 1963. p. 627.

6. Wang JY et al. Kexue (Science) 1948 30(6):176.

7. Pathophysiology Section, Xi'an Medical College. Shaanxi Medical Journal 1978 (1):64.

8. Liang ZL et al. Acta Academiae Medicinae Lanzhou 1962 (1):73.

9. Yunnan Institute for Drug Control. Chinese Traditional and Herbal Drugs Communications 1977 (12):20.

10. Linzhou Farm Hospital of the Production and Construction Corps of Xizang Military Region. Xizang Yiyao (Xizang Medical Journal) 1978 (1):133.

11. Pharmaceutical Department, Hospital of Dongchuan Bureau of Mines, Medical Journal of Dongchuan Copper Mine (Health Division of Dongchuan Bureau of Mines, Yunnan) 1974 (1):54.

12. Pharmaceutical Factory, 71st Hospital of the Chinese PLA. Xinzhoungyi (Journal of New Chinese Medicine) 1977 (4):10.

13. Ye YQ et al. Chinese Traditional and Herbal Drugs Communications 1980 11(1):40.

14. Luo LC. Journal of Traditional Chinese Medicine 1980 (9):37.

15. Zhou YJ et al. Health Journal of Guangxi 1976 (2):39.

16. Zhou YJ et al. Jiangsu Yiyao (Jiangsu Medical Journal) 1978 (9):44.

17. Zhou YJ et al. Medical Literature 1979 (7):70.

18. Wang XY. Chinese Journal of Paediatrics 1959 10(1):83.

19. Wang C. Wuhan Medicine and Health 1959 2(2):150.

20. Chen WB. Acta Academiae Medicinae Sichuan 1959 (4):11.

21. Yuan SN. Chinese Journal of Internal Medicine 1959 7(6):584.

22. Dong HS et al. Wuhan Medical Journal 1964 1(6):446.

23. ECG Room of the Internal Medicine Department, Second Hospital of Shanghai Bureau of Textile Industry. Medical Exchanges 1976 (8):44.

24. Cao WF et al. Health Journal of Guangxi 1976 (2):40.

25. He DY. Xinyiyaoxue Zazhi (Journal of Traditional Chinese Medicine) 1977 (11):15.

26. Gufeng Commune (Xincheng County) Health Centre. Barefoot Doctor of Guangxi 1978 (11):21.

(Deng Wenlong)

CHANGSHAN 常山

<Changshan> is the root of *Dichroa febrifuga* Lour. (Saxifragaceae) whose tender leafy twig called <Shuqi> or <Tiancha> is also used as medicine.

<Changshan> is bitter, slightly "cold", and a little bit toxic. It is an antimalarial.

CHEMICAL COMPOSITION

<Changshan> contains 3 tautomers α-, β- and γ-dichroines, dichroidine, 4-quinazolone and umbelliferone.

The root contains about 0.1% of alkaloids whereas the leaf contains about 0.5%. Febrifugine and isofebrifugine were reported to be isolated from the root and leaf. Subsequently, they were proved to be β-dichroine and α-dichroine, respectively.

PHARMACOLOGY

1. Antimalarial Effect

Plasmodium gallinaceum (chicken malaria) was very susceptible to the aqueous extract of <Changshan> (1) and to a certain extent to the ethanol extract (2). The antimalarial efficacy of the leaf <Shuqi> was five times that of the root (1). Dichroines had been given to chicken with *P. gallinaceum* infection: α-dichroine 20 mg/kg, β-dichroine 0.4 mg/kg, γ-dichroine 0.2 mg/kg, intramuscularly two times a day for 4 days. Quinine was used as control. Similar therapeutic results were obtained with various dichroines, but there was disparity in their efficacies. The most potent alkaloid was γ-dichroine which was about 100 times as potent as quinine; the next, β-dichroine was 50 times as potent; the least potent, α-dichroine, was almost as potent as quinine (1,3–5). Another paper reported that β-dichroine was 100 times as effective as quinine against *Plasmodium lophurae* (duck malaria) (6).

2. Amebicidal Effect

In vitro, β-dichroine was shown to inhibit *Entamoeba histolytica*, with a potency twice that of emetine hydrochloride. The miminal effective dosage of β-dichroine in rats against *Entamoeba coli* was 1.0 mg/kg/day PO; administration of this dosage for 6 days was proved to be more effective than emetine, having a therapeutic index twice that of the latter (7).

3. Antipyretic Effect

Oral administration of the <Changshan> decoction 2 g/kg to rabbits with artificial fever produced an antipyretic effect more marked than that achieved with the root of *Bupleurum chinense* (8). Injection of the ethanol extract at 0.3 g/kg SC to rabbits produced an antipyretic effect equivalent to that of antipyrine 100 mg/kg; increasing the dosage to 0.7 g/kg produced an antipyretic effect longer than that produced by antipyrine (9). The antipyretic effect of the orally administered γ-dichroine in rats was stronger than that of aspirin (10).

4. Effect on the Cardiovascular System

The α-, β-, and γ-dichroines were shown to have a marked hypotensive action in anesthetized dogs, and their efficacy as well as duration of action were dose-dependent. In addition, they also decreased the amplitude of cardiac contraction and increased the splenic and renal volumes. All three dichroines markedly inhibited the isolated rabbit heart. Low concentrations of α-dichroine mostly stimulated the isolated frog heart, whereas high concentrations depressed it. These results indicate that the hypotensive action of the dichroines was consequent to cardiac depression and visceral vasodilation (11). In addition, a new quinidine-like antiarrhythmic drug, changrolin, has been produced by Chinese scientists from structural modification of β-dichroine; its chemical name is 4-(3',5'-bits((N-pyrrolidinyl)methyl)-4'-hydroxyanilino)quinazoline. Administration of this agent 377 mg/kg PO to rats was effective in preventing aconitine-induced arrhythmia. Injection of 5.2 mg/kg IV for a few times was also effective in ouabain-poisoned dogs. Changrolin administered to rabbits or dogs by intravenous injection or infusion produced the following effects; elevation of the threshold of ventricular fibrillation induced by electrical stimulation, initial slight slight increase succeeded by a decrease in the heart rate, prolongation of the PR interval and widening of the QRS complex on the ECG, slow fall in the blood pressure, and slight decrease of cardiac function (12). In experiments with anesthetized dogs, continuous or rapid administration of changrolin gave rise to weak cardiac contraction and conduction block (13). However, milder side effects on the heart was produced if the intravenous infusion was administered at a speed of less than 1 mg/minute (12). It was rather safe when the blood concentration was adjusted below 8 μg/ml despite changes in cardiac electroconduction (13).

5. Effect on Smooth Muscles

All three dichroines caused motor inhibition of the isolated small intestine of rabbits, and α-dichroine also caused inhibition of the isolated small intestine of dogs. Low concentrations of α- and β-dichroines inhibited the isolated guinea pig small intestine and high concentrations usually caused stimulation which at times was preceded by transient inhibition. The response of the *in situ* small intestine of dogs to the three dichroines were inconsistent — sometimes excitation and at other times inhibition (11). The actions of dichroines on the isolated uteri were found to be more complicated: α- and β-dichroines had no significant effect on the isolated uteri of nonpregnant rabbits and guinea pigs; inhibitory effects were mostly observed in the isolated uteri of nonpregnant rats and excitatory effects in the pregnant specimens. The effect of the three dichroines on isolated uteri of pregnant rabbits and on *in situ* uteri of nonpregnant dogs was excitatory (11).

6. Miscellaneous Actions

In vitro, the aqueous extract of <Changshan> inhibited influenza virus PR_8; it was therapeutically effective in mice infected by the latter (14,15). *In vitro* studies proved that β-dichroine was lethal to Ehrlich ascites carcinoma cells and therapeutically effective against various experimental neoplasms; the following tumor inhibition rates were obtained: 50–100% for mouse Ehrlich ascites carcinoma, 45% for mouse Ehrlich ascites carcinoma solid type, 45% for mouse sarcoma 180, 75% for mouse melanoma, 55% for rat ascitic hepatoma, 30% for rat sarcoma 45, and 45% for rat Walker carcinoma (16).

7. Pharmacokinetics

It was proved in experiments with rats that the orally administered β-dichroine was easily absorbed from the gastrointestinal tract. The blood level of the intravenous injection fell rapidly. Drug distribution was highest in the kidneys, next in the heart, liver, muscle, fat, and spleen. The blood level was very low. Only about 16% of unchanged β-dichroine was excreted in urine. Only traces were found in feces, and almost nil in bile (17). The intragastric dose of changrolin was readily absorbed and the peak blood level was attained in 1.5–4 hours. A more rapid and complete absorption was achieved with the intramuscular injection; its peak level was reached within 5 minutes after which it declined. Studies on the ^{14}C-labelled changrolin indicated that it was primarily distributed in the liver, the gastrointestinal tract and its contents (12).

8. Toxicity

The acute LD_{50} of the orally administered alkaloids of <Changshan> were determined to be: α-dichroine, 570 mg/kg; β-dichroine, 6.57 mg/kg; γ-dichroine, 6.45 mg/kg; and total alkaloids, 7.79 mg/kg (4). The acute LD_{50} by intravenous administration in mice were: α-dichroine, 18.5 mg/kg; β-dichroine, 6.5 mg/kg; and γ-dichroine, 5 mg/kg (1). The MLD of β-dichroine in young rats was 20 mg/kg PO (7). Either β- or γ-dichroine administered orally to mice at daily doses of 0.75, 0.25, or 0.075 mg/kg for 14 days inhibited the growth of the animals. In both acute and subacute experiments, the oral dose produced diarrhea and even bloody stool in mice; autopsy revealed gastrointestinal mucosal congestion or hemorrhage and yellowing of the liver and kidneys

(4). In another report, repeated oral administration of γ-dichroine to mice caused hepatic edematous degeneration (10). Nausea, vomiting, diarrhea, and gastrointestinal mucosal congestion and hemorrhage appeared in dogs after oral administration of the aqueous extract of <Changshan>, or intramuscular injection of its ethanol extract, or subcutaneous injection of α-dichroine (2).

α-, β-, and γ-Dichroines given intravenously to pigeons induced emesis; chlorpromazine did not completely relieve but only prolonged the latent period of emesis (18). Dogs were used to elucidate the emetic mechanism of β-dichroine. The experiments revealed that it was not causally related to the medullary emetic chemoreceptor trigger zone (CTZ). Chlorpromazine only inhibited vomiting caused by the threshold dose of β-dichroine, but not that caused by larger doses. Emesis induced by β-dichroine was greatly attenuated by bilateral vagotomy and completely blocked by sectioning of the gastrointestinal vagal and sympathetic nerves. It is deduced from these results that β-dichroine primarily stimulated the vagal and sympathetic nerve endings of the gastrointestinal tract, causing reflex vomiting (19). The acute LD_{50} of changrolin was 377 mg/kg IP in mice (12).

CLINICAL STUDIES

1. Malaria

Dichroa-Pogostemon Tablet given before meals was used to treat 1926 cases. Tertian malaria responded better to this tablet than to chloroguanide hydrochloride and quinacrine hydrochloride. However, all the three drugs were similarly effective against subtertian malaria, though the plasmodia disappeared earlier in the group treated with Dichroa-Pogostemon Tablet (20). Satisfactory results were also reported in 5984 malaria carriers below 10 years of age twice administered the Changshan Injection at an interval of 25 days. The positive plasmodium rate was reduced from the pretreatment 41.4% to 6.3% (21). Many compound formulae consisting of Radix Dichroae, Rhizoma Pinelliae, Radix Bupleuri, Herba Pogostemi or Pericarpium Citri Reticulatae were effective in controlling malaria symptoms and preventing relapses (22,23).

2. Giardiasis

The decoction of <Changshan> 3–9 g per day in 2–3 doses for 7 days was reported to be effective against infection of *Giardia lamblia* (24).

3. Miscellaneous

<Changshan> has been discovered in recent years to have some quinidine-like action and was tried in the treatment of arrhythmia. Satisfactory results were achieved with the orally administered decoction of a compound formula (stir-fried Radix Dichroae and Herba Pyrolae, roasted Radix Astragali, Radix Sophorae Flavescentis, Radix Codonopsis Pilosulae) (22). Moreover, excellent

clinical effects were achieved with changrolin in the treatment of frequent ventricular premature beats and paroxysmal ventricular tachycardia; it was also effective against atrial premature beats, paroxysmal supraventricular tachycardia, and paroxysmal atrial fibrillation. In a clinical trial involving 489 cases of arrhythmia a total of 80.8% benefitted from changrolin treatment (25,26).

ADVERSE EFFECTS

Nausea and vomiting are the major adverse effects. Ancient prescriptions had used <Changshan> as an emetic to treat phlegm retention, etc. (22). The emetic effect may be reduced by stir-frying the herb with ginger juice or yellow wine, or using it with the tuber of *Pinellia ternata*, the whole plants of *Pogostemon cablin*, or *Citrus* peel (20,22). Statistical analysis revealed that in malaria patients the incidence rate of nausea and vomiting on the first day of medication with Dichroa-Pagostemon Tablet was 40.1%, gradually decreasing with the days so that on the fifth days only 20.5% reported these reactions (20).

REFERENCE

1. Zhang CS. Modern Research on Chinese Materia Medica. Chinese Scientific Books and Instruments Company. 1953. p. 139.

2. Pharmacology Department, Fujian Medical College. Acta Academiae Fujian 1959 (1):93.

3. Wang JY. Medicine 1950 3(10):225.

4. Wu YY et al. Abstracts of the 1956 Academic Conference of the Chinese Academy of Medical Sciences. Vol. 1. 1956. p. 20.

5. Tang RY et al. Shanghai Zhongyiyao Zazhi (Shanghai Journal of Traditional Chinese Medicine) 1958 (2):37.

6. Hewitt RI et al. American Journal of Tropical Medicine and Hygiene 1952 1(5):768.

7. Zhang TM et al. Acta Academiae Medicinae Wuhan 1958 (1):1.

8. Sun SX. Chinese Medical Journal 1956 42(10):964.

9. Jin YC. Chinese Medical Journal 1954 40(11):873.

10. Rose CL et al. Chemical Abstracts 1949 43:3929h.

11. Zhang CS et al. Acta Physiologica Sinica 1956 20(1):30.

12. Li LQ et al. Scientia Sinica 1979 (2):723.

13. Qu ZX et al. Acta Pharmaceutica Sinica 1980 15(8):449.

14. Wang SY et al. Kexue Tongbao (Science Bulletin) 1958 (3):90.

15. Wang SY. Kexue Tongbao (Science Bulletin) 1958 (5):155.

16. Verme' BM et al. Voprosy Onkologii 1960 6(7):56.

17. Song ZY et al. Acta Pharmaceutica Sinica 1964 11(7):1.

18. Jiang WD. Acta Academinae Medicinae Primae Shanghai 1957 (3):258.

19. Jiang WD. Acta Physiologica Sinica 1961 24(3–4):180.

20. Yunnan Sanitation and Anti-epidemic Station. Yunnan Medical Journal 1961 (3):8.

21. Yunnan Institute of Malaria. Yunnan Medical Journal 1961 (1):15.

22. Yuan F. Acta Academiae Medicinae Anhui 1976 (1):76.

23. Chongqing First Hospital of Traditional Chinese Medicine. Journal of Traditional Chinese Medicine 1956 (7):466.

24. Xu JF. Jiangsu Zhongyi (Jiangsu Journal of Traditional Chinese Medicine) 1962 (10):17.

25. Coordinating Research Group for Clinical trial of Changrolin. Zhonghua Yixue Zazhi (National Medical Journal of China) 1978 58(2):84.

26. Xu JM. Tianjin Pharmaceutical Industry 1978 (1–2):41.

(Duan Meifen)

BIJIUHUA 啤酒花

<Bijiuhua> is the female inflorescence of *Humulus lupulus* L. (Moraceae). Also called <Shemahua>, it has a bitter flavor and "mild" property. It is reputed for its stomachic, tranquilizing, antitussive and mucolytic actions. It is mainly used in dyspepsia, abdominal distention, bone tuberculosis, and insomnia.

Recently, it has been discovered that the bioactive components of the herb have tuberculostatic action. Consequently, various preparations of the herb have been employed in the treatment of tuberculosis.

CHEMICAL COMPOSITION

<Bijiuhua> mainly contains resin, volatile oil, flavonoids and tannin. The gland on the bracts of the female inflorescence of <Bijiuhua> contains 8–15% of resins, which may be divided into hard and soft ones. The soft resin contains α-acids and β-acids; the α-acids are mainly humulone and isohumulone, whereas the β-acids are essentially lupulone and analogues.

<Bijiuhua> contains volatile oil 0.5% which has tens of components. The main component is myrcene 30–50%, followed by humulene 8–33%, and small amounts of linalool, geraniol and luparenol. The flavonoid components include astragalin, isoquercitrin, rutin and kaempferitin.

PHARMACOLOGY

1. Antibacterial Effect

In vitro, the fluidextract of <Bijiuhua> and its active components, humulone and, in particular, lupulone, were shown to have strong inhibitory actions against various gram-positive bacteria and acid-fast bacilli, but no activity against gram-negative bacteria and fungi. Their MIC against some common bacteria were as follows:

	Lupulone	Humulone
Bacillus anthracis	1:300,000	1:100,000
Bacillus cereus	1:300,000	1:100,000
Bacillus subtilis	1:1,000,000	1:50,000
Corynebacterium diphtheriae	1:1,000,000	1:10,000
Lactobacillus pastorianus	1:100,000	1:40,000
Staphylococcus aureus	1:400,000	1:50,000
Diplococcus pneumoniae	1:300,000	1:20,000
Sarcina Lutea	1:100,000	1:30,000
Streptococcus fecalis	1:500,000	1:30,000

At the concentration of 1:3000, the agents had no bacteriostatic effect on over 10 kinds of gram-negative bacilli including *Escherichia coli, Salmonella typhi*, and *Shigella dysenteriae* (1–3). However, the MIC of Lupulone and humulone against lactobacillus were $10-50$ and 200 $\mu g/ml$, respectively (4). Chinese scientists reported that the MIC of natural lupulone against *Staphylococcus aureus* was 1.25 $\mu g/ml$, and that of synthetic lupulone was 0.6 $\mu g/ml$ (5). There is a great disparity among authors with respect to the inhibitory action of lupulone against *Mycobacterium tuberculosis*. A paper reported that the MIC of the drug against *Mycobacterium tuberculosis* var. *hominis* $H_{37}RV$ strain was 1:40,000 (6), whereas another paper claimed it to be between 1:200,000 and 1:300,000 (3). In China, the following MIC had been reported: <Bijiuhua> fluidextract $10-100$ $\mu g/ml$, lupulone $1-10$ $\mu g/ml$ (7), <Bijiuhua> fluidextract $3.1-25$ $\mu g/ml$, lupulone $1.5-6.2$ $\mu g/ml$ (8). and <Bijiuhua> decoction 7.5 $\mu g/ml$ (9). Although lupulone etc. had been reported to have a very weak inhibitory effect against pathogenic and nonpathogenic fungi, some reports alleged that both lupulone and humulone strongly inhibited plant fungi such as *Rhizopus stolonifer* and *Ceratocystis fimbriata* (10). In addition, lupulone and humulone at 50 $\mu g/ml$ also disrupted the growth of *Ascochyta pisi* (11).

The <Bijiuhua> fluidextract after removal of lupulone and humulone was still bacteriostatic; apart from these two components, azelaic acid which strongly suppressed the fermentation of alcohol was considered another active principle (12). Another paper reported that lactobacillus was strongly inhibited by isohumulone and humulinone (2).

6-Hydrolupulone, obtained by hydrogenation of some synthetic lupulone derivatives, was found to be stable for several months at room temperature. It strongly inhibited *Staphylococcus aureus*. Some of the diketoacylindane derivatives of lupulone were inhibitory against *Staphylococcus aureus* and *Mycobacterium tuberculosis* at MIC as low as 1:3,000,000 and 1:5,000,000, respectively (13–15).

In vitro, lupulone usually synergized with other antibiotics. Penicillin slightly potentiated the inhibitory action of lupulone against *Staphylococcus aureus*, and potentiated that of 6-hydrolupulone by $5-10$ times. On the other hand, erythromycin potentiated the effects of both lupulone and 6-hydrolupulone by about fourfold (14). Many factors could influence the antibacterial activity of <Bijiuhua>, such as storage time, serum and pH. Since lupulone can easily be destroyed by oxidation, the bacteriostatic titer progressively decreased with the increase in storage time. For instance, it was reported that the MIC of the fresh preparation of lupulone solution against *Mycobacterium tuberculosis* $H_{37}RV$ was 1:300,000. After 10 days of storage, this was reduced to 1:80,000 (3). Even storing the drug at $4°C$ for a few days would reduce its efficacy. Ultraviolet ray irradiation, however, had no significant influence (16). The antibacterial activity of lupulone was most strongly influenced by serum. For instance, its MIC against Mycobacterium tuberculosis $H_{37}RV$ in non-serum culture media was 1:200,000, but after addition of 10% horse serum, no antibacterial effect was observed even at the concentration of 1:10,000 (3). In China, it was reported that the addition of 5% serum increased the MIC of lupulone against $H_{37}RV$ from 25 to 200 $\mu g/ml$, representing an eightfold decrease in activity (8). Serum also exerted a similar influence on other bacteria such as

Staphylococcus aureus. A report claimed that the presence of 10% horse serum could lower the antistaphylococcal activity of lupulone by nine-tenths. After precipitating the proteins of horse serum with 48% ethanol, lupulone in the supernatant was still active, suggesting that it was not deactivated by serum (17). The antibacterial activity of lupulone and 6-hydrolupulone could also be blocked by 10% human serum or 1.5% human albumin (14). Experiments also proved that the phospholipids in the serum was one of the components influencing the effect of lupulone (18). pH also affects the antibacterial activity of lupulone; lowering the pH would increase its potency. For example, lupulone had a higher activity at pH 5 or 6 than at pH 7 or 8 (17). A report pointed out that p-aminobenzoic acid had no effect on the antistaphylococcal activity of lupulone (19).

In experimental therapy of albino mice intravenously injected with *Mycobacterium tuberculosis* $H_{37}RV$, it was shown that administration of lupulone 150 mg/kg PO every 12 hours, or daily injection of 60 mg/kg IM, for 30 days, markedly inhibited the multiplication of the tuberculous bacilli, and markedly decreased the number of tuberculous bacilli in the lungs, spleen, liver, kidneys, and heart, as compared to the control. These findings were more pronounced with the intragastric dose. The fact that lupulone has weak antituberculous activity *in vitro* but strong *in vivo* is probably due to its high lipid solubility which allows rapid penetration of the waxy membrane of the tuberculous bacilli, resulting in some sort of special affinity (6). Recent studies indicated that intragastric administration of the <Bijiuhua> fluidextract for 5 days prior to intravenous injection of $H_{37}RV$, then followed by continuous medication, decreased the mortality rate of the infected animals (8,9). However, many therapeutic experiments on animals showed negative results (16,20,21). 6-Hydrolupulone was ineffective in experimental tuberculosis in mice; lupulone was also ineffective in albino mice with *Staphylococcus aureus* infection (3).

2. Sedative Effect

It was reported that low dosage of <Bijiuhua> caused sedation, moderate dosage, hypnosis, and high dosage, paralysis. The hypnotic action was characterized by a slow onset and long duration (22,23). Injection of the <Bijiuhua> extract 625–2500 mg/kg SC to mice resulted in prolonged sleep and, three days later, in death (24). Sedation was believed to be induced by the acidic bitter principle of the herb and not by its volatile oil (25). Meanwhile, some authors believed it to be causally related to the isovaleric acid content (26). Others, however, cast doubts on the presence of this action (27).

3. Estrogenic Effect

<Shemahua> produced strong estrogenic effect. Experiments using the uterus-weight method indicated that the estrogenic activity of one gram of the dried flower was equivalent to 200–3000 units and that each liter of beer contained 10–360 units. This activity comes chiefly from the β-acid portion of the resin, a gram of which corresponded to 15,000 units. The α-acid portion was proven inactive (28–29).

4. Spasmolytic Effect

The <Bijiuhua> fluidextract exerted a very strong spasmolytic action on the smooth muscles, mainly as a direct relaxant effect. On specimens of rabbit jejunum, guinea pig duodenum, and albino rat uterus, it antagonized smooth muscle spasms induced by acetylcholine (2×10^{-5} g/ml), barium chloride (10^{-4} g/ml) and histamine (10^{-4} g/ml) (30).

5. Miscellaneous Actions

The <Bijiuhua> fluidextract markedly inhibited granulation induced by cotton pledgets and was useful clinically in suppressing pleural thickening due to pleurisy (9). A report claimed that this herb therapeutic value in experimental atherosclerosis, and that it slightly lowered the blood pressure in rabbits (31). Moreover, the fluidextract and the volatile oil of <Bijiuhua> injected intravenously to dogs produced a weak and transient hypotensive effect (32), and intravenous injection of lupulone to anesthetized or normal rabbits or monkeys enhanced the animals' respiration (33).

6. Pharmacokinetics

Lupulone given orally to 7 patients at a dose of 1 g every 4 hours from 6 am to 10 pm (5 g daily) for 8 weeks established a blood concentration of only 1.9–6.5 µg/ml (34).

7. Toxicity

<Bijiuhua> has low toxicity. The LD_{50} of its fluidextract in mice were determined as 1.2 g/kg SC, 314 mg/kg IP, and 30.1 mg/kg IV (24). Recent studies in China revealed that the LD_{50} in mice were 115.8 (8). and 175 mg/kg IP (9). The LD_{50} of lupulone in mice were 1.5 g/kg PO and 600 mg/kg IM (6), and that in rats was 330 mg/kg IM (33). Most animals died within 24 hours of medication, with manifestations of excitation and convulsion before death. The cause of death was asphyxia. Autopsy revealed distinct congestion or hemorrhage in the liver, lungs, and kidneys (33).

7.1 *Subacute toxicity studies.* Daily intragastric administration of 150, 300 and 450 mg/kg of lupulone to young rats for 12 days, of 300 mg/kg to guinea pigs for 14 days, of 300 mg/kg to rabbits for 12 days, and of 500 mg/kg to monkeys for 13 days, did not result in any abnormality in the blood picture, ECG, hepatic and renal functions, and pathological examinations (33).

7.2 *Chronic toxicity studies.* Different groups of mice were given feed containing 4, 2 and 1% lupulone (5 g of feed daily) for 40 days; 50% of the animals in the 4% group died on Day 18, 25% of the animals in the 2% group died on Day 13, and only 10% of the animals in the 1% group died on Day 40. There were different degrees of weight loss in all groups as compared with the control. Autopsy revealed distinct pathological changes in the lungs from leukocyte infiltration to pulmonary consolidation. Daily oral administration of 5 g of lupulone in normal subjects or patients for 12 weeks did not result in any alterations in the routine blood examination, liver and kidney functions, blood pressure, and ECG (33,34).

CLINICAL STUDIES

In other countries <Bijiuhua> preparations have long been used clinically. In China the ethanol extract, called "Sanhesu" or "Jiuhuasu" is the most commonly used preparation.

1. Tuberculosis

Different degrees of therapeutic effect had been achieved with various <Bijiuhua> preparations (16,35). One hundred and fifty cases of different types of tuberculosis had been effectively treated with "Edwil" prepared from the residue in beer making (containing <Bijiuhua>, yeast, and barley sprout, etc.). There were symptomatic improvement, increase in body weight, disappearance of shadows in chest X-ray, and negative sputum finding (16). The pure lupulone was also efficacious in 7 cases (34). Preparations of the herb fluidextract, including tablets, pills and emulsion, are used in many places of China to treat various types of tuberculosis, such as primary or relapse pulmonary tuberculosis (36–44), tuberculous pleurisy (45,46), tuberculosis of lymph nodes (47–49), and silicosis complicated with tuberculosis (50). The response of exudative tuberculous pleurisy to the medication was most satisfactory. Thus, in the primary treatment of 105 cases of pulmonary tuberculosis with the tablets or pills at daily doses corresponding to 3.5 g of <Bijiuhua> fluidextract or 14.5 g of the crude drug, the effective and marked effective rates obtained in 3 months were 70.2 and 25.6%, and in 6 months were 71.4 and 46.4%, respectively. Neither synergism nor antagonism to isoniazid were observed (36). Retreatment of 50 cases of pulmonary tuberculosis with these medications afforded a 30.5% effective rate in 3 months and 49.4% in 6 months (37). Out of 103 cases of exudative tuberculous pleurisy so treated, 100 were cured, two improved, and one was unchanged. Eighty out of 95 cases with fever had body temperature normalized within one month, chest pain reduced, appetite increased, and particularly, pleural fluid rapidly absorbed (45). Among 45 cases of pleurisy treated with the herb fluidextract, not a single case relapsed during 7.5 years of follow-up (46).

2. Leprosy

The <Bijiuhua> fluidextract was effective in different types of leprosy. Its therapeutic efficacy on the various types was in the order of: tuberculoid > borderline > lepromatous. The absorption of specific infiltration was most dramatic in tuberculoid leprosy; in the other types, the subsidence of skin lesion was good. In addition, beneficial effects on nerve swelling and histopathology of leprosy and lepra reaction were also achieved (15–56). Out of 153 cases treated, 12 achieved clinical cure, 5 short-term cure, 53 marked effects and 56 improvement; the effective rate was 82.4%. Drug effects also included lowering of the average index and morphological change of the bacteria (51). the ointment prepared from prepared from the herb fluidextract benefitted patients with leprous ulcers. Out of 67 lesions (38 cases), 27 healed, 5 short-term healed, 8 markedly improved, and 24 improved (57).

3. Acute Bacillary Dysentery

Although the inhibitory action of <Bijiuhua> against *Shigella dysenteriae* is not significant, it was reported to be effective clinically in the treatment of bacillary dysentery. For instance, 3 tablets of the <Bijiuhua> fluidextract, 0.4 g each, were given four times daily in 87 cases; 71 cases were cured in 7–10 days and 7 cases benefitted to different extents (58). Further treatment of 78 cases with this tablet cured 67 cases and improved 6 cases (59).

4. Surgical Diseases

The plaster and ointment prepared from the <Bijiuhua> fluidextract had an antibacterial effect and promoted granulation. Satifactory results were obtained with the local use of the ointment and plaster in cases of skin and surgical infections due to *Mycobacterium tuberculosis* and *Staphyloccus aureus*, poor post-operative wound healing, suppurated frostbite, and chronic ulcers (60–65). It was most efficacious in acute skin infection and mastitis, achieving a cure rate of 92.2% and an effective rate of 94.4%. In tuberculous infections such as surgical wound of tuberculous empyema, bone tuberculosis with abscess and fistula, and peripheral tuberculous lymphadenitis with fistula, the cure rate and effective rate obtained were 52.4 and 94.5%, respectively. The cure rate and effective rate in chronic skin ulcer and chronic infections were 58.1 and 92.3%, respectively (60).

5. Silicosis and Asbestosis

Treatment of silicosis and asbestosis with the tablet of <Bijiuhua> fluidextract ameliorated the symptoms. In particular, the appetite increased, the occurrence of common cold minimized, and coughing was reduced, but the clarity of the chest X-ray was only slightly improved (66–68).

6. Miscellaneous

There were also reports on the effective treatment of duodenal ulcer with a compound prescription of <Bijiuhua> (69), and of chronic bronchitis with a compound prescription of the root (70,71).

ADVERSE EFFECTS

The pollen of <Bijiuhua> may cause allergic dermatitis in man; the incidence rate was claimed to be as high as 90–95% (72). Menstruation was induced in most women 2–3 days after contact with the herb during harvest. The side effects of the orally administered preparations of the <Bijiuhua> fluidextract were mild and referrable mainly to the gastrointestinal tract, viz., gastric discomfort, nausea, anorexia, mushy stool, etc. (36–39,45–50). Moreover, drug rash may develop (36,37) and local application may cause local prickling pain (49). Lupulone had very low toxicity; daily administration of 5 g for more than 8 weeks did not produce severe side effects nor any untoward effects on the major organs such as the liver and kidneys, except gastrointestinal irritation (34).

REFERENCE

1. Lewis JC et al. Journal of Clinical Investigation 1949 28:916.

2. Cook AH et al. Journal of the Chemical Society 1950:1873.

3. Salle AJ et al. Proceedings of the Society for Experimental Biology and Medicine 1949 70:409.

4. Robert JF et al. Chemical Abstracts 1953 47:10055i.

5. Chemistry Department, Shandong College of Oceanology. Shandong Pharmaceutical Industry 1974 (3):8.

6. Chin YC et al. Proceedings of the Society for Experimental Biology and Medicine 1949 70:158.

7. Laboratory of Beijing Institute of Tuberculosis. Tuberculosis 1973 (1):27.

8. Materia Medica Section, Bacteriology-Immunology Department. Tuberculosis 1974 (1):3.

9. Beijing Coordinating Research Group on <Jiuhua>. Tuberculosis 1973 (1):29.

10. Michener HD et al. Archives of Biochemistry 1948 19:199.

11. Wallen VR et al. Chemical Abstracts 1952 46:5140e.

12. Zafir M. Chemical Abstracts 1964 60:7142a.

13. Carson JF. Journal of the American Chemical Society 1951 73:1850.

14. Barboriak J et al. Chemical Abstracts 1965 62:5759g.

15. Hassel CH. Experientia 1950 6:462.

16. Erdmann WF. Pharmazie 1951 6:442.

17. Chin YC et al. Journal of Clinical Investigation 1949 28:909.

18. Sacks LE et al. Proceedings of the Society for Experimental Biology and Medicine 1951 76:234.

19. Glistscher EA et al. Pharmazie 1953 8:950.

20. Livaditi C et al. Compt Rend Soc Biol 1949 143:1474.

21. Livaditi C et al. Compt Rend Soc Biol 1950 144:474.

22. Staven-Grouberg A. Chemical Abstracts 1933 27:136(9).

23. Leclere H. Presse Med 1934 42:1652.

24. Strenkovskaya AG. Chemical Abstracts 1970 73:2162k.

25. Rusiecki W. Chemical Abstracts 1938 32:303(8).

26. Zafir M. Chemical Abstracts 1965 63:1130f.

27. Hansel R et al. Arzneimettel Forschung 1967 17(1):79.

28. Chury J. Chemical Abstracts 1961 55:10610a.

29. Bednar J et al. Chemical Abstracts 1961 55:18894i.

30. Fernand C et al. Chemical Abstracts 1970 72:41267x.

31. Nitta G et al. The Journal of Society for Oriental Medicine in Japan 1958 9(3)93.

32. Steidle H. Archives of Experimental Pathology and Pharmacy 1931 161:154.

33. Chin YC et al. Archives Internationales de Pharmacodynamie et de Therapie 1950 82:1.

34. Farber SM et al. Disease of the Chest 1950 18(1):10.

35. Erdmann WF. Pharmazie 1952 7:75.

36. Beijing Coordinating Research Group on Clinical Trial of Jiuhuasu. Tuberculosis 1974 (1):35.

37. Internal Medicine Research Department. Tuberculosis 1972 (1):14.

38. Qingdao Research Group on New Chinese Medicine. Yimeng Yiyao (Yimeng Medical Journal) 1973 (1):25.

39. Guiyang Hospital of Tuberculosis. Medical Information (Guizhou Health Bureau) 1973 (5):24.

40. Beijing Institute of Tuberculosis. Tuberculosis 1973 (1):23.

41. Beijing Coordinating Research Group on <Jiuhua>. Selected Information on Combined Western and Traditional Chinese Medicine. Medical Information Unit of Beijing Health Bureau. 1975. p. 20.

42. Tuberculosis Department, Fushun Third Hospital. Health Journal of Fushun 1974 (3):33.

43. Shanghai Second Hospital of Tuberculosis et al. Shanghai Exhibition on Achievements in Combined Western and Traditional Chinese Medicine. Shanghai Exhibition Group. 1974. p. 185.

44. Dou YF. Yiqiyiyao (Medical Journal of No. 1 Car Factory)(Staff Hospital of No. 1 Car Factory) 1978 (4):51.

45. Qingdao Research Group on New Chinese Medicine. Shandong Yiyao (Shandong Medical Journal) 1972 (3):20.

46. Tuberculosis Department, Staff Hospital of Qingdao Bureau of Textile Industry. Shandong Yiyao (Shandong Medical Journal) 1978 (8):16.

47. Shenyang Second Hospital of Tuberculosis. Medical Information (Shenyang Health Bureau) 1972 (6):7.

48. Qingdao Research Group on New Chinese Medicine. Qingdao Yiyao Keji Jianbao (Qingdao Bulletin of Medical Sciences and Technology) (Qingdao Health Bureau) 1971 (2):20.

49. Information Department of the Chinese Academy of Sciences. Keji Xiaoxi (Scientific and Technological News) 1972 (23):23.

50. Staff Hospital of Longyan Iron Mine (Xuangang, Hebei). Tuberculosis 1974 (1):43.

51. Qingdao Research Group on New Chinese Medicine (Subgroup 2). Dermatological Research Communications 1972 (4):305.

52. Qingdao Research Group on New Chinese Medicine (Subgroup 2). Dermatological Research Communications 1972 (1):37.

53. 908 Hospital of Tonghua (Jilin). Qingdao Yiyao Keji Jianbao (Qingdao Bulletin of Medical Sciences and Technology) 1972 (5):3.

54. Jimo County Leprosarium. Qingdao Yiyao Keji Jianbao (Qingdao Bulletin of Medical Sciences and Technology) 1972 (5):7.

55. Yunmenshan (Shandong) Sanatorium. Qingdao Yiyao Keji Jiangbao (Qingdao Bulletin of Medical Sciences and Technology) 1972 (5):9.

56. Yidu County Leprosarium. Qingdao Yiyao Keji Jianbao (Qingdao Bulletin of Medical Sciences and Technology) 1972 (5):13.

57. Qingdao Research Group on New Chinese Medicine (Subgroup 2). Qingdao Yiyao Keji Jianbao (Qingdao Bulletin of Medical Sciences and Technology) 1972 (7):9.

58. Infectious Diseases Department, Jiulongpo Railways Hospital of Chongqing. Chongqing Yiyao (Chongqing Medical Journal) 1973 (4):25.

59. Infectious Diseases Department, Jiulongpo Railways Hospital of Chongqing. Chongqing Yiyao (Chongqing Medical Journal) 1975 (6):55.

60. Beijing Coordinating Research group on <Jiuhua>. Tuberculosis 1974 (1):39.

61. Communications on New Drug Market Research (New Drug Market Research Department of Shanghai Medical and Pharmaceutical Company) 1976 (1):9.

62. Tang ZM. Communications on New Drug Market Research (New Drug Market Research Department of Shanghai Medical and Pharmaceutical Company) 1972 (2):34.

63. Pharmacy of Traditional Chinese Medicine, Shanghai Second Hospital of Tuberculosis. Pharmaceutical Industry 1972 (2):20.

64. Shanghai Second Hospital of Tuberculosis. Chinese Traditional and Herbal Drugs Communications 1972 (2):45.

65. Shanghai Second Hospital of Tuberculosis. Shanghai Exhibition on Achievements in Combined Western and Traditional Chinese Medicine. Shanghai Exhibition Group. 1974. p. 232.

66. Staff Hospital of Longyan Iron Mine (Xuangang, Hebei). Tuberculosis 1974 (1):42.

67. New Chinese Medicine Department, Staff Hospital of Xuanhua Steel Works. References on Tuberculosis (Beijing Institute of Tuberculosis) 1976 (3):43.

68. Beijing Coordinating Research Group on Jiuhuasu Therapy of Silicosis and Silicotuberculosis. Notes on Science and Technology (236 Logistics Unit of the Chinese PLA) 1975 (3):8.

69. Yang SH. Heilongjiang Yiyao (Heilongjiang Medical Journal) 1979 (3):59.

70. Qingdao Central Research Group on Senile Chronic Bronchitis. Qingdao Yiyao Keji Jianbao (Qingdao Bulletin of Medical Sciences and Technology) 1971 (3):6.

71. Qingdao Research Group on New Chinese Medicine. Qingdao Yiyao Keji Jianbao (Qingdao Bulletin of Medical Sciences and Technology) 1971 (3):17.

72. Mu RW et al. Chinese Journal of Dermatology 1957 (3):201.

(Deng Wenlong)

SHECHUANGZI 蛇牀子

<Shechuangzi> refers to the fruit of *Cnidium monnieri* (L.) Cusson (Umbelliferae). It has a pungent and bitter flavor with a "warm" property. It is noted for its astringent, anthelmintic and antipruritic effects. Thus, it is used to treat leukorrhea in pruritus vulvae, trichomonas vaginitis, eczema, skin pruritus, and impotence.

CHEMICAL COMPOSITION

<Shechuangzi> contains 1.3% of volatile oil which mainly contains 1-pinene, 1-camphene and bornyl isovalerate. It also contains coumarins osthol, columbianetin, cnidimine (edultin) and cnidiadin.

PHARMACOLOGY

1. Antitrichomonal Effect

At the concentration of 1:2 the <Shechuangzi> fluidextract was found to have trichomonacidal activity *in vitro* (1). But other literature reported that no trichomonacidal action was exhibited *in vitro* by osthol, or the 10 and 20% decoctions of this herb (2,3).

2. Sex Hormone-Like Effect

Subcutaneous injection of the herb fluidextract at 20 mg once daily to mice for 32 days prolonged the estrus period and shortened the anestrus period. In case of sterilized mice, daily administration of the same dosage for 21 days led to the return of estrus period and increased the weight of the uterus and ovary (4). By weighing the prostate, seminal vesicle, and levator ani, it was shown that the <Shechuangzi> extract had androgenic effects in mice as evidenced by the increase in weights of these specimens (5).

3. Antifungal and Antiviral Effects

In vitro studies showed that <Shechuangzi> inhibited *Epidermophyton floccosum*, *Microsporum gypseum*, and *Microsporum lanosum* (6). It also prolonged the life of chicken embryos inoculated with the New castle virus for 6 hours (7).

4. Miscellaneous Actions

The <Shechuangzi> powder can kill wrigglers and houseflies (8,9).

CLINICAL STUDIES

1. Trichomonal Vaginitis

Vaginal application of the decoction (10), powder (11), or extract (12,13) of <Shechuangzi> had therapeutic value in trichomonal vaginitis. When used in the treatment of profuse leukorrhea in nontrichomonal vaginitis, the medications reduced leukorrhea, abated cervical erosion and markedly alleviated pruritus.

2. Skin Eczema

The <Shechuangzi> ointment had an astringent effect in infantile eczema (14). One case of skin candidiasis had been effectively treated with the 20% ointment of this herb (15).

REFERENCE

1. Ob-Gyn Section, Hunan Medical College. Bulletin of Hunan Medical College 1958(Inaugural Issue):48.

2. Wang FC et al. Chinese Pharmaceutical Bulletin 1959 7(12):621.

3. Parasitology Section, Henan Medical College. Acta Academiae Medicinae Hunan 1960 (7):23.

4. Folia Pharmacologica Japonica 1959 55(6):153.

5. Miwa T. Folia Pharmacologica Japonica 1960 56(3):96.

6. Zheng WF. Chinese Medical Journal 1952 38(4):315.

7. Gao SY. Science Record 1951 4(1):77.

8. Lin ZL et al. Chinese Pharmaceutical Bulletin 1959 (4):187.

9. Hong BZ. Zhongji Yikan (Intermediate Medical Journal) 1960 (6):72.

10. Gui CH. Journal of Traditional Chinese Medicine 1950 (5):250.

11. Jiang YM. Chinese Pharmaceutical Bulletin 1959 7(8):393.

12. Nanjing College of Pharmacy. Acta Pharmaceutica Sinica 1966 13(2):99.

13. Yu KJ et al. Bulletin of Chinese Materia Medica 1956 (6):229.

14. Guo DJ. Chinese Journal of Dermatology 1957 (2):154.

15. Liu MR et al. Chinese Journal of Dermatology 1959 (6):400.

(Wang Jingsi)

YEBAIHE AND DAZHUSHIDOU 野百合與大豬屎豆

<Yebaihe>, also known as <Nongjili>, refers to the plant and seed of *Crotalaria sessiliflora* L. (Leguminosae). <Dazhushidou> or <Dazhushiqing> refers to the plant and seed of *C. assamica* Benth. The herbs have a bitter and bland flavor with a "mild" property and are toxic. They are ascribed with latent-heat-clearing, antipyretic, diuretic, detoxicant and anti-inflammatory effect. The herbs are prescribed in dysentery, sores, furuncles, and malnutrition in children. Recently, it has been tried in the treatment of cancer.

CHEMICAL COMPOSITION

The seed and whole herb of *C. sessiliflora* and *C. assamica* contain about 7 kinds of alkaloids. The major alkaloids are monocrotalines I and II; the latter is a dipyrridine derivative of retronecine and platynecic acid (trans,2S,3R) (1).

It was preliminarily shown that nongjili alkaloid A (Beijing), monocrotaline (Shandong), dayezhuzhiqing alkaloid (Hubei) and monocrotaline (Zhejiang) all are actually monocrotaline I (1–5) (collectively called monocrotaline thereafter).

The seed of *C. sessiliflora* contains 0.2% of monocrotaline and that of *C. assamica* 3% (1–3). Eight monocrotaline derivatives were recently synthesized; 3 of them were shown to have antineoplastic activity (1).

PHARMACOLOGY

1. Antineoplastic Effect

In vitro experiments showed that monocrotaline 100 μg/ml inhibited the growth of human hepatoma BEL-7402 strain cells, turning them spherical with shrunken and deeply stained nucleus, and producing large and deformed cells (6). It also inhibited the growth of KB cells at an ED_{50} of > 100 μg/ml (7). *In vivo* studies showed that monocrotaline at 5–100 mg/kg IV, IP or IM once or once daily for 3–5 days produced an inhibition rate of 70–100% against Walker carcinoma 256 in rats; the ED_{50} was approximately 8.6–9.8 mg/kg and the chemotherapeutic index was over 16. Daily injection of the same agent 2–3.4 mg/kg IP to mice for 10 days resulted in an inhibition rate of 59–70% against sarcoma 180. A strong inhibitory action was also demonstrated by this agent against sarcoma 37, lymphosarcoma ascitic type L_1, Ehrlich ascites carcinoma, metastatic Lewis lung cancer, melanoma B_{16}, reticulocytic leukemia L_{615}, and lymphocytic leukemia L_{1210} in mice as well as against plasma cell tumor and adenoma 755 in hamster; the chemotherapeutic index was greater than 5 for leukemia L_{1210} and greater than 3 for adenoma 755 (2–7). Several monocrotaline derivatives, including methylsulfonyl monocrotaline, ethyl formyl monocrotaline chloride, and monocrotaline N-oxide exhibited potent inhibitory action against rat Walker carcinoma 256, but they were not recommended for clinical trial on account of their high toxicity (1).

Monocrotaline and similar compounds were converted in the body into their corresponding pyrrolizidine derivatives which selectively alkylated specific areas of the cellular DNA molecule, i.e., cross-linking with DNA molecules, thereby disrupting the advance of the cells from the S to the M phase. Monocrotaline also caused deformities or breaking in the sex chromosomes of fruit flies and also the chromosomes of the root-tip cells of broad beans, producing various biological effects like those induced by ionizing radiation. Monocrotaline also intercalated into specific sites of the DNA molecule to from complexes, thus inhibiting the replication and transcription of DNA.

Monocrotaline also alkylated the nicotinamide of intracellular coenzyme A molecules, causing impairment of cellular oxidation; it also acted on ribosomes, thereby interfering with the biosynthesis of protein. Since its effects were initiated rapidly and significantly both in highly-susceptible cancer and liver cells, damage to normal liver cells by this drug could hardly be precluded (3,4,6,8,9).

2. Effect on the Heart and Blood Vessels

Monocrotaline at 100–500 µg/ml briefly inhibited the isolated rabbit heart. High concentrations caused cardiac arrest. Injection of monocrotaline 2–6 mg/kg IV to dogs rapidly decreased the blood pressure by 15–50%; the degree and duration of hypotension were directly proportional to the dosage employed. Normal readings were restored 10–45 minutes after discontinuation of medication. All the effects on the heart beat and blood pressure were blocked by atropine 1 mg/kg (10).

3. Effect on Smooth Muscles

Monocrotaline 10–20 µg/ml caused increases in the tone and contraction amplitude of isolated rabbit and guinea pig ilea, and in the contraction of guinea pig and rat uteri. These effects could be blocked by atropine, and monocrotaline exhibited no synergism with acetylcholine. At 50–100 µg/ml, monocrotaline rapidly induced prolonged contraction of the dog trachea strip; this action was also blocked by atropine (10).

4. Effect on Respiration

Injection of monocrotaline 2–6 mg/kg IV to dogs briefly and weekly inhibited the rate and depth of respiration (10).

5. Pharmacokinetics

Monocrotaline and its N-oxide appeared rapidly in the blood after administration of monocrotaline to various kinds of animals (rabbit, rat, mouse) intravenously, intramuscularly, or intragastrically. Colorimetry revealed that peak blood level appeared 5 minutes after an intravenous injection and the drug disappeared relatively fast. A similar result was observed following intramuscular injection though the elimination was slower, and the blood level persisted for about 1–2 hours. Following intragastric administration the drug also appeared in the blood quickly, but the peak level was lower and the elimination slow. The drug was still detectable in the blood 72 hours after any of these three routes of administration. Monocrotaline was mainly distributed in the viscera including the liver, lungs, and kidneys and had a very serious cumulative effect. The metabolism of this alkaloid in the body was rather complicated; there were hydrolysis, oxidation and pyrrolizidine metabolites (2). A paper reported that monocrotaline was metabolized in the body into retronecine and dehydroretronecine; the latter can alkylate the mercaptyl group of cysteine and glutathione (11). The original compound, monocrotaline, and its metabolites were excreted mainly in the urine; however, the 72-h urinary excretion accounted for only 8–17% of the administered drug. As late as 22–90 days after discontinuation of medication, the original drug, monocrotaline, and its metabolites could still be detected in the urine of patients (2).

6. Toxicity

The LD_{50} of monocrotaline in mice was 296 ± 51 mg/kg IP and in rats was 130 mg/kg IM. Rabbits given 45–85 mg/kg IM died in 15–18 days. Daily injection of monocrotaline 8–10 mg/kg IV or IM to dogs for 7 days did not result in any significant toxic reactions, but increasing the dosage to 18–80 mg/kg killed the test animals. The toxic symptoms were referrable mainly to the liver: elevation of SGPT, decreased ability to synthesize albumin, increase in copper reserve, ascite formation, hemorrhage and necrosis in liver tissue, cessation of hepatocellular mitosis, formation of large hepatocytes, suppression of hematopoiesis, decrease in WBC and platelet counts, pulmonary hemorrhage, blood stasis, and renal parenchymal damage. The latent period of monocrotaline poisoning was rather long, and toxic symptoms might appear long after discontinuation of treatment. Therefore, caution should be exercised when using the drug clinically (2–5).

Some workers discovered that prolonged (4–12 months) and intermittent injection of monocrotaline 5 mg/kg SC to rats would induce cancer of the liver, lungs and striated muscle, acute granulocytic leukemia, or adenoma of the lungs. A large dose 40 mg/kg injected subcutaneously to rats resulted after 500 days in a very high incidence of cancer of the islets of Langerhans (8,12–15). A metabolite of monocrotaline, dehydroretronecine, was also found to be carcinogenic (15). Therefore, this alkaloid should be used with extreme caution.

Experiments proved that 1-cysteine, dimercapto sodium succinate, glycyrrhetic acid and the "Niuhuang Qingxin Wan" (Bovine Bezoar Sedative Pill) afforded protective and detoxicant effects in monocrotaline poisoning. However, the antineoplastic effect of monocrotaline was affected to certain extents by the mercapto compounds and glycyrrhetic acid (2,3,5).

CLINICAL STUDIES

The crude preparation of <Nongjili> and monocrotaline were mainly used externally to treat 708 cases of various kinds of neoplasms including 194 cases of skin cancer also treated by injection of these drug into the tumor bases (including 120 cases with monocrotaline, 19 cases with the whole plant preparation, and 55 cases with the whole plant plus the alkaloid), and 150 cases of cervical cancer. Both skin and cervical cancers benefitted from the treatment as evidenced by shrinking of the tumor and symptomatic improvement. Individual patients obtained good results. The intramuscular and intravenous injections were also efficacious on cancers of the stomach, esophagus, lungs, rectum, breast, and liver, as well as on hematological neoplasms. However, systemic use of these drugs was contraindicated owing to their extreme toxicity to the liver (2,3,5).

Dosage and administration. External application supplemented by local injection into the tumor base was used in skin and cervical cancers, whereas intravenous or intramuscular injection was useful in other tumors. Monocrotaline ointment, suppository, and crystalline powder, or crushed whole plant can be applied to the tumor surface or cervix. Monocrotaline Injection 50 mg/ampoule or injection containing 4 g of crude drug/ampoule can be injected into the tumor base, or via intravenous or intramuscular route, once a day or on alternate days for 30 days as a course, generally for 2–4 courses. The average total dose of the alkaloid was 3–4 g (3,4,6).

ADVERSE EFFECTS

Systemic use of these drugs triggered serious adverse effects. A statistical study of 284 cases (3.5%) showed 10 cases had serious toxic reactions with prominent symptoms of toxic hepatitis syndrome. Anorexia and abdominal distention appeared first, followed by hepatomegaly, jaundice, ascites, and in severe cases hepatic coma, leading to irreversible liver damage and subsequent death (3,4,6).

REFERENCE

1. Huang L et al. Acta Pharmaceutica Sinica 1980 15(5):278.
2. Shandong Institute of Medical Sciences. Selected Information on Scientific Research (1965–1977). Vol. 3. Shandong Institute of Medical Sciences. 1980. p. 1.
3. Shandong Institute of Traditional Chinese Medicine and Materia Medica. Studies on Traditional Chinese Medicine (Shandong Institute of Traditional Chinese Medicine and Materia Medica) 1976 (10):1.
4. Tumor Research Unit, Wuhan Medical College. Chinese Medical Journal 1973 (8):472.
5. Zhejiang Coordinating Research Group on Tumor. Chinese Traditional and Herbal Drugs Communications 1972 (2):11.
6. Du CZ et al. Zhongliu Fangzhi Yanjiu (Researches on Prevention and Treatment of Cancer) 1979 (6):6.
7. Kupchan SM et al. Journal of Pharmaceutical Sciences 1964 53:343.

8. Mclean EK. Pharmacological Review 1970 22:429.

9. Culvenor CC et al. Nature 1962 195:570.

10. Garg KN et al. Indian Journal of Medical Research 1962 50(3):435.

11. Robertson KA et al. Cancer Research 1977 37:3141.

12. Schoental R et al. Brit Cancer 1955 9:229.

13. Schoental R et al. Cancer Research 1968 28:2237.

14. Clark AM. Nature 1959 183:731.

15. Allen JR et al. Cancer Research 1957 35:997.

(Zeng Qingtian)

YEJUHUA 野菊花

<Yejuhua> refers to the capitulum of *Dendranthema indicum* (L.) Des Monl. (*Chrysanthemum indicum* L.), or *D. boreale* (Makino) Ling (*C. boreale* Mak., *C. lavandulaefolium* Mak.) (Compositae). These plants or their leaves are also used as medicine. <Yejuhua> is also called <Yehuangju>, or <Kuyi>. It is bitter and slightly "cold". <Yejuhua> is reputed to be hepatic-depressing, latent-heat-clearing, antipyretic, detoxicant and anti-inflammatory. It is a useful drug for acute conjunctivitis, headache and vertigo, carbuncle, furuncle, and erysipelas, especially at the onset.

CHEMICAL COMPOSITION

The flower and the whole plant contain volatile oil which is mainly composed of camphor. The volatile oil also contains α-pinene, carvone, limonene, camphene, eucalyptol, borneol, and angelic acid esters. The herb also contains linarin, luteolin glycosides, yejuhua lactone, chrysanthemin, chrysanthemum pigments, coumarins and polysaccharides. The flower bud contains two bitter principles, yejuhua lactone and arteglasin-A.

PHARMACOLOGY

1. Hypotensive Effect

The aqueous solution of the ethanol extract of <Yejuhua> given IP or PO to unanesthetized rats and anesthetized cats and dogs produced a significant hypotensive effect. Intra-intestinal injection of the refined extract of the ethanol extract (containing the crystalline yejuhua lactone, flavonoid glycoside, bitters and some impurities) 50–100 mg to anesthetized cats produced a hypotensive area of 19 to 22% within 2 hours but no significant effect on the heart rate and respiration. A fall in the blood pressure was also triggered by an intragastric dose of 100–150 mg/kg in normal dogs, or by 3 weeks of daily intragastric doses of 100–200 mg/kg in dogs with chronic renal hypertension. The hypotensive action was characterized by a slow onset and prolonged effect, unaccompanied by serious toxic reactions. Studies on the hypotensive action of the 95, 50, and 25% ethanol extracts and the aqueous extract of <Yejuhua> revealed that, in anesthetized cats, the lower the concentration of ethanol, the poorer the effect, whereas the aqueous extract was essentially inactive. The whole plant preparation had a poor hypotensive action (1,2,3).

The intraperitoneal dose of the aqueous solution of the <Yejuhua> fluidextract decreased the blood pressure even in spinal cats; it also inhibited the pressor response to blockade of the carotid arterial blood flow. These studies also proved that this herb had no significant effect on nerve ganglions and muscarinic receptors and that it had adrenergic antagonistic effect. Intraperitoneal administration to anesthetized dogs did not reduce the cardiac output but dilated the blood vessels and lowered the total peripheral resistance and blood pressure. Injection of this solution not exceeding 36 g/kg IP did not modify the ECG of conscious rats. To sum up, the hypotensive effect was not attributable to reduced cardiac output, blockade of the sympathetic ganglions or vagal reflex. It was causally related to adrenergic blockade, dilation of the peripheral blood vessels, and possibly inhibition of the vasomotor center (1,2).

2. Effect on the Cardiovascular System

<Yejuhua> preparations markedly increased the myocardial uptake of ^{131}Cs in dogs with experimental myocardial infarction or myocardial ischemia (4). The ethyl acetate extract of the alcohol-precipitated decoction of this herb (containing mainly flavones, phenols and lactones) 80 mg/kg injected intravenously to anesthetized healthy dogs increased the coronary flow by 49.6% and decreased the coronary resistance by 45.8%. Its effect lasted about 10 minutes. Concurrently, the drug decreased the heart rate, blood pressure and peripheral resistance, increased the cardiac output and stroke volume, and decreased the left ventricular work; these changes were all significant as compared to premedication determinations. In multiple contact points pericardial ECG, using the number of leads with ST elevation and the grand sum of elevation as criteria, with normal saline for both pre- and post-medication and intergroup comparison, the <Yejuhua> extract at the above mentioned dosage protected dogs from myocardial ischemia induced by ligation of the anterior left descending coronary branch. Other hemodynamic alterations resulting from this medication were the same as in healthy dogs, except that the increase in the coronary flow was more conspicuous. In addition, the <Yejuhua> extract also increased the renal blood flow by 51.5% and decreased the renal vascular resistance by 47.1%; its effect lasted more than 20 minutes (5,6). The <Yejuhua> injection at 2 g(crude drug)/kg IV significantly protected dogs from experimental myocardial ischemia; this effect was found to be stronger than that of propranolol 1 mg/kg (7).

3. Antimicrobial Effect

At the concentration of 1:5 the decoction of <Yejuhua> or of the leafy branch of the plant inhibited *Shigella dysenteriae in vitro*; the leafy branch also inhibited *Salmonella typhi* (8). The <Yejuhua> decoction inhibited many other pathogenic bacteria; the MIC was found to be between 1:10 and 1:80. High concentrations exhibited different degrees of inhibitory effect against many skin fungi (9–12). Some compounds or preparations of the herb grown in certain areas inhibited *Mycobacterium tuberculosis* var. *hominis* H_{37}RV strain at the MIC of around 1:1000. Yet, these was no significant therapeutic effect observed from its subcutaneous dose in mice infected with this bacterial strain (13). A stronger bacteriostatic action was exhibited by the whole plant than by the flower, and the fresh herb was more potent than the dried one. Heat treatment (e.g. autoclaving) weakened its effect (8,11).

The <Yejuhua> decoction also delayed the pathological change in the cells of the primary monolayer culture of the epithelial cells of the human embryonic kidney or lung induced by $ECHO_{11}$ virus, herpes virus, and influenza virus Jingke 68-1 strain, but it was inactive against parainfluenza virus (Xiantai strain), adenovirus type 3 and rhinovirus types 17 and 20 (14,15). In addition, <Yejuhua> was found to have a similar inhibitory effect against different types of leptospirae *in vitro*, the decoction being more potent than the ethanol extract (16,17).

4. Enhancement of Leukocytic Phagocytosis

In vitro studies showed that the <Yejuhua> decoction at a concentration of 1:1280 enhanced the phagocytic function of human leukocytes against *Staphylococcus aureus*, but its aqueous distillate was inactive (18).

5. Miscellaneous Actions

Intraperitoneal injection of the alcohol-precipitated decoction of <Yejuhua> 50 or 150 mg to mice, which were poisoned by the venom of many-banded krait (*Bungarus multicinctus*) or cobra (*Naja naja*), reduced the mortality rate as compared to the control, but it had no therapeutic value against poisoning caused by *Agkistrodon acutus* venom (19).

6. Toxicity

The aqueous solution of <Yejuhua> fluidextract injected to conscious rats at a dose < 36 g/kg IP did not change the ECG and animal activity. Increasing the dosage to 52 g/kg produced marked reduction in the heart rate, prolongation of PR and QT intervals, and widening and blunting of T waves. Death occurred 4 hours later. According to a preliminary study, the LD of this agent was ninefold of the ED (2). The acute LD_{50} of the ethyl acetate extract of the alcohol-precipitated decoction of <Yejuhua> injected into the caudal vein of mice was determined to be 1669 ± 188 mg/kg; the poisoned animals developed paroxysmal convulsion and finally died of respiratory paralysis (6). Except occasional vomiting, no serious toxic effects or significant changes in the food intake, body weight, ECG, and serum bromsulphalein sodium retention were resulted by intragastric administration of the refined <Yejuhua> ethanol extract 300 mg/kg daily to dogs for 3 weeks. The blood nonprotein nitrogen was increased to 53 mg% at the end of treatment. Post-treatment pathological examination revealed no significant abnormalities except mild interstitial nephritis, granular degeneration of renal convoluted tubules, and local breaking of the smooth muscle fibres of the tunica media of the renal artery (3). The whole plant preparations were more toxic than the flower extract. Chronic use of this flower would not result in accumulation poisoning (2,20).

CLINICAL STUDIES

1. Hypertension

Preliminary studies of 35 cases of stages I, II and III of hypertension treated with 2 ml of <Yejuhua> fluidextract (equivalent to 4 g of crude drug) thrice daily by mouth revealed excellent effect in 6 cases and improvement in 18 cases. Improvement of symptoms such as insomnia, sensation of head distention, headache, vertigo, etc. was achieved (1). The decoction prepared from <Yejuhua> plus the root of *Uncaria rhyncophylla* and the flower-spike of *Prunella vulgaris*, or with the ripe seed of *Cassia tora* and the whole plant of *Plantago asiatica*, was also useful in stages I and II of hypertension. In recent years, some antihypertensive prescriptions containing chiefly <Yejuhua>, including the most well-known "Juming Antihypertensive Tablet" (21) and "Huaiju Shanzha Yanzhu Decoction" (22), have been reported to lower blood pressure to different extents and to improve symptoms in essential hypertension and chronic renal hypertension.

2. Prophylaxis of Common Cold, Influenza, and Epidemic Cerebrospinal Meningitis.

Administration of <Yejuhua> and the compound prescriptions in which this herb is a major component reduced the incidence and ameliorated the symptoms of common cold and influenza. The decoction and tablets prepared from it are the commonly used oral preparations. Some authors prescribed the herb together with the rhizome of *Imperata cylindrica* var. *major* or with the whole plant of *Bidens bipinnata*. Others used it with the whole plant of *Mentha haplocalyx* and the root of *Platycodon grandiflorum* (23–29). The <Yejuhua> nasal ointment is available for external use (30). Throat culture, conducted on the third day of spraying the throat of 78 meningococcus carriers with 2 ml of the 50% <Yejuhua> decoction, showed 82% to be negative for the bacteria. All the remaining positive cases became negative after another one or two sprayings (31). This treatment was claimed effective as a prophylactic measure against influenza, epidemic meningitis, scarlet fever, and measles (32).

3. Bronchitis

An injection was prepared from the volatile substance from the distillate of the stem and leaf of the plant minus the ethanol-insoluble insoluble portion. It was injected intramuscularly to 100 cases of acute bronchitis, producing excellent effect in 88. It was reported to markedly ameliorate fever, cough and asthma (33). The combination of <Yejuhua> and the vine of *Luffa cylindrica* was shown to be effective in chronic bronchitis of the elderly (34).

4. Furuncle, Abscess, etc.

<Yejuhua>, or the "Wuwei Xiaodu Decoction" (Detoxifying Decoction of Five Herbs) (Flos Chrysanthemi Indici, Flos Lonicerae, Herba Taraxaci, Herba Violae, and Semen Semiaquilegiae),

or <Yejuhua> and the sclerotium of *Poria cocos* or the browned fruit of *Gardenia jasminoides*, the leaf of *Morus alba*, and the whole plant of *Plantago asiatica* are recommended for oral use (35–39). The fresh herb including the stem and leaf may be crushed and applied locally, or its decoction used as a wash (40). The calcinated root of *C. indicum* with small quantities of borneol and tea oil may be applied to furuncles on the face (41). <Yejuhua> decocted with the flower of *Sesamum indicum* and calcinated alum may be used as soaking and washing lotions, and as hot compress in treating eczema (42). The 20% <Yejuhua> oil had been used to treat external bacterial infection or to prevent traumatic wound infection (32).

5. Other Inflammatory Diseases

<Yejuhua> was also used in stomatitis, tonsillitis, parotitis, enteritis, appendicitis, mastitis, epidemic conjunctivitis, hordeolum, and cervical erosion. Better responses were obtained in the acute than in the chronic cases. The herb is often used orally with the whole plant of *Taraxacum mongolicum*, the root of *Clematis chinensis*, the mature spores of *Lygodium japonicum*, the flower bud of *Lonicera japonica*, and the rhizome of *Imperata cylindrica* var. *major*. The extract and fluidextract of the herb, as well as the crushed fresh whole plant may be used locally (38,43–47). The <Yejuhua> suppository was efficacious in pelvic infection (48). It is reported that inflammatory diseases responded to intramuscular or acupoint injection, or local use of the ointment of the crystalline or liquid portion obtained under normal temperature from the volatile oil of the fresh flower, or the whole plant minus the flower (49–53). The effect of the <Yejuhua> injection in the treatment of tuberculosis of lymph nodes or tuberculous pelvic infection was reported to be insignificant (54,55).

ADVERSE EFFECTS

The decoction or ethanol extract of <Yejuhua> given orally produced mild action and few side effects. A few patients may develop digestive symptoms such as gastric discomfort, poor appetite, borborygmus, and mushy stool (8,26,43). The intramuscular injection may occasionally cause mild diarrhea; injection to the posterior fornix vaginae may cause irritation (55).

REFERENCE

1. Shanghai Institute of Hypertension. Compiled Information on Hypertension Research. 1st edition. 1959. pp. 11, 14, 116.

2. Sun QX et al. Acta Physiologica Sinica 1959 23(3):254.

3. Liu JF et al. Acta Pharmaceutica Sinica 1962 9(3):151.

4. Chen KY et al. Zhejiang Zhongyiyao (Zhejiang Journal of Traditional Chinese Medicine) 1979 (10):377.

5. Li LD et al. Abstracts of the First National Symposium on Cardiovascular Pharmacology. 1980. p. 22.

6. Li LD et al. The active constituents of Chrysanthemum indicum flower. II. The effects of the extract of Chrysanthemum indicum flower (CI-2) on the hemodynamics and experimental myocardial infarction in dogs. In: Proceedings of the First National Symposium on Cardiovascular Pharmacology. 1980.

7. Li LD et al. Journal of Traditional Chinese Medicine 1980 21(11):68.

8. Xia XH et al. Chinese Medical Journal 1962 48(3):188.

9. Laboratory Group. Xinzhongyi (Journal of New Chinese Medicine) 1971 (2):30.

10. Senile Chronic Bronchitis Research Group of Suzhou Medical College. Scientific Research Information (Suzhou Medical College) 1971 (5):50.

11. Lingling District Sanitation and Anti-epidemic Station et al. Hunan Yiyao Zazhi (Hunan Medical Journal) 1974 (4):60.

12. Chen FR. Bulletin of Microbiology 1978 5(4):14.

13. Yan BS et al. Chinese Journal of Tuberculosis and Respiratory Diseases 1980 3(2):68.

14. Virus Section, Institute of Chinese Materia Medica of the Academy of Traditional Chinese Medicine. Xinyiyaoxue Zazhi (Journal of Traditional Chinese Medicine) 1973 (1):26.

15. Guangzhou Institute of Medicine and Health. New Medical Communications (Guangzhou Health Bureau) 1974 (1):14.

16. Microbiology Section, Luda Health School. Medicine and Health (Luda Health Bureau) 1973 (2):63.

17. Leptospirosis Research Group. Selected Information (First and Second Teaching Hospitals of Jiangsu College of New Medicine) 1974 (2):78.

18. Hangzhou Second People's Hospital. Notes on Science and Technology — Medicine and Health (Information Institute of Zhejiang Bureau of Science and Technology) 1972 (5):20.

19. Snake Bite Research Unit, Guangxi Medical College. Health Journal of Guangxi (Zhuang Autonomous Region Health Bureau, Guangxi) 1973 (2):23.

20. Pharmacology Section, Shanghai Second Hospital. Abstracts of the Third Symposium of Shanghai Second Medical College. 1959. p. 177.

21. Shiqi Pharmaceutical factory (Guangdong). Chinese Traditional and Herbal Drugs Communications 1970 (2):30.

22. Zhenhai County (Zhejiang) Group for Popularization of Chinese Traditional Drugs. Cardiovascular Diseases 1975 3(3):257.

23. Shijiazhuang (Hebei) Health Bureau. Compiled Information on the Prevention and Treatment of Common Cold and Chronic Bronchitis. 1972. p. 5.

24. Bronchitis Unit, Shenyang Eighth People's Hospital. Medical Research Communications (Tangshan District Health Bureau, Hebei) 1972 (2):88.

25. Yuanyang Pilot Area, Xinxiang District Coordinating Research Group for Compound Lepidium apetalum Seed Ointment. Journal of Barefoot Doctor (Henan Health Bureau) 1975 (12):34.

26. Shenyang Coordinating Research Group for Chrysanthemum indicum flower Therapy of Chronic Bronchitis. Liaoning Yiyao (Liaoning Medical Journal) 1974 (1):5.

27. Health Department, 6731 Unit of the Chinese PLA. People's Military Medicine (Health Division of the Logistics Department of the Chinese PLA) 1974 (7):36.

28. Chinese Traditional Drugs Research Group of Jiefang Commune (Wuxi). Jiangsu Yiyao (Jiangsu Medical Journal) 1976 (1):36.

29. Fu ZX et al. Chinese Journal of Internal Medicine 1976 (new) 1(5):279.

30. Bronchitis Group, Liaodun Teaching Hospital of Shenyang Medical College. Medical Research (Shenyang Medical College) 1977 (3):44.

31. Yan GH et al. Journal of Traditional Chinese Medicine 1960 (6):20.

32. Jiang JL et al. Medicine and Health (Luda Health Bureau) 1976 (1):76.

33. Wuji District (Shuyang County) Hospital. Jiangsu Yiyao (Jiangsu Medical Journal) 1976 (5):55.

34. Jingmen People's Hospital. Hubei Science and Technology — Medicine 1972 (2):11.

35. Yuan F. Acta Academiae Medicinae Anhui 1977 (2):62.

36. Editorial Group of "Clinical Applications of Chinese Traditional Drugs". New Chinese Medicine 1971 (6–7):75.

37. Xu KX. Jiangsu Journal of Traditional Chinese Medicine 1980 (3):41.

38. Zhang ML et al. Hunan Yiyao Zazhi (Hunan Medical Journal) 1976 3(4):55.

39. Bian GS et al. Journal of Traditional Chinese Medicine 1963 (7):277.

40. Bi ZD. Jiangxi Yiyao (Jiangxi Medical Journal) 1966 (6):222.

41. "Red" Medicine Research Group, Fengtang Middle School (Chaoan County, Guangdong). Xinzhongyi (Journal of New Chinese Medicine) 1975 (3):25.

42. Wu CW. Jiangsu Yiyao (Jiangsu Medical Journal) 1976 (5):3.

43. Zhao CB. Journal of Barefoot Doctor 1975 (9):41.

44. Qi XM. Acta Academiae Medicinae Anhui 1974 (4):26.

45. Cooperative Medical Clinic of Shuinan Production Brigade (Chengguan Commune, Yongxing County). Hunan Yiyao Zazhi (Hunan Medical Journal) 1977 4(2):56.

46. Lu DM. Zhejiang Zhongyiyao (Zhejiang Journal of Traditional Chinese Medicine) 1979 (9):322.

47. Dong SY. Chinese Journal of Obstetrics and Gynecology 1958 6(6):537.

48. Wang Q. Studies on Chinese Proprietary Medicines 1980 (1):3.

49. Jingzhu Commune Health Centre (Guangji County, Hubei). Xinzhongyi (Journal of New Chinese Medicine) 1974 (2):32.

50. Jinqiao Production Brigade Health Post (Maji Commune, Yizheng County). Jiangsu Yiyao (Jiangsu Medical Journal) 1976 (6):35.

51. Cooperative Medical Clinic of Heshang Production Brigade (Taiping Commune, Xinjin County). Medicine and Health (Luda Health Bureau) 1975 (1):45.

52. Zhang ZL. Barefoot Doctor (Henan Health Bureau) 1976 (10):56.

53. Red Cross Hospital of Chongqing. New Chinese Medicine 1971 (5):32.

54. Dai GW. Antituberculosis Communications (1976–77). Beijing Hospital of Tuberculosis. 1978. p. 15.

55. Ob-Gyn Department, Capital Hospital of the Chinese Academy of Medical Sciences. Antituberculosis Communications (1976–77). Beijing Hospital of Tuberculosis. 1978. p. 11.

(Dai Guangjun)

YINXING 銀杏

<Yinxing> refers to the fruit of *Ginkgo biloba* L. (Ginkgoaceae). Also called <Baiguo>, the herb is sweet, bitter and puckery. It has a "mild" property and is slightly toxic. It is known for its lung-astringent, antiasthmatic, enuresis-quenching and antileukorrheal actions and is, therefore, used to treat cough and dyspnea (due to lung asthenia), enuresis, and leukorrhea.

CHEMICAL COMPOSITION

The kernel and the outer seed coat contain ginkgolic acid, hydroginkgolic acid, hydroginkgolinic acid, ginkgol, bilobol, ginnol and ginkgotoxin. The kernel contains traces of hydrocyanic acid.

PHARMACOLOGY

1. Effect on the Respiratory System

Intraperitoneal injection of the ethanol extract of <Yinxing> to mice increased phenol red excretion in the respiratory tract, suggesting a possible expectorant action. The intragastric dose had no significant antitussive effect in mice with cough induced by ammonia spray. It exhibited a weak relaxant effect on the isolated smooth muscle of guinea pigs (1). In comparison with the control, Compound Gingkgo Spray, used to treat experimental chronic bronchitis induced in mice by sulfur dioxide, improved the secretory function of the bronchial mucous membrane, and decreased the goblet cells, mucous secretion, and inflammatory affections (2).

2. Effect on the Circulatory System

Bilobol 500 mg/kg was inactive on the frog heart but produced transient hypotension in rabbits. It increased the capillary permeability, most significantly in guinea pigs, and next in rats and rabbits. Perfusion of bilobol into the rat hind limb triggered histamine release, which in turn increased the capillary permeability, causing edema. This action was antagonized by chlorpheniramine (3). The effect of ginkgotoxin on the isolated frog heart was characterized by an initial stimulation succeeded by inhibition, and even cardiac arrest; low doses caused vasoconstriction, and high doses caused the opposite effect (4).

3. Antibacterial Effect

In vitro, the kernel and juice of <Yinxing>, ginkgol and, especially, ginkgolic acid were shown to inhibit *Mycobacterium tuberculosis* var. *hominis* and *M. tuberculosis* var. *bovis* (5–7). These substances were heat-stable; the antituberculous action of ginkgolic acid, however, was significantly weakened by serum (5,6). All parts of <Yinxing>, the oil soaked or non-oil soaked <Yinxing>, and ginkgolic acid had no significant therapeutic effect against experimental tuberculosis in mice (5). Despite its therapeutic effect in guinea pigs infected with *Mycobacterium tuberculosis* var. *hominis*, the <Yinxing> extract has no clinical value because of its toxicity (8,9). Many pathogenic bacteria such as *Staphylococcus aureus*, streptococcus, *Corynebacterium diphtheriae, Bacillus anthracis, Bacillus subtilis, Escherichia coli*, and *Salmonella typhi* were inhibited to different extents by <Yinxing> (6). The aqueous extract of <Yinxing> inhibited common pathogenic fungi to different extents (10).

4. Miscellaneous Actions

The aqueous extract, the active principle of which could be precipitated by methanol, suppressed glucose-6-phosphate dehydrogenase, malate dehydrogenase and isocitrate dehydrogenase (11). The kernel of <Yinxing> had an astringent action (12). The <Yinxing> extract had therapeutic effect on experimental cerebral ischemia in rats (13).

5. Toxicity

Anorexia, weight loss, different degrees of liver damage, glomerulonephritis, and even death were seen in guinea pigs given the oil-soaked <Yinxing> 3 g/kg daily for 95–113 days, or the acidic fraction of the crude extract of kernel 150–200 mg/kg daily for 60 days (9), and also in mice fed with large amounts of the kernel powder (14).

    Ginkgolic acid and ginkgotoxin were found to have hemolytic action (4,12). Ginkgotoxin exerted a paralyzing action on the CNS of frogs. Initial elevation of the blood pressure followed by hypotension, dyspnea, convulsion and death were seen in rabbits injected with ginkgotoxin 0.2 g/kg IV (4). Injection of the neutral fraction of the kernel 6 mg/kg SC to mice also resulted in convulsion and death (15).

CLINICAL STUDIES

1. Chronic Bronchitis

Compound Gingkgo Aerosol No. 1 (Semen Ginkgo, Lumbricus, Radix Scutellariae), Compound Gingkgo Aerosol No. 2 (Semen Ginkgo, Lumbricus, Herba Taraxaci), and Compound Gingkgo Tablet No. 1 (Semen Ginkgo, Lumbricus, Radix Scutellariae) were clinically evaluated in 600 cases of chronic bronchitis; an effective rate of 89–99% was attained. Aerosol No. 1 was more effective than Aerosol No. 2, and since the effect of the former was similar to that of the tablet preparation, the oral dosage is recommended (16). Antiasthmatic Decoction (Semen Ginkgo, Herba Ephedrae,

Rhizoma Pinelliae, Flos Farfarae, Cortex Mori, Fructus Perillae, Semen Armeniacae Amarum, Radix Scutellariae) was also satisfactory in relieving cough, asthma, and expectoration in patients with chronic bronchitis (17).

2. *Pulmonary Tuberculosis*

The oil-soaked <Yinxing> is a folk remedy for pulmonary tuberculosis, but its effect has not been confirmed.

ADVERSE EFFECTS

The juice and the ethanol or ether extract of <Yinxing> are extremely irritating to the skin, causing pruritus, erythema, edema, papules and pustules, which disappeared after 7–10 days, leaving scales resembling pityriasis (18). Strong skin irritation was also produced by ginkgolic acid and bilobol (12). Ginkgotoxin had mylabris-like action. Upon contact with ginkgotoxin, skin and mucous membrane developed serious inflammatory reaction. The oral doses caused severe gastrointestinal irritation and gastroenteritis. Nephritis was associated with its use as it irritated the kidney during excretion (4,12,19). *Poisoning and detoxication.* Overdosage of the kernel may cause poisoning which is more common in young children. The clinical manifestations include foamy salivation, vomiting, diarrhea, high fever and restlessness, twitching and convulsion, tonic spasm of the extremities, asymmetric and variable changes in pupil size, loss of the light reflex, pallor or flushing, and, in infants, protruding forebrain, dyspnea, unconsciousness, and even death. Emergency treatment includes gastric lavage, oral administration of sedatives and diuretics, intravenous infusion of glucose solution, and keeping the patient warm (20–23).

REFERENCE

1. 230th Hospital of the Chinese PLA. Medical Information (230th Hospital of the Chinese PLA) 1973 (1):14.

2. 230th Hospital of the Chinese PLA. Medical Information (230th Hospital of the Chinese PLA) 1973 (1):11.

3. Han DS. Chemical Abstracts 1966 65:7861c.

4. Saito J. The Tohoku Journal of Experimental Medicine 1930 16(5,6):413.

5. Yang ZC et al. Acta Academiae Medicinae Primae Shanghai 1957 (2):117.

6. Zhou YW. Chinese Medical Journal 1950 36(2):549.

7. Wang FL. Chinese Medical Journal 1950 68(5–6):169.

8. Shen QZ. Chinese Medical Journal 1956 42(7):680.

9. Pharmacy Faculty, Central Institute of Health. Kexue Tongbao (Science Bulletin) 1954 (6):43.

10. Cao RL et al. Chinese Journal of Dermatology 1957 5(4):286.

11. Vanni P et al. Chinese Journal of Dermatology 1972 48(23):1031.

12. Watt JM. Medicinal and Poisonous Plants of Southern and Eastern Africa. 2nd edition. 1962. p. 456.

13. Larsen RG et al. Chemical Abstracts 1979 90:115360t.

14. Yi HB. Acta Academiae Medicinae Primae Shanghai 1957 (1):39.

15. Chu WC. Chinese Medical Journal (Chengdu Edition) 1943 61A:171.

16. 230th Hospital of the Chinese PLA. Medical Information (230th Hospital of the Chinese PLA) 1973 (1):8.

17. Hudong Hospital of Yangpu District (Shanghai). New Chinese Medicine 1972 (9):14.

18. Saito J et al. Chemical Abstracts 1930 24:4828(8).

19. Saito J et al. The Tohoku Journal of Experimental Medicine 1930 16(5,6):385.

20. He SF. Chinese Journal of Internal Medicine 1959 7(2):157.

21. Gao YE et al. Chinese Medical Journal 1951 37(9):753.

22. Sen XZ et al. Journal of Tokyo Women's Medical College 1970 40(1–2):56.

23. Meng ZD. Chinese Journal of Paediatrics 1953 (3):192.

(Gong Xuling)

YINXINGYE 銀杏葉

<Yinxingye> is the leaf of *Ginkgo biloba* L. (Ginkgoaceae). It is sweet, bitter and puckery. It has a "mild" property and is slightly toxic. Its actions are considered to be lung-astringent, antiasthmatic, and antileukorrheal. The herb is useful in cough and asthma, leukorrhea, and in various conditions caused by adverse flow of the vital energy (*such as vomiting, nausea, vertigo, dizziness, etc.).

CHEMICAL COMPOSITION

The leaf of *G. biloba* contains flavonoids ginkgetin, isoginkgetin, bilobetin, quercetin, kaempferol, rhamnetin, isorhamnetin, and kaempferol-3-rhamnoglucoside. It also contains bilobalide, rutin, and bitter principles ginkgolides A, B and C. 3'-O-Methylmyricetin-3-rhamnoglucoside was recently isolated (1).

PHARMACOLOGY

1. Effect on the Circulatory System

The flavone compounds in <Yinxingye> could dilate the isolated coronary vessels (2) as well as the *in situ* blood vessels of the hind limb of guinea pigs and that of isolated rat hind limb (2,3). They also increased the blood flow in the carotid and pinnal arteries of rabbits (4). The therapeutic doses had no significant effect on the heart rate, blood pressure, and respiration in rats, guinea pigs, cats, and rabbits (2,5). Doses 100–1000 times the therapeutic dose caused a moderate fall in the blood pressure, acceleration of respiration, and decrease of heart rate (5). The residual extract or the total aglycones of the ethanol extract of <Yinxingye>, "Shuxuening (6911)" antagonized epinephrine-induced vasoconstriction in isolated rabbit ears (6).

2. Effect on Smooth Muscles

2.1 *Bronchial smooth muscles*. The ethanol extract of <Yinxingye> directly related the tracheal smooth muscle; it also relieved the spasmodic response of the isolated guinea pig trachea to histamine phosphate and acetylcholine, and inhibited histamine-induced asthmatic attack in guinea pigs (7). In pulmonary overflow or histamine spray experiment on guinea pigs, the flavones exhibited a bronchodilatory action which could be antagonized by propranolol, suggesting possible involvement of β-receptors (8).

2.2 *Gastrointestinal smooth muscles.* The ethanol extract of the leaf and the flavonoid glycosides had spasmolytic action on isolated intestines of guinea pigs and antagonized spasm induced by histamine, acetylcholine, and barium chloride; its potency was similar to that of papaverine but its effect was longer-lasting (2,5,6). Kaempferol and quercetin had weaker spasmolytic action than papaverine (2). Markedly enhanced intestinal peristalsis was observed in anesthetized rabbits and dogs after administration of Shuxuening (6). The bradykinin-induced stimulant effect on the ileum could be antagonized by ginkgetin (3).

3. Antibacterial Effect

In vitro experiments showed that the <Yinxingye> decoction inhibited *Staphylococcus aureus, Shigella dysenteriae*, and *Pseudomonas aeruginosa* (9).

4. Miscellaneous Actions

Ginkgetin can be used as an emollient. It can increase sebaceous secretion, giving a healthier look to the dry and senile skin (10).

5. Toxicity

Daily injection of Shuxuening to dogs at doses 10 or 40 times the human dose for one week produced gastrointestinal symptoms including salivation, nausea, vomiting, diarrhea, and impaired appetite. Histological examination revealed hypersecretion of the small intestinal mucosa. Local injection of this agent may cause vascular sclerosis, inflammation and organized thrombosis, but no abnormalities were observed in the blood picture and liver function tests (6). The flavones of <Yinxingye> did not cause any morphological changes in the heart, liver, spleen, lungs, kidneys, and arteries during subacute experiments on rabbits, guinea pigs, rats, and mice (2).

CLINICAL STUDIES

1. Atherosclerosis of Coronary Arteries

There are voluminous reports regarding the use of <Yinxingye> preparations, or its compound prescriptions, in the treatment of coronary disease. It is generally conceded that these medications produced different degrees of therapeutic effect (11–19). For instance, 32 cases treated with the Shuxuening tablet (2 mg of the total flavones/tablet), two tablets thrice daily for a course of three months, obtained a short term effective rate of 69% (11). The effective patients felt improvement of chest discomfort, angina pectoris and palpitation, and their ECG were improved.

2. Hypercholesterolemia

"Guanxintong Tablet" composed of the aqueous extract of the leaf, (1.14 mg of flavone/tablet), was used to treat 100 cases of hypercholesterolemia at the dosage of 4 tablets three times daily for 1–5 months; serum cholesterol in 88 cases with an average pretreatment level of 236 mg% was reduced by 39 mg% ($P<0.001$), on the average. This result suggests that the tablet has a significant hypocholesterolemic effect. The tablet also had an incremental effect on phospholipids, thus improving the cholesterol/phospholipid ratio, as shown by the post-treatment elevation of serum phospholipids in 65 cases (20).

Guanxintong also had an antihypertensive action in patients of hypercholesterolemia associated with hypertension (20). Moreover, the <Yinxingye> preparation (9) and the Yinchuan Hong Shu Tablet (17) also showed antihypertensive effect in the treatment of such patients.

3, Chronic Bronchitis

Senile chronic bronchitis responded satisfactorily to treatments with <Yinxingye> decoction, compound <Yinxingye> decoction, Ginkgo-Bile Tablet (Folium Ginkgo, Swine Bile) (21), and the folk prescription Liangye Yijiang Decoction (Folium Ginkgo, Folium Artemisiae Argyi, Rhizoma Zingiberis Recens) (22).

4. Parkinson Disease

The symptoms of the nervous system were improved in 9 cases of Parkinson disease after treatment with the injection containing quercetin, kaempferol, and isorhamnetin, or the oral preparation of <Ynixingye> extract. This was attributed to the increase in cerebral blood flow caused by the medications (23). In addition, <Yinxingye> preparation was also reported to be useful in cerebral thrombosis, cerebrovascular spasm (12), and peripheral arterial circulatory disorder (24).

ADVERSE EFFECTS

<Yinxingye> preparations have mild side effects. Occasional dizziness, headache, lassitude, xerostomia, dry and red tongue, chest discomfort, gastric discomfort, loss of appetite, abdominal distention, constipation, or diarrhea may occur, but generally they do not affect the completion of treatment (12,17,25).

REFERENCE

1. Geiger H. Chemical Abstracts 1980 92:55084k.
2. Peter H et al. Arzneimettel Forschung 1966 16(6):719.
3. Natarajan S et al. Chemical Abstracts 1971 74:62962b.

4. Asano M et al. Chemical Abstracts 1973 79:87548n.

5. Peter H. Chemical Abstracts 1970 72:11142k.

6. Institute of Botany, Chinese Academy of Sciences et al. Chinese Traditional and Herbal Drugs Communications 1972 (4):15.

7. Senile Chronic Bronchitis Group, Jiangxi Medical College. Reports on Senile Chronic Bronchitis. Jiangxi Medical College. 1972. p. 24.

8. Pharmacology Section, Jiangxi Medical College. Xinyiyaoxue Zazhi (Journal of Traditional Chinese Medicine) 1976 (1):43.

9. 153rd Hospital of Henan Military Region. Brief summary of the clinical efficacy of Gingko biloba leaf preparation (internal information). 1972.

10. Rovesti P. Chemical Abstracts 1974 81:126679u.

11. Coronary Disease Research Unit, First Teaching Hospital of Zhejiang College. Notes on Science and Technology — Medicine and Health (Zhejiang Centre of Medical and Health Information) 1972 (6):13.

12. Zhejiang College of Tradtional Chinese Medicine. Notes on Science and Technology — Medicine and Health (Zhejiang Centre of Medical and Health Information) 1972 (6):11.

13. Jinhua District Hospital. Notes on Science and Technology — Medicine and Health (Zhejiang Centre of Medical and Health Information) 1972 (6):17.

14. Internal Medicine Department, Chaoyang Hospital of Beijing. Special Edition on Prevention and Treatment of Coronary Disease. Hebei Institute of Medical Sciences. 1972. p. 84.

15. Editorial. Special Edition on Prevention and Treatment of Coronary Disease. Hebei Institute of Medical Sciences. 1972. p. 80.

16. Friendship Hospital et al. Compiled Information. Beijing Coordinating Research Group on Coronary Disease. 1971. p. 55.

17. Friendship Hospital et al. Compiled Information. Vol. 2. Beijing Coordinating Research Group on Coronary Disease. 1972. p. 33.

18. Coronary Disease Research Unit, Traditional Chinese Medicine Department. Selected Medical Information (General Hospital of the Chinese PLA) 1977 4(Supplement):89.

19. Coronary Disease Research Unit, Traditional Chinese Medicine Department. Selected Medical Information (General Hospital of the Chinese PLA) 1977 4(Supplement):91.

20. General Hospital of Wuhan Military Region of the Chinese PLA. New Chinese Medicine 1973 (1):13.

21. Bronchitis Group, Second Teaching Hospital. Academic Information (Second Military Medical College of the Chinese PLA) 1975 (2):253.

22. Yang JX. Acta Academiae Medicinae Wuhan 1977 (6):81.

23. Hemmer R et al. Arzneimettel Forschung 1967 17(4):491.

24. Kolss P et al. Chemical Abstracts 1973 78:47787n.

25. Health Divison of the Logistics Department of the Chinese PLA. Prevention and Treatment of Coronary Disease (internal information). 1972. p. 22.

(Gong Xuling)

TIANGUADI 甜瓜蒂

<Tianguadi>, also known as <Kudingxiang>, refers to the fruit-stalk of *Cucumis melo* L. (Cucurbitaceae). It is bitter, "cold", and toxic. The herb is an emetic. It is used to treat jaundice. The book "Jin Kui Yao Lue" (Synopsis of Prescriptions of the Golden Chamber) states that `<Guadi> cures all kinds of jaundice'.

CHEMICAL COMPOSITION

The drug contains cucurbitacin B, cucurbitacin E (elaterin, melotoxin), cucurbitacin D, isocucurbitacin B and cucurbitacin B-2-0-β-D-pyranoglucoside. The amount of cucurbitacin B is highest, about 1.4%, and the next is cucurbitacin B-2-0-β-D-pyranoglucoside (1).

PHARMACOLOGY

1. Liver-Protective Effect

Experiments on rats indicated that the subcutaneous or oral doses of cucurbitacins B and E, cucurbitacin B-2-0-β-D-pyranoglucoside, and the crude preparations containing cucurbitacins B and E offered significant protection against carbon tetrachloride-induced and subacute liver damage, as evidenced by the substantial decrease in the number of liver cells with porous, vacuolar, and fatty degenerations, and in the considerable abatement of pathological lesions, rapid repair of the central lobular necrotic areas, lowering of the serum transaminase activity, and increase in glycogen storage (2,3). Cucurbitacin B was proved in histological examination and hydroxyproline determination to markedly inhibit fibroplasia in the damaged liver. Thus, 85.7% of the treated animals were shown to have no fibroplasia, and none had moderate fibroplasia, whereas the number of animals with moderate fibroplasia in the liver damaged control group accounted for 64.3% of the total experimental animals. The chronic experiments also showed significant decrease in the incidence of liver cirrhosis and much milder lesions in the treatment group. Whether or not cucurbitacin B is capable of promoting collagenase activity that causes degradation and absorption of collagen fibers has to be verified by further studies. Moreover, since serum β-lipoprotein increased with the abatement of fatty changes, it appeared that cucurbitacin B could improve the ability of liver cells to synthesize lipoprotein, allowing the excretion of fat in the form of β-lipoprotein from the liver (2).

2. Enhancement of Cellular Immunity

It was observed clinically that in patients with chronic persistent hepatitis the <Guadi> powder nasal spray increased the lymphocyte transformation rate from a mean of 36.3 to 60.6% in 2–3 weeks, and also the absolute lymphocyte count in the peripheral blood. Accompanying these changes were the progressive improvement in the liver function and subsidence of jaundice. The results suggest that <Guadi> enhances the cellular immunity of the body, which appeared to be responsible for its therapeutic effect against hepatitis (4). Similar results were also obtained from oral administration of the crude extract of <Guadi> or cucurbitacin B or E (5). However, the number of effective cases was small; a few cases showed weakened reaction in some cellular immunity tests (5). Hence, this problem has to be further investigated. On the other hand, <Guadi> was found to be ineffective in 4 cases of hepatitis with persistent positive rheumatoid factor and hypergammaglobulinemia, suggesting that in some patients with chronic hepatitis mainly due to autoimmunity, <Guadi> was ineffective because had no suppressive effect on autoimmunity (5). A paper, however, claimed that <Guadi> suppressed autoimmunity (6).

3. Emetic Effect

A strong emetic effect was produced by oral administration of <Guadi> and elaterin 2.5 mg/kg in rabbits; the subcutaneous or intravenous dose had no definite effect. The drug were considered to stimulate the gastric mucosa, reflexively causing stimulation of the vomiting center. In dogs, oral doses exceeding 20 mg/kg also caused strong emesis and finally death due to respiratory paralysis (7).

4. Antineoplastic Effect

A few cucurbitacins were proved in vitro to be cytocidal to human nasopharyngeal and cervical cancer cells. They caused cellular degeneration in Ehrlich ascites carcinoma, solid melanoma, and ascitic melanoma. *In vivo* animal studies had also confirmed the antineoplastic action of the cucurbitacins. A paper, however, claimed that cucurbitacin has no clincal value because of its low antineoplastic efficacy and high toxicity (6).

5. Miscellaneous Actions

Injection of cucurbitacin D to dogs and cats decreased the blood pressure, myocardial contractility and heart rate. It also markedly augmented intestinal peristalsis resulting in diarrhea. The drug was devoid of anesthetic action though it greatly increased the toxicity of thiopental sodium as well as prolonged sleep induced by the latter. It had no effect on the neuromuscular junction and nerve ganglia, but could increase the capillary permeability (8).

6. Toxicity

The LD_{50} of cucurbitacin B by a single intragastric administration a single subcutaneous and 6 subcutaneous injections in mice were determined to be 14±3.0, 1.0±0.07, and 2.2±0.3 mg/kg, respectively. The LD_{50} of a single injection of the mixture of cucurbitacins B and E in mice was 6.6 ± 1.0 mg/kg SC (3). The LD_{50} of cucurbitacin D in mice were 6.3 mg/kg PO, 4.6 mg/kg SC, 1.75 mg/kg IP, and 0.96 mg/kg IV (9).

Cucurbitacins B and E, and their mixture injected to anesthetized dogs at doses of 1, 1 and 2 mg/kg IV, respectively, did not affect the respiration, blood pressure, and heart rate. When the dose of the mixture of cucurbitacins B and E was increased to 6 mg/kg, irregular breathing, hypotension, bradycardia, and weakened respiration occurred. Death ensued with respiratory arrest. Rats given 2 mg/kg PO of the cucurbitacins B and E mixture, once daily for 2 months, were found to remain in good conditions and their physiobiochemical parameters were within normal ranges; histological examination revealed no abnormalities in all organs except a trivial effect on the heart (3).

Experiments with the doses 20, 10 and 5 mg/kg PO (i.e. corresponding to 1000, 500, and 250 times the clinical doses in terms of body weight) of the mixture of cucurbitacins B and E showed that most animals of the 20 mg/kg-dose group died within 30 day, while some of the 10 mg/kg-dose group and individual animals of the 5 mg/kg-dose group also died. Random examination before death revealed no anomalies in the various laboratory tests except a marked increase in the platelet count. The results obtained from histological examination were similar to those observed in the 2 mg/kg-dose group (3).

Administration of the mixture of cucurbitacins B and E 0.12 mg/kg PO to three dogs for three months did not result in any abnormalities in two of them but mild hepatic lesions and testicular degeneration in the other animal. When the dose was raised to 0.3 mg/kg, one dog died on the 75th day of medication due to reduced appetite, weight loss and severe anemia, whereas the other animals appeared normal during 3 months of medication. When the dose was adjusted to 0.9 mg/kg, one dog died of significant weight loss on the 9th day and one dog refused food, became emaciated with severe toxic symptoms. Histological examinations of the animal sacrificed on the 16th day of medication revealed mild hepatic lesions but no significant abnormalities in the other organs. After 50 days of dosing, another dog also died followed loss of appetite, emaciation, and severe anemia. Histological examinations revealed only liver damage (3).

Sodium acetate and glucose-vitamin C significantly protected mice receiving the lowest absolute lethal dose of the B and E mixture. The decremental effect of the B and E mixture on serum transaminase could not be modified by sodium acetate (3).

CLINICAL STUDIES

1. Acute and Chronic Persistent Hepatitis

The extract of 5 g of <Guadi> obtained by soaking it in 100 ml of water for 10 days was given in two doses as a daily dosage to 103 cases of acute hepatitis. Jaundice subsided within 5 days in 70.9% and within 10 days in 95% of the cases. At the time of discharge, all hepatic functional tests were normal. The dosage may be appropriately reduced in clinical applications (9).

An aggregate effective rate of 69.9% and a marked effective rate of 46.6% were obtained in 309 case of chronic persistent hepatitis treated with the tablet of cucurbitacins B and 0.6 or 0.9 mg daily or the No. 22 tablet of the crude extract of <Guadi> 4.5 mg daily in three doses together with sodium acetate 200 mg/dose and vitamin C 200 mg/dose for 7–13 weeks. Satisfactory symptomatic improvement included reduction in hepatomegaly and splenomegaly, subsidence of jaundice, and lowering of transaminase level, as well as improvement in the turbidity tests, correction of the inverted albumin/globulin ratio, and increase in the nonspecific cellular immunity. Good long-term effects were also observed in about 100 cases followed-up (1,5).

The <Guadi> powder nasal spray was reportedly used in treatment of chronic persistent hepatitis (4). The patients had febrile reaction, profuse nasal discharge and loss of a large amount of protein, resulting in poor drug acceptability. Because of its bitter taste and susceptibility to molds, the aqueous extract is not an ideal dosage form.

2. Chronic Rhinitis

A herbalist in the Yuan dynasty, Wang Haogu, had used the <Guadi> powder as the main agent to treat anosmia. The Rhinitis Powder, composed of Pediculus Cucumis 3 g, Rhizoma Coptidis powder 0.9 g and Borneolum Syntheticum 0.3 g, has been formulated in recent years. It has been used to treat chronic rhinitis. It was efficacious in 324 cases (4).

3. Primary Hepatoma

Tablets of cucurbitacins B and E were tried in 33 cases of stages II and III of common and sclerotic types of primary hepatoma. The dosage used was 0.2 mg thrice daily, gradually increased to 0.6 mg thrice daily. Generally after 1–3 weeks of treatment the tumor became 2–6 cm smaller and softer; hepatic pain was markedly reduced, and appetite increased. When the liver ceased to reduce in size after one month of treatment, low doses of radiotherapy or chemotherapy could prevent regrowth of tumor after 1–2 weeks. It is effective in prolonging the survival period of terminal patients; thus, the half-year survival rate was about 40%. In one case the tumor mass reportedly disappeared after 4 months of treatment (6).

ADVERSE EFFECTS AND TREATMENT OF INTOXICATION

The <Guadi> powder nasal spray produces severe reactions and is therefore contraindicated in weak patients and in those with heart disease (4). Sufficient doses of the aqueous extract and cucurbitacins B and E by mouth caused in individual patients transient mild diarrhea, abdominal discomfort, impairment of appetite, and mild dizziness. Brief elevation of transaminase level appeared in some patients, but in most of them it was restored to normal level without discontinuation of medication. No abnormalities in the blood routine examination, platelet count, nonprotein nitrogen and creatinine were observed (5).

Intoxication and death could result from ingestion of more than 30 pieces of <Guadi> (10,11). Toxic symptoms and signs included vomiting, respiratory and circulatory failure, elevated serum transaminase level, and myocardial damage shown in the ECG. The direct cause of death was central respiratory paralysis.

REFERENCE

1. Section 404, Fourth Department of Hunan Institute of Medical and Pharmaceutical Industry. Chinese Traditional and Herbal Drugs Communications 1979 10(3):1.

2. Han DW. Journal of Traditional Chinese Medicine 1979 59(4):206.

3. Hepatitis Group, Pharmacology Department of Hunan Institute of Medical and Pharmaceutical Industry. Chinese Traditional and Herbal Drugs Communications 1979 10(9):30.

4. Shanghai General Hospital of Infectious Diseases. Xinyiyaoxue Zazhi (Journal of Traditional Chinese Medicine) 1976 (9):42.

5. Infectious Diseases Department, First Teaching Hospital of the Third Military Medical University et al. Chinese Traditional and Herbal Drugs Communications 1978 (1):40.

6. Qiu JP. New Medical and Pharmaceutical Communications 1979 (3):41.

7. Inoko K. The Tokyo Journal of Medical Sciences 1894 8(1–7).

8. Edery H et al. Archives Internationales de Pharmacodynamie et de Therapie 1961 130(3–4):315.

9. Li SX. Chinese Journal of Paediatrics 1959 (2):123.

10. Internal Medicine Department, Hospital of Fushun Bureau of Mines. Liaoning Yiyao (Liaoning Medical Journal) 1976 (4):60.

11. Lou XY et al. Xinyiyaoxue Zazhi (Journal of Traditional Chinese Medicine) 1976 (12):15.

(Xue Chunsheng)

ZHULING 豬苓

<Zhuling> refers to the sclerotium of *Grifola umbellata* (Pers.) Pilat (*Polyporus umbellatus* (Pers.) Fr.) (Polyporaceae). It is sweet, bland, and "mild". It has a diuretic and "damp"-clearing action. Thus, it is mainly used in the treatment of dysuria, edema, diarrhea, urinary tract infection, and leukorrhea.

CHEMICAL COMPOSITION

The sclerotium of *G. umbellata* contains ergosterol, α-hydroxytetracosanoic acid, biotin, soluble polysaccharide I (Gu-I) and crude protein.

PHARMACOLOGY

1. Diuretic Effect

Oral administration of the <Zhuling> decoction 8 g (4 times) in healthy subjects increased the 6-hour urine output and chloride excretion by 62 and 54.5%, respectively; the diuretic action was stronger than caffeine, the stem of *Akebia quinata* or the sclerotium of *Poria cocos* (1). The usual clinical dose of the ethanol extract of this herb by mouth, however, produced no diuretic effect in healthy subjects (2). Diuresis was achieved in rabbits by intragastric or intraperitoneal administration of this agent only at doses close to those used in man (2,3). In chronic experiments on dogs with ureteral fistula, injection of the <Zhuling> decoction 0.25–0.5 g/kg IV or IM produced a significant diuretic effect, increasing the urine output by threefold in 4–6 hours, but no effect was observed when the intragastric or intravenous dose was lower than 0.0048 g/kg (4,5). When "Wuling San" (Five-Drug Powder of Grifola, Poria, Rhizoma Atractylodis Alba, Rhizoma Alismatis, Ramulus Cinnamomi) was injected intravenously to dogs, along with the increase in urine output there was increase in the excretion of sodium, potassium and chloride (5). Intragastric administration of the soluble ethanol-extract of <Zhuling> or "Wuling San" initiated marked diuresis in the first hour (6). On the other hand, in adrenalectomized rats, simultaneous administration of the <Zhuling> decoction and deoxycorticosterone resulted in a decrease in the 5-hour urine output, though urinary sodium and potassium were not significantly different from that of the control (7). The determinations of hematocrit, plasma specific gravity, and plasma electrolyte concentration showed no thinning of blood or change of the glomerular filtration rate by <Zhuling> (4). Hence, the diuretic effect of the herb was considered due to inhibition of electrolyte and water reabsorption by the renal tubules (4).

2. Antineoplastic Effect

The polysaccharides of <Zhuling> had antineoplastic activity (8). The soluble ethanol-extract of this herb injected intraperitoneally to mice at 2 g (crude drug)/kg daily for 10 days produced inhibition rates of 62 and 37–54% against sarcoma 180 and hepatoma, respectively; it was, however, inactive against leukemia L_{615} (9). Another paper reported that <Zhuling> extracts (including the crude extract, semi-refined and refined products) given to mice by intraperitoneal, intravenous, and intragastric routes significantly inhibited mouse sarcoma 180 (10). The inhibitory effect achieved by the fermentation liquid and the crude extract of <Zhuling> against sarcoma 180 was similar to that attained by the crude extract of wild <Zhuling> (11).

Histochemical studies of cAMP and phosphodiesterase activities and autoradiography of ^{3}H-TdR incorporation revealed that the <Zhuling> extract "757" could inhibit DNA synthesis in the mouse sarcoma 180 ascitic tumor cells, thereby interfering with the multiplication of tumor cells, and could increase the cAMP level in the tumor cells. These effects were probably due to the inhibition of 3'-5'-cAMP phosphodiesterase activity in the tumor cells (12–15).

3. Effect on Immunologic Function

Both the extract and the soluble ethanol-extract of <Zhuling> could enhance the reticuloendothelial phagocytosis in mice (9,16). The hemolytic plaque test proved that the <Zhuling> extract caused an increase in antibody forming cells in the spleens of tumor-bearing mice (16). However, another paper claimed that the soluble ethanol-extract caused a reduction in the antibody forming cells (9). Experiments on graft-versus-host reaction and thymic weight indicated that the <Zhuling> extract weakly inhibited T cells (16). Further studies are required in order to evaluate whether this effect was consequent to the selective inhibition of active T cells.

In addition, a single or 10 consecutive intramuscular injection of the semi-refined extract of <Zhuling> to healthy subjects increased the T-lymphocyte transformation rate. These results imply a nonspecific immunostimulant action which might be responsible for the antineoplastic effect.

4. Antibacterial Effect

In vitro, the ethanol extract of <Zhuling> inhibited *Staphylococcus aureus* and *Escherichia coli* (17,18).

5. Toxicity

A large dose of the semi-refined <Zhuling> extract, 200–250 mg/kg PO or 500 mg/kg IP, produced no significant toxic reactions in mice. No significant toxicity was observed in mice in a period of one month following daily injection of the semi-refined extract at 1–100 mg/kg IP for 28 days (19).

CLINICAL STUDIES

1. Neoplasms

The <Zhuling> extract "757" has effectively been employed since 1976 in the treatment of cancers of the lung and esophagus, etc. It is preliminarily held that this extract has antineoplastic activity and immunoadjuvant action but no adverse side effects (20).

1.1 *Lung cancer.* The <Zhuling> extract "757" combined with chemotherapy was given to 50 cases of primary lung cancer and the control group was given the "757" extract alone. Evaluation of the short-term therapeutic effect showed that with the combined therapy the percentage of cases with symptomatic improvement was increased to 86.1% as compared to 62.5% of the control; the percentage of cases with stable tumors was up to 70% in contrast to 25% of the control group. This herb could also reduce the side effects of chemotherapy and increase the immunologic function of the body (21).

1.2 *Esophageal cancer.* The therapeutic effect of "757" in 13 cases of esophageal cancer was not satisfactory; cancer continued to advance in nine cases and was stabilized in only four cases. The therapeutic effect was improved when the extract was used in combination with chemotherapy. Among 20 cases so treated, 10 cases benefitted to certain extents, while one cases obtained marked improvement. Since no control group was employed in this experiment, further studies would be necessary to demonstrate if there was any synergism between the extract and chemotherapeutic agents (22). During the combined treatment, the immunological parameters such as lymphocyte transformation rate and macrophage phagocytic rate were elevated in most patients, and in all patients the counts of leucocytes and platelets fluctuated within the normal ranges. These findings indicated that the bone marrow was protected during chemotherapy and the nonspecific immune system of the body was not weakened but strengthened.

2. Cirrhosis of Liver, Ascites, Dysuria, and Urinary Tract Infection

Thirty-nine cases of liver cirrhosis with ascites unresponsive to various treatments were treated with the modified prescription of "Wuling San" (Grifola, Poria, Rhizoma Atractylodis Albae, Rhizoma Alismatis, Ramulus Cinnamomi) or "Wu Pi Yin" (Five-peel Decoction (Pilare Poria, Pericarpium Arecae, Pericarpium Benincasae, Pericarpium Citri Reticulatae, Pilare Zingiberis Recens)). Seventeen of these cases were clinically cured, seven markedly improved and 12 significantly improved (23). The decoction alone can be used at doses of 6–12 g daily to treat dysuria, urodynia, hematuria, and urinary tract infection (24). Also, five cases of chyluria had been treated with the prescription Grifola Decoction (Grifola 12 g, Colla Corii Asini 9 g, Poria 12 g, Rhizoma Alismatis 12 g, Talcum 12 g); four cases obtained good results while one case was ineffective (25).

REFERENCE

1. Shen JW et al. Acta Academiae Medicinae Primae Shanghai 1957 (1):38.

2. Internal Medicine Department, Beijing Medical College. Chinese Medical Journal 1961 47(1):7.

3. Luo ZL et al. Abstracts of the Annual Conference of the Chinese Medical Association (Luda Branch). 1957. p. 116.

4. Wang LW et al. Acta Pharmaceutica Sinica 1964 11(12):815.

5. Wang LW et al. Abstracts of the Symposium of the Chinese Society of Physiology (Pharmacy). 1964. p. 132.

6. Zhu Y et al. Proceedings of the 1962 Symposium of the Chinese Pharmaceutical Association. 1964. p. 327.

7. Luo HW et al. Journal of Nanjing College of Pharmacy (10):69.

8. Ito H et al. Nihon Yakugi Shianpo 1977 2769:43.

9. Pharmacology Department, Institute of Cancer of the Chinese Academy of Medical Sciences. Chinese Traditional and Herbal Drugs Communications 1978 (8):36.

10. Tumor Section, Institute of Chinese Materia Medica of the Academy of Traditional Chinese Medicine. Xinyiyaoxue Zazhi (Journal of Traditional Chinese Medicine) 1979 (2):15.

11. Dai RQ et al. Xinyiyaoxue Zazhi (Journal of Traditional Chinese Medicine) 1979 (2):83.

12. Cell Biology Department, Beijing Institute of Tumor et al. Abstracts of the First National Symposium of the Chinese Society of Pharmacology. 1979. p. 104.

13. Cell Biology Department, Beijing Institute of Tumor et al. Abstracts of the First National Symposium of the Chinese Society of Pharmacology. 1979.p 103.

14. Pharmacology Department, Institute of Chinese Materia Medica of the Academy of Traditional Chinese Medicine. Abstracts of the First National Symposium of the Chinese Society of Pharmacology. 1979. p. 105.

15. Pharmacology Department, Institute of Chinese Materia Medica of the Academy of Traditional Chinese Medicine. Abstracts of the First National Symposium of the Chinese Society of Pharmacology. 1979. p. 106.

16. Immunology Section of the Microbiology Department, Institute of Chinese Materia Medica of the Academy of Traditional Chinese Medicine. Xinyiyaoxue Zazhi (Journal of Traditional Chinese Medicine) 1979 (3):179.

17. Harada T et al. Chemical Abstracts 1952 46:7618g.

18. Kubo H et al. Chemical Abstracts 1954 48:810i.

19. Tumor Section Academy of Traditional Chinese Medicine. Xinyiyaoxue Zazhi (Journal of Traditional Chinese Medicine) 1979 (5):315.

20. Institute of Chinese Materia Medica, Academy of Traditional Chinese Medicine. Xinyiyaoxue Zazhi (Journal of Traditional Chinese Medicine) 1979 (2):73.

21. Dongzhimen Hospital of Beijing College of Traditional Chinese Medicine et al. Xinyiyaoxue Zazhi (Journal of Traditional Chinese Medicine) 1979 (2):75.

22. Guang' anmen Hospital of the Chinese Academy of Traditional Chinese Medicine et al. The References of Traditional Chinese Medicine 1978 (2):27.

23. Chongqing First Hospital of Traditional Chinese Medicine. Chinese Journal of Internal Medicine 19778 (10):1003.

24. Zhongshan Medical College (editor). Clinical Applications of Chinese Traditional Drugs. Guangdong People' s Publishing House. 1975. p. 139.

25. Internal Medicine Department, 159th Hospital of the Chinese PLA. Henan Zhongyi Xueyuan Xuebao (Journal of Henan College of Traditional Chinese Medicine) 1978 (1):48.

(Chen Quansheng)

ZHUDAN 豬膽

<Zhudan> refers to the dried bile and gallbladder of pigs (*Sus scrofa domestica* Brisson) (Suidae). It is bitter an "cold". Latent-heat-clearing, antipyretic, demulcent, detoxicant and anti-inflammatory actions are attributed to it. It is used internally as a remedy in fever due to common cold, thirst and constipation, and, externally, in carbuncles and deep-rooted ulcers.

CHEMICAL COMPOSITION

Pig bile contains bile acids; the major bile acids are hyocholic acid and hyodeoxycholic acid. It also contains bilirubin, mucoprotein, lipids and inorganic substances. The bile acids also include small amounts of chenodeoxycholic acid, 3α-hydroxy-6-oxo-5α-cholanic acid, cholic acid, deoxycholic acid and lithocholic acid. The bile acids are mainly conjugated with glycine (1–3).

PHARMACOLOGY

1. Effect on the Respiratory System

In mice with cough induced by ammonia aerosol, a marked antitussive action was exhibited by: Compound suspension of pig bile (Galla Suis, Radix Platycodi, Rhizoma Pinelliae, Lumbricus), cholic acid, sodium cholate, deoxycholic acid and sodium chenodeoxycholate (1,4–6). Administration of the pig bile powder 0.5–1.0g/kg PO or of sodium cholate 20 mg/kg IV to anesthetized cats suppressed the cough reaction induced by electrical stimulation of the superior laryngeal nerve; sodium deoxycholate and sodium taurocholate were ineffective (7–9). Perfusion of sodium cholate into the isolated guinea pig lungs directly dilated the bronchi, its effect was slow but prolonged. The drug also antagonized bronchospasm induced by histamine-pilocarpine (8). The results of experiments on guinea pigs with bronchospasm induced by drug aerosol showed that the compound suspension of the pig bile, cholic acid, sodium cholate, and sodium chenodeoxycholate had antiasthmatic activity (4–6). Expectorant effects were achieved by the oral doses of the compound suspension of the pig bile, cholic acid and its sodium salt in expectoration experiment on rats using the capillary technique (4). The orally administered hyocholic acid and deoxycholic acid increased phenol red excretion in the brochi of mice, proving its expectorant action (6,10). Intravenous injection of sodium cholate to rabbits prolonged the pulmonary stretch reflex time, indicating a depressant effect on the respiratory center (8).

2. Bacteriostatic Effect

In vitro bacterial inhibition tests indicated that the compound pig bile powder, pig bile linctus, sodium hyocholate, and cholic acid had inhibited to different extents *Diplococcus pneumoniae*, alpha and beta *Streptococcus hemolyticus*, and *Hemophilus influenzae*. Among these agents cholic acid and sodium hyocholate were the most potent (4). On the other hand, hyocholic acid, sodium hyodeoxycholate, sodium chenodeoxycholate, sodium cholate, and sodium deoxycholate inhibited *Staphylococcus aureus*, streptococci, and sarcinae (1,5,10). The pig bile, pig bile powder, sodium deoxycholate, and sodium glycocholate suppressed the growth of *Bordetella pertussis* (7,11,12). Different of bacteriostatic action against *Mycobacterium tuberculosis* were also exhibited by the pig bile, pig bile powder, sodium cholate, sodium taurocholate, sodium α-glycine hyodeoxycholate, and sodium chenodeoxycholate (1). The folk remedy for dysentery, "Hei Hu Dan" (Black Tiger Pill which contains Galla Suis and Semen Setariae Italicae) inhibited *Shigella dysenteriae, Staphylococcus aureus, Salmonellae* and *Escherichia coli*. These informations showed that pig bile and its bile salts have bacteriostatic action against multiple kinds of bacteria; they are considered less efficacious than antibiotics and other specific antibacterial agents. The mechanism of action of the bile salts could be due to reduction of the surface tension. causing rupture of bacterial cell membrane and thus lysis of the bacteria (1).

3. Anti-inflammatory, Anti-allergic, and Detoxicant Effects

Oral administration of the 10% pig bile powder solution produced anti-inflammatory effect against aseptic ear inflammation in rabbits and formaldehyde-induced paw swelling in rats (7). Intracardiac injection of cholic acid 5 mg/kg to guinea pigs sensitized with horse serum enabled the animals to tolerate a second dose of the horse serum injection and markedly decreased the incidence of anaphylactic shock (13). Please refer to the monograph on <Xiongdan> for details of the detoxicant action of sodium chenodeoxycholate and sodium cholate.

4. Effect on the CNS

Crude hyocholates given orally to mice markedly antagonized cocaine-induced convulsion in a more efficacious manner than crude taurocholate. The anticonvulsant action was attributed to central depression and blockade of neuromuscular junctions (14). A marked sedative effect was elicited with the oral doses of <Zhudan> powder in mice (9). Cholates exhibited both sedative and antipyretic actions, details of which may be obtained in the monograph on <Niuhuang>.

5. Effect on the Digestive System

In clinical practice, pig bile used as retention enema can promote intestinal motility, relieve postoperative meteorism, and promote defecation (15). Details on the effects of the bile acids of <Zhudan> on bile secretion and excretion, gallstone dissolution, and alimentary tract motility are discussed in the monograph on <Xiongdan>.

The bile acid salts promoted the digestion and absorption of fat, lipoids, and lipophilic vitamins through three mechanisms; (1) promoting the emulsification of lipids, (2) enhancing lipase activity, (3) combining with the fatty acids from hydrolyzed fat to form soluble complexes, thus facilitating their absorption through the intestinal mucosa (1). Experiments in early years proved that cholic acid, deoxycholic acid, chenodeoxycholic acid, ursodeoxycholic acid, and hyodeoxycholic acid could increase the activity of pancreatic lipase (16,17). Since the bile salts promoted lipid absorption, they also promoted the absorption of carotenes and vitamin D and K (1). Radioisotope tracing experiments proved that taurodeoxycholic acid, glycochenodeoxycholic acid and glycocholic acid could promote calcium absorption by the small intestine (18).

6. Effect on the Cardiovascular System

The refined extract of pig bile (the chief component being glycohyodeoxycholic acid) stimulated the isolated toad heart. Intravenous injection of this agent to anesthetized rabbits resulted in hypotension; it also antagonized the pressor effect of epinephrine. Experiments on the oral doses given to normal rats indicated that the hypotensive effect of the refined extract of the pig bile was not comparable to that obtained with bovine bezoar or calcium cholate (19). Please refer to the monograph on <Xiongdan> for the cardiovascular effects of chenodeoxycholic acid and cholic acid, etc.

7. Toxicity

A single dose of the crude hyocholate 2.0–8.0 g/kg PO was not lethal to mice; administration of 50 or 100 mg/kg daily for 18 days to rats resulted in a slight increase in body weight (14). The LD_{50} of deoxycholic acid in mice determined to be 1.991±0.232 g/kg PO. Hyodeoxycholic acid, owing to its strong hemolytic action, is not recommended for intravenous injection (1). Please consult the monograph on <Xiongdan> for the toxicity of chenodeoxycholic acid and cholic acid.

CLINICAL STUDIES

1. Whooping Cough

The powder, syrup, or fluidextract of pig bile were used to treat 1215 cases of whooping cough; the onset of therapeutic effect was usually 2–4 days. After a course of 5–14 days, the effective rates were 62–97% (20–22).

2. Chronic Bronchitis

The oral doses of the pig bile powder capsule and the tablet prepared from pig bile and starch, or the intramuscular doses of the pig bile injection, were able to achieve antitussive and expectorant effects, and, to a lesser extent, antiasthmatic effect in 315 cases (23–25). Similar results were obtained in the clinical trial of sodium hyocholate in 100 cases (26) and of sodium chenodeoxycholate in 30 cases (5).

3. Prevention of Diphtheria

Fresh pig bile steamed with sugar was reported as effective for preventing diphtheria (27).

4. Acute Bacillary Dysentery and Acute Enteritis

Mungbean-Bile Pill prepared from mungbean powder soaked in pig bile is efficacious against acute bacillary dysentery and acute gastroenteritis. However, pig bile is contraindicated in the acute state of gastrointestinal inflammatory diseases because it irritates the gastrointestinal tract.

5. Acute Infectious Hepatitis

Capsules prepared from the baked and pulverized pig bile were used to treat infectious hepatitis with favorable results in respect of jaundice, restoration of normal liver function, and, particularly, improvement of gastrointestinal symptoms (28,29).

6. Simple Dyspepsia

Seventy-one of 81 cases of simple dyspepsia in young children were cured by the 3% syrup of the pig bile powder (30).

7. Gynecological and Obstetrical Inflammatory Diseases and Postoperative Infection

Out of 137 cases of chronic cervicitis treated with a local spray of the powder prepared from pig bile and alum, 94 cases were cured, 36 improved, and 7 were unresponsive or had relapses; the effective rate was 94.8% (31). Another paper reported that satisfactory results were achieved with an injection prepared from pig bile and scutellarin at 2 ml IM twice daily in the treatment of 200 cases of ovarian tumors, ectopic pregnancy, postoperative infection after sterilization operation, and chronic pelvic infection (32).

8. Tuberculosis of Lymph Nodes

Excellent effects were achieved in 53 cases treated with the pig bile linctus prepared from pig bile, vinegar, and the rhizome of *Nardostachys chinensis* by local application on the tuberculous lymph nodes. This linctus can clear up latent heat, detoxify, relieve stasis, drain the pus, relieve inflammation, and regenerate tissues (33).

9. Eye Diseases

An effective rate of 69.3% was obtained in 814 cases of trachoma treated with the 10% pig bile preparation. It was effective in all stages and grades of the disease and was found to be superior to sodium sulfacetamide at the same concentration (34). The pig bile diluted with normal saline and sterilized was used in 197 cases of acute conjunctivitis, and 190 cases (96.4%) benefitted (35). The pig bile powder was also effective in herpetic conjunctivitis (36).

10. Chronic Suppurative Otitis Media

The Pig Bile-Alum Powder was used in chronic suppurative otitis media with good short-term therapeutic effect. An effective rate of 96% was obtained in a trial of 149 cases. However, long-term follow-ups revealed that 14 cases had relapse (37).

11. Constipation

The autoclaved pig bile used as enema is a good laxative. It is useful in constipation after abdominal surgery and due to pregnancy, postoperative meteorism, and paralytic ileus. Thus, most of the 394 cases treated with this enema were able to defecate within one hour of medication and a few in more than 2 hours (15).

ADVERSE EFFECTS

The pig bile preparations, hyodeoxycholic acid, and chenodeoxycholic acid given orally often caused gastrointestinal reactions such as nausea, gastric upset and diarrhea, but they were mostly mild and tolerable. Dizziness and insomnia may also occur (5,26,28). Injection of the pig bile may cause local irritation such as red swelling and pain which may be relieved by applying hot compress or additional use of procaine (23–25).

REFERENCE

1. Scientific and Technical Information Room, Shenyang College of Pharmacy. Basic Studies and Uses of Bile — A Chinese Traditional Drug. Shenyang College of Pharmacy. 1973. p. 29.

2. Beijing Institute of Chinese Materia Medica. Bulletin of Chinese Materia Medica Research (Beijing Institute of Chinese Materia Medica) 1975 (2):50.

3. Florkin M et al. Comparative Biochemistry. Vol. 3. Part A. Academic Press. 1962. p. 205.

4. Fuyang District Research Group on Chronic Bronchitis. Medical Status in Fuyang (Fuyang Health Bureau) 1972 (2):7.

5. Shenyang Pharmaceutical Factory of Biological Products et al. New Pharmaceutical Communications (Shenyang College of Pharmacy) 1971 (3):27.

6. 236 Logistics Unit of the Chinese PLA. Compiled Research Information on Chronic Bronchitis. 1973. p. 1.

7. Pharmacology Department, Shenyang College of Pharmacy. Preliminary Studies on the Pharmacological Actions of Swine Bile (Sus scrofa domestica). Shenyang College of Pharmacy. 1959.

8. Zhang JQ. Chinese Pharmaceutical Bulletin 1965 (2):92.

9. Research Group of Pharmacology Class 23012. Acta Academiae Medicinae Xi' an 1960 (9):21.

10. Coordinating Research Group on Pharmacological Study of Artificial Bovine Bezoar. Studies on Artificial Bovine Bezoar. National Institute of Scientific and Technological Information. 1972. p. 5–6.

11. Medical Laboratory, Maternal and Child Health Centre Affiliated to Dalian Medical College. Liaoning Medical Journal 1959 2(2):12.

12. Han FJ et al. Chinese Journal of Paediatrics 1959 10(1):15.

13. Ren CW (translator). Chinese Medical Journal 1955 41(11):1078.

14. Cui ZG et al. Collections of Research Information. 5th edition. Sichuan Institute of Chinese Materia Medica. 1966. p. 311.

15. Surgery Department, Shanghai Tenth People' s Hospital. Journal of Traditional Chinese Medicine 1957 (8):431.

16. Shoda M. Chemical Abstracts 1927 21:1280.

17. Shoda M. Chemical Abstracts 1928 22:981.

18. Wabling DD' A. Biochemical Journal 1966 100(3):652.

19. Iwaki R. Folia Pharmacologica Japonica 1964 (60):529.

20. Chinese Academy of Medical Sciences. Medical and Health Express 1959 (10):148.

21. Institute of Epidemiology, Chinese Academy of Medical Sciences (Shaanxi Branch). Shaanxi Journal of Medicine and Health 1959 (4):285.

22. Pediatrics Section of Dalian Medical College. Acta Academiae Medicinae Dalian 1960 (2):60.

23. Dongfu Commune Health Centre. Medical and Health Communications (Xiamen Institute of Medical and Pharmaceutical Sciences) 1972 (1):12.

24. Dongfeng District (Xiamen) Hospital. Medical and Health Communications (Xiamen Institute of Medical and Pharmaceutical Sciences) 1972 (1):16.

25. Changwei District Sanatorium. Barefoot Doctor (Changwei District Health Bureau) 1971 (5):17.

26. Wuhan Coordinating Research Group for Bile Therapy of Senile Chronic Bronchitis. Hubei Science and Technology — Medicine (Hubei Institute of Scientific and Technological Information) 1972 (2):1.

27. Ye GT et al. Guangdong Zhongyi (Guangdong Journal of Traditional Chinese Medicine) 1961 6(2):72.

28. Wang XY. Jiangsu Zhongyi (Jiangsu Journal of Traditional Chinese Medicine) 1965 (7):14.

29. Zhou XF et al. Fujian Zhongyiyao (Fujian Journal of Traditional Chinese Medicine) 1964 (2):91.

30. Zheng YS. Guangdong Zhongyi (Guangdong Journal of Traditional Chinese Medicine) 1960 5(6):303.

31. Zhongshan County Sanitation and Anti-epidemic Station. Health Journal of Guangxi 1972 (3):33.

32. Liaoning College of Traditional Chinese Medicine. Revolution in Medical Education 1971 (1):16.

33. Chen SJ et al. Journal of Traditional Chinese Medicine 1980 (3):38.

34. Nanjing Sanitation and Anti-epidemic Station. Jiangsu Yiyao (Jiangsu Medical Journal) 1975 (5):35.

35. Xiao BF. Acta Academiae Medicinae Wuhan 1976 (4):77.

36. Ophthalmology Department, 322nd Hospital of the Chinese PLA. People's Military Medicine 1975 (12):67.

37. Zhang ZY et al. Chinese Journal of Otorhinolaryngology 1965 11(5):291.

(Duan Meifen)

ZHUMAOCAI 豬毛菜

<Zhumaocai> refer to the whole plant of *Salsola collina* Pall. or *S. ruthenica* Iljin (Chenopodiaceae). It is also known as <Zhapengke>, or <Cipeng>. Sweet, bland, and "cool", it produces hypotension. It is used to treat hypertension and headache.

CHEMICAL COMPOSITION

S. ruthenica contains betaine, succinic acid and polysaccharides. *S. richteri* Karelin, a species of the same genus, has salsoline as the principal constituent which is used in Russia for the treatment of hypertension. However, salsoline is not found in *S. collina* and *S. ruthenica*

PHARMACOLOGY

1. Hypotensive Effect

The aqueous or ethanol extract of <Zhumaocai> injected intravenously to anesthetized animals produced a marked and prolonged hypotensive effect (1–9). Among various test animals, dog was most sensitive to this herb, followed by rabbit, then cat. They did not develop tachyphylaxis (6). Intravenous injection of the aqueous extract of this herb (1:0.66) 1–2 ml to cats lowered the blood pressure by 59–82 mmHg (5). Intragastric administration of the 5% tincture 1 g/kg 4 times daily to dogs with senile (or essential) hypertension for 4–7 days decreased the systolic pressure by 20–40 mmHg and the diastolic pressure by 10–20 mmHg. This effect persisted for about 7–30 days after discontinuation of treatment (2). Another report, however, claimed that administration of the extract 5–16 g/kg PO daily for 2 months to dogs with chronic hypertension did not signifincantly decrease the blood pressure (7). A paper reported that the ethanol fluidextract of this herb inhibited the heart of anesthetized rabbits, resulting in ST segment depression in the ECG, whereas the crude absolute-ethanol extract had weaker cardiac and hypotensive effects than the ethanol fluidextract (9).

The betaine obtained from <Zhumaocai> injected intravenously to anesthetized animals produced a mild hypotension but is was inactive in hypertensive dogs. A kind of saponin obtained by electrophoresis was found to lower blood pressure in anesthetized dogs and hypertensive albino rats (10).

The significant hypotensive effect was found to be accompanied by attenuation or abolition of the pressor reflex induced by pressing the carotid artery or stimulating the afferent sciatic nerve. Perfusion experiments using isolated rabbit ears with intact nerves revealed that the hypotensive action of <Zhumaocai> was due to reflex vasodilation (6). Direct vasodilatory action was also exhibited by the crude absolute-ethanol extract perfused into the isolated hind limb blood vessels of frogs and isolated renal blood vessels of rabbits (9). Based on these experiments, the mechanism of action of <Zhumaocai> was considered to be inhibition of the vasomotor center and direct vasodilation.

Another paper reported that the decoction or ethanol extract of the plantlings of a related species grown in Zhengzhou District of Henan, *S. komarovii* lljin, did not cause hypotension in experimental animals but exhibited a significant pressor effect. The fruit-bearing herb, however, was shown to have a hypotensive effect (11).

2. Effect on the CNS

Subcutaneous injection of the <Zhumaocai> extract to albino mice decreased the spontaneous activity of the animals and prolonged the hypnosis induced by pentobarbital sodium, but did not antagonize the convulsant and lethal effects of the central convulsants pentylenetetrazole and strychnine (6). It was shown in the conditioned avoidance reflex experiment on mice that the herb extract given subcutaneously accelerated the disappearance of the reflex; in other words, it probably intensified cortical depression (6).

3. Toxicity

The LD_{50} of the aqueous extract of <Zhumaocai> in mice was determined to be 56 g/kg SC. The dose 8 g/kg IP was lethal to rats. No toxic reactions were seen in rabbits given the dose 40 g/kg PO, whereas the animals died when the dose was increased to 80 g/kg (6). Intragastric administration of the 1:1 <Zhumaocai> aqueous extract 5 ml to guinea pigs (weighing 500–600 g) or 10 ml to rabbits (weighing 2.4–2.7 kg) once daily for one week (no medication on the third day) did not result in any toxic reactions (4).

CLINICAL STUDIES

Hypertension

<Zhumaocai> or its fluidextract given as beverage at daily dosages of 9–20 g or the herb decoction at daily dosages of 20–40 g (crude drug) was given to 13 cases of hypertension for 5 months. With the disappearance of subjective symptoms such as headache, palpitation, oversensitivity, tension, irritability, insomnia and light sleep, the patients became more relaxed, less deppressed and their blood pressure, particularly the systolic pressure, lowered (12,13).

In another series of 24 cases treated with the Xuekeping Tablet (5 g of crude drug/tablet) 2–3 tablets thrice daily, 15 cases had their blood pressure decreased, of which 8 were restored to normal (14).

ADVERSE EFFECTS

Two hypertensive patients had developed allergic skin rashes which disappeared readily after discontinuation of the treatment (14).

REFERENCE

1. Li GC et al. Abstracts of the First Congress of the Chinese Society of Physiology (Pharmacy). 1956. p. 48.

2. Xia BN et al. Abstracts of the First Congress of the Chinese Society of Physiology (Pharmacy). 1956. p. 49.

3. Pharmacology Section, Xi' an Medical College. Acta Academiae Medicinae Xi' an 1958 (5):20.

4. Sun YL et al. Harbin Zhongyi (Harbin Journal of Traditional Chinese Medicine) 1959 2(3):24.

5. Sun YL et al. Chinese Journal of Internal Medicine 1958 6(12):1141.

6. Sun GZ et al. Acta Pharmaceutica Sinica 1962 9(7):412.

7. Pharmacology Section, Dalian Railways Medical College. Selected Papers of Dalian Railways Medical College. 1960. p. 139.

8. Pharmacology Section, Qiqihar Medical College. Abstracts of the Chinese Society of Physiology (Pharmacology). 1964. p. 115.

9. Lin XL et al. Shaanxi Journal of Medicine and Health 1960 (3):196.

10. Ding GS et al. Pharmacological studies of antihypertensive drugs. In: Collection of Papers of Scientific Achievements in Commemoration of the 10th National Day of the People' s Republic of China (1949–1959). People' s Medical Publishing House. 1959. p. 179.

11. Pathophysiology Section, Henan Medical College. Proceedings of the 10th National Day Symposium of Henan Medical College (internal information). 1959.

12. Fu SY et al. Chinese Journal of Internal Medicine 1959 7(10):977.

13. Liu HD et al. Chinese Journal of Internal Medicine 1958 6(12):1139.

14. Pharmacology Section, Xi' an Medical College. Acta Academiae Medicinae Xi' an 1960 (6):34.

(Chen Gurong)

XUANFUHUA 旋覆花

<Xuanfuhua> refers to the capitulum of *Inula japonica* Thunb., *I. linariaefolia* Turcz., or *I. britannica* L. (Compositae). It is bitter, salty, and slightly "warm".

It is credited with antiemetic, mucolytic, and diuretic actions. It is used to treat dyspnea and cough with excessive sputum, eructation, vomiting, chest tightness and costalgia.

CHEMICAL COMPOSITION

<Xuanfuhua> contains flavonoid glycosides, sterols such as taraxasterol, inulin, quercetin, alkaloids, volatile oil and fixed oil.

The aerial part of *I. britannica* during the flowering season contains the sesquiterpenes britanin and inulicin.

PHARMACOLOGY

1. Antiasthmatic and Antitussive Effects

The flavones of <Xuanfuhua> significantly protected guinea pigs from histamine-induced bronchospastic asthma; it also antagonized histamine-induced spasm of isolated guinea pig bronchi, though the action was slower and weaker than that of aminophylline. However, both the ammonia spray and phenol red excretion experiments on mice proved that the flavones had no antitussive nor expectorant effects (1). Intraperitoneal injection of the 150% <Xuanfuhua> decoction 0.1 ml in mice produced marked antitussive effect in one hour but no significant expectorant effect (2).

2. Antibacterial Effect

In the disc or well diffusion method, the 1:1 decoction of <Xuanfuhua> was shown to strongly inhibit *Staphylococcus aureus*, *Bacillus anthracis* and *Shigella flexneri* IIa strain, but it was weak or inactive against *Streptococcus hemolyticus*, *Escherichia coli*, *Salmonella typhi*, *Pseudomonas aeruginosa*, *Proteus vulgaris* and *Corynebacterium diphtheriae* (2–4). Outside China, the whole plant of *I. britannica* is used as a folk remedy for wounds and ulcers; the lipids and other ether-soluble components contained in its root and aerial part also inhibited some bacteria (15).

3. Miscellaneous Actions

Injection of the dilute-alcohol extract of <Xuanfuhua> to rabbits at 0.5 or 1.0 g(crude drug)/kg IP daily for 5 days produced no significant diuretic effect (6).

4. Toxicity

The acute LD_{50} of the 150% <Xuanfuhua> decoction in mice was determined to be about 22.5 g/kg IP. The intraperitoneal dose 2 ml promptly produced rapid breathing and six minutes later excitation, convulsion, tail erection and tremor of the extremities, and, at the end of 8 minutes, death (2).

CLINICAL STUDIES

1.Acute and Chronic Bronchitis

Excellent therapeutic effects were obtained from the pills prepared from this herb plus the root of *Platycodon grandiflorum*, the whole plant of *Patrinia scabiosaefolia*, 3 g each, and honey 9 g given daily in two doses (morning and evening) for 10 days as a therapeutic course; three courses are recommended with an interval of five days between two courses. Chronic bronchitis may also be treated with the herb in combination with the root bark of *Morus alba*, the root of *Platycodon grandiflorum*, and the plant *Rhus chinensia* (* parts not specified). The old saying "all flowers exacerbate except <Xuanfu>" has prompted the use of <Xuanfuhua> to treat acute and chronic bronchitis with cough, expectoration and dyspnea.

2. Vomiting and Hiccup

This herb is often used together with the rhizome of *Pinellia ternata*, the peel of *Citrus reticulata* and *hematite* as in the Inula Hematite Decoction. In a clinical trial using this decoction to treat 50 cases of vomiting, 34 cases were cured, 14 improved, and 2 unresponsive. This decoction is believed to be useful for gastric distention and hiccup due to "disharmony of the liver and stomach" (7). The symptoms of gastric neurosis, gastric dilatation etc. were alleviated after treatment with the modified prescription of the Inula Hematite Decoction (8,9). The Inula Hematite Decoction and the Six Major Herbs Decoction, modified as needed, plus mega-dose of hematite, resolved 10 cases of intractable vomiting (10).

3. Incomplete Abortion

The Inula Decoction (Flos Inulae, Herba Allii Fistulosi, Radix Rubiae and silk decocted, filtered and mixed with red wine, children urine, and sugar) had been used with some modifications as needed in 30 cases of incomplete abortion. Complete expulsion of the embryo and decidual membrane, cessation of bleeding, relieve of abdominal pain, and cure were achieved (11).

REFERENCE

1. Pharmacology of Bronchitis Drug Research Unit, Second Military Medical College of the Chinese PLA. Preparation and pharmacological experiments of the extract of Flos Inulae (brief summary). 1972.

2. Tangshan District (Hebei) Health School. Medical Research Communications (Tangshan District Health Bureau, Hebei) 1974 (2):45.

3. Lingling District Sanitation and Anti-epidemic Station et al. Hunan Yiyao Zazhi (Hunan Medical Journal) 1974 1(5):54.

4. Antibacterial Section, Institute of Materia Medica of the Chinese Academy of Medical Sciences. Chinese Pharmaceutical Bulletin 1960 8(2):59.

5. Rashba OY et al. Chemical Abstracts 1955 49:10430h.

6. Gao YD. Chinese Medical Journal 1955 41(10):963.

7. Chen SJ. Zhejiang Journal of Traditional Chinese Medicine 1966 9(7):30.

8. Wang FD. Shandong Yiyao (Shandong Medical Journal) 1978 (5):21.

9. Zhang SG et al. Shanghai Zhongyiyao Zazhi (Shanghai Journal of Traditional Chinese Medicine) 1966 (2):63.

10. Nantong Medical College. Selected Information on Scientific Research. 1973; Guangdong Medical College. Chinese Traditional Prescriptions. 1974. p. 139.

11. Zhang ZC. Zhejiang Journal of Traditional Chinese Medicine 1966 9(2):20.

(Dai Guangjun)

MAHUANG 麻黄
(APPENDIX: MAHUANGGEN 附：麻黄根)

<Mahuang> is derived from the stem and branch of *Ephedra sinica* Stapf, *E. equisetina* Bge., and *E. intermedia* Schrenk et C.A. Mey. (Ephedraceae). It is bitter, punget, and "warm", and is known to be diaphoretic, "cold"-discutient, antiasthmatic and diuretic. It is used in common cold due to pathogenic "wind-cold", asthmatic cough, bronchial asthma, bronchitis, and edema.

CHEMICAL COMPOSITION

The whole plant contains 1–2% of alkaloids, of which 40–90% is ephedrine. Other alkaloids include pseudoephedrine and trace amounts of l-N-methylephedrine. d-N-pseudomethylephedrine, l-norephedrine, d-demethylpseudoephedrine, ephedine, catechoflavone and volatile oil. The volatile oil is l-d-terpineol (1). Ephedroxane was isolated from *E. intermedia* (2).

PHARMACOLOGY

1. Sympathomimetic Effect

1.1 Cardiovascular system

1.1.1 *Heart*. Ephedrine strengthens cardiac contractility and increase the cardiac output. In intact animals the alteration in the heart rate was negligible since the direct effect of ephedrine was counteracted by the reflex stimulation of the vagus nerves brought about by the elevated blood pressure. The heart rate, however, was accelerated with vagal blockade (3).
Arrhythmia caused by ephedrine is less frequent than by epinephrine. But it may accidentally develop in patients with severe organic heart disease or in those on digitalis therapy. Large doses depressed the heart (4,5). In addition, the emulsion of <Mahuang> volatile oil depressed the isolated frog heart (6).

1.1.2 *Blood vessels*. Ephedrine caused vasodilation in the heart, brain, and muscles and so reduced the blood flow in them. Ephedrine, however, caused vasoconstriction in internal organs, such as the kidneys and spleen, skin and mucous membranes, reducing the blood flow in them (3). Vascular congestion was relieved by application of ephedrine solution to the mucous membranes and no rebound was resulted (4). It was shown that the vasoconstricting action of ephedrine on the nasal mucosa was stronger and more prolonged than that of pseudoephedrine (7).

1.1.3 *Blood pressure*. Ephedrine increase both the systolic and diastolic blood pressure (0.01–0.2 mg/kg) and the pulse pressure (3). Low doses (0.01–0.02 mg/kg) of ephedrine given to dogs by intravenous injection elevated the blood pressure and maintained it for 10–15 minutes; high doses (6–10 mg/kg) caused cardiac depression, reducing the blood pressure (3,5). The pressor effect of d-pseudoephedrine is about one-half that of l-ephedrine, and that of the synthetic racemic ephedrine is intermediate (8). Ephedine may cause a fall in blood pressure (9).

1.2 Smooth muscles

1.2.1 *Bronchi*. The relaxant effect of <Mahuang> on the bronchial smooth muscle was weaker but more prolonged than that of epinephrine. Perfusion of low concentrations of ephedrine or pseudoephedrine into isolated rabbit lungs and bronchi resulted in bronchial dilation. Both l-ephedrine and d-pseudoephedrine can relieve increased respiratory tract resistance in dogs due to histamine or acetylcholine. Methylephedrine also can dilate bronchial smooth muscles (3,10,11).

1.2.2 *Eyes*. Instillation of ephedrine to eyes could dilate the pupils. Its mydriatic effect was more evident in Chinese who have heavily pigmented irises than in whites whose irises are light colored. Ephedrine has no significant effect on the light reflex, accommodation, and intraocular pressure (3,5).

1.2.3 *Gastrointestinal smooth muscles*. The herb relaxed gastrointestinal smooth muscles, suppressed peristalsis, and delayed the propulsion and evacuation of gastrointestinal content (5). The effect of ephedine on the isolated rabbit intestine was first depression and then stimulation (9).

1.2.4 *Uterus*. Ephedrine increased the tone and contraction amplitude of animal uteri. Such stimulant effects were blocked by ergotamine and enhanced by cocaine. Generally, the effect of ephedrine on the human uterus is inhibitory, and it was used in relieving dysmenorrhea (3,5). In isolated rat uterus at estrus, ephedrine was shown to antagonize serotonin (12). Ephedine produced a contractile response in isolated uterus of guinea pigs (9).

1.2.5 *Urinary bladder*. The herb increased the tone of the deltoid and sphincter muscles of the urinary bladder. Ephedrine reduced the frequency of urination, and, in sufficient dosage, caused urinary retention. It has, therefore, been used to treat enuresis in children (4,5).

2. Effect on the CNS

The central stimulant activity of ephedrine is known to be much stronger than that of epinephrine. Large therapeutic doses stimulated the cerebral cortex and subcortical centers, causing insomnia, restlessness, nervousness, and tremor. It also stimulated the respiratory center and vasomotor center (4). The emulsion of <Mahuang> volatile oil was found to initially stimulate and later depress rabbit respiration. Ephedrine at a certain dosage was shown to antagonize the sedative effect of the volatile oil emulsion in mice (6).

3. Antipyretic and Hypothermic Effects

The emulsion of <Mahuang> volatile oil reduced artificial fever in rabbits. The volatile oil and, particularly, terpineol of <Mahuang> showed a hypothermic effect in normal mice. These two agents did not cause diaphoresis in normal and pyretic cats (6). Both ephedrine and the total alkaloids of <Mahuang> failed to induce perspiration in man. The dose 50–60 mg produced a more powerful and quick-acting diaphoretic effect in subjects who had been exposed to high temperature for as long as 1.5–2 hours than in the unexposed, suggesting that ephedrine has a moderate diaphoretic effect (13).

4. Antimicrobial Effect

In vitro studies proved that the <Mahuang> decoction had different degrees of antibacterial action against *Staphylococcus aureus*, alpha streptococcus beta streptococcus, *Bacillus anthracis*, *Corynebacterium diphtheriae*, *Pseudomonas aeruginosa*, *Shigella dysenteriae*, and *Salmonella typhi* (14,15). In experiments with chicken embryos, the volatile oil was shown to inhibit the type A Asian influenza virus (6); it showed a therapeutic effect against the type A influenza virus PR_8 strain in mice (16,17). The MIC of the <Mahuang> decoction against the type A Asian influenza virus *in vitro* was determined to be 2 mg/ml (18). Another report claimed that application of 0.1 ml of the 50% <Mahuang> decoction to each chicken embryo was inactive against the type A influenza virus PR_8 strain (19). This negative result might probably be due to the influence of the protein in the allantoic fluid or to insufficient dosage which should be higher than the *in vitro* one. The Ephedra-Prunus-Gypsum-Glycyrrhiza Decoction was shown in experiments on chicken embryos to have inhibitory action against the influenza virus Shaanzhong 61-1 strain; the main active component in the prescription was <Mahuang> (20).

5. Miscellaneous Actions

The oral or intraperitoneal dose of the aqueous extract of <Mahuang> was shown to have antitussive effect (21).

Generally, ephedrine inhibits gastrointestinal secretion. It caused a weak and unstable hyperglycemic effect in dogs. Ephedrine caused a marked and persistent increase in the tone of exhausted skeletal muscles (4). It was also shown to antagonize generalized muscular paralysis in rabbits induced by the emulsion of <Mahuang> volatile oil (6). A diuretic effect was achieved by pseudoephedrine in dogs (22). The release of allergy mediators could be suppressed by the aqueous or ethanol extract of <Mahuang> (23).

Ephedroxane isolated from *E. intermedia* was found to have an anti-inflammatory action (2).

6. The Mechanism of Action of Ephedrine

Ephedrine belongs to the type of sympathomimetic amines with mixed actions.

6.1 The chemical structure of ephedrine resembles that of epinephrine. It can directly combine with α- and β-adrenergic receptors to produce sympathomimetic effects. This fact was confirmed in experiments using rabbit aorta strips (24–26).

6.2 Ephedrine also acts on adrenergic nerve endings, leading to the release of norepinephrine. In experiments on reserpinized spinal cats the ED_{50} of ephedrine in producing effects on the nictitating membrane, blood pressure, and heart rate were higher than those in nonreserpinized animals (25,27), thus confirming its norepinephrine-releasing action. Both ephedrine and pseudoephedrine were shown to inhibit norepinephrine uptake by nervous and nonnervous tissues. The most powerful action was exhibited by l-ephedrine in experiments on the isolated rabbit heart (28). *In vitro* ephedrine inhibited monoamine oxidase (MAO) (29).

In addition, ephedrine also interacts with serotonin and histamine receptors (26).

7. Tachyphylaxis to Ephedrine

Repeated use of ephedrine within a short period progressively attenuated its effect which was, however, restored in a few hours after discontinuation of the medication. The development of tachyphylaxis was attributed to the following factors: (1) Saturation of the receptors, for the direct effects, and (2) exhaustion of transmitters, for the indirect effect (30). Another paper claimed absolute tachyphylaxis developed faster in experimental cats with intact medulla oblongata-inferior colliculi than in those animals with the latter areas sectioned. Consequently, it was considered that the development of tachyphylaxis was related to central regulation (31). On the other hand, tachyphylaxis to deoxyephedrine was not altered by destruction of the reticular nuclei in the lateral midbrain (32).

8. Toxicity

The LD_{50} of the aqueous extract of <Mahuang> in mice was determined to be 650 mg/kg IP (21), and that of the volatile oil was 1.35 ml/kg (6). The MLD of ephedrine, racemic ephedrine and pseudoephedrine in various animals are listed in the table below (33).

MLD of ephedrine, dl-ephedrine, and pseudoephedrine.

Animal	Route of Administration	MLD (mg/kg) Ephedrine	dl-Ephedrine	Pseudoephedrine
frog	lymph sac	540	630	770
vole	IP	350	310	310
grey rabbit	SC	230	360	400
grey rabbit	IV	80	90	100
albino rabbit	IV	50	70	130
dog	IV	70	100	130

CLINICAL STUDIES

1. Hypotension

Hypotension resulting from extradural and spinal anesthesia can be prevented and treated with ephedrine. *Dosage and administration*: 15–30 mg injected intramuscularly or subcutaneously before anesthesia. If hypotension had already occurred, a dose of 30–60 mg can be injected intramuscularly (34).

2. Bronchial Asthma

Intramuscular injection or oral administration of ephedrine may alleviate or prevent the attack of bronchial asthma (34). Satisfactory therapeutic effects were obtained in 20 children with bronchial asthma treated with a decoction prepared from roasted <Mahuang> and sugar, each 30 g. Antibiotics were used in addition to control infection (35).

3. Chronic Bronchitis and Asthmatic Bronchitis

Therapeutic effects were achieved in chronic asthmatic bronchitis treated with the "San Ao Decoction" (Herba Ephedrae, Semen Armeniacae Amarum, Radix Glycyrrhizae, Fructus Perillae, and Lumbricus) modified to suit individual manifestations (36). The Ephedra-Prunus-Gypsum-Glycyrrhiza Decoction was reported to be effective in chronic bronchitis in aged persons (37).

4. Pneumonia of Children

The concentrated crude ethanol extract of the Lung-Clearing Decoction (Herba Ephedrae, Fructus Forsythiae, Semen Armeniacae Amarum, gypsum, Flos Lonicerae, Radix Scutellariae, Folium Isatidis, Semen Lepidii seu Descurainiae, Rhizoma Cynanchi Stauntonii, Fructus Aristolochiae, Fructus Perillae, and Radix Glycyrrhizae) given by mouth was effective in bronchopneumonia of children. Except for symptomatic treatment given to severe cases, no antibiotics were prescribed, yet therapeutic effects were achieved in all patients (38). The Ephedra-Prunus-Gypsum-Glycyrrhiza Decoction was also effective in pneumonia of children (39,40).

5. Whooping Cough

Satisfactory results were obtained in 288 cases of whooping cough, mostly between 3 to 5 years old, treated with the Ephedra-Prunus-Gypsum-Glycyrrhiza Decoction (Herba Ephedrae, Semen Armeniacae Amarum, gypsum, Radix Glycyrrghizae, Radix Stemonae, Semen Lepidii seu Descurainiae, Fructus Jujubae, maltose). It was relatively effective in catarrhal and spastic stages

(41). Whooping cough of children had also been effectively treated with the modified "Wenfei Huayyin Tang" (Lung-warming and Mucolytic Decoction, used to be called "Xiaoqinglong Tang" (42).

6. Diseases of the Skin and Mucous Membrane

The modified Ephedra-Cicada Decoction (Herba Ephedrae, Periostracum Cicadae, Flos Sophorae, Rhizoma Coptidis, Herba Spirodelae, and Radix Glycyrrhizae), or the modified Ephedra-Forsythia-Phaseolus Decoction (Herba Ephedrae, Fructus Forsythiae, Semen Phaseoli, Semen Armeniacae Amarum, Radix Glycyrrhizae, Rhizoma Zingiberis Recens, Fructus Jujubae, and Cortex Catalpae Radicis), was effectively used in treating urticaria, eczema, drug rash, allergy to paint, varicella, and pityriasis rosea (43–46). The Ephedra-Prunus-Coix-Glycyrrhiza Decoction was useful in multiple warts (47). The intramuscular dose of ephedrine was effective in alleviating allergic cutaneous and mucosal symptoms of urticaria and angioneurotic edema. The 0.5–1.0% ephedrine nose drops relieved mucosal congestion and swelling in rhinitis, thus relieving nasal obstruction.

7. Common Cold

The Ephedra Decoction (Herba Ephedrae, Ramulus Cinnamomi, Semen Armeniacae Amarum, and Radix Glycyrrhizae) was effectively used in the treatment of influenza (48). Good therapeutic effects were also reported of the <Mahuang> volatile oil (49).

8. Miscellaneous

8.1 *Lethargy.* The Ephedra-Aconitum-Asarum Decoction was reported to be effective (50).

8.2 *Nephritis.* Acute nephritis of children 120 cases was effectively treated with the Ephedra Decoction plus Atractylodes (51).

8.3 *Rheumatoid arthritis.* Effective treatment with the modified Yang-Harmonizing Decoction has been reported (52). Ephedrine was also used to treat myasthenia gravis (3).

ADVERSE EFFECTS AND EMERGENCY TREATMENT OF POISONING

The acute toxic reactions are headache, restlessness, insomnia, chest discomfort, palpitation, lacrimation, rhinorrhea, general malaise, fever, hyperhidrosis, upper abdominal discomfort, xerostomia, nausea, vomiting, tinnitus, elevation of body temperature and blood pressure, as well as tachycardia and extrasystole. Large doses may cause cardiac depression and bradycardia (53–56).

Intoxication from oral administration of this herb should be treated with emetics, gastric lavage, and purgatives in order to reduce absorption. Severe nervousness and spasm should be treated with barbiturates or chloral hydrate. Other measures include fluid replenishment and supply with oxygen (54–56).

(APPENDIX: MAHUANGGEN 附: 麻黄根)

<Mahuanggen> refers to the root and rhizome of *E. sinica, E. equisetina*, or *E. intermedia*. It has a sweet taste and a mild property. It is an anhidrotic useful in checking spontaneous profuse sweating, and night sweat. In recent years a pressor principle, 1-tyrosine betaine, was isolated from <Mahuanggen> and named maokonine (57). Two hypotensive principles isolated from this herb were ephedradine A (58) and ephedradine B (59). Ephedradine A hydrochloride or hydrobromide injected to rats at 1.5–1.8 mg/kg IV markedly decreased the blood pressure (58).

REFERENCE

1. Liu GS. Acta Pharmaceutica Sinica 1963 10(3):147.

2. Zhu DY. Guowai Yixue (Medicine Abroad) — Pharmacy 1980 2:123.

3. Goodman LS et al. The Pharmacological basis of Therapeutics. 6th edition. 1980. p. 163.

4. Goodman LS et al. The Pharmacological Basis of Therapeutics. 2nd edition. 1955. p. 505.

5. Sollmann T. A Manual of Pharmacology. 8th edition. 1957. p. 500.

6. Wei DQ et al. Abstracts of the Symposium of the Chinese Society of Physiology (Pharmacology). 1964. p. 103.

7. King T et al. Chinese Journal of Physiology 1929 3(1):95.

8. Pak C et al. Chinese of Physiology 1928 2(4):435.

9. Chen KK et al. Chinese Journal of Physiology 1935 9(1):17.

10. Pak C et al. Chinese Journal of Physiology 1930 4(2):141.

11. Akiba K et al. Chemical Abstracts 1980 92:88025v.

12. Mikawa U et al. Kampo Kenkyu 1978 11:425.

13. Kuno Y et al. Chinese Journal of Physiology 1937 11:47.

14. Lingling District Sanitation an Anti-epidemic Station et al. Hunan Yiyao Zazhi (Hunan Medical Journal) 1974 (5):49.

15. Medical Laboratory, 178th Hospital of the Chinese PLA. Medical Information (Health Division of the Logistics Department of Fuzhou Military Region) 1976 (3):54.

16. Wang SY. Kexue Jiyao (Science Record) 1958 2(7):301.

17. Wang SY. Kexue Jiyao (Science Record) 1959 3(3):93.

18. Liu GS et al. Acta Microbiologica Sinica 1960 8(2):164.

19. Microbiology Laboratory, Hubei Sanitation and Anti-epidemic Station. Chinese Medical Journal 1958 (9):888.

20. Ma ZY et al. Abstracts of the 1962 Symposium of the Chinese Pharmaceutical Association. Chinese Pharmaceutical Association. 1963. p. 345.

21. Shoji T et al. Chemical Abstracts 1978 88:115366h.

22. Pak C et al. Chinese Journal of Physiology 1929 3(3):287.

23. Zhang BH. Chinese Pharmaceutical Bulletin 1979 14(5):224.

24. Trendelenburg U et al. Journal of Pharmacology 1962 138:181.

25. Li WS et al. Acta Pharmaceutica Sinica 1964 11(4):252.

26. Li WS et al. Acta Physiologica Sinica 1966 29(2):205.

27. Trendelenburg U et al. Journal of Pharmacology 1962 138:170.

28. Chanh PH et al. Chemical Abstracts 1979 90:114933v.

29. Pei MY. Acta Pharmaceutica Sinica 1964 11(12):834.

30. Yang ZC et al. Acta Physiologica Sinica 1963 26(4):306.

31. Tao JY et al. Acta Physiologica Sinica 1960 24(1):22.

32. Tao JY et al. Abstracts of the Symposium of the Chinese Society of Physiology (Pharmacy). 1964. p. 35.

33. Pak C et al. Chinese Journal of Physiology 1929 3(1):81.

34. Shanghai First Medical College et al. Medical Pharmacology. People's Medical Publishing House. 1977. p. 401.

35. Gao LZ. Journal of Barefoot Doctor 1978 (3):13.

36. Fu SF. Heze Yiyao (Heze Medical Journal) (Heze District Health Bureau, Shandong) 1979 (3):3.

37. Donglou Health Centre (Hexi District, Tianjin) et al. Tianjin Medical Journal 1975 (12):626.

38. Pediatrics Department, Teaching Hospital of Qingdao Medical College. Shandong Yiyao (Shandong Medical Journal) 1978 (1):6.

39. Ding JH. Barefoot Doctor (Changwei District Institute of Medical Sciences, Shandong) 1977 (1):14.

40. Zheng NS et al. New Chinese Medicine 1977 (9):452.

41. Research Group of Oujiangcha Commune Health Centre (Yiyang, Hunan). Jiangxi Zhongyiyao (Jiangxi Journal of Traditional Chinese Medicine) 1960 (10):25.

42. Zhumushan Health Centre (Hanshou County, Hunan). New Chinese Medicine 1978 (2):104.

43. Wang JY. Journal of Traditional Chinese Medicine 1964 (7):7.

44. Gong ZF. Zhejiang Journal of Traditional Chinese Medicine 1966 9(4):36.

45. Zhu Y. Journal of Traditional Chinese Medicine 1964 (2):29.

46. Xia ZF. Chinese Medical Journal 1956 42(10):939.

47. Fan CF. Xinyiyaoxue Zazhi (Journal of Traditional Chinese Medicine) 1978 (1):30.

48. Traditional Chinese Medicine Group, Health Clinic of Shangzhuang Coal Mine (Fengcheng Bureau of Mines). Information on New Chinese Medicine (Jiangxi College of Traditional Chinese Medicine) 1975 (4):32.

49. Guo PG. Pharmaceutical Industry 1960 (4):47.

50. Jiang KM. Shanghai Zhongyiyao Zazhi (Shanghai Journal of Traditional Chinese Medicine) 1979 (6):37.

51. Chen PJ. Zhejiang Journal of Traditional Chinese Medicine 1964 (11):15.

52. Xiao ZX. Health Journal of Youjiang (Baise District Health Bureau, Guangxi) 1979 (2):38.

53. Shangguan KF. Chinese Journal of Internal Medicine 1963 11(5):350.

54. He BK. Chinese Journal of Internal Medicine 1964 12(5):477.

55. Yuan SY et al. Chinese Journal of Internal Medicine 1959 7(2):179.

56. Fang YC. New Chinese Medicine 1973 (4):212.

57. Zhu YQ. Guowai Yixue (Medicine Abroad) — Pharmacy 1979(4):245.

58. Tamada M et al. Chemical Abstracts 1979 91:157966w.

59. Tamada M et al. Chemical Abstracts 1979 91:123916q.

(Gong Xuling)

LURONG 鹿茸

<Lurong> refers to the noncornified young horn of *Cervus nippon* Temminck or *C. elaphus* L. (Cervidae). It is sweet and salty with a "warm" property. It has "kidney"-warming, yang-fortifying, sperm-generating, blood-nourishing, muscle-fortifying and marrow-tonifying actions. It is prescribed in emaciation due to tuberculosis, vertigo, anemia, soreness of lumbar and knees, impotence, spermatorrhea, and metrorrhagia due to asthenia and "cold".

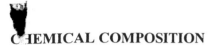

CHEMICAL COMPOSITION

<Lurong> contains 50.13% of amino acids, dry weight. The amino acids include tryptophane, lysine, threonine, valine, leucine, isoleucine, phenylalanine, histidine, arginine, proline, hydroxyproline, aspartic acid, serine, glutamic acid, glycine, alanine, cystine, methionine and tyrosine (1).

It also contains sphingomyelin, ganglioside (2), chondroitin A sulfate (3,4), PGE_1, PGE_2, PGF_{1a}, PGF_{1b} (5), androgens, estrogens, cholesterol, choline analogues, calcium phosphate and calcium carbonate. Pantocrine is an alcohol extract of the young horn.

PHARMACOLOGY

1. Tonic Effect

Various amino acids contained in <Lurong> were shown to have a tonic effect on the human body by increasing the capacity to work, reducing fatique, improving sleep, increasing appetite (6), correcting malnutrition and protein metabolic disorder (1), and improving glycolysis and Krebs cycle. This herb is believed to be capable of improving low tissue respiration occurred in yang-deficient states (7,8,9). <Lurong> also improves the health of aged and asthenic persons and promotes convalescence from disease (1). <Lurong> added into feed of mice and rats rapidly increased the body weight and accelerated the growth of tadpoles (2,10). Administration of pantocrine to animals for a certain period increased erythrocytes, hemoglobin, reticulocytes (2) and leukocytes (11). <Lurong> also markedly increased the oxygen consumption of the brain, liver, and kidneys of rats (12), suggesting increasing tissue metabolism.

2. Effect on the Circulatory System

Experiment on the blood pressure, isolated heart and blood vessels of various animals revealed that large doses of pantocrine decreased the myocardial contraction amplitude and heart rate, caused peripheral vasodilation and lowered the blood pressure; moderate doses caused marked activation of the isolated hearts, increase in the myocardial contraction amplitude and heart rate, and consequently increased the stroke volume and cardiac output. The action was particularly evident in the recovery of stressed heart. It could restore normal rhythms of the isolated heart. Small doses, on the other hand, had no marked cardiovascular effect. In clinical pediatrics, pantocrine turned the faint heart sound clear, strengthened weak pulse, elevated the blood pressure, and shortened the ECG PQ interval (6).

3. Sex Hormone-Like Effect

The prostate and seminal vesicle weighing method in orchidectomized rats and mice and the vaginal smear method in ovariectomized mice failed to find any sex hormone-like effects in the mixed ethanol and normal saline extracts of the young horn of *C. elaphus*. The aqueous extract could not cause ovulation in nonpregnant rabbits nor ejaculation of male toads; therefore, it exhibited no gonadotropic effects (10). Pantocrine slightly reduced the weight of the prostate and seminal vesicle of orchidectomized adult rats (13). However, the subcutaneously injected pantocrine increased the weights of the prostate and seminal vesicle of young rats, but it was less potent than testosterone propionate (14).

4. Effect on Wounds

Pantocrine could promote the regeneration of intractable ulcers and wounds and the healing of fractures (6). In rabbits and rats with wounds and injuries, cerebrospinal glycolysis appeared abnormal and the activities of hexokinase, aldolase, glycerophosphatase, glutamic oxaloacetic transaminase, glutamic pyruvic transaminase, and alkaline phosphatase were found inhibited. Treatment of these injured animals with pantocrine satisfactorily corrected all these abnormalities, and in rabbits improved the anomalous EEG (7,8).

5. Miscellaneous Actions

<Lurong> was shown to enhance the kidney function and gastrointestinal motility and secretory function. It also increased the tone and strengthened the rhythmic contraction of isolated uteri (6). <Lurong> is probably an immunoactivator because it was found to promote lymphocyte transformation in healthy subjects (15). Another paper stated that minute quantities of <Lurong> accelerated multiplication of cancer cells (16). Administration of pantocrine in rats increased the latent period and decreased the severity of audiogenic convulsion, mainly due to lowering of the excitability of related cortical regions (17).

CLINICAL STUDIES

1. Hematopoietic Diseases

The 20% "Lurong Xuejiu" prepared from the marrow of fresh <Lurong> and white wine 10 ml was given three times a day to treat thrombocytopenia, leukopenia, aplastic anemia, and blood dyscrasia due to chronic benzene poisoning. Different degrees of improvement in the blood picture and symptoms were achieved (18).

2. Ailments due to Asthenia

This herb is useful in treating all kinds of diseases due to asthenia including visceral asthenia and impotence in male, atrophy and weakness of low-back and knee, vertigo, spermatorrhea, metrorrhagia, metrorrhea, and chronic circulatory disorder with hypotension. It is also useful for restoring body strength after sickness, and as tonic for the old and weak subjects. The "Shenrong Weisheng Wan" (Ginseng-Antler Health Pill) is useful in old or weak persons.

REFERENCE

1. Fan YL et al. Chinese Traditional and Herbal Drugs Communications 1979 (8):4.

2. Pan LS (abstract translator). Fujian Medical Journal 1980 (2):64.

3. Kim et al. Chemical Abstracts 1977 87:99331q.

4. Fan HZ et al. Chinese Traditional and Herbal Drugs Communications 1979 (5):6.

5. Kim YE et al. Chemical Abstracts 1978 88:126250s.

6. Reshetnikova AD. Sovetskaia Meditsina 1954 (2):23.

7. Takigawa K et al. Folia Pharmacologica Japonica 1972 68(4):473.

8. Takigawa K et al. Folia Pharmacologica Japonica 1972 68(4):489.

9. Liu YG. Xinzhongyi (Journal of New Chinese Medicine) 1979 (1):50.

10. Xu YX. Acta Pharmaceutica Sinica 1959 7(7):283.

11. Chen HZ. Notes on Military Medicine (Medical Information Compiling Group of the 59170 Unit of the Chinese PLA) 1977 (2):1.

12. Biochemistry Section, Harbin Medical College. Heilongjiang Medical Journal 1959 (10):66.

13. Kit SM. Farmakologiia I Toksikologiia 1962 (5):629.

14. Iida T et al. Japan Centra Revuo Medicina 1966 219:497.

15. Qian RS. Journal of Traditional Chinese Medicine 1980 21(3):75.

16. Sato A. Kampo Kenkyu 1979 (2):51.

17. Dobrokhotova LP. Chemical Abstracts 1967 66:1486d.

18. Editorial Group. Notes on Science and Technology (236 Logistics Unit of the Chinese PLA) 1972 (1):14.

(Gong Xuling)

LUXIANCAO 鹿銜草

<Luxiancao>, also called <Luticao>, refers to the whole plants of *Pyrola rotundifolia* L. subsp. *chinensis* H. Andres, *P. decorata* H. Andres, or *P. rotundifolia* L. (Pyrolaceae). It is bitter and "warm". It has muscle- and bone-fortifying, antirheumatic, "kidney"-tonifying, lumbar-fortifying and hemostatic actions. Thus, it is used as a remedy for tuberculosis, cough, hemoptysis due to internal injury, rheumatism, low-back pain due to asthenia of the "kidney", and metrorrhagia.

CHEMICAL COMPOSITION

Methylhydroquinone, called luticaosu, is the active antibacterial component (1). The whole plant also contains arbutin, chimaphillin, ursolic acid, sucrose, invertase and small amounts of emulsin.

The young leaf contains tannin, volatile oil and bitter substances.

PHARMACOLOGY

1. Antibacterial Effect

<Luxiancao> has a relatively strong broad-spectrum bacteriostatic activity (1–4). The herb decoction was shown to inhibit *Staphylococcus aureus*, *Shigella flexneri*, *Salmonella typhi*, and *Pseudomonas aeruginosa* (4). Methylhydroquinone inhibited *Staphylococcus aureus*, *Salmonella typhi*, *Pseudomonas aeruginosa*, *Proteus vulgaris*, *Shigella sonnei*, and *Escherichia coli* at the MIC of 12.5, 12.5–50, 25–50, 50, 50 and 100 µg/ml, respectively (1).

2. Effect on the Cardiovascular System

Despite its weak action on the isolated frog heart, the herb extract enhanced myocardial contractility and antagonized arrhythmia in weak frog hearts. It also strengthened the myocardial contractility, dilated the blood vessels and lowered the blood pressure in dogs and rabbits. The leaf is more potent than the root and stem (5). Perfusion of the injection preparation of this herb (0.25 g/ml) to isolated rabbit ears, limbs, and hearts increased the blood flow; its vasodilatory effect was stronger on the coronary vessels than the ear and limb vessels of rabbits. Perfusion of the <Luxiancao> injection preparation also antagonized the vasoconstricting action of norepinephrine and caused vasodilation (6). In studies using myocardial ^{86}Rb uptake in mice as a parameter, the ether extract, the ethanol extract, crystal III of the ether extract and No. V and VI fractions of the ether extract of <Luticao> were found to increase to different extents the ^{86}Rb uptake, indicating their efficacy in improving myocardial blood flow (7).

3. Contraceptive Effect

When adult female mice were given the 20% <Luxiancao> decoction (species not specified) at 0.06 ml/10 g PO for 10 days and caged with male mice starting on the fifth day of medication for one month, all test animals were prevented from concention. The contraceptive action is presumed to be due to the inhibition of the estrous phase and causing atrophy of the uterus and particularly of the ovaries (8).

4. Miscellaneous Actions

Arbutin given orally rapidly hydrolyzes in the body to produce hydroquinone which conjugates with glucuronic acid. Administration of large doses of arbutin to subjects who had alkaline urine led to release of free hydroquinone which has bactericidal action. However, urinary tract infection was not quite responsive to this agent (9,10). An active transport system common for uvaol (xiongguofen) and glucose was found in the small intestine of voles and chicks; the affinity between this system and these substances was enhanced by Na^+ and inhibited by K^+ (11).

5. Pharmacokinetics

Within 10 minutes of injection of ^{14}C-methylhydroquinone to mice through the tail vein at the dose of 50 mg/kg (around 0.4 μCi/animal), drug concentration was found highest in the kidneys and liver, and lower in the heart and spleen. The drug was also found in the brain tissue. However, it had a short half-life in blood, only 15 minutes. The drug was excreted quickly mainly through the kidneys, mainly as metabolites (12).

6. Toxicity

The LD_{50} of methylhydroquinone in mice was determined to be 0.227±0.037 g/kg IV. When dogs were orally given 5 or 15 mg/kg of methylhydroquinone daily for 14 days, no abnormalities in the blood picture, routine urinalysis, liver and kidney functions, ECG, and pathohistological examination were found apart from mild vomiting in the high-dose group (1).

CLINICAL STUDIES

1. Pulmonary Infections

Out of 18 cases of pulmonary infection treated with methylhydroquinone, 16 were cured and 2 ineffective. The usual dosage was 200 mg daily by intravenous infusion plus intramuscular injection of 10 mg four times a day. In some cases the dosage was increased to 400 mg by IV infusion plus 100 mg IM daily (1).

2. Intestinal and Urinary Tract Infections

Satisfactory results were achieved with methylhydroquinone in 36 cases of infantile and children diarrhea, 16 cases of acute bacillary dysentery in young children, and 30 cases of acute bacillary dysentery in adults. The dosage of methylhydroquinone for mild diarrhea and simple bacillary dysentery in children was 40 mg PO 3–4 times a day, or 40 mg IM 2–3 times a day. In cases of severe diarrhea and severe bacillary dysentery in children, the dosage is 100–300 mg by intravenous infusion in two doses initially, and upon improvement of the patients's condition it was switched to intramuscular or oral administration. The adult dosage consisted of 200 mg four times daily by mouth, concurrently with daily intravenous infusion of 400 mg and intramuscular injection of 40 mg every 8 hours. The infusion was stopped after three days, and medication discontinued three days after disappearance of all symptoms (13). In another study using methylhydroquinone to treat 24 cases of enteric and urinary tract infections, fever was controlled in around 5 days in 18 out of 21 febrile cases. The drug was more ideal in controlling the acute symptoms of urinary tract infections but was less effective in rendering the urine tests negative. The dosage used was the same as for pulmonary infections (1).

3. Liver Abscess

One case of multiple liver abscess refractory to various antibiotics following operation was treated with methylhydroquinone alone at 200 mg by IV infusion twice daily together with 50 mg IM every 6 hours for 3 days. Treatment was subsequently switched to 100 mg IM every 6 hours for 9 days. The body temperature approached normal and symptoms were alleviated on the third day; the patient was cured and discharged from hospital after three months (14).

4. Miscellaneous

Methylhydroquinone was used to treat three cases of severe thromboangiitis obliterans with excellent results. It was also effective in 6 cases of hypertension and coronary disease. One of the cases had hypertension complicated with coronary disease; the blood pressure was restored to normal and remained stable. The coronary insufficiency and clinical symptoms were markedly improved; the ECG was also improved. The other 5 cases were acute myocardial infarction; the patients had marked improvement is symptoms and ECG after the treatment (6).

ADVERSE EFFECTS

No adverse reactions were known from daily intravenous infusion of 400 mg or intramuscular injection of 100 mg of methylhydroquinone (1).

REFERENCE

1. Chinese Traditional Drugs Research Group, Shuguang Teaching Hospital of Shanghai College of Traditional Chinese Medicine. Chinese Traditional and Herbal Drugs Communications 1976 (7):12.

2. Microbiology Section, Heilongjiang College of Traditional Chinese Medicine. Heilongjiang Zhongyiyao Xuebao (Heilongjiang Journal of Traditional Chinese Medicine) 1977 (2):20.

3. Wuhan Sanitation and Anti-epidemic Station. Hubei Information on Combined Western and Traditional Chinese Medicine. Hubei Institute of Scientific and Technological Information. 1974. p. 209.

4. Suzhou Medical College. Hubei Science and Technology — Medical Series (Hubei Institute of Scientific and Technological Information) 1971 (2):21.

5. Fang HS et al. Kexue (Science) 1946 28(6):266.

6. Wang SZ et al. Shaanxi Zhongyi Xueyuan Xuebao (Journal of Shaanxi College of Traditional Chinese Medicine) 1978 (1):35.

7. Zhuang PE et al. Abstracts of the First National Symposium on Cardiovascular Pharmacology. 1980. p. 14.

8. Gao YD et al. Abstracts of the Symposium of the Chinese Society of Physiology (Pharmacology). 1964. p. 69.

9. Frohne D. Chemical Abstracts 1970 72:41331p.

10. Winter AG et al. Chemical Abstracts 1958 52:2252h.

11. Alvarado F. Chemical Abstracts 1966 64:2514h.

12. Song S et al. Chinese Traditional and Herbal Drugs Communications 1979 (9):27.

13. Pediatrics Department, Shuguang Teaching Hospital of Shanghai College of Traditional Chinese Medicine. Shanghai Medical Journal 1978 (7):57.

14. Digestion Department, Zhongshan Teaching Hospital of Shanghai First Medical College. Medical Exchanges 1976 (10):51.

(Liang Yongyu)

Shanglu 商陸

<Shanglu> is the root of *Phytolacca acinosa* Roxb. or *P. americana* L. (Phytolaccaceae). Also known as <Yeluobo>, the root is bitter, pungent and "cold"; it is slightly toxic. It has diuretic and detoxicant actions. It is prescribed for oliguria, edema, and ascites. Externally, it is useful in trauma, hemorrhage, carbuncle, and in pyogenic infections of the skin.

CHEMICAL COMPOSITION

<Shanglu> contains oxyristic acid, jaligonic acid, acidic steroidal saponins, phytolaccine, phytolaccatoxin and large amounts of potassium nitrate.

PHARMACOLOGY

1. Diuretic Effect

Perfusion of the toad kidney with the <Shanglu> extract caused a marked increase in the urine output; instillation of the extract into the kidney or web of frogs caused capillary dilation and increase of blood flow. It is postulated that it acts by stimulating the vasomotor center leading to dilation of the glomerular capillaries, acceleration of circulation and finally diuresis in frogs. The action was dose-dependent; low dosage caused diuresis, but high dosage reduced the urine output (1).

2. Expectorant Effect

The phenol red excretion test on rabbits proved that the <Shanglu> decoction administered either intragastrically or intraperitoneally had marked expectorant effect. The dose 3 g/kg IP was more powerful than the dose 10 g/kg PO. Vagotomy did not modify this effect (2). Phenol red excretion experiment on mice also showed that the extract, tincture, and decoction of this herb given orally produced marked expectorant effect. The decoction preparation was most potent, comparable to that of the decoction of the root of *Platycodon grandiflorum*, whereas the tincture and aqueous extract had weaker effects (3). Small dose of the decoction 0.01 ml injected directly into the trachea increased the phenol red excretion which could be antagonized by atropine (2). The capillary permeability enhanced by egg white injection in rats could be decreased by the ethanol extract of this herb (4). Experiment on mucus transport speed of the intratracheal cilia of rabbits showed that the herb decoction could enhance ciliary movement (2). This result suggests that the expectorant effect may be due to direct stimulation of the respiratory mucous membrane, enhancement of ciliary movement and thus promoting expectoration. It can also decrease capillary permeability, thus alleviating bronchomucosal edema and reducing exudation. The active expectorant components were proved to be phytolaccagenic acid and methyl phytolaccagenate (5).

3. Antitussive Effect

As demonstrated in concentrated ammonia water spray method, the decoction and tincture of this herb had a weak antitussive action. Injection of this herb at 20 g/kg SC produced only slight antitussive effect in mice, and intragastric administration of its chloroform extract and saponins to mice also produced an insignificant effect. In contrast, the alkaloid fraction administered intragastrically to mice produced pronounced antitussive effect (6).

4. Antiasthmatic Effect

In asthma induced by histamine aerosol, the dose of 5 g/kg SC of the decoction or tincture did not produce anti-asthmatic effect. The drug exhibited antiasthmatic effect only at doses as high as 8 g/kg (approaching the lethal dose) (3).

5. Antibacterial Effect

The decoction and tincture of this herb were shown in disk diffusion method to inhibit some strains of *Hemophilus influenzae* and *Diplococcus pneumoniae* (3). They were highly effective against *Shigella flexneri* and *S. sonnei* and moderately effective against *Shigella shigae*. The aqueous extract also inhibited some skin fungi including Schlemm's *Dermatomyces favosa* and *Microsporum audouini* (7). A kind of glycoprotein present in the herb juice was shown to be active against tobacco mosaic virus (8).

6. Effect on Inflammation and the Adrenocortical Function

A single or multiple intragastric doses of the ethanol extract of this herb significantly inhibited the formaldehyde-induced paw swelling in rats. This effect disappeared after bilateral adrenalectomy. This herb also caused thymic atrophy in young rats and mice; a single intragastric dose significantly reduced the vitamin C content in rat adrenal glands, but failed to prolong the life of adrenalectomized young rats. Prednisolone completely blocked the decremental effect of <Shanglu> on the vitamin C level in rat adrenal glands, but it was unable to block the action of corticotropin under the same condition. In contrast, the action of corticotropin was completely blocked by pentobarbital sodium. These events imply that the herb has no corticotropic action but is capable of activating the pituitary-adrenocortical system through its influence on the CNS (9).

In addition, a triterpenic acid obtained from this herb also exhibited an anti-inflammatory action as potent as hydrocortisone on rat paw swelling (10).

7. Miscellaneous Actions

In vitro, the acidic steroidal saponin isolated from this herb was shown to have a spermicidal action (11). The 5% aqueous extract of <Shanglu> killed the wrigglers of *Culex pipiens pallens* (mosquitoes) (8). Antiradiation effect was provided by the 100% <Shanglu> decoction as evidenced by the reduced loss and quick recovery of platelets in rats received 600 rads of radiation (12). In addition, this herb was found to have emetic, purgative and taeniafugal actions (11).

8. Toxicity

The LD_{50} of the aqueous extract, decoction, and tincture of this herb administered orally to mice were determined to be 26.0, 28.0, and 46.5 g/kg, respectively. In terms of the lethality to mouse, the red herb is twice as toxic as the white herb. Boiling for two hours could greatly reduce the toxicity of both varieties of the herb. No abnormalities were observed in pathological examination of the heart, liver, lungs, and kidneys in rats fed with the decoction 5 g/kg for 3 weeks and in those fed with the ethanol extract 3.6 g/kg/day for 30 days. The ethanol extract did not aggravate toxic hepatitis lesions due to carbon tetrachloride. Oral administration of this agent to cats at doses of 2.5–10 g/kg resulted in vomiting; the severity of vomiting increased with the dosage. Oral doses of 1 g/kg also induced vomiting in dogs and reduced their activities (3,4).

CLINICAL STUDIES

1. Nephritis, Edema and Ascite

<Shanglu> produced excellent diuretic effect, and was very effective in acute, chronic nephritis of various origins, in cardiogenic edema, and ascites (13,14).

2. Chronic Bronchitis

The therapeutic effect of various preparations and extracts of <Shanglu> had been confirmed in more than 1790 patients from different regions and treated in different seasons. The medications were more efficacious as expectorant and antitussive than as antiasthmatic remedies, and were more effective in bronchitis of the simple type than in the asthmatic type. The tablet of the ethanol extract of this herb could enhance patients' adrenocortical function. In 682 cases treated with the honey syrup and honey pill for 30 days, the effective rate and short-term control rate were 89.4 and 57%, respectively. The ethanol extract tablet used in 1117 cases for 30 days afforded an effective rate and short-term control rate of 87–94.6% and 59–74%, respectively. Sixty cases were effectively treated with the crude total sapogenins (15).

3. Thrombocytopenic Purpura

All 21 cases, except one, were benefitted from treatment with the 100% herb decoction, as evidenced by the gradual disappearance of petechiae in 2–4 days, alleviation of epistaxis and gum bleeding, restoration of platelet count in 50% of the cases, and remission of bone marrow abnormality. This agent was also quite effective in anaphylactic purpura and hemoptysis (16).

4. Psoriasis

The <Shanglu> tablet was effective in 35 out of 43 cases of various types of psoriasis; it was more efficacious in arthritic psoriasis and simple psoriasis than in acute punctate psoriasis. *Dosage and administration*: 9 g a day divided into 3 doses orally for adults; dosage scaled down for children (17).

ADVERSE EFFECTS

<Shanglu> is toxic. Large oral doses of the dried herb caused diarrhea, central nerve paralysis, respiratory and cardiac disorders, and death. The causative agent was phytolaccatoxin. The adverse effects of the herb could be greatly decreased by processing and treatment. For instance, by prolonged decoction of the fresh herb and by preparation of the dried herb into honey pill, honey syrup, and ethanol extract. No pronounced ill effects were seen in 189 cases of chronic bronchitis given the honey pill and in 424 cases given the ethanol extract tablet for three courses. Only a few patients developed dryness of the nasopharynx and gastrointestinal symptoms, which usually disappeared spontaneously in 3–5 days. There was no significant toxicity on the liver, kidneys, heart and blood vessels (6,8).

REFERENCE

1. Masuzawa H. Chemical Abstracts 1943 37:1772(9).
2. Pharmacology Section, Xi' an Medical College. Acta Academiae Medicinae Xi' an 1976 (1):27.
3. Shaanxi Coordinating Group for Basic Clinical Research of Chronic Bronchitis. Shaanxi Medical Journal 1973 (3):31.
4. Xianyang District (Shaanxi) Science and Technology Group. Xianyang Science and Technology — Special Edition on Prevention and Treatment of Chronic Bronchitis with Yeluobo Gen 1975 (4):90.

5. Xianyang District (Shaanxi) Science and Technology Group. Xianyang Science and Technology — Special Edition on Prevention and Treatment of Chronic Bronchitis with Yeluobo Gen 1975 (4):103.

6. Shaanxi Coordinating Group for Basic Clinical Research of Chronic Bronchitis. Chinese Traditional and Herbal Drugs Communications 1973 (1):13.

7. Cao RL et al. Chinese Journal of Dermatology 1957 (4):286.

8. Foster JW. Chemical Abstracts 1948 42:7840c.

9. Xianyang District (Shaanxi) Science and Technology Group. Xianyang Science and Technology — Special Edition on Prevention and Treatment of Chronic Bronchitis with Yeluobo Gen 1975 (4):95.

10. Sick WW. Chemical Abstracts 1974 80:141071n.

11. Watt JM. Medicinal and Poisonous Plants of Southern and Eastern Africa. 2nd edition. 1962. p. 185, 833, 834.

12. Radiomedicine Section, Basic Sciences Division of Shenyang Medical College. Medical Research (Shenyang Medical College) 1975 (4):47.

13. Xue ZR. Journal of Traditional Chinese Medicine 1956 (11):586.

14. Liu BG. Journal of Barefoot Doctor 1975 (5):27.

15. Xianyang District (Shaanxi) Science and Technology Group. Xianyang Science and Technology — Special Edition on Prevention and Treatment of Chronic Bronchitis with Yeluobo Gen (Internal Information). 1975.

16. Jiangsu College of New Medicine. Encyclopedia of Chinese Materia Medica. Vol. 2. Shanghai People's Publishing House. 1977. p. 2245.

17. Dermatology Department, Second Teaching Hospital. Academic Information (Shanghai Second Military Medical College) 1975 (2):171.

(Gu Shiying)

YINYANGHUO 淫羊藿

<Yinyanghuo> refers to the whole plant of *Epimedium sagittatum* (Sieb. et Zucc.) Maxim., *E. brevicornum* Maxim. and *E. macranthum* Morr. et Decne (Berberidaceae). It is pungent and "warm" and has "kidney yang"-tonifying, muscle- and bone-fortifying as well as antirheumatic actions. It is used for impotence, atrophy and weakness of the low-back and knee, numbness of limbs, neurasthenia, amnesia and climacteric hypertension.

CHEMICAL COMPOSITION

The stem and leaf of *E. sagittatum* contain icariin, des-O-methylicariin, β-anhydroicaritin and magnoflorine. The underground part contains the flavone des-O-methyl-β-anhydroicaritin, icariins A, B, C, D and E, and 4 kinds of lignan (1).

PHARMACOLOGY

1. Effect on Endocrine Secretion

The aqueous extract of <Yinyanghuo> given to dogs intragastrically did not cause erection (or mounting behaviour) though it promoted semen secretion. The rank of potency of the various plant parts was leaf and root > fruit > stem (2). The weight-increase experiment on mouse prostate, seminal vesicle, and levator ani proved that the injection of the <Yinyanghuo> extract 20–40 mg was as efficacious as androgen 7.5 µg (3). A significant rise in the mean 24-hour urinary 17-ketosteroids even exceeding the normal level in healthy subjects was induced by administration of the herb to patients with chronic bronchitis, but no significant change in the 24-hour 17-hydroxycorticosteroid excretion was obtained. These results suggest that <Yinyanghuo> has gonadotropic effects (4).

2. Antitussive, Expectorant, and Antiasthmatic Effects

The phenol red excretion method proved that, except for the methanol extract, the fresh herb crude extracts "A", "B", and "C" as well as the ethyl acetate extract of the dried herb exhibited expectorant actions in mice. The methanol and ethyl acetate extracts were shown to have antitussive effect in mice with cough induced by sulfur dioxide. Likewise, cough in cats induced by electrical stimulation of the superior laryngeal nerve was completely suppressed by the methanol extract, suggesting a central action (5,6). In addition, the methanol extract protected guinea pigs from histamine-induced asthma (6).

3. Antimicrobial Effect

<Yinyanghuo> markedly inhibited *Staphylococcus albus, Staphylococcus aureus*, and, to a lesser extent, *Neisseria catarrhalis, Diplococcus pneumoniae*, and *Hemophilus influenzae* (7). At 1% concentration, the herb inhibited the growth of *Mycobacterium tuberculosis in vitro* (8). *In vitro*, this herb was showed to inhibit *Poliomyelitis virus*, ECHO virus types 6 and 9, and Coxsackie virus types A_9, B_4 and B_5. It directly deactivated these viruses (9).

Experiments also showed that the methanol extract of this herb could enhance the phagocytic ability of cells in inflammatory exudates of mice (6).

4. Effect on the Cardiovascular System

4.1 *Blood pressure*. Either the decoction or the ethanol-fractionated decoction of <Yinyanghuo> injected intravenously to rabbits (2.5 ml/kg), cats (2 ml/kg), or rats (4 ml/kg) produced a hypotensive effect; it was most conspicuous in rabbits (10–12). Some of the cats given intraperitoneal injection of the methanol extract developed hypotension in 1–2 hours; the blood pressure was recorded to be 30–60% of the original reading. In some cats, however, no significant changes in the blood pressure occurred (6). Intraduodenal injection of the "Erxian Mixture" (Herba Epimedii, Rhizoma Curculiginis, Radix Morindae Officinalis, Cortex Phellodendri, Rhizoma Anemarrhenae, and Radix Angelicae Sinensis) 6 g/kg to cats decreased the blood pressure starting 30 minutes after medication; the blood pressure was reduced by a mean of 30% at the end of two hours. The dose 6 g/kg IP of the same mixture caused an abrupt fall in the blood pressure and decrease in cardiac index but no significant peripheral vasodilation (13). Administration of the methanol extract 10 g/kg PO to rats with renal hypertension markedly decreased the blood pressure. The reading rose again after discontinuation of the medication (11). In experiments where dogs with renal hypertension were given the "Erxian Mixture" twice daily, at 9 g/kg PO daily for 10 days, 18 g/kg daily for additional 10 days and no medication for the next 10 days, the 30-day mean reduction in blood pressure was determined to be 10 mmHg (8%) and the mean "largest reduction" achieved in a 5-day period was 16 mmHg (12%) (12). Studies on the acute effect of the herb on rabbit blood pressure revealed that <Yinyanghuo> inhibited the pressor response to bilateral carotid arterial blockade but did not block the pressor effect of norepinephrine. Atropine injection did not significantly affect the hypotensive effect of this herb in cats but it surely markedly inhibited contraction of the nictitating membrane due to electrical stimulation of the preganglionic sympathetic fibers, but not that due to electrical stimulation of the postganglionic fibers. Consequenetly, it is considered that the hypotensive action of <Yinyanghuo> was not causally related to the α-adrenergic and muscarinic receptors but was primarily related to the blockade of sympathetic ganglions (12).

4.2 *Action on the heart*. Perfusion of isolated rabbit hearts with the ethanol extract of this herb or the non-amino acid fraction obtained from the tablet of its 200% aqueous extract (No. 5–1–1) markedly increased the coronary flow by 75.3% (14,15). Perfusion of isolated guinea pig heart with 0.5 ml of the 200% <Yinyanghuo> decoction precipitated a mean increase of 126.6% in coronary flow (16). Injection of No. 5–1–1 1 g/kg IV to anesthetized dogs did not significantly alter the heart rate, but markedly increased the coronary flow and decreased the coronary resistance. Injection of No. 5–1–1 1 g/kg IV to anesthetized rabbits produced a transient and slight drop in the left ventricular diastolic pressure and the difference between systolic and diastolic pressure of the left ventricle (15). In rats with pituitrin-induced acute myocardial ischemia, injection of the ethanol extract of this herb 3 g/kg IV failed to improve the first-phase T wave peak but significantly improved the second-phase T wave depression on the ECG (14). No. 5–1–1 could protect rats against pituitrin-induced acute myocardial ischemia, and also markedly shortened the duration of arrhythmia induced by K-strophanthin and epinephrine in guinea pigs although it failed to antagonize them completely (15). Determination of the oxygen consumption of rat myocardial homogenate with the Warburg's apparatus showed that No. 5–1–1 2 mg markedly increased the oxygen consumption of the myocardium within one hour of medication (15).

5. Effect on the Tolerance of Mice to Normobaric Hypoxia

Compared with the control mice, test mice given the 100% <Yinyanghuo> decoction 0.1–0.15 ml IP were protected from the lethal effect of hypoxia (16). However, the 100% ethanol extract 10 ml/kg had no effect on the tolerance of mice to hypoxia (14).

6. Effect on Blood Lipids

Intragastric administration of the 100% <Yinyanghuo> decoction to rabbits with experimental hyperlipidemia at 5 ml twice daily for 30 days lowered β-lipoprotein and cholesterol levels on the 10th, 20th, and 30th treatment days, and, on the 10th day, reduced triglycerides which rose slightly on the 20th and 30th treatment days (17).

7. Effect on Blood Glucose

In rats with experimental hyperglycemia, the extract of <Yinyanghuo> 10 mg/kg PO caused a marked lowering of the blood glucose level, which lasted over 60 minutes (18).

8. Anti-inflammatory Effect

Injection of the methanol extract of this herb 50 mg/kg SC to rats markedly reduced the severity of egg white-induced paw swelling (6). Oral administration of the same preparation to rabbits at 15 g/kg reduced the increase in capillary permeability induced by histamine (6).

9. Miscellaneous Actions

A significant sedative effect was observed in mice receiving the dose 20 ml/kg IP of the 10%

\<Yinyanghuo> decoction (16). Injection of the aqueous extract of this herb 0.5 ml IP to mice enhanced the immunological function of the animals (19).

10. Toxicity

The LD_{50} of \<Yinyanghuo> extract in mice was determined to be 36 g/kg IP (14). The LD_{50} of No. 5–1–1 in mice was 56.8 ± 2.7 g/kg IV (15). The methanol extract is low in toxicity; the dose 450 g/kg PO did not alter the normal activity of mice or produce any toxic effects in 3 days of observation (6). In an experiment in which dogs were orally given the "Erxian Mixture" at doses of 18, 54 or 72 g/kg for 20 days, dogs given the 54 g/kg-dose developed vomiting and passed watery stool after 7 days, while dogs given the 72 g/kg-dose had vomiting, anorexia and reduced activity on the third day. Microscopic examination of the animals sacrificed on the 15th day revealed mild hepatic fatty changes (13).

CLINICAL STUDIES

1. Chronic Bronchitis

An aggregate effective rate of 74.6% was achieved in 1066 clinical cases treated with the Herba Epimedii Pill alone. The effective rate obtained in cough (549 cases), expectoration (543 cases) and asthma (149 cases) were 86.8, 87.9 and 73.8% respectively. These results indicate that the drug has good expectorant and antitussive actions but poorer antiasthmatic effect (20). Clinical trials proved that the "Yanghuo" Ganchuan Ping" Tablet (Herba Epimedii, crude Concha Ostreae, Os Sepiae, Radix Polygoni, Herba Rubiae, Fructus Foeniculi, lycorine, clorprenaline glycyrrhizinate) was effective in asthmatic bronchitis, chronic bronchitis with emphysema, and particulary in bronchial asthma; it had very few side effects (21).

2. Coronary Disease

The Herba Epimedii Tablet was effectively used in 104 cases, 61 of which had angina pectoris. *Dosage and administration*: 4–6 tablets (0.3 g/tablet) twice daily. Each course lasts one month, intervals of 7–10 days between courses (22).

The injection of the fraction No. 5–1–1 caused different degrees of reduction in the cholesterol, β-lipoprotein, and triglyceride levels in 20 cases. The effect was more pronounced for the latter two lipid levels. *Dosage and administration*: No 5–1–1 Injection (2 ml/ampoule, from 4 g of the crude drug), 2 ml intramuscularly twice daily for 15 days as a course (23).

3. Hypertension

The Herba Epimedii Extract Tablet was tried in the treatment of 1115 cases of hypertension at a dose of 30 g(crude drug)/day in three doses for 1 month as a course. The maximal blood pressure reduction achieved by this treatment was 80/40 mmHg; better responses were seen in stage I patients (24). The "Erxian Decoction" (1:15) 15–30 ml twice daily was tried in 57 cases of hypertension. It was more effective in 14 cases with stage III hypertension, and also benefitted hypertension due to "yin" deficiency and "yang" excessiveness as well as that due to deficiency of both "yin and yang" (25). The drug was more satisfactory in treating menopausal syndrome and climacteric hypertension (26).

4. Poliomyelitis

Clinical trials showed that <Yinyanghuo> had therapeutic value in acute stage of poliomyelitis (26 cases). *Dosage and administration*: 10% Herba Epimedii Injection 2 ml IM once daily for 10 days as a course (27). A second paper reported that the "Anti-paralytic Injection" (Herba Epimedii and Ramulus Loranthi) was efficacious in the acute stage as well as sequelae of poliomyelitis. *Dosage and administration*: Acute stage — 100% Anti-paralytic Injection 2 ml IM twice daily for 20 days. Sequelae — 4 ml IM every other day (28).

5. Neurasthenia and Sexual Neurasthenia

Out of 104 cases of neurasthenia treated by iontophoresis with preparation of this herb, 22 were cured, 21 greatly improved, 44 improved, and 15 ineffective (29). In case of sexual neurasthenia, patients can be given a decoction prepared from 3–9 g of the herb orally daily, or small oral doses of the herb maceration (60 g of herb in 1 liter of wine) (30).

REFERENCE

1. Liu BQ. Chinese Traditional and Herbal Drugs 1980 (5):201.

2. Hashimoto R. Jikken Yakubutsugaku Shi 1937 14(2,3):195.

3. Miwa T. Japan Centra Revuo Medicina 1960 160:142.

4. Hubei Coordinating Research Group on Bronchitis. Selected Research Information on Chinese Materia Medica (Hubei Health Bureau) 1975 (6):48.

5. Scientific Research Group, Hubei Medical College. Scientific and Technical Information (Hubei Medical College) 1972 (1):9.

6. Hubei Coordinating Research Group on Bronchitis. Selected Research Information on Chinese Materia Medica 1976 (6):44.

7. Microbiology Section, Hubei Medical College. Scientific and Technical Information (Hubei Medical College) 1972 (1):14.

8. Guizhou Hospital of Tuberculosis. Chinese Journal of Prevention of Tuberculosis 1959 (6):37.

9. Zheng Y. Chinese Medical Journal 1964 50(8):521.

10. Hypertension Research Group, Pharmacology Section of Dalian Medical College. Compiled Information on Medical Research (Dalian Medical College. 1959. p. 363.

11. Liu GX et al. Abstracts of the Symposium of the Chinese Society of Physiology (Pharmacology). 1964. p. 115.

12. Pharmacology Section, Zhejiang Institute of Traditional Chinese Medicine. Scientific Research Compilation. Beijing Institute of Traditional Chinese Medicine. 1979. p. 109.

13. Chen WZ. et al. Acta Pharmaceutica Sinica 1960 8(1):35.

14. Pharmacology Section, Zhejiang Institute of Traditional Chinese Medicine. Scientific Research Compilation. Zhejiang Institute of Traditional Chinese Medicine. 1979. p. 112.

15. 234th Hospital of the Chinese PLA and Epimedium Research Unit of Shenyang College of Pharmacy. Journal of Shenyang College of Pharmacy 1975 (7):86.

16. Stage 42 Epimedium Research Unit of Shenyang College of Pharmacy. Journal of Shenyang College of Pharmacy 1977 (8):90.

17. Pharmacology Section, Jinzhou Medical College. Science and Technology of Jinzhou Medical College (Jinzhou Medical College) 1977 (6):19.

18. Hirayama S et al. Japan Centra Revuo Medicina 1971 276:344.

19. Military Medical School of Beijing Military Region et al. Compiled Medical Information (Beijing Military Region) 1978 (1):62.

20. Enshi District Office for Prevention and Treatment of Chronic Bronchitis. Health Journal of Hubei 1972 (7):15.

21. Shanghai Institute of Scientific and Technological Information. Shanghai Compilation of New Drugs. Shanghai Institute of Scientific and Technological Information. 1977. p. 80.

22. Coronary Disease Unit. 234th Hospital of the Chinese PLA. Journal of Shenyang College of Pharmacy 1977 (8):85.

23. Coronary Disease Unit, 234th Hospital of the Chinese PLA. Journal of Shenyang College of Pharmacy 1975 (7):92.

24. Cardiovascular Diseases Research Section, Zhejiang Institute of Traditional Chinese Medicine. Zhejiang Zhongyiyao (Zhejiang Journal of Traditional Chinese Medicine) 1977 (6):11.

25. Zhang BN et al. Chinese Journal of Internal Medicine 1965 13(6):501.

26. Guo YQ. Acta Academiae Medicinae Shandong 1978 (3):68.

27. Guangzhou Hospital of Infectious Diseases. New Medical Communications (Guangzhou Health Bureau) 1975 (6):12.

28. Zhengzhou Chinese Medicine Factory. Chinese Traditional and Herbal Drugs Communications 1972 (2):28.

29. Cai N et al. Jiangsu Zhongyi (Jiangsu Journal of Traditional Chinese Medicine 1962 (11):23.

30. Zhu Y. Pharmacology and Applications of Chinese Medicinal Materials. People's Medical Publishing House. 1958. p. 261.

(Yuan Wei)

DANZHUYE 淡竹葉

<Danzhuye> refers to the aerial part of *Lophatherum gracile* Brongn. (Gramineae). It is sweet, bland, and "cold" and has latent-heat-clearing, antipyretic and diuretic actions. It is prescribed for dry mouth in fever, and oliguria with yellow urine.

CHEMICAL COMPOSITION

The root, stem and leaf of *L. gracile* contain triterpenes and the steroids arundoin, cylindrin, friedelin, β-sitosterol, stigmasterol, campesterol, and taraxasterol.

PHARMACOLOGY

1. Antipyretic Effect

The aqueous extract of <Danzhuye> administered intragastrically to rats relieved fever induced by injection of an yeast suspension; the antipyretic principle was found to be soluble in water and dilute hydrochloric acid but not quite soluble in ethanol and ether (1). In fever of cats and rabbits induced by *Escherichia coli*, the antipyretic efficacy of this herb 2 g/kg was determined to be 0.83 times that of phenacetin 33 mg/kg (2).

2. Miscellaneous Actions

The <Danzhuye> Decoction 10 g administered to normal subjects produced a weak diuretic effect but increased the chloride excretion in urine (3). *In vitro*, the herb decoction inhibited *Staphylococcus aureus* and *Streptococcus hemolyticus* with MIC of 1:10 (4). Preliminary screening using mice with transplanted tumor showed that daily administration of the crude herb extract 100 g(crude drug)/kg for 14–20 days inhibited sarcoma 180 by 43.1–45.6%. It had no inhibitory action against cervical cancer U_{14} and ascitic lymphosarcoma-1 (5). In addition, this herb exerted a hyperglycemic action (2).

3. Toxicity

The LD_{50} of <Danzhuye> in mice was 64.5 g/kg (2).

CLINICAL STUDIES

1. Fever, Thirst, and Oliguria Due to Acute Infections
The decoction of 3–9 g of <Danzhuye> can be used as tea. It is, however, mostly employed in compound formulae such as the Zhuye Liu Bang Decoction and Lophatherum Gypsum Decoction.

2. Hordeolum and Serpiginous Corneal Ulcer

It was reported that a 95% cure rate in 57 cases of hordeolum was achieved by local application of the juice. Three out of 5 cases of serpiginous corneal ulcer treated with this juice were cured, 1 improved, and 1 was unresponsive (6).

3. Urolithiasis and Infection

Fourteen cases of urinary tract infections and one case of ureteral lithiasis were cured or alleviated by the use of the modified "Dao Chi Powder" (Folium Lophatheri, Radix Rehmanniae, Caulis Aristolochiae Manshuriensis, and Radix Glycyrrhizae) (7).

REFERENCE

1. Hutchins LG et al. Chinese Journal of Physiology 1937 11:35.

2. Zhu HB et al. Abstracts of the First Congress of the Chinese Society of Physiology (Pharmacy). 1958. pp. 65–67.

3. Shen JW et al. Acta Academiae Medicinae Primae Shanghai 1957 (1):38.

4. Laboratory of Guangdong College of Traditional Chinese Medicine. Xinzhongyi (Journal of New Chinese Medicine) 1971 (2):30.

5. Tumor Research Section, Institute of Materia Medica of the Academy of Traditional Chinese Medicine. Selected Information on Science and Technology. Information Department of the Academy of Traditional Chinese Medicine. 1972. p. 136.

6. Ge XM. Jiangsu Yiyao (Jiangsu Medical Journal) 1976 (5):46.

7. Internal Medicine Department, Yulin Special Zone Hospital of Traditional Chinese Medicine. Fujian Zhongyiyao (Fujian Journal of Traditional Chinese Medicine) 1965 10(6):43.

(Dai Guangjun)

LINGYANGJIAO 羚羊角

<Lingyangjiao> is the horn of the antelope *Saiga tatarica* L. (Bovidae). It is salty and "cold". It has hepatic-depressant, anticonvulsant, latent-heat-clearing, antipyretic, detoxicant and anti-inflammatory actions. It is, therefore, used for the treatment of coma and convulsions in febrile diseases, delirium, headache and vertigo, epilepsy or convulsion precipitated by fear, cramps, acute conjunctivitis, and corneal opacity.

CHEMICAL COMPOSITION

The antelope horn contains keratin, calcium phosphate and vitamin A. The amount of keratin is highest.

PHARMACOLOGY

1. Sedative and Anticonvulsant Effects

Intraperitoneal injection of the ethanol extract or injection of the antler to mice reduced the spontaneous activity of animals (1,2). The cortical extract of the antler decreased the orientating motor response and shortened the induction period of barbital and ether anesthesia in mice (3). Similar effects were achieved with the intraperitoneally injected ethanol extract 10 g/kg, decoction 2 g/kg, and hydrolysate 80 mg/kg of <Lingyangjiao>, i.e., they all markedly prolonged the thiopental sodium-induced sleep in rats (1,4). The hydrolysate injection 80 mg/kg significantly prolonged sleep induced by pentobarbital sodium (2). These results imply that hydrolysis increased the sedative activity of <Lingyangjiao> (4).

In addition, injection of the 10% antler decoction 0.1 g into toad lymph sac did not significant decrease the incidence of caffeine-induced convulsion but markedly increased the recovery rate. In mice given the decoction 10 g/kg PO, the caffeine-induced convulsion rate was significantly decreased and the recovery rate was increased; however, it had no significant anticonvulsant effect on strychnine-induced convulsion (5). The dose 80 mg/kg IP of Antler Injection antagonized strychnine-induced convulsion (2).

2. Antipyretic Effect

A prominant antipyretic effect was achieved by intravenous injection decoction and ethanol extract of antler 2 g/kg each, or the hydrolysate 40 mg/kg, or the injection 800 mg/kg in rabbits with experimental fever (1,2,4). The dose of the antler decoction 4 g/kg PO reduced experimental fever of rabbits in 2 hours, and normal body temperature was gradually restored after 6 hours (5).

3. Effect on the Circulatory System

Injection of the 50% decoction 2 ml/kg IV to anesthetized cats decreased the blood pressure, but the hypotensive action was somewhat attenuated after bilateral vagotomy, suggesting a central action (1). In isolated toad hearts, low dosage of the decoction or ethanol extract increased the cardiac contractility; moderate dosage caused conduction block, and high dosage decreased the heart rate and contraction amplitude, leading to cardiac arrest (1).

4. Miscellaneous Actions

In vitro tests showed that the Antler Injection had no inhibitory action against various gram-positive and gram-negative pathogens (6). The extract of the antler cortex increased the tolerance of mice to hypoxia and also produced an analgesic effect (3).

5. Toxicity

After intravenous injection of the 4% antler hydrolysate 8 ml/kg (equivalent to 100 times the adult dose) to mice, no abnormalities were observed apart from a slight decrease in activity in 3 hours (4). The oral dose 2 g/kg of the 10% antler decoction given to mice for 7 days produced no significant effect except a slight decrease in the increase of body weight (5).

CLINICAL STUDIES

1. Hyperpyrexia

The Antler Injection (from hydrolysate) was used as an antipyretic given intramuscularly to 100 cases, including 38 cases of influenza, 22 measles, 19 pneumonia in children, and 21 other febrile diseases. Marked effects were obtained in 41 cases, and moderate effects in 45; there were 14 cases ineffective (4).

2. Convulsion due to Hyperpyrexia in Infectious Diseases

The antler was claimed to clear up heat and stop convulsion. It is often used in formulae with the hook bearing branches of *Uncaria rhyncophylla*, the root of *Rehmannia glutinosa* and the flower of *Chrysanthemum morifolium*, e.g., the Antelope-Uncaria Decoction. In eclampsia of pregnancy with deficiency of the "liver-yin", the antler can be used with the seed of *Ziziphus jujuba*, the root of *Ophiopogon japonicus*, the branch and leaf of *Loranthus parasiticus*, the gelatin of ass skin, and the shell of *Ostreae rivularis*, e.g., the modified "Antler Powder" (7).

3. Primary Thrombopenic Purpura Hemorrhagica

Twenty-two patients had been treated with the "Lingyang Sanhuang Decoction" (Cornu Antelopis, Radix Rehmanniae, Flos Lonicerae, Cortex Moutan Radicis, Pericarpium Citri Reticulatae, Cortex Phellodendri, Rhizoma Coptidis, Fructus Gardeniae, Radix Paeoniae Alba, Rhizome Imperatae, Radix Glycyrrhizae, and Colla Corii Asini). Three of them had a short 3-day course of the disease. Except for one who received 300 ml of blood transfusion because of profuse epistaxis, all cases received no other drugs. Hemorrhage stopped after 3–7 days in all cases with subsidence of purpura. Platelet count in one case which had the lowest measurement of 25,000 was increased to over 128,000 without relapse in two years. On the other hand, of the 18 cases with course over six months, 6 had pretreatment platelet level below 40,000 and 12 between 40,000–80,000. Most of them had bleeding stopped in 3–13 days after the treatment. The platelet count rose to 95,000 in one case and to over 122,000 in the other 17 cases. Bleeding time was restored to normal range in all cases (8).

4. Glaucoma Pain, Dizziness, Headache, Blurred Vision with Nausea and Vomiting due to "Upward Disturbance of Liver-Fire".

The antelope horn is often used with the seed of *Plantago asiatica*, the root of *Scutellaria baicalensis*, the root of *Scrophularia ningpoensis*, the rhizome of *Anemarrhena asphodeloides*, the sclerotium of *Poria cocos*, the root of *Ledebouriella divaricata* and the whole plant of *Asarum heterotropoides* var. *mandshuricum*. The antelope horn can be made into powder (Antelope Horn Powder) to be taken with water, or cut into pieces to be decocted for one hour and taken by mouth, or as pill and powder preparations (7).

A paper reported the effectiveness of the horn powder in treating infantile eczema (8).

REFERENCE

1. Drug Control Laboratory, Nanjing Medicinal Materials Company et al. Jiangsu Yiyao (Jiangsu Medical Journal) 1976 (4):57.

2. Li YG et al. Chinese Traditional and Herba Drugs Communications 1979 (5):12.

3. Brekhman II. Farmakologiia I Toksikologiia 1971 34(1):36.

4. Heilongjiang Health School. Chinese Traditional and Herbal Drugs Communications 1977 (1):17.

5. Qu SY et al. Harbin Zhongyi (Harbin Journal of Traditional Chinese Medicine) 1963 (3):38.

6. Qian Q et al. Abstracts of the Academic Conference of Nanjing Medical College. Volume 2. Nanjing Medical College. 1979. p. 109.

7. Zhongshan Medical College. Clinical Applications of Chinese Traditional Drugs. 1957. p. 463.

8. Yang QB. Chinese Medical Journal 1974 (6):364.

(Yuan Wei)

BANMAO 斑蝥

<Banmao> refers to the Chinese cantharide *Mylabris phalerata* Pallas (*M. sidae* Fab.) or *M. cichorii* Fab. (Meloidae). It is pungent, "cold", and toxic. It has antivirulent, antiulcerative, hemostasis-eliminative (anticoagulant), and discutient actions. It is mainly used to treat malignant sores, abdominal mass, lymph node tuberculosis, thyroid tumor, and rabies, and to induce abortion.

CHEMICAL COMPOSITION

The Chinese cantharide contains cantharidin 1–1.2%, fats 12%, wax, formic acid and pigments. A series of cantharidin derivatives were recently synthesized in China; those having antineoplastic activity were sodium cantharidinate, hydroxycantharidinimide, methylcantharidinimide and propenylcantharidinimide (1–3).

PHARMACOLOGY

1. Antineoplastic Effect

In 1933, it was discovered abroad that 3–4 doses of cantharidin caused the disappearance of tar-induced cancer in rabbits (4). In-depth studies undertaken in recent years by Chinese workers revealed that cantharidin was capable of inhibiting ascitic malignant hepatoma and reticulosarcoma ARS in mice. It was found that injection of the agent at the tolerance dose 1–1.25 mg/kg IM daily for 7 days to mice with ascitic hepatoma prolonged the animals' survival by 63.5–208%, and in mice with ascitis ARS by about 56%. However, this effect depended on the number of inoculated cancer cells and the dosage employed. Thus, no significant effect was observed whenever the dosage was reduced or the number of inoculated cancer cells was increased to over 2×10^6 per animal (5). On the other hand, cantharidin showed no significant inhibitory effect on other tumors in mice, such as sarcoma 180, reticulosarcoma L_2, sarcoma S_{AK}, reticular leukemia L_{615}, Ehrlich ascites carcinoma, and Walker carcinoma 256 in rats (5,6). Cantharidin was also reported to cause marked atrophy, degeneration and cytoplasmic vacuolization of ascitic hepatoma cells in mice. Experiments proved that cantharidin initially inhibited protein synthesis of cancer cells and later the biosynthesis of RNA and DNA, resulting in inhibition of the growth and mitosis of cancer cells (7).

Intraperitoneal injection of hydroxycantharidinimide 60–100 mg/kg (6,8), methylcantharidinimide 170–230 mg/kg (6), propenylcantharidinimide 60–80 mg/kg (6), or sodium cantharidinate 1–2 mg/kg (2,9,10) once daily for 7–9 times inhibited ascitic hepatoma and ascitic reticulosarcoma ARS in mice. Their antineoplastic activities resembled that of cantharidin. Among these derivatives hydroxycantharidinimide showed the highest chemotherapeutic index (11). Sodium cantharidinate, however, had a wider antineoplastic spectrum; it inhibited not only ascitic hepatoma and ARS but also sarcoma 180, cervical cancer U_{14}, and solid Ehrlich ascites carcinoma in mice. *In vitro*, it was also inhibitory to HeLa cells, human squamous carcinoma of the esophagus CaEs-17 cells and human hepatoma BEL-7402 cells. Electron microscopy revealed that ^{3}H-sodium cantharidinate directly penetrated the nuclei and nucleoli of ascitic hepatoma cells in mice. Biochemical techniques also showed that sodium cantharidinate reduced the DNA and RNA contents of the cancer as well as incorporation of DNA and RNA precursors into cells. These findings showed that the drug inhibited the nucleic acid metabolism of cancer cells and caused morphological and functional changes, consequently killing the cancer cells (2,9).

In addition, the results of the concomitant immunity studies on mice with reticulosarcoma ARS, the graft-versus-host reaction (GVHR) tests, and determination of the phagocytic ability of macrophages in tumor-bearing animals proved that cantharidin and its derivatives had no influence on these immunities (2,5,8,10,12). Methylcantharidinimide, however, was shown to inhibit the cutaneous delayed hypersensitivity induced by DNCB in normal mice and in mice with ascitic hepatoma (13).

2. Antiviral Effect

A cure rate of over 90% was achieved with the lipophilic <Banmao> extract 0.6–1.0 mg in the treatment of acute Newcastle disease in chickens. In contrast, the mortality rate of the untreated fowls or the those treated with the soluble <Banmao> extract was found to be 90–100% (14).

3. Increase of Leukocytes

By stimulating the bone marrow, the Chinese cantharide increased white blood cells. In nine persons poisoned by inadvertent ingestion of the beetles, the WBC counts mostly lied between $10,000-20,000/mm^3$, the highest WBC count being $50,000/mm^3$. Test animals given cantharidin showed active leukocyte multiplication in bone marrow. A similar phenomenon was observed with sodium cantharidinate (2).

4. Local Irritation

Chinese cantharides may cause reddening and blistering of the skin in both animals and man, the active agent is cantharidin (15,16). The beetle is commonly said to be an aphrodisiac; this may be due to its irritating effect on the urethral musosa which induces penile erection when it is excreted in the urine (15).

In recent years many hospitals in China have a good method of obtaining large numbers of macrophages for the determination of their phagocytic function. This method involves producing blisters on the wrist skin by a 10% tincture of the Chinese cantharide (17).

5. Gonadotropic Effect

Intragastric administration of cantharidin (1–20 mg/ampoule) to female rabbits for 20–45 days resulted in dose-dependent increases in the urinary estrogens and progesterone (18). One paper, however, reported that only the semi-pure preparations of the Chinese cantharides had some estrogenic effect, whereas the pure preparation was inactive (19).

6. Miscellaneous Actions

In vitro, the 1:4 aqueous extract of <Banmao> was shown to inhibit 12 kinds of pathogenic skin fungsi including *Trichophyton violaceum* (20). It could also kill larvae of filaria. Moxibustion with the Mylabris Pill produced a significant detumescent effect in experimental ankle arthritis in rabbits (21).

7. Pharmacokinetics

The results of studies on the obsorption, distribution, and excretions of the tritiated cantharidin, sodium cantharidinate, hydroxycantharidinimide, and methylcantharidinimide are listed in Table 1. The pharmacokinetic indices of hydroxycantharidinimide and methylcantharidinimide are shown in Table 2.

8. Toxicity

Among cantharidin and its derivatives, the former is the most toxic, next sodium cantharidinate, whereas hydroxycantharidinimide and methylcantharidinimide are very low in toxicity. Table 3 shows the results of toxicological studies.

Early literature reported that the lethal dose of cantharidin for man is 30 mg PO; the lethal doses for cat and dog, for rabbit and for hedgehog are 2.5, 45 and 3000 times higher than that for man, respectively (4).

Both acute and subacute toxicity tests indicated that the kidney is highly sensitive to cantharidin. Dogs given the lethal dose (1 mg/kg) of cantharidin developed very serious cloudy swelling of renal glomerular epithelial cells followed by leukocytosis, albuminuria, cylindruria, hematuria and elevation of serum nonprotein nitrogen (25). Cloudy swelling of the renal tubular epithelial cells was seen in both acute and subacute toxicity tests. Renal toxicity was more marked in the subacute than in the acute test, and more severe in high-dosage than in the low-dosage group. The intoxicated dogs and mice might also develop hepatocellular cloudy swelling, fatty change, hepatic lymphofiberous damage, hepatocellular necrosis, myocardial cloudy swelling, and pulmonary congestion (4,5). Cantharidin has also been reported to be carcinogenic. In 60.3% of mice locally treated with the 0.016% solution of cantharidine in benzene, skin tumor, skin cancer, reticulocytosis and malignant lymphoma developed 16 months later. The drug synergized with small dose of the carcinogen 20-methylcholanthrene (26).

Table 1

Drug	Route of adminis-tration	Experimental animal	Absorption	Distribution	Excretion	Reference
^{3}H-Canthari-din	IP PO	Mice with ascitic hepatoma	Blood level peaked at 1 hr after an oral dose. Absorption and elimination was faster by IP than PO	Highest in bile and GI content next in the liver, kidneys and tumor tissues	Mainly urinary	(2,5)
^{3}H-Sodium canthari-dinate	IP PO	Mice with Ehrlich ascites carcinoma and ascitic hepatoma	Blood level peaked at 2 hr after oral dose. Eliminated in 72 hr. Absorption was faster by IP than PO	High in bladder, gallbladder kidneys, liver, and tumor tissues	Mainly urinary	(2,9)
^{3}H-Hydroxy-canthari-dinimide	IV	Normal mice and mice with ascitic hepatoma	T½β was 4.5 min	Highest in kidneys next in the liver and tumor tissues After 6 hr, evenly distributed in various organs	Mainly urinary	(2,8)
^{3}H-Methly-canthari-dinimide	PO	Mice with solid ascitic hepatoma	Blood level peaked 20 min after an oral dose; eliminated in 24 hr	Highest in the bile and liver, next in tumor tissues	Mainly urinary; rapid	(22)

Table 2

Drug		^{3}H-Hydroxycanth-aridinimide		^{3}H-Methylcanth-aridinimide	
Animal		Rat		Mouse	
Route of Administration		IV	PO	IV	PO
Pharmaco-kinetic indices	Absorption t$_{1/2}$Ka (hr)		2.99		0.083
	Distribution t$_{1/2\alpha}$ (hr)	0.067		0.03	0.25
	Elimination t$_{1/2\beta}$ (hr)	2.208		0.51	0.72
	Bioavailability F (%)		94.15		87.90
	Theoretical peak time, t'max (hr)		0.90		
	Volum of distribution Vd* (1/kg)	1.237		0.31	
	Elimination rate (1/hr/kg)	0.388		0.986	
Reference		(23)		(24)	

* Area method

Table 3

| Drug | Acute toxicity in mice | | Subacute toxicity | | | | Refer-ences |
	Route of administ-ration	LD_{50} (mg/kg)	Animal	Dose (mg/kg)	Route × days	Main toxic reactions	
Canthari-dine	I P	1.71 1.25*	Mouse	0.375–0.5	IP × 10	Mainly organic damage of heart and kidneys	(5,25)
Sodium canthari-dinate	PO I P IV	3.8±0.23 3.4±0.26 2.67±0.22	Mouse	0.25–1	IP × 12	Mild affection in renal tubular epithelium and lumen	(10)
Hydroxy-canthari-dinimide	IV	1037	Rat Dog	200–300 18–36	IP × 13 IV ×12	Rare mild inflamma-tory affection in urinary system	(8)
Methyl-canthari-dinimide	IV PO	818 375	Rat	100–300	PO × 35	Rare very mild affection in kidneys	(12)

* Data from referene 24

Injection of sodium cantharidinate to test animals at doses of 0.25 and 1 mg/kg IP daily for 7 days did not produce any significant pathological changes in various internal organs in the low dose group but, in the high dose group, mild porous changes in the epithelial cells of renal convoluted tubules and considerable accumulation of suspension in the tubular lumen, as well as mild pathological changes in the liver and lungs. In general, the toxic reactions were milder than those of cantharidin (10).

The subacute toxic reactions of hydroxycantharidinimide and methylcantharidinimide were relatively mild. Except occasional pathological changes in the urinary system in the high-dosage group (300 mg/kg), no pronounced toxic reactions in rats and mice were observed (8,12).

CLINICAL STUDIES

1. Primary Hepatoma and Other Neoplasms

Chinese cantharides cooked with chicken eggs or powder of Chinese cantharides and eggs (5–6 cantharides with the head, wings, and legs removed were introduced into the egg, baked to dryness by low heat, pulverized, and divided into two packs) had been administered by mouth one pack 1–3 times daily. The longest course was 14 months. It allegedly caused remission of the symptoms and prolonged the patients' life (2).

The "Compound Cantharidin Tablet" chiefly composed of cantharidin (each tablet containing cantharidin 0.25 mg; plus Rhizoma Bletillae powder, aluminum hydroxide, and magnesium trisilicate) was usually administered orally at 2–6 tablets daily in 3 doses. Most cases started with small doses and gradually increased to the usual dose. According to criteria established in China, this medication was effective 45–60% of over 800 cases of primary hepatoma. Some cases had tumor shrinkage, symptomatic improvement, and prolongation of survival period. The one-year survival rate was 12.7%. It was also effective in neoplasms of the rectum, colon, and esophagus (2).

Hydroxycantharidinimide is available in injection and tablet dosage forms. The usual dose of the injection is 80 mg daily, which can be administered intramuscularly or by intravenous infusion. The usual dosage of the tablet is 75–300 mg/day divided into 3 doses. One therapeutic course lasts one to several months. The aggregate effective rate in 142 cases of primary hepatoma, according to Chinese criteria, was 56.3%; the survival rate was up to 36%; α-fetoprotein became negative in some patients. The drug was preliminarily shown to be effective against cancers of stomach and esophagus. No significant toxic effects and side effects were known with its use (2,27).

The usual oral dose of methylcantharidinimide is 30–200 mg. It was effective against primary hepatoma. It use was associated with 8–9 months of survival, tumor shrinkage and alleviation of symptoms. It has marginal toxicity and side effects (28,29).

2. Viral Hepatitis

The Lipophilic Cantharidin Tablet (cantharidine 0.1 mg, edible vegetable oil 20 mg) at 0.02 mg/kg daily by mouth, or external application of an oil gauze of cantharidin 1:10,000 over the liver area 5–20 cm^2/kg very 1–2 days, had been used to treat 100 cases of hepatitis A (50 cases each of icteric and nonicteric types); 70% of the cases obtained symptomatic relief in 2–5 days and the remaining 30% in 6–8 days; 65% achieved normal liver function 14–20 days and the remaining 35% in 21–30 days. It is a must to continue treatment for additional 1–2 weeks after the initial cure. The systemic and topical uses of this drug in combination were of utility in the management of acute and chronic hepatitis B (14).

3. Allergic Rhinitis

Significant symptomatic relief was achieved in 150 cases of allergic rhinitis topically treated with the Chinese cantharide powder to the "Yintang" acupoints bilaterally (30).

ADVERSE EFFECTS

Oral administration of 0.6 g of Chinese cantharides to normal subjects may cause serious toxic reactions, and the oral doses 1.3–3 g can cause death. Toxic symptoms include: burning sensation of the oral cavity, thirst, dysphagia, swelling and blistering of tongue, dyspnea, salivation, nausea, vomiting, gastric bleeding, intestinal colic, inflammatory diarrhea and abdominal pain, urinary symptoms including urodynia, polyuria, proteinuria, cylindruria, hematuria and paroxysmal pain, and other symptoms such as weak pulse, shock, and prostration (4). Deaths due to attempts to induce abortion by administering large numbers of Chinese cantharides were not uncommonly reported; however, abortion was never succeeded (2,31).

Cantharidin produced toxic and side reactions in most patients treated for primary hepatoma. The manifestations were due to irritation of the urinary and digestive systems. The urinary symptoms included frequency and urgency of urination, hematuria, dysuria, and in a few patients albuminuria and cylindruria; the digestive symptoms included nausea, vomiting, diarrhea, etc. Individual patients may develop paroxysmal tachycardia, focal numbness of fingers and face. The toxic reactions can be relieved by taking green tea which has a diuretic effect and with herbal medicines reputed to reinforce the "spleen" and soothe the "stomach". Upon discontinuation of medication, serious side effects usually remitted or disappeared quickly. Cantharidin tablet is contraindicated in cardiac and renal insufficiency, severe gastrointestinal ulcer, persons with bleeding tendency, and pregnancy (2;4,32).

REFERENCE

1. Liu JY. Acta Pharmaceutica Sinica 1980 15(5):271.

2. Wang GS. Chinese Pharmaceutical Bulletin 1980 15(5):23.

3. Phytochemistry Department, Institute of Materia Medica of the Chinese Academy of Medical Sciences. Acta Pharmaceutica Sinica 1979 14(12):746.

4. Sollmann T. A Manual of Pharmacology and Its Applications to Therapeutics and Toxicology. 8th edition. W. B. Saunders Company. 1951. p. 160.

5. Chen RT et al. Zhonghua Yixue Zazhi (National Medical Journal of China) 1977 57(8):475.

6. Tianjin Institute for Drug Control and Tianjin Institute of Materia Medica. Compiled Information. Tianjin Institute for Drug Control and Tianjin Institute of Materia Medica. 1975. p. 120.

7. Cancer Nucleic Acid Research Section, Shanghai Institute of Experimental Biology. Studies on the inhibitory action of cantharidin on transplanted tumor of mice. Shanghai Institute of Experimental Biology. 1974.

8. Li DH. National Medical Journal of China 1980 60(7):410.

9. Lu BL. Acta Pharmaceutica Sinica 1980 15(2):78.

10. Fu NW et al. Chinese Journal of Oncology 1980 2(2):96.

11. Chen JH et al. Chinese Traditional and Herbal Drugs 1980 11(1):1.

12. Du DJ et al. Research Information on Chinese Traditional Drugs (Sichuan Institute of Chinese Materia Medica) 1978 (12):14.

13. Zeng QT et al. The effects of methylcantharidinimide on delayed hypersensitivity reaction of normal mice and of mice with hepatoma. Sichuan Institute of Chinese Materia Medica. 1980.

14. Wang RW. Ziran Kexue (Natural Sciences) 1980 3(6):458.

15. Goodman LS et al. The Pharmacological Basis of Therapeutics. 4th edition. U.S.P. New York: 1955. p. 1022.

16. Zhang CS. Pharmacology. People's Medical Publishing House. 1962. p. 122.

17. Xu YW. Techniques of Experimental Immunology. Science Press. 1979. p. 121.

18. Bertani M. Chemical Abstracts 1953 47;8262e.

19. Steidle H. Chemical Abstracts 1952 46:637b.

20. Cao RL. Chinese Journal of Dermatology 1957 5(4):286.

21. Editorial Group. National Collection of Chinese Materia Medica. Vol. 1. People's Medical Publishing House.1975. p. 821.

22. Zheng ZY. Collections of Research Information (Sichuan Institute of Chinese Materia Medica) 1979 (16):31.

23. He SX. Chinese Pharmaceutical Bulletin 1980 15(4):39.

24. Zheng ZY. Studies on the Metabolism and Pharmacodynamics of Methylcantharidinimide. Sichuan Institute of Chinese Materia Medica. 1980.

25. First Teaching Hospital of Zhejiang Medical College. Zhejiang Oncology Communications 1972 (4):59.

26. Laerum OD et al. Cancer Research 1972 32:1463.

27. Secretariat of the Conference on the Identification of Hydroxycantharidinimide. Chinese Traditional and Herbal Drugs Communications 1977 (7):48.

28. Chongqing Third People's Hospital et al. Sichuan Jianbao (Sichuan Tumor Bulletin) (Sichuan Office for Prevention and Treatment of Tumor) 1977 (Supplement):67.

29. Wang KB. Acta Academiae Medicinae Luzhou 1978 (3):23.

30. Shao ZD. Popular Science 1975 (5):28.

31. Liu SS. Abstracts of Research Literature on Chinese Traditional Drugs. Science Press. 1962. p. 692.

32. Huanghe Pharmaceutical Factory (Shanghai). Pharmaceutical Industry 1975 34(1):36.

(Zheng Qingtian)

BOLUOHUI 博落回

<Boluohui> refers to the root, stem, leaf, fruit or whole plant of *Macleaya cordata* (Willd.) R. Br. (Papaveraceae). Also known as <Haotonggan>, the herb is bitter, "cold", and highly toxic. It has detumescent, detoxicant, anti-inflammatory and anthelmintic actions. It is used in the treatment of malignant sores, goiter, tumor, polyps, vitiligo, tympanites due to parasitic infection, and diseases caused by unhygienic water. The root, which can easily cause poisoning, is a folk medicine for wounds and injuries.

CHEMICAL COMPOSITION

M. cordata, especially the fruit, contains many alkaloids. Five alkaloids were isolated in China: sanguinarine, chelerythrine, protopine, α-allocryptopine and β-allocryptopine. During the isolation process, upon crystallization with ammoniated ethanol, sanguinarine and chelerythrine were converted into ethoxysanguinarine and ethoxychelerythrine, respectively (1). The root and aerial part contain sanguinarine, chelerythrine, bocconine, protopine, α-allocryptopine, coptisine, berberine, corysamine and alkaloids A, B and C. Bocconoline was recently isolated (2).

PHARMACOLOGY

1. Antibacterial Effect

The herb decoction was shown to be a potent inhibitor of various gram-positive and gram-negative bacteria (3) and leptospirae (4). The "Haotong Injection" prepared from the whole plant was reported to have a strong inhibitory action against *Staphylococcus aureus*, *Staphylococcus albus*, *Shigella shigae*, *Proteus vulgaris*, *Salmonella typhi*, *Shigella sonnei*, *Bacillus anthracis*, *Shigella flexneri*, and, to a lesser extent, against *Shigella boydii*, *Escherichia coli* and *Bacillus coli similis*, but inactive against *Pseudomonas aeruginosa* (5). The active antibacterial component was proved to be alkaloids. The MIC of the mixed alkaloids (possibly a mixture of ethoxysanguinarine and ethoxychelerythrine) obtained from the seed against *Bacillus subtilis*, *Staphylococcus aureus*, *Diplococcus pneumoniae*, *Escherichia coli*, *Shigella flexneri*, *Shigella sonnei*, and *Pseudomonas aeruginosa* were determined to be 2.5, 5, 5, 25–50, 50, 100 and > 100 μg/ml, respectively (6). Ethoxysanguinarine and ethoxychelerythrine were proved to be more active than berberine in inhibiting *Bacillus subtilis*, *Staphylococcus aureus*, and *Diplococcus pneumoniae*. Different degrees of inhibitory action were also exhibited by chelerythrine, sanguinarine, and bocconine against *Staphylococcus aureus*, *Bacillus subtilis*, Sarcina, *Escherichia coli*, *Proteus vulgaris*, *Pseudomonas aeruginosa* and some fungi (8,9). Ethoxychelerythrine had a very strong leptospiricidal activity *in vitro* (10).

2. Vermicidal Effect

<Boluohui> exhibited a powerful lethal effect against *Trichomonas vaginalis*. All trichomonal organisms were rapidly killed upon contact with <Boluohui> extract on the slide (11). Sanguinarine, chelerythrine, and bocconine were lethal to *Enterobius vermicularis* (8).

3. Lethal Effect on Maggots

<Boluohui> is a folk insecticide used to kill maggots. It was shown to cause excitation and subsequently paralysis and death of the larvae. It also seemed to be active in suppressing hatching of fly ova. It was found that the most potent effect was exhibited by the leaf and the rind; the stem is weaker and the root weakest. Drying did not modify its potency. The active component was determined to be alkaloids (12,13).

4. Miscellaneous Actions

The mixture of ethoxysanguinarine and ethoxylchelerythrine could suppress pneumococcus-induced fever in rabbits (7). Sanguinarine could inhibit cholinesterase and markedly increase the sensitivity of the frog musculi rectus abdominis, leech dorsal muscle, and the intestinal tract of rabbits and cats to acetylcholine. It could also markedly increase the tension of the intestinal tract of cats and rabbits and that of the uterine smooth muscle of pregnant cats. Sanguinarine was reported to have antihistaminic action; its effect on isolated guinea pig intestinal tracts was reported to be very weak. Thus, sanguinarine at the concentration of 10^{-4} could only partially inhibit the intestinal spasm induced by histamine at 10^{-7}. At 5 mg/kg IV, sanguinarine failed to modify the effect of histamine on blood pressure. Also, sanguinarine had cardiotonic, sialogogic, diuretic and sympatholytic actions (14,15). On the other hand, protopine and allocryptopine showed depressant effect on isolated guinea pig hearts (16). It was reported that sulfates of the total alkaloids of <Boluohui> had a more potent local anesthetic activity than procaine (17). Protopine at 0.5–1 µg/ml could markedly contract the uterus (18).

5. Toxicity

The safety dose of the mixture of ethoxysanguinarine and ethoxychelerythrine in albino mice was 5 mg/kg IP and the LD_{50} mg/kg IP. Injection of this agent 4–5 mg/kg/day IV for 7 days to rabbits and dogs produced no toxic reactions but local irritation which might cause vascular obstruction at the site of injection (6). The LD_{50} of ethoxysanguinarine in oil was 125 mg/kg SC in mice. Ethoxysanguinarine citrate at 70–80 mg/kg IV caused ECG changes, which consisted of sinoatrial node inhibition, sinus asystole and myocardial ischemic patterns in rats and ventricular, arrhythmia such as ventricular premature beat and ventricular tachycardia in rabbits (7). The LD_{50} of sanguinarine in mice was 19.4 mg/kg IV; intoxication might lead to convulsion (14).

CLINICAL STUDIES

1. Trichomonal Vaginitis, Cervical Erosion, etc.

<Boluohui> has good therapeutic value in trichomonal vaginitis. It can be used as a decoction, fluidextract and suppositories of its alkaloids (19,20). One hundred and thirty-two cases of trichomonal vaginitis had been treated by local application of 25 g/ml extract from fresh young stem and leaf 1–2 times daily. After a course of 7–10 days, symptomatic relief and negative microscopic examination were achieved in all cases (11).

<Boluohui> is also of utility in the treatment of cervical erosion. It was reported that 726 cases had been treated with the suppository, and that 336 cases were cured (46.28%), 165 markedly improved and 187 significantly improved, the aggregate effective rate being 94.77%. The medication was more effective in moderately severe and mild cases. *Dosage and administration*: Intravaginally on alternate days, usually 3–5 times in mild cases, 7–8 times in moderate cases, and around 10 times in severe cases. Sixteen other cases with interstitial lesions of the cervix were cured by the same method (21). Follow-up of 100 cases for 2–8 months showed an effective rate as high as 92%. Furthermore, all patients positive for *Staphylococcus aureus, Monilia albicans*, and *Escherichia coli* were found to be negative in the vaginal bacterial culture after the treatment (22).

2. Neoplasms

Thirty-two cases of thyroid adenoma, thyroid tumors, thyroglossal cyst, and mixed parotid cancers benefitted from the injection of <Boluohui> alklaoids. Treatment of cervical cancer with the herb also showed bright prospects (21).

3. Infectious Diseases

The "Haotong Injection" was satisfactorily used to treat more than 300 cases of infections including lobar pneumonia, pneumonia in children, acute tonsillitis, and upper respiratory infection with high-grade fever (4). The same injection was also effective in the treatment of 126 cases of chronic bronchitis, especially for the relief of cough (23).

4. Lethal Effect on Maggots

Pieces of the aerial part of *M. cordata* thrown into manure pits (5–10 catties for each small manure pit) should be good for 20–25 days.

ADVERSE EFFECTS

Caution should be exercised when using <Boluohui> internally because of its high toxicity. Poisoning by this herb is not rare. Reports of deaths due to <Boluohui> poisoning are available (24–29). The toxic symptoms were chiefly cardiogenic: premature beat, paroxysmal arrhythmia, complete atrial block and Stokes-Adams syndrome. Other reactions including central symptoms were mania, depression, and coma. Cardiac toxicity could often be relieved clinically by large doses of atropine (25,27). Vaginal application might cause local irritation in some patients (11). Intramuscular injection might cause severe pain over the injection site (6). In addition, the Boluohui Injection may also cause dizziness, xerostomia and numbness of the extremities.

REFERENCE

1. Hu ZB et al. Acta Pharmaceutica Sinica 1979 14(9):535.

2. Hisashi I et al. Chemical Abstracts 1978 88:191182K.

3. Sichuan Institute of Chinese Materia Medica. A table of the antibacterial actions of Chinese traditional drugs. 1976.

4. Leptospirosis Research Group. Research Information on Chinese Traditional Drugs (Sichuan Institute of Chinese Materia Medica) 1972 (6):32.

5. Pharmaceutical Factory, Hengfeng County People's Health Centre. New Medical Information (Jiangxi School of Pharmacy) 1970 (3):19.

6. Dexing Team of Shanghai Institute of Materia Medica. Compiled Information on the National Seminar on Chinese Materia Medica. Dexing County Health Bureau. 1972. p. 44.

7. Shanghai Institute of Materia Medica. Antibacterial and animal experiments on Macleaya cordata. 1977.

8. Onda M et al. Chemical Abstracts 1965 63:18964n.

9. Mitscher LA et al. Lloydia 1972 35(2):157.

10. Deng WL. Studies on some natural compounds with anti-leptospira activity. 1979.

11. Hainan (Guangzhou) et al. New Chinese Medicine 1971 (6–7):45.

12. Zhang SX. Bulletin of Chinese Materia Medica 1957 3(2):60.

13. Ye DN. Bulletin of Chinese Materia Medica 1958 4(9):308.

14. Nikolvska BS. Farmakologiia I Toksikologiia 1966 29(1):76.

15. Kelentey B. Arzneimettel Forschung 1960 10(2):135.

16. Alles GA et al. Journal of Pharmacology and Experimental Therapeutics 1952 104:253.

17. Goto K et al. Journal of the Pharmaceutical Society of Japan (Tokyo) 1949 69:307.

18. Goto M et al. Taketa Kenkyiyo Ho 1957 16:21.

19. Pharmacy of Hunan People's Hospital. Compiled Information (Hunan People's Hospital) 1972 (2):103.

20. Ob-Gyn Department, Teaching Hospital of Hengyang Medical School. Medical Practice (Teaching Hospital of Hengyang Medical School) 1974 (1):33.

21. Clinical efficacy of Macleaya cordata pessary in cervical erosion and anaplasia. In: Clinical Information on Macleaya cordata Pessary. Shanghai No. 2 Chinese Medicine Factory. 1977.

22. Li XQ et al. Shanghai Journal of Barefoot Doctor 1978 (4):60.

23. Chronic Bronchitis Group, 366th Hospital of the Chinese PLA. Selected Information on Combined Western and Traditional Chinese Medicine. (Health Division of the Logistics Department of Hunan Military Region) 1976 (2):35.

24. Ye TG. Chinese Journal of Internal Medicine 1958 (6):617.

25. Jia LW. Chinese Journal of Internal Medicine 1963 (5):399.

26. Li FC. New Medical Information (Jiangxi School of Pharmacy) 1972 (1):49.

27. Wuxuan County Hospital. Health Journal of Guangxi 1974 (1):55.

28. Zhu YR. Clinical Medical Information (Hangzhou First People's Hospital) 1980 (1):17.

29. Fang N. Notes on Science and Technology — Medicine and Health (Information Institute of Zhejiang Bureau of Science and Technology) 1972 (12):34.

(Deng Wenlong)

MIANHUAGEN AND MIANZI 棉花根與棉籽

<Mianhuagen> refers to the root or root-bark of *Gossypium hirsutum* L. or *G. herbaceum* L. (Malvaceae). The seed of these plants may also be used as medicine.

<Mianhuagen> has a sweet flavor and a "warm" property. It has tonifying (for the spleen, stomach, and vital energy), antitussive and antiasthmatic actions. It is a remedy for gastrointestinal disorders, and splenic hypofunction as well as for cough and dyspnea due to asthenia of the vital energy.

<Mianhuazi> has a pungent flavor and a "hot" property. It is tonifying for the liver and "kidney" and has a fortifying effect on the low-back and knee. It is used in epigastric and abdominal pain, hemorrhage and for promoting lactation.

CHEMICAL COMPOSITION

The root bark, stem bark and seed all contain gossypol. The root bark contains the highest amount of gossypol, 0.56–2.05%. The root bark also contains asparagine, resin mixtures, and arginine.

The flower contains quercimeritrin. The root bark of *G. herbaceum* contains gossypol, whereas the flower contains kaempferol, herbacitrin, quercetin, isoquercetin, gossypetin, and gossypitrin.

PHARMACOLOGY

1. Antifertility Effect

Intragastric administration of feed containing 5% of the cotton seed powder, or of gossypol or gossypol acetate for 2–4 weeks to male rats abolished the animals' fertility. The onset of the antifertility effect was dose related. The antifertility effect persisted for 3–5 weeks after discontinuation of medication; thereafter, the fertility gradually recovered (1). The antifertility effect of gossypol is attributed to damage of spermatids in the convoluted seminiferous tubules with the more mature sperms displaying greater sensitivity of gossypol (1–3). Under the electron microscope the acrosome and head of the spermatid appeared swollen, detached and cracked. The mitochondria of the spiral fiber of the middle piece became disordered, swollen and with fewer cristae. Increasing the dosage and prolong medication caused damage, detachment and death of spermatocytes, resulting in decreased or finally zero sperm count. No significant change, however, was seen in the structure of testicular interstitial cells (1,4–6). The gossypol-treated rats did not differ significantly from the control group with respect to the serum luteinizing hormone (LH) level and the response of the pituitary gland to luteinizing hormone releasing hormone (LHRH). Neither did it alter the plasma testosterone content in rats and monkeys, nor significantly modify the copulation behaviour and secondary gonadal function in rats (3,7). After discontinuation of medication and recovery of reproductive ability, all rats had progenies with normal growth and reproductive function (7). No significant difference was observed between the control group and gossypol-treated rats with respect to the rate of appearance of polyploid cells as observed in the chromosomes of spermatogonia (1).

The gossypol commonly used in laboratory and clinical practice is a racemate. Since d-gossypol had neither significant antifertility nor toxic effects, l-gossypol was considered to be responsible for these effects (7). Gossypol acetate had a more potent antifertility effect and higher toxicity than gossypoln formate (8). The antifertility action was lost if the aldehyde or hydroxyl group of gossypol was replaced by other groups (7).

2. Antitussive, Expectorant, and Antiasthmatic Effects

Intragastric administration of the root of *G. hirsutum* or its constituents, asparagine and gossypol, in mice produced an antitussive effect (9–11). Studies in rats indicated that both the decoction and extract of the root had strong expectorant effect, especially the ethanol extract and the resin fraction (9,11). Intragastric administration of the resin fraction of the crude root bark extract to guinea pigs relieved asthma induced by the histamine-acetylcholine mixture (11). These effects might be exerted by different fractions of the extracts. Both the decoction of the root bark and gossypol were able to alleviate inflammatory cellular infiltration in chronic bronchitis (11,12).

3. Antibacterial and Antiviral Effects

In vitro studies showed that the root decoction, the resin fraction of the extract and gossypol were inhibitory to certain bacteria (9,13) but not to fungi (14). Long-term administration of gossypol preparations could upset the balance of the intestinal bacterial flora (13). Chicken embryo experiment showed that gossypol could suppress the multiplication of the type A influenza virus PR-8 strain with a potency higher than that of amantadine (15). Nose drops of gossypol 10–1000 μg was shown to prevent death in mice inoculated with 1–10 lethal doses of the type A influenza virus PR-8 strain; administering the nose drops for 8 days to mice with experimental pneumonia caused by this virus also afforded a curative effect (16).

4. Antineoplastic Effect

Contact with gossypol significantly inhibited the Jitian sarcoma; among the transplanted tumors, Ehrlich ascites carcinoma in mice showed high susceptibility to the drug which was also effective against solid tumors such as Walker carcinosarcoma 256 in rats and breast cancer in mice (17). Gossypol applied locally could dissolve melanoma yet was not deleterious to normal tissues (18). According to one source the antineoplastic effect of gossypol could be attributed to its being a low-toxicity quinone derivative which can be converted by thyrozinase, an enzyme present in considerable amounts in tumor cells, into a highly toxic quinone which inhibits tumor cells (17).

5. Effect on the Uterus

Gossypol stimulated isolated uteri of both pregnany and nonpregnant guinea pigs (19). The root bark has been used by folks in other countries to induce abortion (20); it has a weak oxytocic action, but much weaker than that of ergot.

6. Miscellaneous Actions

Animal studies showed that the root extract caused thymic atrophy and increased the weight of the adrenal glands in mice, suggesting an enhancing effect on adrenocortical function. However, the antifatigue and hypoxia tolerance studies on mice did not demonstrate that the root could strengthen body resistance (11).

7. Pharmacokinetics

As shown in animal studies, most of the ingested gossypol was directly excreted in feces; only a small fraction was absorbed from the gastrointestinal tract after being transformed into a fat-soluble phthalein. Gossypol was chiefly distributed in the liver, blood, muscle and kidneys. The highest concentration was found in the liver (1). After 1–2 days of a single oral dose of ^{14}C-labelled gossypol 94 μCi/35 mg in rats, the labelled compound was mainly distributed in the stomach, intestines and liver; 4–9 days after administration, the corresponding peak levels were reached in the heart, spleen, lungs, kidneys, pancreas, testes, epididymis, accessory gonads, adrenal glands, pituitary gland, thymus, saliva, bone marrow, lymph nodes and muscle. Thereafter, the labelled compound gradually spread to the whole body, and 14 days after medication the radioactivity significantly declined. By Day 19, radioactivity became difficult to trace. No prolonged accumulation was found in any specific site. The absorption and distribution did not differ whether the drug be given in one or multiple doses. No cellular pathological changes were observed in organs with high radioactivity; nevertheless, the testicles which showed moderate radioactivity had marked cellular damage in the convoluted seminiferous tubules, showing higher sensitivity of the spermatogenic epithelial cells to gossypol relative to other organs (21,22).

8. Toxicity

The contraceptive dosage of gossypol has no significant toxicity (1). The LD_{50} of gossypol in mice and rats were determined to be 315 and 2250–3340 mg/kg PO, respectively. Among a variety of experimental animals, rabbit showed highest sensitivity to this agent, followed by guinea pig, mouse and rat in decending order. The low sensitivity of rats to gossypol is probably due to high microsomal oxidase activity in the liver of the animal, which detoxicates gossypol. Feed containing 0.02% of gossypol could poison pigs (23).

Daily administration of gossypol to dogs at doses 3–30 mg/kg PO caused vomiting, diarrhea, decrease of appetite, weight loss, diminution of erythrocytes and hemoglobin. When treated for 4–8 weeks, all the animals died one by one due to acute circulatory and respiratory failure. Autopsy revealed myocardial cloudy swelling, liver damage, ecchymoma in visceral organs, anomalies in testicular spermatogenic epithelium and spermatozoa (23,24). Rats orally given 7.5 mg/kg of gossypol for one year showed no changes in blood picture, bone marrow, GPT level, blood urea nitrogen level and ECG; neither pathological changes in major organs (except the convoluted seminiferous tubules of testes) nor morphological changes in testicular interstitial cells were revealed by autopsy. In comparison with the control, no significant difference in the microstructure of the interstitial cells of rat testes was observed after oral administration of gossypol 30 mg/kg daily for 30 days. Oral administration of gossypol to rats at 10 mg/kg daily, 6 days per week for a period of 6 months, produced no change in the blood picture, bone marrow, morphology of various major organs, and microstructure of hepatocytes. Oral administration of the agent at 20 mg/kg daily to rats for 9 months or at 30 mg/kg daily for 2 months did not result in significant morphological changes in the major organs except the testes (1,7,25,27). Gossypol acetate at contraceptive dosage produced no significant change in mutation rate of human lymphocytic chromosomes (36). The root bark decoction can cause flattening of T wave, ST depression, or prolongation of QT interval on the ECG of rabbits (9). No significant changes could be observed on the ECG and cardiac histology of rabbits if the dose of gossypol did not exceed 16 mg/kg (26). Increasing the protein content in animal feed reduced the toxicity of gossypol and lowered the gossypol level in tissues. This is probably due to conjugation of gossypol with protein (amino group) leading to an increase in the excretion of gossypol. Since iron was able to complex with gossypol and calcium preparations accelerated their complexation, both iron and calcium could reduce its toxicity but could not completely prevent its accumulation (23).

CLINICAL STUDIES

1. Male Contraception

Gossypol has been tried clinically in over 4000 male subjects for contraceptive purpose. The drug was administered for at least 6 months, and more than half of the subjects had taken the drug for 2 years, the longest being four years. Administration of 20 mg of gossypol for about 2 months decreased the sperm count of 99.89% of the subjects to the contraceptive level. When this level is reached, the maintenance dosage of 150–220 mg per month in divided doses (generally twice weekly) was given. The effect is reversible and fertility is not affected (1,28).

2. Chronic Bronchitis

Gossypol 1 mg/kg PO was proved effective for symptomatic treatment in 87 cases of chronic bronchitis (29). A compound formula of the root tried in 72 cases of chronic bronchitis afforded good antitussive and expectorant effects but relatively poor antiasthmatic and anti-inflammatory effects (30).

3. Gynecological Diseases

Gossypol Tablet, 4.5 mg each, 2 tablets twice daily for one month as a therapeutic course, may be administered according to the patients condition for 1–4 months. It was shown to be markedly effective in myoma of the uterus, endometriosis, and dysfunctional uterine bleeding (31).

4. Epididymal Stasis

Five cases benefitted from gossypol treatment for more than two months, resulting in marked reduction of the size of swollen epididymis in some (32).

ADVERSE EFFECTS

Clinically, gossypol has a low toxicity and few side effects. Transient, mild lassitude at the early phase of medication occurred in 12.8% of patients. Recovery was spontaneous, requiring no treatment. About 1.2% of patients developed nausea and gastrointestinal upset, and a few subjects complained of mild reduction in sexual desire, though sexual function itself was not affected. These symptoms generally did not interfere with gossypol treatment. Some patients required symptomatic treatment or counselling before they resume medication (1,28,31). In some places, hypokalemia occurred in patients taking this drug, but no such abnormality was observed in more than 1000 cases in another region. Hence, whether or not hypokalemia is caused by gossypol requires further study; in fact, it is being studied in animals (1,33–35).

REFERENCE

1. National Coordinating Research Group on Male Contraceptives. National Medical Journal of China 1978 58(8):455.
2. Jiangsu Coordinating Research Group on Male Contraceptives. Studies on Gossypol — A Male Contraceptive. 1972.
3. Shandong Coordinating Research Group on Chinese Traditional Contraceptives. Studies on the Antifertility Effect of Gossypol in Rats. 1973.

4. Dai RX et al. Compilation of the Achievements of Shanghai Institute of Experimental Biology in 1973–75 (II). 1977. p. 137.

5. Radiomedicine Section, Hebei College of New Medicine. Research of New Traditional Chinese Medicine 1979 (1):17.

6. Dai RX et al. Acta Experimentalis Biologiia 1978 11(1):27.

7. Wang YE et al. Acta Pharmaceutica Sinica 1979 14(1):662.

8. Yu MQ et al. Selected Information on Scientific Research (Wuhan Medical College) 1979:53.

9. Materia Medica Research Group of Nanjing Military Region of the Chinese PLA. Chinese Traditional and Herbal Drugs Communications 1972 (4):30.

10. Jiangsu Coordinating Research Group on Bronchitis. Chemical and Pharmacological Studies on <Siguadun> and Gossypium Root. 1972.

11. Pharmacology Section, Tangshan Coal Mine Medical College. Research Communications on Medical Education (Tangshan Coal Mine Medical College) 1973 (2):19.

12. Pharmacology Section, Tangshan Coal Mine Medical College. Research Communications on Medical Education (Tangshan Coal Mine Medical College) 1973 (2):12.

13. Magalith P. Applied Microbiology 1967 (15):952.

14. Vichknova SA. Antibiotiki 1968 13:828.

15. Goriunoba LV. Farmakologiia I Toksikologiia 1969 32:615.

16. Vichknova SA. Antibiotiki 1970 15:1071.

17. Vermeli EM. Voprosy Onkologii 1963 9(12):39.

18. Vermel EM. Acta Unio Inter Contra Cancrum 1964 20(1–2):211.

19. Ding QX. Zhejiang Yixueyuan Yixue Tongxun (Communications of Zhejiang Medical College) 1959 (4):3.

20. Guerra MO et al. Contraception 1978 18(2):191.

21. Xue Sp et al. Acta Experimentalis Biologiia 1979 12(3):179.

22. Abou-Donia MB. Toxicology and Applied Pharmacology 1971 18:507.

23. Nanjing Institute of Materia Medica. Pharmacological Effects and Clinical Use of Gossypol. 1974.

24. Shandong Coordinating Research Group on Chinese Traditional Contraceptives. Toxicity studies of gossypol in dogs. 1973.

25. Shandong Coordinating Research Group on Chinese Traditional Contraceptives. Toxicity studies of gossypol in the major organs of rats. 1973.

26. Shandong Coordinating Research Group on Chinese Traditional Contraceptives. Toxicity studies of gossypol in rabbits. 1973.

27. Lei HP. National Medical Journal of China 1979 59(6):330.

28. Shandong Institute of Traditional Chinese Medicine and Materia Medica. Summary of the Clinical Evaluation of Male Contraceptives at Stage 42. 1975.

29. Jiangsu Coordinating Research Group on Prevention and Treatment of Chronic Bronchitis. Analysis of the efficacy of chronic bronchitis treatment and study of its chemopharmacology. 1972.

30. Bronchitis Research Group, Tangshan Coal Mine Medical College. Research Communications on Medical Education (Tangshan Coal Mine Medical College) 1973 (2):1.

31. Research Institute of Family Planning, Wuhan Medical College. Selected Information on Scientific Research. Wuhan Medical College. 1979. p.43.

32. Shandong Institute of Traditional Chinese Medicine. Preliminary observations of six cases of epididymis stasis treated with gossypol. 1975.

33. Nanjing Institute of Materia Medica. Jiangsu Yiyao (Jiangsu Medical Journal) 1978 4(1):29.

34. Feng ZQ. Abstracts of the Academic Conference of Nanjing Medical College. Volume I. 1979.

35. Qian SZ et al. Acta Pharmaceutica Sinica 1979 14(9):513.

36. Wu LF et al. Acta Academiae Medicinae Sichuan 1980 (3):190.

(Zhou Shiqing)

KUANDONGHUA 款冬花
(APPENDIX: KUANDONGYE 附: 款冬葉)

<Kuandonghua> is the flower bud of *Tussilago farfara* L. (Compositae). It is pungent and "warm". Mucolytic, antitussive and antiasthmatic actions are attributed to it. It is a remedy for chronic and acute asthma, and blood-tinged sputum. In Europe, it is a folk medicine for cough, hoarseness, bronchitis and bronchial asthma (1).

CHEMICAL COMPOSITION

<Kuandonghua> contains faradiol and its isomer arnidiol, taraxanthin, volatile oil, triterpenoid saponins and phytosterols. An alkaloid, senkirkine, was recently isolated.

PHARMACOLOGY

1. Antitussive, Expectorant, and Antiasthmatic Effects

The 40% <Kuandonghua> decoction 4 ml/kg administered intragastrically to dogs produced a marked antitussive effect (2). No significant antitussive action was observed in mice with the dose 5 g/kg, but a very prominent effect was achieved one hour after the dose 10 g/kg (3). The herb had an expectorant effect in cats, which was weaker than that achieved with the root of *Platycodon gransiflorum* or the whole herb of *Plantago asiatica* (4). The ethyl acetate extract of this herb had an expectorant effect, whereas its ethanol extract had an antitussive action (5). The active antitussive and expectorant constituents were believed to be the volatile oil and potassium nitrate, respectively (1).

Perfusion of the isolated trachea-lung specimen of rabbits and guinea pigs with low dosages of the ether extract of <Kuandonghua> slightly dilated the bronchi; at higher dosages it produced the opposite effect. No definite spasmolytic action was observed in guinea pigs with histamine-induced bronchospasm (6). The <Kuandonghua> decoction was also devoid of bronchodilatory action (5).

2. Respiratory Stimulant Effect

Intravenous injection of the ethanol extract or the ether extract of <Kuandonghua> to anesthetized cats and rabbits stimulated respiration, but transient respiratory arrest sometimes occurred before or after the stimulant effect. These effects could be attenuated by hexamethonium (6,7). This stimulant effect of the herb on respiration resembled that of nikethamide. Thus, the herb could antagonize morphine-induced respiratory depression (8).

3. *Effect on the Cardiovascular System*

Intravenous injection of the ethanol extract or decoction of <Kuandonghua> to cats caused transient mild hypotension, followed by rapid rise in blood pressure which sustained for a longer period of time. Trials with the ether extract in cats, rabbits, dogs and rats generally did not show any first-phase hypotension but a more pronounced pressor response. In cats with hemorrhagic shock, a very prominent pressor response was observed following administration of 0.2 g(crude drug)/kg of the ether extract. The average elevation being 120 mmHg. This pressor effect was elicited with low dosage, was pronounced, had a rapid onset, and was prolonged. Repeated medication did not result in tachyphylaxis (9).

The pressor effect was also achieved in decerebrated cats, but it became very weak when the spinal cord was sectioned at the level of the second cervical vertebra. Administration of the herb preparation into the vertebral artery or the cisterna magna also elicited a pressor response. Thus, the pressor effect is considered primarily due to stimulation of the medullary vasomotor center. α-Receptor blockers could only slightly weaken this effect, and injection of the herb preparation into the femoral artery also elicited a pressor response, showing a peripheral pressor effect. Neither reserpinization nor cocainization could modify this effect. Ephedrine had no synergistic effect. These findings indicate that the action is not mediated by the release of sympathetic neurotransmitters and that it is not uptake by the sympathetic nerve terminal. It is also possible that the herb can stimulate the sympathetic ganglions because hexamethonium and nicotine can weakly antagonize its pressor effect (9).

4. *Effects on Gastrointestinal and Uterine Smooth Muscles*

The ether extract of <Kuandonghua> inhibited the gastrointestinal smooth muscles and antagonized the intestinal contraction induced by barium chloride. Small doses had stimulant effects on the *in situ* and isolated uteri, whereas large doses produced inhibitory effects or initial stimulation succeeded by inhibition (7,10).

5. *Miscellaneous Actions*

Intravenous injection of <Kuandonghua> preparations increased the blood pressure and concurrently the pupil size, lacrimal and bronchial secretions and muscular tone of the extremities (9). However, no mydriatic effect was achieved with the ether extract instilled into the eyes (10).

6. *Toxicity*

The ether extract of <Kuandonghua> injected into te lymph sac of frogs or toads at doses of 1.05 or 1.75 g, or intraperitoneally to rats, mice and guinea pigs at doses of 70, 80, and 10.7 g/kg, respectively, or intravenously to rabbits at 0.4 g/kg, caused irritability and restlessness, respiratory stimulation, tense muscles, tremor, clonic seizure and finally death from convulsion. Convulsion ensued from strong stimulation of the brain stem below the diencephalon, extending down to the spinal cord. The convulsant effect of <Kuandonghua> could be prevented or reduced by central depressants such as chlorpromazine and barbital sodium. However, death could not be precluded. Scopolamine and small doses of thiamine afforded protection against <Kuandonghua>-induced convulsion and death (8).

In mice the LD_{50} of the <Kuandonghua> decoction was determined to be 124 g/kg PO, that of the ethanol extract 112 g/kg PO, and that of the ether extract, 43 g/kg IP (8).

The alkaloid senkirkine contained in this herb was proved to be hepatotoxic (11).

CLINICAL STUDIES

1. Cough Due to Acute and Chronic Bronchitis and Other Factors

<Kuandonghua> is often used with the root and rhizome of *Aster tataricus*, to be given as an oral decoction, 5–10 g each time. In 68 cases of chronic bronchitis treated intramusculary with the Compound Tussilago farfara Injection (Flos Farfarae and Lumbricus) once daily, cough, expectortion, and dyspnea were markedly alleviated after 3–4 days of medication. After 10 days, 8 cases achieved short-term control, 32 cases marked effects, and 4 cases no effect. Concurrent fall in the blood pressure was also observed (12); this might be induced by Lumbricus (earthworm) (12).

2. Bronchial Asthma and Asthmatic Bronchitis

The ethanol extract of <Kuandonghua> 5 ml (equivalent to 6 g of crude drug) three times daily was used in treating 36 cases. It was effective in 27 cases, including 8 and 19 cases obtained marked improvement in 1–2 and 3 days, respectively. It was considered that the extract had antiasthmatic effect but when used alone was ineffective in severe asthmatic attack, in that it could only be used as an adjuvant (6).

ADVERSE EFFECTS

The most commonly seen ill effects were gastrointestinal. Of the 36 asthmatic patients mentioned above, 10 cases developed nausea. In individual patients medication had to be discontinued. Two other cases developed irritability and insomnia (6).

(APPENDIX: KUANDONGYE 附: 款冬葉)

<Kuandongye>, the leaf of *T. farfara*, contains bitter glycosides, phytosterols, polysaccharides, β-sitosterol, vitamin C, and tussilagine. Since early times this herb has been used as medicine among the Soviet and European peoples to bring about expectoration and to mitigate stimulations (13). The aqueous and the ether extracts, as well as the distillate of <Kuandongye> exerted a spasmolytic action on the isolated small intestines; its volatile components could also paralyze the small intestine. No pharmacological activity was exhibited by the ethyl acetate extract. The methanol extract could cause spasm of the small bowel; it displayed mutual antagonism with the ether or aqueous extract (14). An author recommended the use of <Kuandongye> as an antidote for tetrodotoxin (15). However, this proposition is still debatable since tetrodotoxin is known to paralyze the central and peripheral nerves and muscles, by blocking the fast Na$^+$ channel of the cell membrane.

REFERENCE

1. Auster F et al. Arzneipflanzen. Tussilago farfara L. 1957. p. 35.
2. Huang QZ. Chinese Medical Journal 1954 40:849.
3. Herbal Drugs Research Group, Teaching Hospital of Jiangxi Medical College. Reports on Senile Chronic Bronchitis (Jiangxi Medical College) 1971 (1):8.
4. Gao YD et al. Chinese Medical Journal 1954 40:331.
5. Wuhan Institute for Drug Control. Wuhan Journal of New Traditional Chinese Medicine 1972 (1):16.
6. Shao CR et al. Shanghai Zhongyiyao Zazhi (Shanghai Journal of Traditional Chinese Medicine 1964 (10):12.
7. Wang JM. Abstracts of the Symposium of the Chinese Society of Physiology (Pharmacy). 1964. p. 117.
8. Wang JM. Chinese Traditional and Herbal Drugs Communications 1979 (3):28.
9. Wang JM. Acta Pharmaceutica Sinica 1979 14(5):268.
10. Wang JM. Scientific Papaers of Shanghai College of Traditional Chinese Medicine 1963 (6):149.
11. Culvenor CCJ et al. Australian Journal of Chemistry 1976 29:229.
12. Weihai City and Commune Health Centre. Yantai Medical Communications 1971 (3):12.
13. Zimlinskii SE. Lekarstevennye Rasteniia SSSR. Lis. Megruz: 1958. p. 192.
14. Borkowski B et al. Acta Poloniae Pharmaceutica 1959 16:347.
15. Ye JQ. Modern Practical Chinese Traditional Drugs. 1952. p. 288.

(Xue Chunsheng)

GEGEN 葛根

<Gegen> is the root of *Pueraria lobata* (Willd.) Ohwi, or *P. thomsonii* Benth. (Leguminosae). It is also known as <Tiange>, <Fen' ge> etc. It is sweet and pungent, and has a "mild" property. It is spasmolytic, antipyretic, secretory, and antidiarrheal. It is also thought to induce the eruption of measles at the early stage. The herb is used to treat fever, headache, stiffness of back and neck, dry mouth in diarrhea or dysentery, and early-stage measles.

CHEMICAL COMPOSITION

<Gegen> contains the flavonoids daidzin, daidzein, puerarin, daidzein-4',7-diglucoside, puerarin-7-xyloside and 4',6'-0-diacetylpuerarin (1).

PHARMACOLOGY

1. Coronary and Cerebral Vasodilatory Effects

The decoction or ethanol extract of <Gegen>, its total flavones, daidzin, and puerarin administered to rats intraperitoneally or subcutaneously antagonized acute myocardial ischemia induced by pituitrin (2). Injection of the total flavones into the coronary artery or vein on anesthetized dogs, or intravenous injection of puerarin caused a marked increase in the coronary flow and decrease in vascular resistance. During intravenous injection, the blood flows of the internal carotid and femoral arteries were also increased though not as markedly as that in the coronary vessels. The inability of reserpine to modify the action of the total flavones and puerarin on coronary circulation indicates a direct relaxant action on the vascular smooth muscle. A similar action was achieved with the ethanol extract of <Gegen>. Puerarin was more potent than the total flavones. Intravenous injection of the total flavones or puerarin in anesthetized dogs decreased the heart rate and the total peripheral resistance, slightly decreased the left ventricular work, reduced the myocardial oxygen consumption, and increased the myocardial efficiency; the cardiac output was not significantly altered. These effects were beneficial to the maintenance of equilibrium between myocardial oxygen demand and supply (3). In anesthetized dogs with acute myocardial infarction induced by ligation of the anterior descending coronary artery, intravenous injection of the total flavones caused a significant fall in the blood pressure, slowing of the heart beat, slight decrease in blood flow in the infarcted area, no significant change in the arterial blood oxygen but significant increase in the venous blood oxygen at the coronary sinus and infarcted area. The oxygen utilization and consumption as well as lactic acid content in both normal and infarcted areas were markedly decreased, whereas lactic acid utilization was markedly increased. These results indicate that <Gegen> has excellent effect on the metabolism of the infarcted myocardium (4).

Injection of the total flavones of <Gegen> 1 mg/kg to the internal carotid artery of anesthetized dogs caused a dose-dependent increase in the cerebral blood flow and decrease in cerebral vascular resistance. It was, however, less potent than papaverine. On the other hand, injection of the total flavones 30 mg/kg IV caused no significant change in the cerebral blood flow but decreased the vascular resistance (5).

2. Hypotensive Effect

Oral administration of the <Gegen> decoction 20 g daily for 14 days to three dogs with renal hypertension resulted in a slight fall in blood pressure in two of them. The ethanol extract orally administered for 12 days to 4 dogs with renal hypertension triggered a drop in the blood pressure in 3 of the animals. Intravenous injection of the total flavones caused a sudden drop in the blood pressure of most normotensive anesthetized dogs which recovered in 4–8 minutes. In unanesthetized dogs, the same drug administered via the same route caused a very brief elevation followed by a fall in blood pressure which lasted 15–18 minutes. In hypertensive dogs, the pressor response to norepinephrine and the hypotensive effect of acetylcholine could be attenuated by administering the ethanol extract of <Gegen> but not by the total flavones (5). <Gegen> has a direct vasodilatory action which decreases the peripheral vascular resistance (3,5). It can also decrease the blood catecholamine level (6) and vascular reactivity (5).

3. Inhibition of Platelet Aggregation

ADP-induced rat platelet aggregation was inhibited to different extents by 0.25, 0.5, and 1.0 mg/ml of puerarin *in vitro*. Intravenous injection of puerarin is also effective. At doses of 0.5–3.0 mg/ml, puerarin also inhibited, *in vitro*, aggregation of rabbit and sheep platelets and those of normal subjects induced by ADP or serotonin. Puerarin 0.5 mg/kg could also inhibit serotonin release from platelets (7); this is favourable to the prevention and treatment of angina pectoris and myocardial infarction.

4. β-Adrenergic Blocking Effect

In various isolated tissues with β-adrenergic receptors, the <Gegen> extract exhibited different degrees of significant antagonism against the effect of isoproterenol. This fact suggests that the herb is a wide-spectrum β-blocker. The <Gegen> extract at doses as low as 15 mg markedly attenuated the stimulant effect of 5 μg of isoproterenol on the isolated heart, whereas tenfold the above dose had practically no direct inhibitory effect on normal hearts, nor did it influence the cardiotonic effect of digitalis glycosides. These findings suggest that the herb has selectivity on the β_1-receptors. The β_2-receptor blocking action was found to be weak because doses up to 150 mg was required to antagonize bronchodilation and peripheral vasodilation induced by isoproterenol (8).

5. Miscellaneous Actions

Oral administration of the ethanol extract of <Gegen> to rabbits produced a marked antipyretic effect in rabbits with fever induced by the typhoid vaccine, whereas the herb decoction had negligible effect (9). The total flavones neither had significant sedative and analgesic actions nor any effect on the conditioned avoidance reflex of rats (10). Daidzein exhibited a prominent spasmolytic action on the isolated intestinal tract of mice by antagonizing acetylcholine-induced intestinal spasm with a potency one-third that of papaverine (11,12). The herb decoction had a weak hypoglycemic action in normal rabbits (13). Thirteen constituents were recently isolated from this herb by successive extraction with acetone, methanol, and water; pharmacological studies revealed a number of pharmacologically antagonistic substances present in the crude drug, and that the various extracts have low toxicity (14).

6. Pharmacokinetics

The orally administered puerarin in rats was rapidly but incompletely absorbed; 37.3% of the administered dose was recovered in the gastrointestinal content and feces at the end of 24 hours. In rats, intravenously injected puerarin was found highest in concentration in the kidney and lower in plasma, liver, and spleen, and lowest in the brain. It was proved *in vitro* that puerarin was minimally destroyed in the gastrointestinal tract, that it was metabolized in the blood, liver, and kidneys, and that it could bind to the proteins of liver, kidneys, lungs, and plasma. The 24-h urinary and fecal excretion of the oral dose of puerarin accounted for 1.85 and 35.7%, respectively; the amounts excreted in the urine, feces and bile after an intravenous injection were 37.62, 7.39 and 3.65%, respectively. The pharmacokinetic data obtained after the intravenous injection of puerarin in rats revealed wide distribution, rapid elimination, and low accumulation. In normal subjects, only 0.78% of the original oral dose was excreted in the urine in 36 hours, whereas 73.3% was excreted in the feces in 72 hours (15), indicating marginal absorption after oral administration.

Daidzein or ^{14}C-daidzein given to rats by mouth was slowly and incompletely absorbed. The amount recovered from the gastrointestinal content and feces represented 49.1% by chemical analysis and by isotope tracing technique 74.5%. The highest drug level was detected in kidneys and liver and a lower level in the brain after an intravenous injection. The 24-h urinary excretion of the oral and intravenous doses in rats determined by chemical methods accounted for 0.73 and 10.99%, and by tracing technique 34.3 and 71.2%. respectively. The 6-h biliary excretion determined by chemical methods after an intravenous injection in rats represented 0.87% and by isotope tracing technique 43.5%. Apparently, there is a great difference between the results obtained by chemical methods and those by tracing technique. This is probably due to the fact that the chemical methods could only detect the original drug and that substances detected by the tracing techniques included, apart from the original drug, metabolites. It was concluded that daidzein is rapidly metabolized in the body (16,17).

7. Toxicity

Oral administration of the dried ethanol extract 10 and 20 g/kg daily for 3 days to mice did not result in any toxic effects. Likewise, no toxic effects were exhibited by the total flavones. The LD_{50} of the dried ethanol extract in mice was 2.1 ± 0.12 g/kg IV and that of the total flavones 1.6 ± 0.06 or 2.1 ± 0.12 g/kg. Oral administration of the ethanol extract 2 g/kg daily in mice for 2 months did not cause pathological changes in the solid organs. Likewise, administration of the ethanol extract to hypertensive dogs at 2 g/kg daily for 14 days by mouth produced no toxic effects (10).

CLINICAL STUDIES

1. Coronary Disease and Angina Pectoris

One hundred and ninety-one cases were treated with the Radix Puerariae Tablet (10 mg of the total flavones per tablet) 3–4 tablets three times daily. The tablet was effective in the relief of anginal pain and in improving the ECG (2,10,18). Another 110 cases of coronary disease were treated with the "Xinxuening Tablet", the extract of Radix Puerariae and Fructus Crataegi (6:1); 90% of the cases had relief of the anginal pain and 43% had marked effects (19).

2. Hypertension

The <Gegen> decoction 10–15 g can be given orally daily in 2 doses. The total flavones 100 mg daily in 2 doses was given for a course of 2–8 weeks to 222 cases of hypertension with pain and stiffness of the neck; 78–90% of the cases reported relief of neck symptoms. In 90% of the cases drug effect appeared after one week of medication, persisting for 1–2 weeks, and in some patients there were no relapses during a period of 3–9 months after discontinuation of therapy. The treatment alleviated symptoms of headache, dizziness, tinnitus, and numbness of extremities but did not significantly lower the blood pressure (2,10). Patients with hypertension and coronary disease had plasma catecholamine lowered after intravenous injection of puerarin (6).

3. Sudden Deafness at Early Stage

The tablet of the ethanol extract of <Gegen>, each equivalent to 1.5 g of the crude drug, was used at dosage of 1–2 tablets thrice daily with the injection of the total flavones, 100 mg IM twice daily, and in some patients also supplementary vitamin B complex, to treat 176 cases for a course of 1–2 months. Hearing power was improved in 79.5% of the cases (2,10,20).

4. Migraine

Symptomatic improvement was achieved in 35 out of 42 cases of migraine treated with the root of

Pueraria lobata (10). Intramuscular injection of the total flavones 200 mg to hypertensive patients complicated with arteriosclerosis improved the cerebral blood flow, lowered the vascular resistance and shortened the influx time in about half of the patients (2,21).

REFERENCE

1. Fang QC et al. Chinese Medical Journal 1974 (5):271.

2. Institute of Materia Medica of the Chinese Academy of Medical Sciences. Medical Research Communications 1972 (2):14.

3. Fan LL et al. Zhonghua Yixue Zazhi (National Medical Journal of China) 1975 (10):724.

4. Zhou YP et al. Zhonghua Yixue Zazhi (National Medical Journal of China) 1977 (9):550.

5. Zeng GY et al. Zhonghua Yixue Zazhi (National Medical Journal of China) 1974 (5):265.

6. Zeng GY et al. National Medical Journal of China 1979 59(8):479.

7. Pharmacology Department, Institute of Materia Medica of the Chinese Academy of Medical Sciences. Research Information on Cardiovascular Diseases (Information Institute of the Chinese Academy of Medical Sciences) 1979 (12):1.

8. Lu XR et al. Acta Pharmaceutica Sinica 1980 15(4):218.

9. Sun SX. Chinese Medical Journal 1956 42(10):964.

10. Institute of Materia Medica of the Chinese Academy of Medical Sciences. Chinese Traditional and Herbal Drugs Communications 1975 (2):34.

11. Shibata S et al Journal of the Pharmaceutical Society of Japan (Tokyo) 1959 79(7):863.

12. Tan HG. Guowai Yixue (Medicine Abroad) — Traditional Chinese Medicine and Materia Medica 1979 (1):39.

13. Luo HW et al. Journal of Nanjing College of Pharmacy 1957 (2):61.

14. Masatoshi H et al. Chemical and Pharmaceutical Bulletin 1975 23(8):1798.

15. Zhu XY et al. Acta Pharmaceutica Sinica 1979 (6):349.

16. Yue TL et al. Scientia Sinica 1977 (2):182.

17. Su CY et al. Acta Pharmaceutica Sinica 1979 (3):129.

18. Beijing Railways Hospital et al. Proceedings of the Symposium of Stage-IV Research Summary of Beijing District Coordinating Research Group on Coronary Diseases 1972 (2):36.

19. Anshan No. I Pharmaceutical Factory. Chinese Traditional and Herbal Drugs Communications 1978 (2):20.

20. Auditus Section, Beijing Institute of Otorhinolaryngology. Chinese Medical Journal 1973 53(10):591.

21. Hypertension Research Unit, Fuwai Hospital of the Chinese Academy of Medical Sciences. Cardiovascular Diseases 1972 (1):29.

(Huang Liangyue)

XISHU 喜樹

<Xishu> is derived from the fruit, root bark, stem bark or leaf of *Camptotheca acuminata* Decne. (Nyssaceae). It is bitter, "cold" and toxic. As an antineoplastic agent, it is used to treat various cancers.

CHEMICAL COMPOSITION

<Xishu> contains many alkaloids. Alkaloids having antineoplastic activity are camptothecine, 10-, 11- or 12-hydroxycamptothecine, 9-, 10- or 11-methoxycamptothecine, 12-chlorocamptothecine, venoterpine and deoxycamptothecine.

The fruit of *C. acuminata* contains the highest amount of camptothecine, about 0.02%, followed by the root bark, about 0.016%, and even less in the bark and leaf (1–6).

Since camptothecine and its derivatives have strong, antineoplastic activity, many of them were synthesized in China and other countries. China has synthesized dl-10-hydroxycamptothecine and dl-10-methoxycamptothecine. China also biooxidized camptothecine with the mould T-36 to form 10-hydroxycamptothecine (4,6).

PHARMACOLOGY

1. Antineoplastic Effect

The ethanol extracts of the root, stem, leaf, and fruit of *C. acuminata* were inhibitory to transplanted tumors in animals (1,7). Camptothecine was shown to have a very strong antineplastic activity *in vivo* and *in vitro* against a great variety of animal tumors (1,8–11). Except for minor differences the antineoplastic spectra of the camptothecine derivatives were essentially similar to that of camptothecine. 10-Hydroxycamptothecine and 10-methoxycamptothecine were found to be quite potent, producing an antineoplastic effect at one-thirtieth and one-sixth the dose of camptothecine, respectively (6,12). The synthetic dl-10-hydroxycamptothecine was also superior to camptothecine (12).

In vitro studies proved that camptothecine had pronounced inhibitory effect on leukemia L_{1210} and DON cells; the ID_{50} were determined to be 1.36×10^{-4} and 3.4×10^{-4} μM/ml, respectively. It was also inhibitory against HeLa cells and other tumor cells (8,10). *In vivo* studies proved that injection of camptothecine 0.25–25 mg/kg IP daily for 7–10 days to mice with leukemia L_{1210}, $L_{5178}y$, K_{1964}, or P_{388} at least doubled the survival period of the animals (8–10); it also prolonged the survival period of mice with leukemia L_{615} or ascitic hepatoma and markedly inhibited many solid tumors such as Lewis lung cancer, melanoma B_{16}, brain tumor B_{22}, solid Ehrlich ascites carcinoma in mice and Walker carcinoma 256 and Jitian sarcoma in rats (9,10,12,13). The therapeutic effect could be increased by changing the therapeutic regimen, for instance, injection of camptothecine 40 mg/kg IP every 4 days for 3 times, or injection of 30, 40 or 50 mg/kg IP on the 1st, 5th and 9th days were better than daily dosing at 25 mg/kg. The modified regimens not only prolonged the survival period of mice with leukemia L_{1210}, $L_{5178}y$, K_{1964}, and P_{388} by 1.85–10 times, but also reduced the toxic and side effects (8,10). Similar results were obtained in other tumors (9). On the other hand, camptothecine was also effective against resistant strains of mouse leukemia L_{1210} and P_{388} (resistant to nitrosourea nitrogen mustard, arabinoside, 6-mercaptopurine, and vincristine) (8). Combined therapy could enhance the therapeutic effect of camptothecine. For example, the aqueous extract of the root of *Salvia miltiorrhiza* markedly increased the efficacy of campotethecine against leukemia L_{615} in mice (13), while propylenediamine tetraacetylimide and ethylenediamine tetraacetylimide markedly enhanced its inhibitory effect against mouse sarcoma 180 (14).

10-Hydroxycamptothecine at 1–2 mg/kg IP once daily for 7–9 days prolonged the survival period of mice with leukemia P_{388}, L_{1210}, Ehrlich ascites carcinoma, ascitic hepatoma, and ascitic reticulosarcoma, and of rats with ascitic Jitian sarcoma by 119–280%. It was also capable of inhibiting the growth of solid tumors such as sarcoma 180, sarcoma 37, and cervical cancer U_{14} in mice, and Walker carcinoma 256 in rats. Various treatment regimens were shown to have antineoplastic effect but a single large dose (20 mg/kg) was the most effective (2,15).

Camptothecine and 10-hydroxycamptothecine caused morphological changes in cancer cells; degeneration, necrosis, nuclear shrinkage, deep staining, chromatin aggregation, vacuolization in cytoplasm, and giant cells. They also caused subcellular changes in both cancer cells and host liver cells: reduction in nucleoplasmic density, swelling and opening of mitochondria, enlargement of endoplasmic reticulum and Golgi bodies, marked increase and degeneration of vacuoles and liposomes, and eventually dissolution, destruction and death of cancer cells (7,16). Morphological and subcellular changes of cancer cells were consistent with biochemical changes. Camptothecine chiefly acted on and killed cells at the S phase of DNA synthesis, but had weaker effect on the G_1 and G_2 phases. It delayed the transition of cells from G_2 to M phase. Higher concentrations (10 µg/ml) inhibited mitosis. The drug was inactive against the cells at the resting (G_0) phase (8). Thus, camptothecine is different from vinblastine and colchicine which selectively acted at the M phase. The inhibitory effect of camptothecine on polynucleotides was greater than that on protein. By inhibiting DNA polymerase it inhibited the biosynthesis of DNA; it can directly destroy DNA or combine with the latter, rendering it vulnerable to endonuclease, thus inhibiting RNA and protein syntheses, leading to death of cancer cells (8,10,11,17).

Experiments have proved that camptothecine 1 mg/ml inhibits the DNA and RNA synthesis of HeLe cells and $L_{5178}y$ cells *in vitro*, but at the same concentration cannot inhibit the mitochondria of rat liver and brain cells. These results indicate that camptothecine has a greater influence on cancer cells than on normal cells and thus is favourable for the treatment of neoplastic diseases (10,17). Studies on structure-activity relationship revealed that the active antineoplastic group in the camptothecine molecule is the lactone on the E ring, and that the 20-hydroxyl group is also indispensible. A specific feature of camptothecine which may account for its antileukemic activity is that it contains a planar ring which allows intercalation with DNA (2).

2. Immunosuppressive Effect

A short therapeutic course consisting of 1–2 injections of camptothecine 0.5–1.0 mg/kg IP had no signifincant effect on the concomitant tumor immunity (CTI) of ascitic hepatoma and ascitic reticulosarcoma (ARS) in mice. When challenged with a large bolus dose 40 mg/kg IP, CTI was only marginally inhibited. On the other hand, the long-term course using the tolerance dose, 1 mg/kg IP per for 9 days, markedly inhibited CTI which could recover in 9 days after discontinuation of treatment (18). 10-Hydroxycamptothecine also inhibited the CTI of these two tumor strains and tumor allografts, though to a much lesser extent than camptothecine. However, the treatment regimen definitely affects the antineoplastic effect. For instance, the degrees of immunosuppression in the 12-mg/kg groups treated for 1, 5, and 9 days were lower than the group receiving a large bolus dose of 40 mg/kg (18,19).

3. Antiviral Effect

In vitro, 10-methoxycamptothecine 10–20 μg/ml inhibited the herpes virus by 89–100%. A similar effect was achieved with camptothecine (20).

4. Anti-early Pregnancy Effect

Early-stage pregnancy was terminated in all of the test animals by camptothecine 5 mg/kg PO or SC once daily for 1–3 days; the drug was administered in rats 7–9 days after copulation, and 7 days in the case of rabbits (7).

5. Pharmacokinetics

5.1 *Absorption, distribution, and excretion of camptothecine and its sodium salt.* Under alkaline conditions, with the opening of its ring, camptothecine becomes a water-soluble sodium salt; it can also be converted in the body into a lactone (10). The fluorescence and enzymatic methods showed that camptothecine was rapidly cleared from the blood, liver, and kidneys of mice after an IV injection of the drug; the half-life was calculated to be 30 minutes in contrast to the clearance half-life of 210 minutes from the gastrointestinal tract (22). In rats, the blood level peaked in 15 minutes after an intraperitoneal dose of camptothecine, its half life being 27 minutes (7). A bimodal descending curve was observed in man after a single intravenous dose of camptothecine. Yet its pharmacokinetics in the human body is not completely understood (23).

Camptothecine has a very high affinity to the mammalian and human plasma protein. Thus, 70 and 98% of the drug was found to bind with the plasma protein of mouse and man, respectively (10,23). The thin-membrane ultrafiltration technique showed that camptothecine can bind to the serum α-globulin and β-lipoprotein of various animals; the drug displayed the highest affinity to α-globulins of bovine serum (10,13).

After intraperitoneal injection, camptothecine was found rapidly distributed in the alimentary tract, liver, kidneys, bone marrow, and spleen of rats and mice, but was undetectable in the brain. The slow decline of the drug level in gastrointestinal tract suggested enterohepatic circulation (7,23). Camptothecine was found in various body tissues in the original form (23).

Bile is the main route of excretion of camptothecine. Over half of the dose intravenously injected into rats with renal ligation was excreted in bile within 90 minutes, wherein the drug concentration was found to be 300-fold of that in the blood. Its serious gastrointestinal toxicity could therefore be traced to its route of elimination (22,23). Since camptothecine was also excreted in urine, it often irritated the urinary tract causing hematuria, polyuria, and urinary urgency. In clinical trials, it was found that whenever urinary output was high (average 1929 ml/day) after camptothecine injection, the hematological reactions to this drug would be milder and vice versa, i.e., hematological reaction was markedly increased when urinary output was low (average 568 ml/day). These findings suggest a parallel relationship between the urinary output and renal toxicity of camptothecine (10).

5.2 Distribution and excretion of camptothecine suspension. Radioisotope tracing showed higher radioactivity in the gallbladder, liver and stomach of mice with ascitic hepatoma 1, 3, and 24 hours after intravenous injection of ^{3}H-camptothecine suspension compared with radioactivity in the same organs attained by injection of ^{3}H-camptothecine sodium; the opposite was true in the tumor tissues. The amounts of the 24-h urinary excretion of both drugs were the same, about 20%, but that of the fecal excretion of the suspension was lower. In normal mice where the labelled drugs were intravenously administered, the suspension achieved a higher blood level than the sodium salt solution. Therefore, the former may be more toxic to the hematopoietic system than the latter agent (26).

5.3 Distribution and excretion of 10-hydroxycamptothecine. Isotope tracing showed that after injection of ^{3}H-hydroxycamptothecine 10 mg/kg IV, the blood level declined in a biphasic manner. The distribution half-life was determined to be 4.5 minutes and the elimination half-life, 29 minutes.

Following intravenous injection of ^{3}H-hydroxycamptothecine at the same dosage to mice with ascitic hepatoma, the highest radioactivity after one hour was detected in the bile and small bowel contents; lower levels were found in the large intestine, heart, brain, muscles, thymus and spleen.

After four hours, the radioactivity in bile was markedly increased whereas that in the bone marrow, liver and intestinal contents was significantly decreased. On the other hand, no significant changes in radioactivity were detected in the cancer cells, whilst the heart, muscle and large intestine showed slight increase.

After 24 hours, radioactivity in bile approximated the level attained one hour after the medication. High levels persisted in the intestinal contents and cancer cells, but low levels were detected in the other tissues, especially in the brain and spleen. ^{3}H-Hydroxycamptothecine is mainly eliminated in feces; 47.8% of the administered dose was excreted in feces within 48 hours, but only 12.8% was excreted in urine (19).

6. Toxicity

6.1 *Acute toxicity.* The LD_{50} of camptothecine in mice was 68.4–83.6 mg/kg IP. The LD_{50} of sodium camptothecine were 57.3 mg/kg IV and 26.9 mg/kg PO in mice, and in rats were 234.1 mg/kg IV and 153.2 mg/kg PO. Apparently, the oral dose of camptothecine was more toxic than the intravenous dose.

The minimal lethal dose of camptothecine in dogs was 80 mg/kg IV. Death occurred within 10 days (7). The LD_{50} of 10-hydroxycamptothecine in mice was 104 ± 11 mg/kg IP (10).

6.2 *Subacute toxicity.* The LD_{50} of sodium camptothecine, 10-hydroxycamptothecine, and dl-10-hydroxycamptothecine in mice were determined to be 2.3 mg/kg (9), 3.6 ± 0.7 mg/kg, and 7.6 ± 1.8 mg/kg (15), respectively, given IP daily for 10 days. The MLD of sodium camptothecine administered in dogs for 14 days was 0.625 mg/kg IV, the toxicity of which was 100 times that of a single dose (28). The different regimens of sodium camptothecine given intravenously in dogs showed great variation in terms of MTD. The MTD was 0.156 mg/kg when given daily for 14 days, 2.5 mg/kg when given once a week for 6 weeks and 40 mg/kg when given once weekly for 2 weeks (10,28). In monkeys, the MLD of sodium camptothecine given intravenously daily for 14 days was less than 1 mg/kg, whereas the MLD of the injection given once every 4 days for 4 times was 10 mg/kg (28). The results showed lower toxicity from high dose short course relative to the low dose long course.

The subacute toxic symptoms in dogs and monkeys included: (1) Identical gastrointestinal symptoms in dogs and monkeys. Following intravenous injection of sodium camptothecine, anorexia, dehydration, weight loss, vomiting, and different degrees of diarrhea occurred. Some animals died due to bloody diarrhea. The most serious pathological lesion was seen in the intestinal tract, and occasionally in the esophagus and stomach. The principal histological changes were epithelial metaplasia, accumulation of necrotic debris in dilated glandular fossae, necrosis of overlying epithelium, mucosal and submucosal hemorrhage (10,28). (2) Hematological changes. Dogs survived the MTD developed reversible anemia, neutropenia and lymphopenia, and, during the recovery phase of the blood picture, mild transient monocytosis (28). Before death, monkeys given the MLD had increases in hemoglobin, elevation of serum alkaline phosphatase, SGOT, and SGPT, but pancytopenia in the bone marrow (28). (3) Toxic symptoms of the gallbladder, liver, and kidneys. Dogs given the MLD developed necrotic cholecystitis and monkeys given the MLD had marked renal tubular damages, and focal necrosis of the liver in a few of them. These were some of the factors responsible for the death of the animals (28).

The toxic effects of 10-hydroxycamptothecine in dogs given at 0.24 mg/kg IV once daily for 9 days, or at 0.8 mg/kg were similar to those of camptothecine, but it was less toxic to the kidneys. The MLD of this alkaloid given intravenously daily for 10 days was 0.08 mg/kg (15).

CLINICAL STUDIES

1. Malignant Tumors

Good therapeutic effect was obtained with camptothecine therapy of neoplasms of the alimentary tract such as stomach and rectum cancers. More than 600 cases of cancers of stomach, intestine, and rectum were treated with sodium camptothecine (10 mg/2 ml in 20 ml of normal saline) at adult doses of 10 mg daily or 20 mg every other day by IV injection or infusion for a total of 100 mg, the maximum being 300 mg. According to the criteria established in China, the effective rate obtained was about 60%. The medication improved the symptoms and reduced tumor size. However, the remission period was short and relapse easily occurred upon discontinuation of treatment, and resuming the treatment was usually ineffective. This drug is also effective for ovarian cancer, malignant hydatidiform mole, chorioepithelioma, lymphosarcoma, and chronic granulocytic leukemia (7).

Adult doses of 2.5–5 mg of camptothecine lactone suspension in 5–10% glucose solution given intravenously once daily or every other day for a course of 25–55 mg, and hepatic arterial infusion of 5–10 mg once daily or every other day for a course of 25–35 mg were used to treat 100 cases of primary hepatoma. In 98% of the cases hepatoma shrunk by more than 2 cm. Increasing the dosage to 50 mg or higher did not, however, increase the therapeutic effect. Not a single case showed complete disappearance of the tumor mass. After treatment, pain over the liver area was reduced, and mental state improved, appetite increased, and fever due to the cancer abated. Better results were obtained when the drug was given prior to operation than management of the ailment with the drug alone (29).

10-Hydroxycamptothecine 4–8 mg by intravenous injection or infusion every day for a course with a total dose of 50–360 mg was tried in 19 cases of primary hepatoma; when effective, a second course was initiated. Based on the criteria established in China, the effective rate was 42.1%, and in 28 cases of malignant tumors of the head and neck region (24 cases of salivary gland cancer and 4 cases of malignant lymphoma), the effective rate was 39.8%. It was also of therapeutic value in acute lymphocytic leukemia, acute granulocytic leukemia, cardia cancer, and bladder cancer (15).

2. Skin Diseases

In 297 cases of the common psoriasis, pityriasis rosea, local neurodermatitis, and epidermophyton infections topically treated with the 75% ethanol extract of the fruit of *C. acuminata*, 187 cases were cured, and 7 cases were improved; 39 cases were ineffective (30).

ADVERSE EFFECTS

The adverse effects of sodium camptothecine injection at doses exceeding 100 mg included: (1) Digestive system — impairment of appetite, nausea, vomiting, gastroenteritis, and, in individual patients, intractable diarrhea leading to water and electrolyte imbalance, enteroparalysis and death. Therefore, treatment has to be stopped as soon as watery diarrhea appears. (2) Hematopoietic system — bone marrow suppression causing decreases in leukocytes, platelets and hemoglobin. (3) Urinary system — hemorrhagic cystitis, polyuria, urodynia, and hematuria. (4) Miscellaneous such as buccal mucosal infection and alopecia (7,28). The adverse effect of 10-hydroxycamptothecine were found to be similar to those of camptothecine except that the former had milder effects on the urinary system (15).

REFERENCE

1. Wall ME et al. Journal of the American Chemical Society 1966 88:3888.

2. Wall ME et al. Annual Review of Pharmacology and Toxicology. 1977 17:117.

3. Lin LZ et al. Acta Chimica Sinica 1977 35(3,4):227, 229.

4. Lin LZ et al. Guowai Yixue (Medicine Abroad) — Pharmacy 1980 (4):222.

5. Phytochemistry Section, Institute of Materia Medica of the Chinese Academy of Medical Sciences. Acta Pharmaceutica Sinica 1979 14(12):746.

6. Shanghai No. 5 Pharmaceutical Factory et al. Kexue Tongbao (Science Bulletin) 1977 22:269.

7. Institute of Blood Transfusion and Hematology, Chinese Academy of Medical Sciences. Tianjin Medical Communications 1971 (6):1; (10):1.

8. Gallo RC et al. Journal of the National Cancer Institute 1971 46:789.

9. Tumor Section of the Pharmacology Department, Shanghai Institute of Materia Medica of the Chinese Academy of Sciences. Zhonghua Yixue Zazhi (National Medical Journal of China) 1975 55(4):274.

10. Cai JC et al. Pharmaceutical Industry 1973 (8):34.

11. Li LH et al. Cancer Research 1972 32(12):2643.

12. Song CQ et al. Guowai Yixue (Medicine Abroad) — Pharmacy 1978 (2):105.

13. Experimental Leukemia Section, Sixth Department of the Chinese Academy of Medical Sciences (Branch). Proceedings of the Mid-Southern and Southwestern Regional Symposium on Cooperative Research in Leukemia. Information Department of the Chinese Academy of Medical Sciences (Branch). 1975. p. 76.

14. Henan Medical College. Proceedings of the Mid-Southern and Southwestern Regional Symposium on Cooperative Research in Leukemia. Information Department of the Chinese Academy of Medical Sciences (Branch). 1975. p. 104.

15. Shanghai Institute of Materia Medica. Chinese Academy of Sciences. National Medical Journal of China 1979 59(10):598.

16. Wang ZW. Chinese Journal of Oncology 1980 1(3):183.

17. Shamma M. Journal of Pharmaceutical Sciences 1974 63(2):163.

18. Yang JL et al. Acta Pharmaceutica Sinica 1979 14(1):12.

19. Yang JL et al. Acta Pharmacologica Sinica 1980 1(1):44.

20. Tatus S et al. The Journal of Natural Products 1976 39(4):261.

21. Shanghai Centre of Medical and Pharmaceutical Industrial Design. Trends on Contraceptive Drug Research. Shanghai Centre of Medical and Pharmaceutical Industrial Design. 1970. p. 7.

22. Hart LG et al. Cancer Chemotherapy Reports 1969 53(4):211.

23. Hunt DE et al. Applied Microbiology 1963 16(6):867.

24. Guarino AM et al. Med Proc 1970 29:543.

25. Suson MS et al. Cancer Treatment Reports 1976 60(8):1135.

26. Chen RT et al. Acta Pharmacologica Sinica 1980 1(2):109.

27. Scheappi N et al. Chemical Abstracts 1969 70:105040m.

28. Scheappi N et al. Cancer Chemotherapy Reports 1974 5(1):25.

29. Surgery Department, Teaching Hospital of Guangxi Medical College. Medical Exchanges (Guangxi Health Bureau) 1978 10(1):5.

30. 169th Hospital of the Chinese PLA. Selected Information. 54014 Unit of the Chinese PLA. 1976. p. 72.

(Zeng Qingtian)

ZIZHU 紫珠

\<Zizhu\> refers to the leaf of *Callicarpa pedunculata* R. Brown (Verbenaceae). In some localities, it is derived from *C. dichotoma* (Lour.) K. Koch, *C. nudiflora* Hook. et Arn., *C. japonica* Thunb., *C. macrophylla* Vahl. and *C. cathayans* H. T. Chang. It is bitter, puckery, and "mild". Its actions are hemostatic, stasis-discutient, and detumescent. It is use to treat hematemesis, hemoptysis, epistaxis, bloody stool, metrorrhagia, and wound bleeding.

CHEMICAL COMPOSITION

\<Zizhu\> contains flavonoids, condensed tannins, neutral resin, carbohydrates, hydroxyl compounds, magnesium, calcium and traces of iron salts.

PHARMACOLOGY

1. Hemostatic Effect

The Callicarpa Injection increased the platelets and shortened the bleeding time, clotting time, and prothrombin time in man and rabbits (1–3). It also markedly inhibited the fibrinolytic system (4). Whether by local application, intramuscular injection, or intravenous injection this herb produced a good hemostatic effect in rabbits (1,2). For instance, local application of the dried powder of the Callicarpa leaf onto the partially sectioned rabbit femoral artery coupled with gentle compression achieved an excellent hemostatic effect. Blood flow from the wound could be slowed by the leaf powder. Hemostasis was effected when a thrombus-like substance was formed by cells accumulating in a kind of network of homogenous rubbery fiberous substance in the vascular lumen at the incision site (a narrow passage filled with a blood remained in the vascular lumen opposite the incision). The \<Zizhu\> liquid impregnated cotton balls pressed onto the cut surface of rabbit liver (0.3×1 cm^2) stopped bleeding in 2 minutes. In contrast, it took normal saline 4 minutes to stop bleeding in a control rabbit which had relapse bleeding (2). The Callicarpa Injection caused constriction of the frog mesenteric blood vessels (3).

2. Antibacterial Effect

The flower, leaf, root, bark and stem of *Callicarpa* were all shown to have bacteriostatic effect, the leaf being the most active. Disc diffusion test showed that *Staphylococcus aureus* and *Staphylococcus albus* were sensitive to the 100% *C. nudiflora* leaf decoction whereas *Pseudomonas aeruginosa*, *Salmonella typhi*, *Salmonella enteritidis*, *Shigella dysenteriae*, *Escherichia coli* and *Neisseria meningitidis* were more sensitive, and *Streptococcus* and *Proteus vulgaris* were slightly sensitive (5). Serial dilution test showed that the MIC of the decoction of *C. nudiflora* against *Staphylococcus aureus, Pseudomonas aeruginosa, Escherichia coli*, or *Shigella dysenteriae* was 1:16 and that against *Salmonella typhi, Proteus vulgaris*, or *Bacillus alcaligenes* was 1:32. The test strains were all isolated from burn wounds (5). The MIC of the decoction of <Zizhu> from Guangdong for *Staphylococcus aureus* was 1:320, for *Streptococcus hemolyticus*, 1:160, *Shigella flexneri* 1:80, *Salmonella typhi* 1:40, and *Pseudomonas aeruginosa* 1:20 (6).

3. Toxicity

The 10% <Zizhucao> solution (200 mg of crude drug/kg) injected intraperitoneally to rabbits at fivefold the hemostatic dose did not cause abnormal activity nor any toxic manifestations. The LD_{50} of the aqueous solution of zizhusu (obtained by leaf salt method) in albino mice was determined to be 237.5 mg/kg IV (1). The 300% *C. nudiflora* injection at 75 g/kg IP was not lethal to 5 mice, but at 180 g/kg killed one in 30 hours and another in 36 hours (5). The 300% injection of *C. nudiflora* was given to 6 dogs at 2 ml/kg IV twice daily for 5 days; no abnormalities were discovered in the blood, urine, and hepatic and renal functions examined for 8 days (5). Intravenous injection did not cause abnormal changes in the heart and blood pressure of rabbits and cats (1).

CLINICAL STUDIES

1. Hemostasis

1.1 *Bleeding from wounds.* Hemostasis can be achieved by local application of the crushed fresh leaf of *Callicarpa* washed properly with the tap water, or of the dried leaf ground into fine powders, then dressed with gauze. Likewise, applying pressure over the bleeding site with gauze impregnated with the <Zizhu> injection, or concurrently with the intramuscular dose, is deemed to be effective (3).

1.2 *Prolonged bleeding following tooth extraction.* The hemostatic effect of the leaf of *Callicarpa* has been confirmed and was found to be devoid of side effects in 469 cases wherein the dried powder of the leaf, or the powder of the aqueous extract, was either directly applied or applied with cotton and gauze to the bleeding site (3,7,8).

1.3 *Epistaxis.* The <Zizhu> nose drops (aqueous extract of the drug <Zizhuye>) instilled into nose 3–4 times a day is useful in treating nose bleeding and bleedings of the eye, ear, throat, and skin. It is also useful in rhinitis. The dried leaf powder 6 g can be mixed with egg white and given by mouth or inserted into nostrils (2,3,7).

1.4 *Hemostasis in surgery.* In 88 cases of operation of the neck, abdomen, face, ankle, and other sites, the gauze packing soaked with 5–10% sterillized <Zizhucao> liquid was applied over the incision sites with gentle pressure, or the herb solution was directly instilled onto the incision sites.

Bleeding from the capillaries and in blood vessels of less than 0.5 mm in diameter was usually stopped in 1–3 minutes. The average hemostatic time was 1 minute and 21 seconds, the shortest being 35 seconds and the longest 1 minute and 30 seconds (1). Ligation was still necessary for small blood vessels. Hemostasis was achieved in 6 cases of post-tonsillectomy hemorrhage (3).

1.5 *Bleeding in internal medicine, ophthalmology, gynecology and obstetrics.* Internal medicine: peptic ulcer with bleeding, hemoptysis due to mitral stenosis and heart failure in rheumatic heart disease, hemoptysis in bronchiectasis, hemoptysis in cavernous pulmonary tuberculosis, hematemesis due to ruptured esophageal varicose in cirrhosis of liver, hematuria and bloody stool. Ophthalmology: bleeding in the anterior chamber after operations for glaucoma and cataract, bleeding in corneal rupture, anterior chamber bleeding due to laceration of the vitreous body. Gynecology and obstetrics: uterine bleeding, bleeding following therapeutic obortion, bleeding after cesarean section, profuse bleeding after removal of old hematoma of ectopic pregnancy and various hemorrhagic conditions. Excellent hemostatic results were obtained in 362 cases treated. For instance, 83.6% of 103 cases of bleeding peptic ulcer became negative for occult blood in stool examination within 6 days of medication (2). Another report claimed that 90% of 30 cases of peptic ulcer responded to treatment with the Callicarpa Mixture without resorting to other hemostatic agents, except in severe cases replenishment of fluid to maintain the blood volume (9).

Preparations and Dosages. The Callicarpa powder or the powder of equal amounts of the herb and the tuber of *Bletilla striata*, 6 g three times daily; the Callicarpa tablet (prepared best from the dried powder of the aqueous extract), 0.3 g/tablet, 3–4 tablets twice or thrice daily (7); the Callicarpa Injection (2%), 2–4 ml IM twice daily (1).

2. Burns

One hundred and seventeen cases of burns from various causes, involving 11–81% of the body surface, were treated with this herb; 112 of them (95.73%) were cured. No intoxication due to drug absorption was known (5). In another report, the compound Callicarpa Liquid (prepared from the powder of Folium Callicarpae, Folium Hibisci, Folium Loropetali, Ramulus Cunninghamiae Lanceolatae) exhibited satisfactory effect in II degree and deep burns. Good effects were also achieved in the treatment of patients with III degree burns of limited area and of those with mixed degrees of burns (10).

Callicarpa therapy has the following advantages: (1) good and wide spectrum antibacterial effect; (2) strong astringent effect, can control wound exudation and thus reducing fluid replenishment; (3) promotion of epithelial growth and acceleration of wound healing; and (4) no significant local and systemic toxicity (5).

3. Hemorrhoid

The Callicarpa Hemorrhoid Solution (100 ml contains Folium Callicarpae 250 g, alunite 3 g and procaine 1–2 g) can be used as an injection to treat internal hemorrhoid, mixed hemorrhoid and circular hemorrhoid. The cure rate in 614 treated cases with complete records was 97.1% (596 cases). The cure rate for internal hemorrhoid was 99.6%, for mixed hemorrhoid 95.1% and for circular hemorrhoid 93.2%. Of the 570 cases with number of treatment recorded, 527 cases (92.35%) were cured after one treatment. In most cases of mixed and circular hemorrhoids, however, the treatment was repeated. In severe cases where treatment was separated to minimize the reactions, a cure was usually obtained after 2–3 treatments. This method is specifically useful in elderly subjects and patients with parenchymatous organic diseases who could not tolerate other treatments. It is to be used with caution in pregnant women and contraindicated in portal hypertension (11).

REFERENCE

1. 168th Hospital of the Chinese PLA. Cultivation, Preparation and Uses of Various Species of Callicarpa. 1970. p. 2.

2. Popularization of Chinese Traditional Drugs Group, Hangzhou First Hospital. Discussion on the Clinical Uses of Callicarpa and Its Hemostatic Mechanism. 1971. p. 3.

3. 459th Hospital of the Chinese PLA. Proceedings of the Symposium on Medical and Health Research. Hengyang (Hunan) Revolutionary Committee. 1972. p. 156.

4. Hematology Research Unit of the Surgery Department, First Teaching Hospital of Hunan Medical College. Medical Research Information (Hunan Medical College) 1976 (3):68.

5. Burns Research Group. 162nd Hospital of the Chinese PLA. Zhonghua Yixue Zazhi (National Medical Journal of China) 1975 (5):343.

6. Revolutionary Committee of Zhongshan Medical College. Xinzhongyi (Journal of New Chinese Medicine) 1971 (3):30.

7. 168th Hospital of the Chinese PLA. Chinese Traditional and Herbal Drugs Communications 1970 (3):40; (4):33.

8. Dentistry Department, Xiamen University (Branch). Chinese Journal of Stomatology 1960 8(3):148.

9. Shiling Health Centre (Lianjiang County, Guangdong). New Chinese Medicine 1973 2:156.

10. Yuanling County (Hunan) People's Hospital. Zhonghua Yixue Zazhi (National Medical Journal of China) 1976 56(3):207.

11. General Hospital of Fuzhou Military Region. People's Military Medicine 1975 (2):57.

(Huo Shaolan)

ZIWAN 紫菀

\<Ziwan\> refers to the root of *Aster tataricus* L. f. (Compositae). It is bitter, pungent, and slightly "warm". It has antitussive, mucolytic, antiasthmatic and antipyretic and antipyretic actions. It is prescribed for purulent and bloody sputum, dyspnea and palpitation, fever (occurring in summer in children), deficiency syndrome and for affections caused by the adverse upward flow of vital energy (*such as asthma, eructation etc.).

CHEMICAL COMPOSITION

\<Ziwan\> contains astersaponin, shionone, shionol, quercetin and epifriedelinol.

PHARMACOLOGY

1. Expectorant Effect

Significant expectorant effect lasting more than 4 hours was demonstrated in anesthetized rabbits after intragastric administration of the \<Ziwan\> decoction 1 g/kg (1). The orally administered crude extract of this herb also significantly increased the bronchial secretion in rats (2). Three kinds of crystals, probably shionone, astersaponin and shionol, obtained by successive extraction of this herb with benzene and methanol, were also proved to have expectorant action (3). Likewise, two other nitrogenous compounds exhibited expectorant activity (2).

2. Antitussive Effect

The \<Ziwan\> decoction had no antitussive effect in cats (4). But shionone isolated from the \<Ziwan\> extract at 5 mg/animal IP produced satisfactory antitussive effect against ammonia aerosol-induced cough (5).

3. Antibacterial Effect

In vitro studies revealed that \<Ziwan\> had different degrees of inhibitory action against *Escherichia coli, Shigella sonnei, Proteus vulgaris, Salmonella typhi, Pseudomonas aeruginosa, Vibrio cholerae*, and common dermatophytes (6,7). However, there is a great disparity in the reports (8,9). A paper reported that \<Ziwan\> at 1:50 inhibited *Mycobacterium tuberculosis* var. *hominis, in vitro*, and had therapeutic effect against experimental tuberculosis in mice (10). But another worker failed to find any antituberculous effect (11). The <Ziwan> decoction markedly inhibited influenza virus in the allantois of chicken embryo (12).

4. Miscellaneous Actions

Quercetin contained in <Ziwan> has a diuretic action (13). Epifriedelinol was shown to have antineoplastic activity against Ehrlich ascites carcinoma (14).

5. Toxicity

Astersaponin has a strong hemolytic action; its crude preparation is not recommeded for intravenous injection.

CLINICAL STUDIES

1. Acute and Chronic Bronchitis, Cough and Expectoration of Various Causes

<Ziwan> 6–9 g was often used with the flower bud of *Tussilago farfara* as a decoction to be administered orally in divided doses, or Aster-Ardisia Tablet (ether extract of Radix Asteris, methanol extract of Herba Ardisiae Japonicae, ethanol extract of Rhizoma Dioscoreae Nipponicae, and hyocholic acid) was effectively used in treating chronic bronchitis (12).

2. Pulmonary Tuberculosis with Cough

The decoction consisting of <Ziwan>, the bulb of *Fritillaria cirrhosa*, the rhizome of *Anemarrhena asphodeloides*, the fruit of *Schisandra chinensis*, ass-skin gelatin, licorice, and the root of *Platycodon grandiflorum* may be given orally.

REFERENCE

1. Gao YD et al. Chinese Medical Journal 1956 42(10):959.
2. Beijing Institute for the Control of Drugs and Biological Products. Extraction of the active principles of Aster tataricus (internal information). 1972.
3. Wuhan Institute for Drug Control. Wuhan Journal of New Traditional Medicine 1972 (1):16.
4. Huang QZ. Chinese Medical Journal 1954 40(11):849.
5. Research Laboratory, Hunan Institute of Traditional Chinese Medicine. Hunan Information on Science and Technology 1972 (11):91.
6. Zhang WX. Chinese Medical Journal 1949 67:648.

7. Li SH et al. Abstracts of the Chinese Pharmaceutical Association (Beijing Branch). 1957. p. 77.

8. Microbiology Section. Acta Academiae Medicinae Shandong 1959 (8):42.

9. Traditional Chinese Medicine and Materia Medica Research Unit of the Internal Medicine Department, First Teaching Hospital of Chongqing Medical College. Acta Microbiologica Sinica 1960 (1):52.

10. Guo J et al. Chinese Journal of Prevention of Tuberculosis 1964 5(3):481, 488.

11. Wang SY. Kexue Tongbao (Science Bulletin) 1958 (12):379.

12. Editorial Group. National Collection of Chinese Materia Medica. Vol. 1. People's Medical Publishing House. 1975. p. 848.

13. Zeng GF. The National Medical Journal of China 1936 22:397.

14. Hano K. Japan Centra Revuo Medicina 1967 224:505.

(Xue Chunsheng)

XIJIAO 犀角

<Xijiao> is the horn of *Rhinoceros unicornis* L., or *R. sondaicus* Desmarest, or *R. sumatrensis* (Fischer) Cuvier (Rhinocerotidae). It has a sour and salty taste and a "cold" property. The horn is credited with latent-heat-clearing, antipyretic, detoxicant, anti-inflammatory and anticonvulsant activities as well as the ability to remove pathogenic "heat" from the blood. It is administered in coma and delirium of febrile diseases, erythema, hematemesis, and epistaxis.

CHEMICAL COMPOSITION

The principal constituent of the rhinoceros horn is keratin. The amino acid constituents include cystine, 8.7%, and 3 alkaline amino acids histidine, lysine and arginine in ratio of 1:5:12. Thus, it resembles wool and cattle horn in mainly composed of eukeratin. In addition, the horn contains other proteins, peptides, free amino acids, guanidine derivatives, and sterols.

PHARMACOLOGY

1. Antipyretic Effect

Intravenous injection of the rhinoceros horn extract relieved rabbits of experimental fever induced by *Escherichia coli* (1). In contrast, others reported on significant antipyretic action in rabbits from oral administration of either the 50% rhinoceros horn decoction or rhinoceros horn-acasia gum solution (2–4). These divergent results might be due to different methods of administration.

2. Anticonvulsant Effect

Administration of the rhinoceros horn suspension 3 g/kg PO to mice, twice daily for 3 days did not significantly modify the effect of pentylenetetrazole and caffeine but prolonged the latent period of strychnine-induced convulsion and the survival period of the animals. Furthermore, it lowered the animals' convulsion reaction and mortality rates. In addition, the drug also prolonged pentobarbital sodium-induced sleep in mice (5).

3. Cardiovascular Effects

In experiments of isolated toad hearts, instillation of 30–50 drops of the 5% rhinoceros horn decoction to the chloral hydrate-inhibited heart resulted in gradual recovery of the heart beat, strengthening of contractility, increase in contraction amplitude and minute cardiac output. The drug also had a cardiotonic effect on the normal toad heart and similarly the *in situ* toad heart. Perfusion of the 2% rhinoceros horn decoction into the isolated rabbit heart inhibited by chloral hydrate caused gradual recovery of the heart beat, acceleration of the heart rate and increase in the contraction amplitude. Increasing the concentration to 5% initially produced cardiac stimulation and late-phase inhibition with the heart stopping at the diastolic phase. Five minutes after injection of the 10% decoction of rhinoceros horn 2 ml/kg IV in rabbits, the heart rate decreased, and normal heart rate was restored after 30 minutes. The R wave was lower than normal (6). Another report alleged that the rhinoceros horn had no significant effect on normal hearts (4). Most anesthetized dogs and rabbits given the 1–10% rhinoceros horn decoction 1 ml/kg IV showed blood pressure flutuations characterized by an initial slight increase, followed by decrease, normalization and again progressive elevation, for 20–30 minutes. Bilateral vagotomy or premedication with atropine did not modify the effect of the decoction on blood pressure, indicating no involvement of the vagal center and cholinergic receptors (6). Perfusion of the rhinoceros horn decoction into the lower limb blood vessel of toads, initially caused a slight constriction and thereafter dilation of the blood vessels, which is consistent with the initial increase and later fall in blood pressure. The possible mechanism of the prolonged pressor effect even after normalization of the blood pressure may be attributed to the strong cardiac stimulant effect overwhelmed vasodilation. Consequently, modification of blood pressure by the rhinoceros horn is thought to have resulted from its combined effect on the heart and blood vessels (6).

4. Miscellaneous Actions

Intravenous injection of the 30% extract of rhinoceros horn 0.5 ml to mice induced spasm, irregular respiration, and exophthalmos, which disappeared within 5 minutes and were followed by hypnosis lasting 5–6 hours. This agent caused mild mydriasis in rabbits and excitation of the isolated intestines and uteri of rabbits (1). The rhinoceros horn was proved *in vitro* to have no antibacterial activity (2).

CLINICAL STUDIES

1. Hyperpyrexia and Hemorrhage in Serious Febrile Infectious Diseases

In serious cases of encephalitis B and epidemic meningitis with persistent high fever, confusion, delirium, insomnia and restlessness, or with convulsion and rashes, the rhinoceros horn may be given with gypsum, mirabilite, etc. such as in the Aster-Hemsleya Pill. With the appearance of skin rashes, hemorrhage (hematemesis, epistaxis, etc.) the herb may be given with the root of *Rehmannia glutinosa* and the root bark of *Paeonia suffruticosa* such as in the Rhinoceros Horn-Rehmannia Decoction (7).

2. Hemorrhagic Diseases

Rhinoceros Horn-Rehmannia Decoction may also be used to treat thrombocytopenic purpura with symptoms of epistaxis, gum bleeding, hematemesis and bloody stool (5). One case of hemorrhagic capillary intoxication was reportedly cured with a modified Rhinoceros Horn-Rehmannia Decoction; cyanosis of the lower extremities resolved significantly and turned pink after one dose, and completely disappeared after 3 more doses; no relapse occurred during the 5-month follow-up period (8).

REFERENCE

1. Ogata et al. Japan Centra Revuo Medicina 1962 172:838.

2. Ye DJ et al. Jiangsu Zhongyi (Jiangsu Journal of Traditional Chinese Medicine) 1962 (11):2.

3. Huang HQ et al. Wuhan Medicine and Health 1959 2(3):340.

4. Yuan SF. Nanman Yixuehui Zazhi (Journal of the Nanman Medical Society) 1923 11(9):517.

5. Guangzhou Institute for Drug Control. Proceedings of the Seminar on the Clinical Pharmacology of Buffalo Horns. 1974. p. 1.

6. Gao YD et al. Shanxi Medical and Pharmaceutical Journal 1958 2(1):78.

7. Editorial Group of "Clinical Applications of Chinese Traditional Drugs" (Zhongshan Medical College). New Chinese Medicine 1971 (12):40.

8. Zhao QL. Guangdong Medical Journal 1964 (3):25.

(Yuan Wei)

BIMAZI 蓖麻子

<Bimazi> refers to the seed of *Ricinus communis* L. (Euphorbiaceae). It has a sweet and pungent taste and a "mild" property, and is toxic. Detumescent, detoxicant, and purgative actions are attributed to this herb. It is indicated in carbuncle, furuncle, lymph node tuberculosis, laryngitis, scabies, tinea, edema and abdominal distention, as well as in constipation.

CHEMICAL COMPOSITION

The seed of *R. communis* contains 40–50% of ricinic oil composed of glycerides of ricinoleic acid, isoricinoleic acid, oleic acid, linolenic acid and stearic acid. The molecular weight of ricin (a toxic protein) is 60,000 and that of *R. communis* hemagglutinin 120,000. It also contains ricinine, trace amounts of cytochrome C, lipase and other enzymes.

Ricin has been studied all over the world for more than a century. Before 1970, ricin was actually a substance of unknown composition which includes *R. communis* hemagglutinin. The former is very toxic, whereas the latter is basically nontoxic (1–4). Besides ricin D, an acidic ricin and a basic ricin can be obtained by fractional purification of crude ricin with DEAE-cellulose. The amino acid compositions of these 3 proteins are similar, with only minute difference in structure (1,5).

Ricin D is a glycoprotein composed of 493 amino acids and 23 saccharide molecules; it is a dipeptide linked by a disulfide bridge (6). The N-terminals are formed by alanine and isoleucine, and the C-terminals are formed by phenylalanine and serine (7).

PHARMACOLOGY

1. Cathartic Effect

Ricinic oil is an oily irritant which by itself has no cathartic effect. Saponification of ricinic oil by lipase in the duodenum yields sodium ricinate and glycerin. The former irritates the small intestine, casues reflexive peristalsis and intensifies the propulsion of intestinal contents towards the colon. Semiliquid stool is evacuated 1–2 times two to six hours after medication. The cathartic effect is not accompanied by intestinal colic, and increasing the dosage would not increase the cathartic effect. Ricin is thus considered to be a safe purgative (8–10).

Used as an adjuvant after anthelmintics, recinic oil can reduce the absorption of santonin (11).

A pathological model of "Taiyang-Yangming" combined syndrome" in mice was established wherein persistent diarrhea and low rectal temperature, etc. were induced by orally administering ricinic oil (12).

2. Antineoplastic Effect

2.1 *Effect on experimental cancers.* In vitro, many strains of cancer cells and variant cells are very sensitive to ricin, which at concentrations of 0.002–0.3 μg/ml was shown to inhibit the growth of lymphoma SI, BW_{5147}, MBC_2, EL_2, myeloma P_3, C_1, RBC_5, S_{117}, S_{194}, J_{588}, $MOPC_{315}/P$ and myeloid leukemia C_{1498} (13). Ricin also inhibited normal cells and various animal cancer cells *in vitro* (1,4,14). Experiments proved that virus-induced fibrinocyte variant (SV_{3T3}) was more susceptible to ricin than normal 3T3 cells (3).

Ricin exhibited definite effectiveness against transplantable animal tumors such as mouse Ehrlich ascites carcinoma, ascitic hepatoma, cervical cancer U_{14}, sarcoma 180 and leukemia. Injection of 7.5 μg/kg IP on the first and third days after tumor inoculation completely inhibited the growth of Ehrlich ascites carcinoma cells in mice and prolonged their survival period. Forty-eight hours after an injection of ricin 25 μg/kg IP decreased cancer cells by 90%; and 96 hours later, almost all cancer cells showed the following morphological changes: cellular swelling, vacuoles in nucleus, cessation of mitosis, heavy staining of cytoplasm, and appearance of scattered vacuoles in cytoplasm (7,15,17).

2.2 *Mechanism of action.* The action of ricin on various cancer cells is characterized by strong inhibition of protein synthesis, moderate inhibition of DNA synthesis, and slight inhibition of RNA synthesis (1,14). Ricin also strongly inhibited the cell-free protein synthesis of the lysate of rabbit reticulocytes, indicating that ricin does not modify carbohydrate metabolism in or amino acid uptake by the cancer cells but strongly inhibits the eukaryotic ribosomal protein synthesis (1,18,19).

Ricin has two peptide chains joined by a disulfide bridge. It is activated by splitting the disulfide bridge to release the A- and B-chains, the former is called the effectomer and the latter haptomer. The B-chain combines with carbohydrate receptors on the cell surface, carrying the free A-chain or the whole ricin molecule through the plasma membrane into the cytoplasm where they interact with the 60-S ribosomal subgroup. The result is inhibition of the binding of aminoacyl t-RNA to the ribosomal enzyme, thereby reducing the elongation factor of nucleic acids, deactivating nucleic acids and inhibiting protein synthesis which lead to cell death (1,18–29).

Abrin, another compound structurally-similar to ricin (*acturally a mixture of phytalbumose and paraglobulin), combines with the same monosaccharide receptors or lactose residue on the cell surface at more than two sites. Treating the cells with neuraminic acid may increase the number of binding sites. It was proven that the monosaccharide chain on the surface of tumor cells differ from that of normal cells in that its glycoprotein contains excessive sialic acid and its glycolipids often contain incomplete chains which readily bind with toxoproteins. This mechanism serves as an explanation of the antineoplastic activity of toxoproteins (21).

3. Cell Agglutination

Huge volume of literature in the past indicated that ricin has a rather strong agglutinating action *in vitro* on animal and human erythrocytes, small bowel mucosal cells, hepatocytes and other cells, as well as tissue suspension. Recent studies discovered that the active agglutinating substance is the nontoxic *R. communis* hemagglutinin and that ricin is inactive (1,3,4). The speed of hemagglutination of *R. communis* hemagglutinin depends not only on the quantity of the hemagglutinin and erythrocytes, but also on the pH. Alkaline medium favors hemagglutination. *R. communis* hemagglutinin needs serum complements for its action. These complements are interchangeable between species; for example, between goat and guinea pig (4,30).

Apart from serum complements, some reducing agents such as cysteine and ascorbic acid may also activate this reaction (31). The hemagglutination of *R. communis* hemagglutinin was found to be accompanied by papain-like proteolysis which may be caused by receptor destroying enzymes (30,31).

4. Pyrogenic Effect

Ricin is a very potent pyrogen in various mammals including human being. It can induce fever at $0.05-0.2$ µg/kg. It has a stronger and more prolonged effect with a longer latent period than any known pyrogens. Subcutaneous injection of 20 µg/kg of recin in rats caused elevation of the body temperature after 3.5 hours and lasting for more than 6 hours (32–35). Repeated injection resulted in tolerance not cross tolerant to bacterial pyrogens (35). The resulting fever can be relieved with aspirin and phenacetin. It can therefore be used as a tool in antipyretic studies (4,33).

5. Immune Reaction

Ricin is highly antigenic. Administration of ricin through various routes in man and various mammals induced production of antibodies and allergic reaction (4,36). Farmers cultivating *R. communis* were found to have ricin antibodies in their blood. These stable antibodies can increase the level of nonspecific antibodies in the body (4). This finding is witnessed by alterations in the plasma composition: the albumin level drops becauses of hepatotoxicity; with hepatic regeneration the albumin level gradually rises, α-globulins also increase, and β-globulins decrease. These findings suggest that antibodies may attenuate the specific destructive effect of ricin on protein synthesis and also suppress the pyrogenic reaction (37). Being cytotoxic, ricin can inhibit immunocytes such as macrophages (36,38).

R. communis hemagglutinin can precipitate immunoglobulins. It can completely precipitate IgM, and 10% of IgG of which IgG_3 was vulnerable while IgG_1 was not (39).

6. Effect on the Cardiovascular and Respiratory Systems

The critical dose of ricin to produce cardiac, hepatic and renal toxicity in anesthetized rabbits was determined to be 3.2 µg/kg IV. Doses lower than this had no significant influence on the cardiovascular and respiratory systems (36). Injection of 250 to 500 µg/kg of ricin to anesthetized cats caused a rise of the blood pressure, acceleration of pulse and respiration, and increase in the tidal volume (40). When the dose was increased to 30 µg/kg, the blood pressure dropped to zero, heart stopped at the diastolic phase, and eventually death occurred due to periodic breathing. The ECG showed prolonged R-R interval, missing P wave, and inverted T wave (36). Ricin at 250–500 µg/kg IV in anesthetized cats slightly antagonized the β-agonist isoproterenol. Injection of veratrine 25 µg/kg followed by injection of ricin attenuated all the pharmacological actions of epinephrine, norepinephrine, acetylcholine, angiotensinamide and histamine. Ricin also diminished the Bezold-Jarish reflex elicited by veratrine and nicotine (40), and in laboratory animals decreased the blood pressure and caused respiratory depression probably by its cyanide group (41).

The decoction of *R. communis* leaf was shown to increase the contraction amplitude of the isolated normal frog heart and of frog hearts intoxicated by chloral hydrate, ergot fluidextract, acetylcholine, atropine, quinine, or potassium chloride. The same decoction also lowered the blood pressure of dogs and caused vasodilation in rat hind limbs (11).

7. Miscellaneous Actions

Ricin can influence the respiration of different kinds of white blood cells, *in vitro*. At concentrations of 0.3–3.3 µg/ml, it decreased the oxygen consumption of monocytes, and increased that of lymphocytes; at 16.6–33.2 µg/ml, it decreased the oxygen consumption of lymphocytes and increased that of neutrophils; when the concentration was increased to 66.6 µg/ml, the respiration of neutrophils was also inhibited (42).

8. Pharmacokinetics

Ricin is not readily hydrolysed in the body by various enzymes and so remains active for a relatively long period, but once hydrolyzed it is quickly eliminated. Within 5 hours of intraperitoneal or intravenous injection in mice, ^{125}I-ricin has high concentration in various tissues and organs; the highest being in the spleen, followed by the kidneys, heart, liver, and thymus in descending order. Thereafter, drug levels rapidly declined and it disappeared from the liver in 10 to 12 hours and from other organs and tissues in 10 to 30 hours. This drug is chiefly excreted in the urine with peak excretion at 5–7 hours (43).

9. Acute and Subacute Toxicity

Roughly speaking, lethal doses (g/kg) of <Bimazi> in various animals are: hen 14, duck 4, goose 0.4, rabbit 0.9, piglet 2.3, pig 1.3, milking cow 2, young goat 0.5, goat 5.5, sheep 1.25, and horse 0.1 (4).

The LD_{50} of ricin by a single injection in mice was 6–12 µg/kg IV (7,44), but others reported much higher values, which is due to variations in the purity of the drug used (36,43). The LD of ricin samples purified by DEAE-cellulose was determined to be 50–150 µg/kg IV in rats (45). The LD_{50} of ricin manufactured by Jianmin Pharmaceutical Factory of Wuhan city in mice was 47.97 µg/kg IV, the MTD in rabbits was 3.2 µg/kg IV. The MTD of this product given to rabbits daily for 16 days was 1.6 µg/kg IV (36).

Mice died from 10 hours to a few days after intraperitoneal or intravenous injection of a lethal dose of ricin. The onset of intoxication was relatively long; generally test animals became unsteady at 12 hours after the medication and lying sideways after 24 hours. Convulsion, dyspnea, opisthotonus and central disturbances developed occasionally. The animals died from respiratory paralysis 30 minutes after the first episode of convulsion. Intoxication was frequently accompanied by severe diarrhea which probably was one of the lethal factors (4).

In acute and subacute toxicity studies of ricin, functional and morphological changes appeared in most organs and tissues of the intoxicated animals (rat, mouse, guinea pig and rabbit). The chief toxicity was confined to the liver, small intestine, and endocrine glands. The drug damaged the endoplasmic reticula and caused mild mitochondrial changes of hepatocytes leading to hepatic degeneration and necrosis. Severe damage on the small intestine is the main cause of diarrhea. The endocrinal organs and tissues are very sensitive to ricin. Hemorrhagic necrosis and regressive degeneration occurred in animals' hypothalamic cells, adrenal gland, pituitary, thymus, testicle, ovary, pancreas, and lymph tissues (4,36,45). It also damaged the reticuloendothelial system and destroyed the chromatins of peripheral neurons in the maxillary ganglion and thoracic plexus (4).

In the ricin-intoxicated animals coagulation time was lengthened because the drug interfered with glycolysis and decreased prothrombin and thrombokinase. Ricin also increased the total red blood cell count and total white blood cell count, increased the blood levels of glucose and urea, decreased the blood concentration of magnesium ion and increased that of calcium ion, and changed the ratio of Ca^{++} to Mg^{++} from 2:1 to 7.75:1, which may be related to the pyrogenic reaction (4,46,47). In animals with acute ricin intoxication, the blood glucose level, liver glycogen, total protein, and hematocrit were decreased, whereas the lactose, nonprotein nitrogen, amino acid, inorganic phosphate, acidic phosphates, lactic acid and pyruvic acid were increased. There was also derangement of the liver function (SGOT, SGPT, LDH) (4). Hematological changes in acute intoxication were only slightly different from those in chronic intoxication.

CLINICAL STUDIES

1. Constipation

Ricinic oil is a relatively safe purgative, but is contraindicated in menstruating or pregnant women because it may cause mild congestion of pelvic organs. *Dosage and administration*: children 4 ml; adults 5–20 ml. Emulsion 30 ml. They should be given in the morning on an empty stomach (8–10).

2. Neoplasms

It was reported that ricin is effective for cancers of the craniocervical region (19,48,49). Cream or ointment containing 3–5% of ricin and 3% of dimethyl sulfoxide can be applied locally to cervix cancer once daily, 5–6 times weekly for a course of 1–2 months. In 8 cases of cervix cancer at middle and late stages managed with the said method plus extracorporal irradiation, 4 obtained a short-term clinical cure, 1 improvement and 3 no effect. The 3–5% ricin ointment or cream was used as a dressing once daily to treat 6 cases of skin cancer; 2 cases (one case each of adenoma and squamous carcinoma) achieved a clinical cure, 2 (one case each of adenoma and squamous carcinoma) had marked effect and 2, no effect. Ricin is therefore for both adenoma and squamous carcinoma (50).

3. Gastroptosis

Ricinus Galla Plaster (Semen Ricini 98%, Galla Chinensis 2%) applied to the acupoint "Baihui" for a period of 5 days each time was employed in 61 cases, In some cases gastroptosis was corrected and in others subjective symptoms were improved (51).

4. Facial Nerve Paralysis

Three cases were reportedly cured within 10 days of treatment with crushed kernel of *R. communis* applied on the mandibular joint and corner of the mouth once daily (11).

5. Miscellaneous

Ricinic oil may also be used as an emollient (11). The root of *R. communis* may be used to treat epilepsy, tetanus, and bronchitis in children (11).

ADVERSE EFFECTS

Poisoning with <Bimazi> by mouth has a latent period and shows toxic symptoms of headache, gastroenteritis, fever, leukocytosis, left shift of blood picture, anuria, cold sweating, frequent spasm, prostration, and even death (4,11). Death due to injudicious oral ingestion of about 20 pieces of <Bimazi> in adults and 2–7 pieces in children was reported (52).

<Bimazi> contains many toxic constituents. Ricinine 160 mg or ricin 7 mg is lethal in adults. The toxicity of ricin was reported to be 22 times greater than that of hydrogen cyanide; 1 g of it is sufficient to kill 3600 persons (4,52).

Local application of ricin cream or ointment on the cervix may cause abdominal pain, pruritus vulvae, and systemic pruritus, eczema, urticaria, hoarseness, itchiness of the throat, laryngeal edema, desquamation of the palm and sole, chills, and fever, which may be relieved by timely symptomatic treatment (50).

REFERENCE

1. Olsnes S et al. Nature 1974 249(6):627.

2. Baenziger J et al. Journal of Biological Chemistry 1979 254(19):9795.

3. Nicolson GL et al. Toxicology 1974 2(1):77.

4. Balint GA. Toxicology 1974 2(1):77.

5. Funatsu M et al. Japanese Journal of Medical Sciences and Biology 1970 23(4):264; 23(5):342.

6. Funatsu M et al. Chemical Abstracts 1972 76:110323j.

7. Lin JY et al. Nature 1970 227:292.

8. Goodman LS et al. The Pharmacological Basis of Therapeutics. 2nd edition. U.S.P. 1955. p. 1503.

9. Zhang CS. Pharmacology. People's Medical Publishing House. 1962. p. 199.

10. Iwao I. Japan Centra Revuo Medicina 1961 169:690.

11. Jiangsu College of New Medicine. Encylopedia of Chinese Materia Medica. Vol. 2. Shanghai People's Publishing House. 1975. p. 2446.

12. Xue RX. Xinzhongyi (Journal of New Chinese Medicine) 1978 (5):back cover.

13. Ralph P et al. Journal of the National Cancer Institute 1973 51(3):883.

14. Lin JY. Cancer Research 1971 31(7):921.

15. Lin JY. Toxicon 1973 11(4):379.

16. Fodstad 0 et al. Cancer Research 1977 37:4559.

17. Phytochemistry Department, Hubei Institute of Botany. Health Journal of Hubei (Hubei Health Bureau) 1975 (6):52.

18. Lugnier AJ et al. Chemical Abstracts 1976 85:154853x.

19. Olsnes S et al. Journal of Biological Chemistry 1976 251(3):3985.

20. Hughse RC et al. European Journal of Biochemistry 1977 72(2):265.

21. Xu B. Antineoplastic Drugs Research (Materials received from the participants to the 2nd international symposium on cancer). 1978.

22. Hedblom ML et al. Chemical Abstracts 1976 85:187478g.

23. Fernandez-Puentes C. Biochemistry 1976 15(20):4364.

24. Benson S et al. European Journal of Biochemistry 1975 59(2):573.

25. Sperti S et al. Biochemical Journal 1975 148(3):447.

26. Olsnes S et al. European Journal of Biochemistry 1975 60(1):281.

27. Youle RJ et al. Journal of Biological Chemistry 1979 254(21):11089.

28. Nolam RD et al. European Journal of Biochemistry 1976 64(1):69.

29. Refsnes k et al. Journal of Experimental Medicine 1976 143(6):1464.

30. Waldschmidt-Leitz E et al. Chemical Abstracts 1969 71:88411j.

31. Waldschmidt-Leitz E et al. Chemical Abstracts 1972 76:111505g.

32. Kcoja N et al. Chemical Abstracts 1975 82:26883h.

33. Hache J et al. Chemical Abstracts 1968 70:113658j.

34. Eperjessy ET et al. Chemical Abstracts 1966 64:4099a.

35. Kcoja N et al. Chemical Abstracts 1975 82:11992u.

36. Huang MM et al. Acta Academiae Medicinae Wuhan 1980 9(2):60.

37. Balint GA et al. Chemical Abstracts 1975 82:84364a.

38. Koga T et al. Chemical Abstracts 1971 74:138652y.

39. Saltvedt E et al. Chemical Abstracts 1975 83:112231w.

40. Balint GA. Chemical Abstracts 1968 69:50616a.

41. Lin QS. Chemical Studies of Chinese Traditional Drugs. Science Press. 1971. p. 706.

42. Balint GA. Chemical Abstracts 1967 67;106984x.

43. Fodstad O. British Journal of Cancer 1976 34:418.

44. Giirtler LG. Biochimica et Biophysica Acta 1973 295:582.

45. Waller GR et al. Proceedings of the Society for Experimental Biology and Medicine 1966 121(3):685.

46. Dirheimer G et al. Chemical Abstracts 1967 67:62653g.

47. Balint GA. Med Pharmacol Exp 1967 17(2):183.

48. Hsu GT et al. Journal of Formosan Medical Association 1974 73:526.

49. Tung TC et al. Journal of Formosan Medical Association 1971 70:569.

50. Tumor Department, Second Teaching Hopital of Wuhan Medical College. Acta Academiae Medicinae Wuhan 1977 (6):35.

51. Chen DX et al. Xinyiyaoxue Zazhi (Journal of Traditional Chinese Medicine) 1974 (2):26.

52. Zhang JM et al. Chinese Journal of Paediatrics 1958 (5):487.

(Zeng Qingtian and Du Deji)

PUHUANG 蒲黄

<Puhuang> is the pollen of *Typha angustifolia* L., or *T. orientalis* Presl. (Typhaceae). The pollens of the other species such as *T. angustata* Bory et Chanberd, *T. latifolia* L., *T. minima* Hoppe and *T. davidiana* Hand.-Mazz are also used medicinally as <Puhuang>. Sweet and of "mild" property, the crude <Puhuang> is reputed to be blood-stimulant, stasis-eliminative, hemostatic and analgesic. The roasted <Puhuang> is astringent and hemostatic. This herb is recommended in hemoptysis, hematemesis, hematuria, postpartum abdominal pain due to blood-stasis, dysmenorrhea, uterine hemorrhage, and in bleeding from wounds and injuries.

CHEMICAL COMPOSITION

<Puhuang> contains α-typhasterol, α-sitosterol, volatile oil, flavonoids (including isorhamnetin) and alkaloids. Leucine, valine, alanine and 6-aminopurine were recently isolated from the soluble fraction of the pollens (1).

PHARMACOLOGY

1. Effect on the Cardiovascular System

Low concentration of the ethanol extract of <Puhuang> increased the contractility of isolated toad hearts, but high concentrations had the opposite effect (2,3). The ethanol extract also decreased the rate of isolated hearts of rabbits and guinea pigs, large doses of it inhibited the heart, precipitating cardiac arrest at the diastolic phase. At doses slightly smaller than that required to inhibit the myocardium, the ethanol extract increased the coronary flow in isolated rabbit hearts with or without electrically induced fibrillation, by 43 and 35%, respectively. This effect which was accompanied by ECG improvement was especially prominent when coronary constriction was induced by pituitrin injection; the coronary flow was increased by 76% (3). Intramuscular injection of <Puhuang> fluidextract 0.6 g (crude drug) increased the ^{86}Rb uptake of the mouse myocardium by 27.9% (P < 0.01), but reducing the dose to one-half or orally administering 2.5 times this dose for 10 days produced no significant influence on the myocardial microcirculation of the animals (4).

The portion of the alcohol-precipitated aqueous extract adsorbed onto the strong acid cation exchange resin (heretofore called the adsorbed agent) had significant cardiovascular effects. In the lung-heart specimen of dogs, the adsorbed agent increased the cardiac output per unit time, increased the aortic pressure, lowered the central venous pressure, accelerated the heart beat, improved the T wave on the ECG and increased the index of cardiac function, but it did not significantly change the stroke volume. Blockade of the β-receptors by alprenolol, however, abolished the effect of the adsorbed agent on the heart rate of the lung-heart preparation of dogs; the stroke volume was markedly increased while the other effects remained unchanged. These findings indicate a possible connection between the positive chronotropic action and β-receptor stimulation. Nevertheless, the adsorbed agent injected intravenously was found to decrease the heart rate of anesthetized dogs, and this negative chronotropic effect could be annulled by atropine or hexamethonium bromide, suggesting that the drug inhibits the heart of intact animals through the vagus nerve ganglion or vagus center. It was also shown that the negative chronotropic action of the drug overcame its direct positive chronotropic effect; thus, it is inferred that the drug has diametrically opposed effects in intact animals and isolated hearts (5).

<Puhuang> extract has vasodilatory effect on the rabbit ear (6). Intraperitoneal injection of the fluidextract increased the arteriorlar blood flow and the number of open capillaries in the hamster cheek pouch, but did not significantly alter the caliber of arterioles (4). The ethanol extract 30 mg/kg injected into the femoral artery of anesthetized dogs increased the femoral arterial blood flow by 75–570% and decrease the peripheral resistance coefficient by a mean of 62.7% (3). Likewise, the adsorbed agent caused vasodilation which was not blocked by alprenolol, implying no relationship with β-receptors (5). The alcohol-fractionated aqueous extract directly caused weak peripheral vasodilation (7).

Intravenous injection of the <Puhuang> decoction, ethanol extract, or the adsorbed agent to anesthetized cats, rabbits, and dogs decreased the blood pressure and heart rate; intraperitoneal injection of these agents also caused mild hypotension in dogs. Hypotension, bradycardia, and decreased vascular resistance of hind limbs elicited by <Puhuang> were partially or completely abolished by blocking the muscarinic receptors or nerve ganglions with atropine or hexamethonium bromide injection. It is postulated that the hypotension and lowering of the vascular resistance were probably linked to the cholinergic receptor and central reflex regulation, and that vasodilation might be the chief cause of acute hypotension (2,3,5,6). Within the range of therapeutic dosages, however, the orally administered <Puhuang> showed no clinical effect on normal blood pressure (8).

Moreover, intraperitoneal injection of large doses of the <Puhuang> preparation increased the tolerance of mice to hypobaric hypoxia (9).

The injection of "Shi Xiao Powder" (equal amounts of Pollen Typhae and Faeces Trogopterori) increased the tolerance of mice to hypobaric hypoxia, antagonized pituitrin-induced acute myocardial ischemia in rats, suppressed the spontaneous activity of mice and lowered the blood pressure of conscious rabbits which was weaker and shorter than that induced by hexamethonium bromide (10).

2. Hypocholesterolemic and Antiatherosclerotic Effects

In studies where rabbits were fed initially with high fat feed plus <Puhuang> 16 g/animal/day for 12 weeks and then with ordinary feed plus <Puhuang> for another 4 weeks, it was discovered that the treatment group had markedly lower serum cholesterol level and milder aortic plaque formation and coronary atherosclerosis lesions than the control group. Electron microscopy revealed that majority of the animals in the treatment group had intact and smooth aortic endothelium, normal subendothelium, and occasionally marginal cellular infiltration and lipid deposition. In contrast, most of the animals in the control group had markedly thickened aortic subendothelium, large amounts of intracellular and extracellular lipid deposits, and large numbers of foam cells and smooth muscle cells penetrating the subendothelium through the cracks in the internal elastic lamina. Further studies revealed that in the treatment groups, the fecal cholesterol was greatly increased and the absorption of the orally administered ^{131}I-cholesterol was rather slow, but they had no correlation with the serum cholesterol level. Consequently, the hypolipemic mechanism is believed to involve the inhibition of intestinal absorption of exogenous cholesterol, and reabsorption of cholic acid and endogenous cholesterol, thus promoting the excretion of cholesterol and cholic acid into the bile and intestinal lumen. Active studies are on-going to determine whether or not <Puhuang> influences cholesterol synthesis in the liver (11,12).

3. Anti-inflammatory Effect

External application with concentrated <Puhuang> decoction produced a striking anti-inflammatory effect on scalds of rat hind limbs and also hastened the resolution of the intradermally injected Evans blue in rabbits. A detumescent effect was also achieved by intraperitoneal injection of the alcohol-fractionated decoction of the herb in rats with egg white-induced paw swelling; it reduced vascular permeability increased by local injection of histamine in rats and mice. In summing up the effects of <Puhuang> including that on the microcirculation of the hamster cheek pouch, it is preliminarily held that the detumescent effect was due to improvement of local circulation, facilitation of reabsorption, and lowering of capillary permeability (13).

4. Coagulant Effect

The <Puhuang> decoction was proved *in vitro* to promote the coagulation of human blood (14). Intragastric administration of the aqueous extract or the 50% ethanol extract of this herb to rabbits significantly shortened the clotting time (6). The clotting time was also shortened following intragastric administration of the herb decoction to rabbits, especially on the first day (15). The crude <Puhuang> by mouth also reduced the clotting time in rabbits and the bleeding time in mice. Oral administration of carbonized <Puhuang> was even more effective than administration of the crude drug (16,17). Subcutaneous injection of the <Puhuang> extract to rabbits increased the platelet count and shortened the prothrombin time (6). Hemostasis was achieved by external application of the <Puhuang> powder to experimental bleeding from femoral artery of anesthetized dogs (18). The bioactive principle responsible for shortening the clotting time and initiating hemostasis is thought to be isorhamnetin (19).

5. *Effect on Uterus*

The decoction, tincture, and ether extract of <Puhuang> had stimulant effect on isolated uteri of guinea pigs, rats, and mice, and at large doses caused spastic contraction. More pronounced effect was achieved on nonpregnant than on pregnant uteri (2,6,8). The ethanol extract also caused rhythmic contraction of the isolated uterus of pregnant rabbits and increased the tonicity of the isolated uterus of the nonpregnant animals (3). Experiments on *in situ* uteri of anesthetized dogs and rabbits and uterine fistulae of rabbits showed that the <Puhuang> decoction, tincture, or ether extract at doses of 0.05–0.2 g/kg IV produced uterine excitation (2). The herb increased the uterine contractility or tonicity in postpartum women (8).

6. *Effect on Intestinal Tract*

The <Puhuang> extract enhanced peristalsis of the isolated rabbit intestine, increased the tone and its rhythmic contraction of the isolated duodenum of rats or guinea pigs. These effects can be blocked by atropine (3,6). On the other hand, with potency of 57% of that of papaverine, isorhamnetin isolated from this herb produced a spasmolytic effect on the isolated intestine of mice (20).

7. *Miscellaneous Actions*

Intravenous injection of the ethanol extract of <Puhuang> to anesthetized dogs produced a choleretic effect (21). Crude or carbonized <Puhuang> was proved to be inactive against hemolytic *Staphylococcus aureus* and various dysentery bacilli *in vitro* (17). An early paper reported that the 1:100 <Puhuang> decoction inhibited growth of *Mycobacterium tuberculosis in vitro* and the intragastrically administered decoction had definite effectiveness in guinea pigs with experimental tuberculosis (22). In addition, clinical observation showed that <Puhuang> has diuretic (23,24) and antiasthmatic effects (13).

8. *Toxicity*

No death of mice occurred after injection of the ethanol extract of <Puhuang> 500 mg/kg IV (6). In experiments with the lung-heart specimen of dogs, myocardial inhibition or arrhythmia were not observed in 2 hours after perfusion with 152 g (crude drug)/800 ml (blood volume) of the absorbed agent. The results indicated that the herb has a low toxicity and a wide safety range (5).

CLINICAL STUDIES

1. *Coronary disease and Hyperlipidemia*

Clinical trials proved that the crude <Puhuang> not only lowered the serum cholesterol level but also markedly decreased the platelet adhesion rate in hyperlipidemic patients (11,12). The sugar-coated tablet of <Puhuang> was used to treat 66 cases of coronary disease and 106 cases of hyperlipidemia. The aggregate effective rates for symptomatic relief were 89.4 and 76.5% and for ECG improvement were 48.8 and 85.7%, respectively. On the other hand, the effective rate for lowering serum total cholesterol and triglycerides was around 70% in both diseases (25).

In 285 cases of hypercholesterolemia complicated with hypertension or coronary disease, the granule infusion or tablet prepared from this herb showed a pronounced anticholesterolemic effect (11). "Xinshu No. 3 Tablet" (crude Pollen Typhae, Radix Codonopsis Pilosulae, Flos Carthami, Rhizoma Curcumae Longae or Rhizoma Zedoariae, Lignum Dalbergiae Odoriferae) administered to 400 cases of cardiovascular diseases was found to be as effective as the sugar-coated tablet of <Puhuang> in treating coronary disease and hyperlipidemia. Furthermore, it produced excellent effect for first and second stage hypertension in about 90% of the cases (26). A number of recent reports from different localities claimed that the variously modified Shi Xiao Powder has some effectiveness against angina pectoris (27–30).

2. Postpartum Blood Retention and Abdominal Cramp

Although the orally administered crude <Puhuang> did not strikingly reduce the size of the uterus and the amount of lochia in 31 puerperal women, it was better than Yimugao used in the control (8).

<Puhuang> is often used with the feces of *Trogopterus xanthipes* in postpartum blood retention and abdominal cramps to improve blood circulation, eliminate blood stasis, relieve distending pain, and clear up lochia. <Puhuang> together with charred ginger had a good hemostatic effect in hemorrhage due to insufficient uterine contraction during the puerperal period. Elimination of blood retention or initiation of hemostasis is mainly achieved through the uterus contracting action of the herb (23).

3. Functional Uterine Bleeding, Hematuria, Bloody Stool, etc.

<Puhuang> stopped or reduced bleeding in over 80 cases of bleeding conditions: hemoptysis with blood-stained sputum, bloody stool, hematuria, epistaxis, uterine bleeding and leukorrhea (24,31). <Puhuang> is often prescribed with the aerial part of *Cephalanoplos segetum* and talc, or charred <Puhuang> with the processed root of *Rehmannia glutinosa* and the browned leaf of *Biota orientalis*, for the treatment of functional uterine bleeding. Hematuria, dysuria, and urodynia due to cystitis or urethritis can be treated with Pollen Typhae Powder (Pollen Typhae, Semen Malval Verticillatae, and Radix Rehmanniae Crudae in equal amounts). Bloody stool, bloody and purulent stool, and dull abdominal pain of chronic colitis, may be treated with stir-fried <Puhuang> plus the feces of *Trogopterus xanthipes*, baked root of *Pueraria lobata* and baked seed of *Myristica fragrans* (23).

4. Miscellaneous

All 30 cases of eczema treated locally with a dressing of the powder of crude <Puhuang> were cured in 6–15 days (32). Local application of the crude herb was also effective against fungal infection of the oral cavity due to medication with various antibiotics (33). The sterile solution of <Puhuang> was given extra-amniotically to induce labor in 40 cases of mid-term pregnancy. Twenty-seven cases had abortion 33.3 hours after one dose, 13 cases also had abortion after 2–3 doses of the agent plus oxytocin (34).

ADVERSE EFFECTS

No significant side effect were reported with the therapeutic dosage of <Puhuang>. However, it is contraindicated in pregnant women because it contracts the uterus (8,23). Extra-amniotic administration of the sterile solution of the herb was reported to produce transient chilliness and elevated body temperature ($< 39°C$) in some patients, which recovered spontaneously (34). Individual patients taking the compound formulae such as Xinshu No. 3 Tablet developed dizziness and diarrhea or urticaria at the beginning of treatment but these reactions disappeared by themselves in 1–2 weeks without disrupting the treatment. No other side effects were encountered. ECG showed that the herb did not aggravate the condition of patients with severe heart diseases (26).

REFERENCE

1. Xu QF et al. Hunan Yiyao Zazhi (Hunan Medical Journal) 1978 (3):45.

2. Li BH. Acta Academiae Medicinae Jiangxi 1956 (1):6.

3. Pharmacology Section, Research Department of Hunan Institute of Traditional Chinese Medicine and Materia Medica. Hunan Yiyao Zazhi (Hunan Medical Journal) 1976 (2):48.

4. Chen ZZ et al. Hunan Yiyao Zazhi (Hunan Medical Journal) 1979 (5):58.

5. Pharmacology Section, Research Department of Hunan Institute of Traditional Chinese Medicine and Materia Medica. Hunan Yiyao Zazhi (Hunan Medical Journal) 1976 (5):49.

6. Luo G et al. Acta Academiae Medicinae Jilin 1960 (1):80.

7. Xu LN et al. Xinyiyaoxue Zazhi (Journal of Traditional Chinese Medicine) 1976 (5):38.

8. Lei YZ et al. Shanghai Zhongyiyao Zazhi (Shanghai Journal of Traditional Chinese Medicine) 1963 (9):1.

9. Huang QX et al. Hunan Yiyao Zazhi (Hunan Medical Journal) 1979 (4):48.

10. Cardiovascular Research Unit, Shanxi Medical College. Xinyiyaoxue Zazhi (Journal of Traditional Chinese Medicine) 1976 (5):41.

11. Ding T et al. Shanghai Medical Journal 1980 (8):53; Pathophysiology Section, Shanghai Second Medical College et al. Abstracts of Papers on Experimental Atherosclerosis of Rabbits Treated with Typha Pollen. 1979.

12. Shanghai Second Medical College. Trends on the studies of the blood-stimulant and stasis-eliminative actions of Typha pollen. In: Development in Scientific Research. Vol. 5. 1975.

13. Huang SY et al. Hunan Yiyao Zazhi (Hunan Medical Journal) 1978 (2):54.

14. Song SJ et al. Health Journal of Hubei 1978 (1):46.

15. Sun HQ et al. Shandong Medical Journal 1961 (10):38.

16. Pharmacology Section, Shandong Institute of Traditional Chinese Medicine and Materia Medica. Chinese Pharmaceutical Bulletin 1965 11(12):562.

17. Chinese Materia Medica Processing and Pharmacology Sections, Shandong Institute of Traditional Chinese Medicine and Materia Medica. Research Information on Traditional Chinese Medicine (Shandong Institute of Traditional Chinese Medicine and Materia Medica) 1975 (8):69.

18. Mabu Production Brigade Cooperative Medical Clinic (Mabu Commune, Xiajiang County) and Jiangxi Institute of Medical Sciences. Jiangxi Medical Information 1972 (1):17.

19. Wang WM. Tianjin Medical Journal 1964 6(5):404.

20. Shibata S et al. Journal of the Pharmaceutical Society of Japan (Tokyo) 1960 80:620.

21. Hunan Institute of Traditional Chinese Medicine and Materia Medica. Discussion on the therapeutic principle — stimulation of vital energy and blood circulation. In: Comprehensive Studies on Typha Pollen (I). Hunan Institute of Traditional Chinese Medicine and Materia Medica. 1978. p. 23.

22. Guo J et al. Chinese Journal of Prevention of Tuberculosis 1964 5(3):490.

23. Editorial Group of "Clinical Applications of Chinese Traditional Drugs". New Chinese Medicine 1972 (7):42.

24. Zhu Y. Pharmacology and Applications of Chinese Medicinal Materials. 1st edition. People's Medical Publishing House. 1958. p. 242.

25. Clinical Research Department, Hunan Institute of Traditional Chinese Medicine and Materia Medica et al. Hunan Information on Science and Technology — Medicine and Health 1979 (3):5.

26. Third Section, Clinical Research Department of Hunan Institute of Traditional Chinese Medicine and Materia Medica. Hunan Yiyao Zazhi (Hunan medical Journal) 1977 (6):20.

27. Jiang YB et al. Journal of Traditional Chinese Medicine 1959 (5):48.

28. Coronary Disease Group, First Teaching Hospital of Shanxi Medical College. Cardiovascular Diseases 1973 1(3):4.

29. Coronary Disease Research Unit, Ruijin Teaching Hospital of Shanghai Second Medical College. Clinical observations of Compound Shixiao Powder in angina pectoris. In: Proceedings of the 1973 National Seminar on Coronary Disease in Nanjing. 1973.

30. Shuguang Teaching Hospital, Shanghai College of Traditional Chinese Medicine. Special Issue on Prevention and Treatment of Coronary Disease. Information Unit of Hebei Institute of Medical Sciences. 1972. p. 101.

31. Yu YX. Yiyao Shijie (Medical World) 1949 2(5):23.

32. Zhu HM. Xinyiyaoxue Zazhi (Journal of Traditional Chinese Medicine) 1977 (9):22.

33. Wang HQ. Tianjin Medical Journal 1979 (8):353.

34. Ob-Gyn Department and Pharmacy, Neimenggu Medical College. Report on sixty-two cases of abortion of mid-term pregnancy induced by Typha pollen (abstract) (internal information). 1979.

(Dai Guangjun)

PUGONGYING 蒲公英

<Pugongying> is the plant *Taraxacum mongolicum* Hand.-Mazz. (Compositae). Many *Taraxacum* species are also used as <Pugongying>. <Pugongying> is sweetish with bitter aftertaste and a "cold" property. The herb is latent-heat-clearing, antipyretic, detoxicant, anti-inflammatory, detumescent, anticarbuncle and discutient. It is, therefore, used in the treatment of acute mastitis, deep-rooted ulcer, carbuncle and various infections.

CHEMICAL COMPOSITION

The whole herb contains taraxasterol, taraxacerin, taraxicin and resin. The milky juice contains taraxacerin, taraxicin, inositol and taraxol. The root contains taraxasterol, taraxerol, taraxicin and caffeic acid. The flower contains flavoxanthin.

PHARMACOLOGY

1. Antimicrobial Effect

The decoction or aqueous extract of <Pugongying> markedly inhibited *Staphylococcus aureus*, *Streptococcus hemolyticus* and *Neisseria catarrhalis*, the MIC against *Diplococcus pneumoniae*, *Neisseria meningitidis*, *Corynebacterium diphtheriae*, *Proteus vulgaris*, *Shigella dysenteriae*, and *Pseudomonas aeruginosa* ranged from 1:10 to 1:640. They had a very weak or virtually no inhibitory action against other common pathogenic bacteria and many skin fungsi (1–11). The injection prepared from the ethanol-soluble fraction of its decoction was shown to have essentially the same antibacterial spectrum *in vitro* as the decoction or aqueous extract (12,13). A paper reported that the crystal, obtained by crystallization of the dilute acid extract of the herb in chloroform, at concentration of 1:400 or higher suppressed the growth of *Mycobacterium tuberculosis* var. hominis $H_{37}R_v$ strain (14). Controlled study showed that 30 of 35 strains of *Neisseria meningitidis* were inhibited by the 25% decoction of <Pugongying> and that all 35 strains survived the challenge of the 10% decoction, but the 1% decoction of <Huanglian> inhibited all 35 strains (15). The <Pugongying> decoction did not significantly inhibit 200 strains of *Shigella dysenteriae* (including *S. shigae, S. sonnei,* and *S. flexneri*) except *S. flexneri* type 4 (16). Thus, this herb is not suitable for the treatment of meningitis and for dysentery without testing for sensitivity. Recent studies confirmed that <Pugongying> decoction can synergize with trimethoprim (TMP); the best combination recommended was Herba Taraxaci 2.5 g(crude drug): TMP 10 mg (17). *In vitro* studies showed that the 12.5% crude <Pugongying> inhibited over 10 types of *Leptospira icterogenes*, the decoction was more potent than the ethanol extract (18,19). Another report claimed that the ethanol extract at the concentration of 31 mg/ml killed leptospirae and at 15 mg/ml only had transient inhibitory effect (20). In tissue culture experiments the decoction or aqueous extract of <Pugongying> delayed the pathological changes induced by $ECHO_{11}$ and herpes virus in primary monolayer culture of human embryonic kidney or lung cells, but did not inhibit the influenza virus Jingke 68−1 strain, parainfluenza virus Xiantai strain, adenovirus type 3, and rhinovirus type 17 (21,22).

2. Enhancement of Immunologic Function

In vitro, the <Pugongying> decoction markedly increased the human peripheral lymphoblast transformation rate, indicating that the herb activates the immunological function (23).

3. Cholerectic, and Liver-Protective Effects

Administration of the <Pugongying> injection (5 g crude drug/ml) 3 ml/kg, or the ethanol extract of the herb 0.1 g to the duodenum of anesthetized rats increased the bile secretion by over 40%. The same result was obtained when the same experiment was repeated after cholecystectomy, implying a direct action on the liver. Moreover, it was noted that the <Pugongying> injection had a more pronounced choleretic effect than the decoction of the stem and leaf of *Artemisia capillaris* (24,25). Experiments on dogs with gallbladder fistulae revealed that the major choleretic component of <Pugongying> is the resin, that the volatile oil has weak and inconsistent effect, and that the alkaloids and glycosides were inactive (26). In rats with carbon tetrachloride-damaged liver, the <Pugongying> injection at 1 ml/day IM or the 200% decoction at 1 ml/day PO for 7 days markedly lowered SGPT level and reduced the fatty degeneration of liver cells for 7 days markedly lowered SGPT level and reduced the fatty degeneration of liver cells (25).

4. Miscellaneous Actions

Low concentrations of the <Pugongying> preparation directly stimulated the isolated frog heart, whereas high concentrations inhibited it (13). The <Pugongying> decoction increased the tone and contractility of the isolated rabbit duodenum (27). The herb was shown clinically to have stomachic and laxative activities (28,29). The ethanol extract, however, produced the opposite effect on the isolated rabbit intestine (26). <Pugongying> was also reported to induce diuresis (29,30); however, an author has casted doubt on its putative diuretic effect in man but confirmed such effect in patients with hepatogenic (portal) water retention which might be due to the high potassium content of the herb (13). In addition, <Pugongying> was claimed to be active against human lung cancer (31), but it had no significant effect on transplanted tumors in mice (32).

5. Pharmacokinetics

In experiment where rats were given the <Pugongying> decoction 30 g/kg PO daily for 4 days, the urine collected on each day still has an antibacterial effect, implying excellent absorption of the herb (1).

6. Toxicity

<Pugongying> has a low toxicity. The LD_{50} of the decoction given orally in mice could not be determined. Apart from mild cloudy swelling of hepatocytes and renal tubular epithelial cells and narrowing of renal tubules, no other changes were observed in rabbits given the decoction at 30 g/kg PO for 3 days; no abnormalities in the total WBC count was noted after 7 days' dosing (1). The acute LD_{50} of the <Pugongying> injection in mice was 156.3 ± 9.0 g(crude drug)/kg IP and 58.9 ± 7.9 g(crude drug)/kg IV. The subacute toxicity study in mice and rabbits showed a few cats in the urine and cloudy swelling of renal tubular epithelial cells (12).

CLINICAL STUDIES

1. Upper Respiratory Tract Infections, Tonsillitis, Pharyngolaryngitis

<Pugongying> 30–60 g may be given as decoction; for more rapid effect, it may be decocted together with a little bit of white wine. It may also be used together with the whole plant of *Viola yedoensis*, the leaf of *Perilla frutescens*, ginger, the flower of *Chrysanthemum indicum*, and the leaf and root of *Isatis tinctoria*. The available preparations include Taraxacum mongolicum Tablet and Taraxacum mongolicum Syrup, etc. Taraxacum mongolicum Tablet (1.5 g crude drug per tablet, 4–8 tablets every 6–8 hours) was used to treat 100 cases of upper respiratory tract infections; body temperature was restored in 80 cases in 48 hours. Similar therapeutic effects were achieved in 102 cases of acute tonsillitis and acute pharyngitis as well as in 6 cases of acute bronchitis (33). Twenty-eight out of 35 cases of acute tonsillitis were improved or cured after treatment with Chrysanthemum Decoction (Herba Taraxaci, Flos Chrysanthemi, Radix Isatidis, Radix Ophiopogonis, Radix Platycodi, Radix Glycyrrhizae) (34).

2. Acute Mastitis

<Pugongying> is of utility in early non-suppurative cases.

2.1 Decoction of <Pugongying> 30 g (doubled if the fresh herb is used) 1–2 times daily; or juice of 500 g fresh herb, warmed over low heat and taken with a certain amount wine; the herb may also be taken with the flower of *Chrysanthemum indicum* or with the flower of *Lonicera japonica*, the fruit of *Forsythia suspensa*, the root of *Trichosanthes kirilowii*, the peel of the unripe fruit of *Citrus reticulata*, fried pangolin scales, and the root of *Bupleurum chinense*. Concurrently, the infection site may be applied with the crushed fresh or with its residue plus some alum. Good therapeutic effects were achieved rapidly (35,36).

2.2 <Pugongying> macerated in dry in 1:5 ratio for 5–7 days may be taken orally at 15 ml thrice daily. Forty-two cases of acute mastitis were so treated. It was effective in 36 cases with a disease course less than 4 days and less effective in those with disease course over 5 days (37).

2.3 Decoction of <Pugongying> 36 g and adequate amount of degelatinized deer horn taken with some weak rice wine and concurrently local application of the drug residue daily were the treatment in 20 cases of mastitis; 16 were markedly improved, 2 slightly improved, and 2 unchanged after 3–5 days of treatment (38). <Pugongying> may also be used to promote lactation (33).

3. Acute Local Infections Such as Furuncle, Carbuncle, and Abscess

Good therapeutic effects were achieved with the decoction of the herb alone or with other herbs, or external application of the crushed fresh <Pugongying> (28,29,39).

3.1 The milky juice from the fresh herb may be instilled into the ears to threat otitis media (13).

3.2 The decoction of this herb and the inflorescence of *Chrysanthermum morifolium* or *Chrysanthemum indicum* is given orally and the luke warm second decoction may be used as an eye wash for the treatment of simple conjunctivitis, blepharitis, and hordeolum (28,33,40,41).

3.3 Mild burns or scalds may be treated locally with the juice of the fresh root (42).

3.4 The fresh <Pugongying> by itself or with the whole plant of fresh *Viola yedoensis*, crushed together and mixed with egg white to form paste, may be used to treat parotitis (43,44).

3.5 Submaxillaritis, submaxillary soft tissue inflammation, cellulitis of the neck and back and other acute soft tissue infections, as well as nodules resulting from intramuscular injections may benefit from local application of the paste of the crushed fresh herb or ointment of the powdered rhizomes (13,45).

3.6 A solution of <Pugongying> and the whole plant of *Commelina communis* or the powder of the herb and placenta is useful for cervical erosion (46,47).

4. Cholecystitis and Acute Icteric Hepatitis

The <Pugongying> extract was clinically used in other countries to increase the bile flow and alleviate pain in chronic gallbladder spasm and cholelithiasis. Chinese reports claimed that <Pugongying> used with the spores of *Lygodium japonicum*, whole plant of *Glechoma longituba*, the rhizome of

Curcuma longa, the fruit of *Media toosendan*, and whole plant of *Bidens bipinnata* in concert with acupuncture or small doses of antispasmodics was effective in the treatment of acute cholecystitis, and that the herb plus the fruit spike of *Prunella vulgaris*, whole plant of *Plantago asiatica*, and young shoots of *Artemisia capillaris* were effective for chronic cholecystitis (13,29). It was reported that the recovery of hepatic function and icterus index was markedly accelerated in 86 cases of acute icteric hepatitis and 24 cases of non-icteric hepatitis treated by the <Pugongying> decoction or injection (25,48). The compound Taraxacum mongolicum Syrup and Artemisia-Taraxacum Injection were reported to be effective in the management of acute infection hepatitis (49,50).

5. Gastritis, Appendicitis and Peptic Ulcers

Chronic gastritis was reportedly cured with <Pugongying> 15 g decocted twice with one tablespoonful of rice wine; the pooled decoction was given by mouth in 3 doses postprandially (29,30). For acute appendicitis, <Pugongying> is often prescribed with the whole plant of *Portulaca oleracea*; other commonly used prescriptions are Patrinia-Taraxacum Decoction and "Lanwei Qinghua Decoction" (Appendicitis Resolvent Decoction) (Herba Taraxaci, Flos Lonicerae, Radix et Rhizoma Rhei, Cortex Moutan Radicis, Radix Paeoniae Rubra, Fructus Meliae Toosendan, Semen Persicae, Radix Glycyrrhizae). However, the effect of these drugs on chronic or recurrent appendicitis is reported to be unsatisfactory (30,31,51). Also, Taraxacum mongolicum root powder at a dose of 1.5 g thrice daily after meals has been used to treat gastric and duodenal ulcers (13).

6. Miscellaneous

<Pugongying> is useful in osteomyelitis (33). Its milkly juice was tried in congenital angioma (13). The herb is often combined with the flower of *Lonicera japonica*, the root back of *Lycium chinense*, the root back of *Paeonia suffruticosa*, and the rhizome of *Anemarrhena asphodeloides* to treat pyelonephritis (33,52). Moreover, <Pugongying> combined with the root or whole herb of *Cirsium japonicum*, the whole plant of *Portulaca oleracea*, the feces of *Trogopterus xanthipes*, and the root of *Phytolacca acinosa* was reported effective for snake bites (pit viper) (30).

Clinical trial of Taraxacum mongolicum Injection in over 700 cases of diseases in internal medicine, surgery, infections, EENT, obstetrics and gynecology and pediatrics showed its effectiveness for ailments caused by gram-positive bacteria, drug-resistant *Staphylococcus aureus*, and *Streptococcus hemolyticus*. The injection was inhibitory to *Salmonella typhi*, but not to *Pseudomonas aeruginosa*. It can therefore be used clinically to reduce the dose of antibiotics (53).

ADVERSE EFFECTS

<Pugongying> at therapeutic doses has few side effects. The decoction only occasionally caused gastrointestinal symptoms such as nausea, vomiting, abdominal discomfort and mild diarrhea. Some

patients experienced heartburn after taking the tablet (33). The wine prepared with the herb may cause dizziness, nausea and hidrosis due to the alcohol content, and in some patients urticaria, and in individual cases urticaria complicated with conjunctivitis which disappear promptly after discontinuation of the drug (37). The Taraxacum mongolicum Injection administered intramuscularly may cause local pain (12,53), and by intravenous infusion, it may cause chilliness, pallor, cyanosis or mental symptoms in individual patients (13,53).

REFERENCE

1. Wang J. Selected Medical Information (Boyang County People' s Hospital, Jiangxi) 1973 (3):1.

2. Lingling District (Hunan) Sanitation and Anti-epidemic Station. Hunan Yiyao Zazhi (Hunan Medical Journal) 1974 (5):49.

3. Microbiology Department. Journal of Nanjing College of Pharmacy 1960 (5):10.

4. Traditional Chinese Medicine and Materia Medica Research Unit of the Internal Medicine Department, First Teaching Hospital of Chongqing Medical College. Acta Microbiologica Sinica 1960 (1):52.

5. Microbiology Section. Acta Academiae Medicinae Shandong 1959 (8):42.

6. Antibacterial Section, Institute of Materia Medica of the Chinese Academy of Medical Sciences. Chinese Pharmaceutical Bulletin 1960 (2):59.

7. Pathological Biology Section. Selected information (Zhangjiakou District Medical School) 1972 (1):21.

8. Section 4, Class 62. These of Anhui Medical College 1960 (2):20.

9. Senile Chronic Bronchitis Scientific Research Group, Suzhou Medical College. Scientific Research Information (Medical Education Section of Suzhou Medical College) 1971 (5):50.

10. Cao RL. Chinese Journal of Dermatology 1957 (4):286.

11. Guiyang Hospital of Tuberculosis. Chinese Journal of Prevention of Tuberculosis 1959 (6):37.

12. Shanghai No. 10 Pharmaceutical Factory et al. Information on the Identification of Taraxacum mongolicum. 1971.

13. Jiangsu College of New Medicine. Encyclopedia of Chinese Materia Medica. Shanghai People' s Publishing House. 1977. p. 2459.

14. Jinzhou Hospital of Tuberculosis. Liaoning Medical Journal 1960 (7):26.

15. Yangxin County (Hubei) Sanitation and Anti-epidemic Division and Centre of Schistosomiasis Control. Studies on Epidemic Prevention 1976 (4):319.

16. Jinzhong District (Shanxi) Sanitation and Anti-epidemic Station. Studies on Epidemic Prevention, 1976 (2):133.

17. Sun SQ. Chinese Traditional and Herbal Drugs Communications 1979 (6):11.

18. Microbiology Section, Luda Health School. Medicine and Health (Luda Health Bureau) 1973 (2):63.

19. Leptospirosis Research Group. Selected Information (First and Second Teaching Hospitals of Jiangsu College of New Medicine) 1974 (2):78.

20. Xuzhou Medical College. Information on New Chinese Medicine (Xuzhou Medical College) 1971 (1):27.

21. Virus Section, Institute of Materia Medica of the Academy of Traditional Chinese Medicine. Xinyiyaoxue Zazhi (Journal of Traditional Chinese Medicine) 1973 (1):26.

22. Guangzhou Institute of Medicine and Health. New Medical Communications (Guangzhou Health Bureau) 1974 (1):14.

23. Medical Laboratory, Second Teaching Hospital. Medical Research (Shenyang Medical College) 1975 (4):41.

24. Bohm K. Arzneimettel Forschung 1959 9(6):376.

25. Shi HG. Journal of Traditional Chinese Medicine 1979 (12):55.

26. Sanochikov AV et al. (Zhang GZ, abstract translator). Medical Abstracts (III) 1964 7(3):4.

27. Acute Abdomen Research Unit, Zunyi Medical College. Xinyiyaoxue Zazhi (Journal of Traditional Chinese Medicine) 1975 (10):36.

28. Editorial Group of "Clinical Applications of Chinese Traditional Drugs". New Chinese Medicine 1972 (2):40.

29. Yuan F. Acta Academiae Medicinae Anhui 1976 (1):75.

30. Guangdong College of Traditional Chinese Medicine. Studies on Chinese Traditional Prescriptions. Guangdong College of Traditional Chinese Medicine. 1973. p. 167.

31. Editorial Group. National Collection of Chinese Materia Medica. Vol. 1. People's Medical Publishing House. 1975. p. 872.

32. Tumor Section, Institute of Chinese Materia Medica of the Academy of Traditional Chinese Medicine. Selected Information on Science and Technology (Information Department of the Academy of Traditional Chinese Medicine). 1972. p. 136.

33. Editorial Group. South Zhejiang Herbal. New edition. Wenzhou Health Bureau, Zhejiang. 1975. p. 396.

34. Second Teaching Hospital, Hunan Medical College. 1970 Information on New Chinese Medicine and Acupuncture (Hunan Medical College) 1971 (2):67.

35. Xu XC. Journal of Traditional Chinese Medicine 1965 (6):39.

36. Bai RD. Journal of Barefoot Doctor 1974 (3):41.

37. Wang CY. Liaoning Medical Journal 1960 (7):21.

38. Jingyuan Commune (Yongjia County) Health Centre. Zhejiang Journal of Traditional Chinese Medicine 1964 (11):17.

39. Tu XX. Journal of Traditional Chinese Medicine 1965 (11):29.

40. Qi XM et al. Acta Academiae Medicinae Anhui 1974 (4):26.

41. Jiang QX. Journal of Traditional Chinese Medicine 1966 (6):30.

42. Huang ZQ. Journal of Traditional Chinese Medicine 1965 (10):17.

43. Liang ZS. Yantai Medical Communications 1974 (1):88.

44. Health Division of Northern Military Subregion (Qinghai). New Chinese Medicine 1972 (10):49.

45. Nursing Group of the Cardiovascular Ward, Internal Medicine Department of the First Teaching Hospital of the Second Military Medical College. Academic Information (Second Military Medical College) 1978 (1):70.

46. Editorial Committee. China's Pharmacopoeia. Part 1. 1977 edition. People's Medical Publishing House. 1978. p. 791.

47. Jiaxing Hospital of Obstetrics and Gynecology. Notes on Science and Technology — Medicine and Health (Information Institute of Zhejiang Bureau of Science and Technology) 1972 (4):22.

48. Infectious Diseases Ward, Xinan 416 Hospital et al. Preliminary report of twenty-four cases of acute infectious hepatitis treated with Taraxacum mongolicum (internal information). 1972.

49. Linyi District Sanitation and Anti-epidemic Station et al. Yimeng Yiyao (Yimeng Medical Journal) (Linyi District Health Bureau, Shandong) 1973 (2):27.

50. Jingmen County People's Hospital. Health Journal of Jingmen 1975 (4):24.

51. Qin F. Communications on Combined Western and Traditional Chinese Therapy of Acute Abdomen (Nankai Medical College, Tianjin) 1976 4(1):26.

52. Chen JM. Barefoot Doctor (Changwei District Health Bureau, Shandong) 1972 (8):6.

53. Shanghai No. 10 Pharmaceutical Factory et al. Pharmaceutical Industry 1971 (6):27.

(Dai Guangjun)

LEIWAN 雷丸

<Leiwan> is the dried sclerotium of *Mylitta lapidescens* Hor. (*Omphalia lapialia* Schroet) (Polyporaceae). It is bitter, "cold", and slightly toxic. <Leiwan> is anthelmintic and is used for tapeworm infection.

CHEMICAL COMPOSITION

The major constituent is a hydrolytic protease, called mylittine. It is effective for cestodiasis and the activity can be destroyed by heating. The content of the enzyme is about 3%.

PHARMACOLOGY

1. Teniacidal Effect

<Leiwan> is an effective agent against tapeworms. It was evaluated *in vitro*. Proglottides of tapeworms were placed into the 5–30% <Leiwan> extract, normal saline, and distilled water at 37°C, respectively. Proglottides in the <Leiwan> extract died in from 2 hours and 40 minutes to 9 hours, while after 9 hours, those in normal saline were still alive and appeared normal, they usually survive for additional 40–62 hours; those in distilled water lived for 24–30 hours (1). <Leiwan> exhibited an anthelmintic action in man infected with unarmed (Taenia saginata) or armed (Taenia solium) tapeworms, or dog tapeworm (Echinococcus granulosus). Most of the expelled worms were already deactivated and the expelled proglottides particularly the small ones were destroyed. Histological examination revealed severe destruction of the nucleus of dermal and deep-layer cells, which was not observed in worms expelled by medication with the rhizome of *Dryopteris crassirhizoma* or the seed of *Areca catechu* (2). Therefore, unlike the mode of action of these two agents, the action of <Leiwan> is not to paralyze the worms but to destroy them. The proteolytic activity of mylittine is maximal in alkaline medium (pH 8) but was inactive in acidic medium. Thus, mylittine digests proglottides in the intestinal tract and eventually achieves an anthelmintic effect (3). Since mylittine is heat labile (generally at >60°C), the herb cannot be decocted; it is usually taken in powder form (4).

2. Ascaricidal Effect

In vitro, the aqueous extract of <Leiwan> was inactive against ascaris, but its ethanol extract significantly inhibited the parasite. As mylittine is insoluble in ethanol, the herb might contain ascaricidal components other than mylittine (4).

3. Antitrichomonal Effect

In a culture medium containing a 5% decoction of <Leiwan>, granulation appeared after 5 minutes in most *Trichomonas vaginalis*, though a few remained active (5).

4. Antineoplastic Effect

Either intramuscular or intraperitoneal injection of mylittine inhibited mouse sarcoma 180 by 33.3–69.3% (6).

CLINICAL STUDIES

1. Teniasis

The <Leiwan> powder 18–20 g made into paste with water and small amounts of sugar may be taken by mouth thrice daily for 3 days. Mylittine 0.3 g thrice daily for 3 days, followed by sodium sulfate 15–20 g on the 4th day (optional as <Leiwan> itself contains large amounts of magnesium ion which has a laxative effect) may be given alternatively. In clinical studies of 54 cases (2,7,8), these medications showed strong anthelmintic activity against *T. solium*, and relatively good effect against *T. saginata*, dwarf tapeworm (*Hymenolepis nana*), and rat tapeworm (*Hymenolepis diminuta*). The anthelmintic effect was further confirmed by the fact the no regenerated proglottides were found in the stool during a period of 76–150 days (2). These drugs are low in toxicity and so hospitalization is not required (2,7,8).

2. Oxyuriasis

Powder of <Leiwan> 2 g, the rhizome of *Rheum palmatum* 3 g, and the seed of *Pharbitis nil* 9 g was given with water to 188 cases early in the morning on an empty stomach. Except 2 cases, all of them benefitted (9).

3. Ancylostomiasis and Filariasis

The <Leiwan> powder in glucose solution may be used to treat ancylostomiasis. The adult dose is 40–60 g in one or three doses. Inconsistent therapeutic effects were reported by different authors. One report claimed that in 20 cases, a high percentage was found negative for the ova after treatment (10). Another paper reported a lower percentage in 27 cases so treated (11). It was also reported that 19 cases given the herb powder twice did not expel worms (12). One case of filariasis with microfilariae in blood achieved negative result in 3 consecutive blood examinations following oral administration of the decoction of <Leiwan> 30 g for 7 days (13).

4. *Intestinal Trichomoniasis*

<Leiwan> decocted under low heat until boiled may be given to adults at 12 g daily for a course of 3 days. Another course may be given if the first was ineffective. In 94 cases so treated, 85 were cured after one course, and the remaining 9 cases were given a second course 4 days after the first. Six more cases were cured. The aggregate cure rate was 95.7% (14).

ADVERSE EFFECTS

With very few side effects, <Leiwan> is a safe and effective agent for teniasis (7). There may be occasional transient nausea and upper abdominal discomfort (10).

REFERENCE

1. Jing HD. Chinese Journal of New Medicine 1951 2(10):753.

2. Liang Z et al. Manzhou Yixue Zazhi (Manzhou Medical Journal) 1937 26(3):799.

3. Liang Z et al. Manzhou Yixue Zazhi (Manzhou Medical Journal) 1938 28:1181.

4. Wu YR et al. The National Medical Journal of China 1948 34(10):347.

5. Pharmacology Section, Henan Medical College. Acta Academiae Medicinae Henan 1960 (7):23.

6. Yao YH et al. Acta Academiae Medicinae Ningxia 1979 (1):50.

7. Liu GS et al. Journal of Traditional Chinese Medicine 1955 (3):28.

8. Xu ZW. Chinese Medical Journal 1956 41 (6):556.

9. Hebei Sanitation and Anti-epidemic Station. Zhongji Yikan (Intermediate Medical Journal) 1960 (7):35.

10. Li RZ et al. Shanghai Zhongyiyao Zazhi (Shanghai Journal of Traditional Chinese Medicine) 1957 (5):22.

11. Hexi (Yongxiu County) Pilot Area for Pest and Disease Eradication. Jiangxi Zhongyiyao (Jiangxi Journal of Traditional Chinese Medicine) 1960 (5):14.

12. Liang RZ. Guangdong Zhongyi (Guangdong Journal of Traditional Chinese Medicine) 1959 (1):27.

13. Shanghai Seventh Hospital. Shanghai Zhongyiyao Zazhi (Shanghai Journal of Traditional Chinese Medicine) 1959 (1):41.

14. Internal Medicine Department, Jiangkou Hospital (Putian County, Fujian). Zhonghua Yixue Zazhi (National Medical Journal of China) 1977 57(7):435.

(Chen Quansheng)

LEIGONGTENG 雷公藤

<Leigongteng>, also called <Caichongyao> or <Huangteng>, etc., is derived from the root of *Tripterygium wilfordii* Hook. f. (Celastraceae). Pungent and of "cool" property, the drug is antirheumatic, detumescent, analgesic, and channel-deobstruent. It is used as an anthelmintic, pesticide for maggots, and rodenticide. Externally, it is employed as an anti-inflammatory and detoxicant agent in the treatment of snake bites and rheumatic arthritis. Recently, the herb was found to contain antineoplastic constituents.

CHEMICAL COMPOSITION

<Leigongteng> contains: (1) *Tripterygium* alkaloids wilfordine, wilforgine, wilfortrine, wilforzine and wilforine. Hydrolysis of these alkaloids yields wilfordic acid and hydroxywilfordic acid. (2) Macrocyclic alkaloids celacemine, celabenzine and celafurine. (3) Epoxyditerpenes triptolide, tripdiolide, triptonide, triptonolide and hypolide. Reduction of triptonide forms triptolide. Hypolide is probably one of the precursors of other epoxyditerpenoids. (4) Tripterin (celastrol) and dulcitol (1–10).

PHARMACOLOGY

1. Anti-inflammatory Effect and Effect on Body Immunity

The terpenes or insoluble substance isolated from the decoction of the whole root prevented paw swelling induced by egg white in rats. The insoluble substance markedly inhibited formaldehyde-induced paw swelling, and the terpenes inhibited cotton ball-induced granuloma of rats; the soluble substance was inactive. Significant preventive and curative effects were achieved with the terpenes used to treat adjuvant-induced multiple arthritis in rats, whereas only a significant preventive effect was exhibited by the insoluble substance. The decoction of the whole root, terpenes, and insoluble substance did not markedly affect the thymus of young mice, but large doses of the total alkaloids caused thymic atrophy in these animals (11). Experiments on ^{3}H-thymidine incorporation and lymphocyte transformation revealed that tripdiolide markedly inhibited the T-lymphocyte transformation as well as rosette formation. At a concentration of 100 μg/0.2 ml whole blood, it virtually suppressed all T-cell transformation, and the inhibition rate was around 90% at 10 μg/0.2 ml whole blood. This activity appeared not due to cytotoxicity (12). *In vivo* studies showed that 0.25 mg/kg of triptolide had insignificant inhibitory effect on the graft-versus-host reaction; it did not affect the concomitant tumor immunity (13,14). Moreover, the whole root decoction or terpenes greatly enhanced the phagocytic activity of mouse peritoneal macrophages on chicken erythrocytes. The decoction of the whole root, terpenes, and total alkaloids were shown to antagonize trichosanthin-induced allergic reaction in mice (11).

2. Antineoplastic Effect

A strong antineoplastic activity was exhibited by the ethanol extract of <Leigongteng>, triptilide or tripdiolide 50–400 µg/kg against mouse leukemia L_{1210} (16); the ED against mouse L_{1210} and P_{388} was determined to be 0.1 mg/kg (5,9). At doses of 0.25 and 0.2 mg/kg, triptolide was very effective against leukemia L_{615}, prolonging the survival period of the animals by over 159.8 and 87.8%, respectively, and allowing some animals to live for an indefinite period of time. Challenge of the long surviving animals once monthly with L_{615} splenocytes for 3 months did not cause cancer nor shorten their survival (9,14). Triptolide inhibited mouse sarcoma 37, hepatoma and solid rat Walker carcinoma 256 by 38, 46.7, and 50%, respectively. However, the effect was unstable. Triptonide is a cytotoxin; its ED_{50} against human nasopharyngeal cancer KB cells was determined to be 0.1–1 ng/ml *in vitro* (5). The antineoplastic activity of the epoxyditerpenes contained in this herb could be due to strong nucleophilic attack through opening of the 9,11-epoxy ring by 14β-hydroxy group, allowing one or more electrophilic groups of the molecule to alkylate nearby nucleophilic groups in the biomacromolecules (17). Macrocyclic alkaloids in this herb such as celacemine also had antileukemic activity (6).

3. Insecticidal Effect

The aqueous and ethanol extracts of the root, stem or leaf can kill *Illiberis pruni* and pear leaf-roller (18). <Leigongteng> seems to be a gastrotoxin and a contact toxin. Its ether extract was found to be lethal to silkworms (19). The insecticidal activity probably emanates from the ester groups of <Leigongteng> alkaloids; for instance, wilforgine which has an ester group more than wilforzine is much more toxic to the larvae of diamond-back moth than the latter (20).

4. Miscellaneous Actions

In vitro studies indicated that the <Leigongteng> decoction is inhibitory against *Staphylococcus aureus* (9). The decoction of the root or terpenes increased the contraction amplitude and tension of the isolated rabbit intestine; this effect could not be completely antagonized by atropine (11). Triptolide had no significant effect on the frog and rabbit hearts *in situ* nor any effect on the activity of the rabbit small intestine *in situ* (22). Hemadromography of the extremities and brain indicated that <Leigongteng> could dilate peripheral arterioles, increase the blood flow, and thus caused brief hypotension (23).

5. Toxicity

<Leigongteng> is a well-known toxic plant; the whole plant is toxic. The toxicity is correlated to the contents of alkaloids and the cytotoxic epoxyditerpenes. The root bark is more toxic than the root core, and the fresh root bark is more toxic than that stored for one year (20,24–27). The acute LD_{50} of the root decoction in mice was determined to be 18.40–26.55 g/kg PO and 4.81 g/kg IP; the LD_{50} of the root bark and root core were 3.92 and 7.25 g/kg IP, respectively. The MLD of the decoction in rats was 10 g/kg SC, (28) and that of the ethanol extract of the insoluble substance was 32.26 g/kg PO. The insoluble substance caused no death of rats even at doses as high as 100 g/kg SC, the rat appeared to be in excellent condition (11). The MLD of the terpenes was 62.30 mg/kg SC or 169 mg/kg Po, and that of the total alkaloids, 277 mg/kg IP. The acute LD_{50} of triptolide in mice was 1.407 (1.191–1.66)mg/kg IP.

Injection of triptolide 0.2 and 0.4 mg/kg IP to rats once daily for 10 days did not significantly change the hemoglobin, platelet, GPT, and blood urea nitrogen. Five days after administration with large doses of triptolide, the leukocyte count was slightly lowered but it was promptly reversed upon discontinuing the drug (14). The toxic reactions vary among various animal species; on poisoning was known in goldfish, rabbits, cats, and sheep, but strong toxic effects were observed in insects, dogs, pigs, and man (29).

During the experiment, mice showed increase in hair loss and eye secretion. In an acute toxicity study, the whole root preparation caused sudden dose-dependent drop in body temperature in dogs (11). Oral administration of the decoction to dogs caused strong gastric irritation leading to gastric mucosal congestion, edema, hemorrhage, necrosis, and detachment, as well as neutrophilic infiltration into the submucosal and muscular layers. The absorbed herb decoction damaged the CNS, resulting in serious dystrophy of the optic thalamus, midbrain medulla oblongata, cerebellum, and spinal cord; it also impaired the myocardium, liver and kidneys, resulting in hemorrhage and necrosis of these organs. The herb inhibited the isolated frog heart after cardiac stimulation. Intravenous injection of larger doses of the root bark decoction in dogs caused bradycardia, prolongation of the P-R interval on the ECG, and hypotension. Intoxication in dogs was first manifested as vomiting, diarrhea, and bloody stool; death occurred with respiratory arrest preceded by cardiac arrest (26–29).

In culture of human embryonic renal cells, the crude alkaloid solution of <Leigongteng> caused cellular shrinkage and desquamation, and vacuolization of remnant cells and marked increase in cytoplasmic granules (27,30). Autopsy of patients poisoned by <Leigongteng> revealed extensive gastrointestinal hemorrhage, myocardial hemorrhage, congestion in the liver and lungs, and renal tubular necrosis. Death due to high doses may be caused by myocardial damage which precipitated acute cardiogenic cerebral ischemia, or due to myocarditis resulting in severe pulmonary edema; slow death associated with lower doses may have resulted from renal failure (28,29, 31–34).

CLINICAL STUDIES

1. Rheumatoid Arthritis

Numerous reports are available regarding the treatment of rheumatoid arthritis with <Leigongteng> (35–42). The effective rates were about 90%. All patients obtained different extents of improvement in arthralgia, swelling, and joint function and decrease of erythrocyte sedimentation rate, whereas some patients had negative latex agglutination test for rheumatoid factors. It was more effective during the active than nonactive stage of the ailment. Advanced cases with joint deformation, rigidity, and muscular atrophy should be treated with this herb combined with other herbal medicines or electroacupuncture to increase the therapeutic effect. The drug should be given intermittently for a long period; the course should be adjusted according to the severity of illness, individual variation, and therapeutic response. In general, treatment starts with low doses, and if ineffective in half a month the dosage may be increased. If after one month it is still ineffective, the medication should be withdrawn and the treatment deemed unsuccessful. Maximal effect is usually obtained after 3 months of medication; thereafter, a maintenance dose (one-third to one-half the initial dose) is given for at least one year. Relapse cases are still reponsive to this drug.

1.1 *Dosage and administration*

1.1.1 Decoction: The root core after removal of two cortical layers 15–25 g, decocted twice over low heat into 400 ml of pooled decoction to be taken postprandially in two doses daily for a course of 7 days with the next course to be started after an interval of 3–4 days.

1.1.2 Fluidextract: The dry fluidextract of <Leigongteng> or the ethanol extract of this dry extract as a 25% solution, 20–40 ml thrice daily orally.

1.1.3 Tablet: Made of the fluidextract of this herb and excipients, each contains 1.5 g of the crude drug, to be given orally at 3–4 tablets thrice daily.

1.1.4 Mixture: The root of *T. wilfordii* 250 g, root tuber and rhizome of *Aconitum carmichaeli* each 60 g, root of *Angelica sinensis*, flower of *Carthamus tinctorius*, bark of *Cinnamomum cassia*, root of *Achyranthes bidentata*, root and rhizom of *Notopterygium forbesii*, bark of *Eucommia ulmoides*, and root bark of *Lycium chinense*, each 18 g, decocted to 1000 ml, filtered, added with half-catty of brown sugar, cooled and finally added with 2 catties of wine. The preparation is to be give orally 30–50 ml thrice daily for adults; dosage to be adequately reduced in elderly patients and children.

1.1.5 Tincture: The root of *T. wilfordii* 60 g macerated in 1 catty of white wine for 7–10 days. Adult dose: 10–15 ml thrice daily.

Oral administration of the 1.3% total lactones in 40% ethanol solution relieved rheumatoid arthritis. The lactones were believed to be the active components. The total alkaloids was ineffective (38). Dulcitol was also reported to be effective for rheumatoid arthritis (15).

2. Lepra Reaction

Satisfactory therapeutic effects on lepra reaction were achieved with the use of <Leigongteng> (43–47). Leprosy cases with neuralgia and nodular lesions (2569 person-times) were treated with <Leigongteng> 6–15 g or its compound formula (Radix Tripterygium 6 g, Flos Lonicerae 15 g, Cortex Phellodendri 12 g, Radix Scrophulariae 9 g, Radix Angelicae Sinensis 15 g); the herbs were decocted twice and the pooled decoction was given in 2 doses daily. Satisfactory therapeutic effects were achieved which included long-term improvement of clinical signs, especially of neuralgia. The corresponding doses for mild, moderate, and severe lepra reaction were 10–20 g, 21–40 g, and 41–60 g.

Type II lepra reaction (284 case-times) was treated with the following extracts: "741" 1% syrup, 30 mg (25 g crude drug) in 2 doses daily by mouth; "420", 40 ml (80 g crude drug) in 2 doses daily by mouth; "104", 40–60 ml (80–120 g crude drug) in 2–3 doses by mouth; "124", 40–60 mg (160–240 g crude drug) in 2–3 doses by mouth. Symptomatic relief was obtained in 257 case-times, and improvement in 24 case-times. For control, thalidomide 100–250, 275–400, and 400 mg were respectively given in 2–3 doses by mouth to 113 case-times of mild, moderate and severe lepra reaction; 97 cases were relieved of symptoms and 12 were improved. There was no significant difference between the two drugs under study with respect to the onset and duration of action.

Type I lepra reaction (34 case-times) was managed with the <Leigongteng> decoction; 32 case-times reportedly benefitted. The average onset of action for skin lesions was 4.5 days, neuralgia 6.3 days, edema 3 days, and fever 4 days. Thalidomide, on the other hand, was ineffective in type I lepra reaction. The total alkaloids of this herb not only had a lower effective rate in 50 case-times of type II lepra reaction, but also caused the deterioration of some cases. Therefore, the alkaloids are believed not the active principles of the herb for lepra reaction (43).

3. Skin Diseases

Satisfactory therapeutic effects were obtained in systemic lupus erythematosus after 1–4 courses (each lasted one month) of the syrup of <Leigongteng> 1 g (crude drug)/ml at 10 ml thrice daily. In improved patients, symptoms subsided or disappeared, and abnormal immune tests and hepatic function were improved. Drug effects usually appeared after 1–3 weeks' treatment; steroids were either discontinued or its dosage reduced (48). The <Leigongteng> tablet given orally also produced satisfactory results (49). For example, treatment of 182 cases of psoriasis with the tablet resulted in cure basically in 44 cases, marked improvement in 28 cases, and some improvement in 42 cases (50,51). Tripterygium II capsule/tablet (total alkaloids) at daily doses of 40–60 mg (ideally 1 mg/kg/day) for adults by mouth after meals was effective in all 101 confirmed cases, including Sweef syndrome, extensive eczema, erythroderma, intractable pruritic rashes, palmar and plantar pustulosis, allergic angiitis, solar dermatitis multiforme, Behcet's syndrome, psoriatic arthritis, and lupus erythematosis. These indicate that Triptergium II was not only effective in ailments responsive to corticosteroids, but also has the following advantages: (1) quicker and stronger anti-inflammatory action than the corticosteroids, (2) effective in those cases poorly responsive or unresponsive to steroids, (3) effective substitute for steroids in long-term treatment of psoriatic arthritis, where the latter agents are proved to produce side effects, and when discontinued or reduced may cause rebound. Being a potent and quick-acting anti-inflammatory agent which tends to produce quick withdrawal relapse, Trypterygium II Capsule/Tablet is thought to act on the last stage of disease process and in case of allergic diseases the effective period (52). Satisfactory results were also obtained using this herb and transfer factor in the treatment of pustular psoriasis (53).

4. Neuralgia

Satisfactory analgesia was obtained in 91 cases of rheumatic arthritis, sciatica, hypertrophic arthritis, myofibrositis, radiculitis, traumatic pain, trigeminal neuralgia, periarthritis, and shoulder-neck syndrome with the decoction of the dried root 500 g added to 2 catties of while wine to make 2000 ml, given at 2.5–10 ml 3–4 times a day by mouth (23).

5. Nephrotic Syndrome in Children

Tablets of the active principle extracted from <Leigongteng>, 10 mg/tablet, was used at 1 mg (0.8–1.4 mg)/kg/day PO in two to three doses for a course of 6 weeks to treat 7 children with nephrotic syndrome; two of them were responsive to corticosteroids, 3 resistant, and 2 dependent. Albuminuria was either reduced or disappeared and edema subsided after treatment. Relapse albuminuria was successfully controlled by resuming medication (54). Albuminuria in patients with chronic nephritis was also reduced by <Leigongteng> (15).

6. Miscellaneous

Most patients with pulmonary tuberculosis or other chronic chest diseases treated with the <Leigongteng> decoction experienced different extents of amelioration of cough, expectoration, fever, and asthma (55). Salutary effects were likewise obtained in cases of thromboangiitis obliterans and cerebral thrombosis. The herb was also effective in menorrhagia, chronic disease of the breast (fibroadenoma), myoma of the uterus, impotence, tinea capitis, tinea manuum and tinea pedis (23).

7. Insecticide

Powder of sun-dried root bark, or the fresh leaf can be used to treat manure pits and sewage to kill maggots and wrigglers. *Method of preparation*: The powdered root bark 1 catty is cooked together with 5 catties of water for 30 minutes, then into which grass and wood ashes and clay, half catty each, are added. This mixture can be applied in oncomelania-infested areas to eradicate the snail. The effect of the mixture could be much improved by adding an equal amount of tobacco powder. The powdered root bark. 1 catty cooked with 5 catties of water for 30 minutes and the decoction mixed into baits can be used as a poison to rats. Sprays prepared by cooking the root powder 1 catty and water 30 catties for 10 minutes, or soaking it in cold water for 24 hours, was at least 80% effective against larvae of *Pieris rapae*, beetles, *Lema oryzae, Diclodispa armigera*, and pine moth (54).

ADVERSE EFFECTS

<Leigongteng> taken by mouth may produce gastrointestinal symptoms such as nausea, upper abdominal discomfort, mild pain, poor appetite, vomiting and occasionally borborygmus and diarrhea. Other reactions included dizziness, xerostomia, palpitation, lacrimation, erosion and bleeding of lips and buccal mucosa, sore throat, skin pruritus, skin rashes, desquamation of cheeks, pigmentation, menstrual disturbance or amenorrhea, leukopenia, etc. Cases of atrioventricular block and allergic reaction to the injection have also been reported. Similar side effects were produced by the <Leigongteng> extract. Reactions are more with large doses, and in elderly or weak patients. Generally, they are reversed 5–7 days after discontinuation of medication. In order to minimize the ill effects, two cortical layers should be removed completely and only the xylum should be used. The herb should be decocted for at least 3 hours. Gastrointestinal upset can be reduced if the drug is taken after meals or combined with Gastropin (antacid tablet) or vitamin B_6. Periodical examination of the blood picture is mandatory during the treatment, and whenever necessary the drug ought to be discontinued followed by administration of vitamins B_4 and C. Precaution should be exercised in patients with disease of the heart, liver, stomach, kidneys, or spleen and in young women; it is contraindicated for pregnant women (23,24,31,39,43,50,52,54,56).

Acute poisoning and emergency measures. <Leigongteng> is highly toxic. Poisoning following oral ingestion of 2–3 pieces of leaf has been reported (57); 7 tender buds (around 12 g) (58), or 30–60 g of the root bark (59,60) is fatal. Poisoning may even result from consuming honey derived from the flowers (30,31,61). Toxic symptoms usually appear 2 hours after ingestion, but may appear earlier and more severe if alcoholic drinks were also taken concurrently. Acute symptoms included severe vomiting, abdominal pain, diarrhea, bloody stool, chest discomfort, shortness of breath, weak heart beat, weak and thready pulse, hypotension, cyanosis, hypothermia, shock, and respiratory failure. Two to three days later, alopecia, edema, uremia, and acute renal failure appeared. The patients generally died in about 24 hours and not later than 4 days after poisoning. Prognosis will be more favorable if they can survive over 5 days. In case of acute poisoning, the conventional emergency measures of symptomatic treatment are applicable. In addition, the patient should be on low salt diet. Oral administration of 200–300 ml of fresh sheep blood is the common folk treatment. Some authors claimed that rabbit stomach is useful for detoxication, however, these claims have yet to be confirmed by further studies (24,26–33,60,61).

REFERENCE

1. Fred A. J Amer Chem 1950 72(4):1608.

2. Beroza M. J Amer Chem 1951 73(8):3656.

3. Beroza M. J Amer Chem 1952 74(6):1585.

4. Beroza M. J Amer Chem 1953 75(5):2136.

5. Kupchan SM. J Amer Chem 1972 94(20):7194.

6. Kupchan SM. J of Chem Commun 1974 (9):329.

7. Kupchan SM. Chemical Abstracts 1977 86:136583a.

8. Phytochemistry Department, Yunnan Institute of Botany et al. Kexue Tongbao (Science Bulletin) 1977 (10):458.

9. Wu DG. Acta Botanica Yunnanica 1979 1(2):29.

10. Deng FX et al. Fujian Medical Journal 1980 (2):27.

11. Tripterygium wilfordii Coordinating Research Group of Hubei, Institute of Combined Western and Traditional Chinese Medicine et al. Health Journal of Hubei 1979 (1):72.

12. Clinical Immunology Unit of the Clinical Trials Department, General Hospital of Nanjing Military Region. Jiangsu Yiyao (Jiangsu Medical Journal) 1979 (10):3.

13. Wu DG et al. Selected Information (Kunming Medical College) 1978 (3):33.

14. Zhang TM et al. Chinese Pharmaceutical Bulletin 1980 15(5):46.

15. Shen JS. Proceedings of the Regional Symposium on Pharmacy (Botany). Chinese Pharmaceutical Association (Shanghai Branch). 1978. p. 54.

16. Kupchan SM. Chemical Abstracts 1976 85:83219g.

17. Cordell GA et al. The Journal of Natural Products 1977 40(1):1; Song CQ et al. References on Medicine Abroad — Pharmacy 1978 (2):98.

18. Hu TS et al. Chemistry 1935 2(3):615; Liu SS. Abstracts of Research Literature on Chinese Traditional Drugs (1820–1961). Science Press. 1963. p. 717.

19. Chen TS. Huaxue Gongye (Chemical Industry) 1934 9(2):22; Liu SS. Abstracts of Research Literature on Chinese Traditional Drugs. (1820–1961). Science Press. 1963. p. 717.

20. Wu RQ (reviewer). Medical Information (Sanming District Second Hospital, Fujian) 1977 (1):27.

21. Gaw HZ. Science 1949 (116):11.

22. Pharmacology Section. Selected Information (Kunming Medical College) 1979 (4):12.

23. Traditional Chinese Medicine Department, Second Teaching Hospital. Acta Academiae Medicinae Wuhan 1979 (2):61.

24. Tripterygium wilfordii Research Group. Medical Information (Sanming District Second Hospital, Fujian) 1974 (1):4.

25. Internal Medicine Department. Medical Information (Sanming District Second Hospital, Fujian) 1974 (1):51.

26. Internal Medicine Section, First Teaching Hospital of Hunan Medical College. Communications on Health and Epidemic Prevention (Hunan Sanitation and Anti-epidemic Station) 1975 (4):80.

27. Fujian Coordinating Research Group on Honey Poisoning. Communications on Health and Epidemic Prevention (Hunan Sanitation and Anti-Epidemic Station) 1975 (4):38.

28. Yang DH. Chinese Medical Journal 1941 (60):222.

29. Xu HY et al. Acta Academiae Medicinae Zhejiang 1958 1(4):365.

30. Jiangxi Institute of Apiculture. Communications on Health and Epidemic Prevention (Hunan Sanitation and Anti-epidemic Station) 1975 (4):64.

31. Jiangxi Institute of Apiculture. Communications on Health and Epidemic Prevention (Hunan Sanitation and Anti-epidemic Station) 1975 (4):54.

32. Jinhua District Hospital. Jinhua Science and Technology — Medicine and Health (Jinhua District Centre of Medical and Health Information) 1973 (4):36.

33. Internal Medicine Department, Jinhua District Hospital. Jinhua Science and Technology — Medicine and Health (Jinhua District Centre of Medical and Health Information) 1973 (4):40.

34. Fujian Coordinating Research Group on Honey Poisoning. Communications on Health and Epidemic Prevention (Hunan Sanitation and Anti-epidemic Station) 1975 (4):6.

35. Sanming District (Fujian) Second Hospital. Chinese Traditional and Herbal Drugs Communications 1974 (3):48.

36. Gou JL et al. Medical Research Information 1980 (8):6.

37. Tripterygium wilfordii Research Group. Medical Information (Sanming District Second Hospital, Fujian) 1978 (1–2):140.

38. Phytochemistry Section, Hubei Institute of Combined Western and Traditional Chinese Medicine. Chinese Traditional and Herbal Drugs Communications 1978 (11):8.

39. Rheumatoid Arthritis Coordinating Research Group, First Teaching Hospital. Acta Acedemiae Medicinae Wuhan 1977 (6):51.

40. Joints Department, Zhongxiang County (Hubei) People's Hospital. Journal of Barefoot Doctor 1978 (10):14.

41. Honghu County People's Hospital. Health Journal of Hubei 1976 (2):40.

42. Xu XY. People's Military Medicine 1980 (3):38.

43. Institute of Dermatology, Chinese Academy of Medical Sciences et al. Acta Academiae Medicinae Sinicae 1979 1(1):71.

44. Fujian Coordinating Research Group on Tripterygium wilfordii Therapy of Leprosy. Fujian Medical Journal 1979 (6):27.

45. Fujian Hospital of Skin Diseases et al. Mindong Yiyao (Eastern Fujian Medical Journal) 1972 (3):4; Medical Information (Sanming District Second Hospital, Fujian) 1977 (1):34.

46. Jiangsu Coordinating Research Group on Tripterygium wilfordii. Medical Research Communications 1976 (4):23.

47. Fujian and Jiangsu Coordinating Research Group on tripterygium wilfordii. Dermatological Research Communications 1977 (4):213.

48. Dermatology Department, Huashan Hospital of Shanghai First Medical College et al. Proceedings of the 1977 Shanghai Annual Symposium on Dermatology. Chinese Medical Association (Shanghai Branch). 1978. p. 62.

49. Liao WQ et al. Dermatological Research Communications 1980 (3):14.

50. Fuzhou Hospital of Skin Diseases. Medical Information (Fuzhou Institute of Medical Sciences) 1978 Supplement:28.

51. Pan HY et al. Barefoot Doctor (Fujian Health Bureau) 1978 (4):78.

52. Tripterygium wilfordii Research Section, Institute of Dermatology of the Chinese Academy of Medical Sciences. Acta Academiae Medicinae Sinicae 1979 1(2):136.

53. Pan HY et al. Dermatological Research Communications 1979 (1):29.

54. Liu SS et al. Abstracts of Research Literature on Chinese Traditional Drugs (1962–1974). Science Press. 1979. p. 787.

55. Hunan Hospital of Tuberculosis. Clinical Data. 1971. p. 40; Medical Information (Sanming District Second Hospital, Fujian) 1977 (1):35.

56. Wei RJ. Guangxi Zhongyiyao (Guangxi Journal of Traditional Chinese Medicine) 1979 (1):32.

57. Technical Department of Fujian Bureau of Public Security. Internal Information 1964; Medical Information (Sanming District Second Hospital, Fujian) 1977 (1):35.

58. Internal Medicine Department, Changsha Second Hospital. Changsha Yiyao (Changsha Medical Journal) 1978 (1):34.

59. Shen SF et al. Acta Academiae Medicinae Wuhan 1979 (2):64.

60. Liao NG et al. (reviewers). Zhongji Yikan (Intermediate Medical Journal) 1981 (1):16.

61. Cai RY et al. Medical Information (Sanming District Second Hospital, Fujian) 1974 (1):15.

(Liao Nengge)

XISHENGTENG 錫生藤

The rhizome of *Cissampelos pareria* L. (Menispermaceae) is the Chinese drug <Xishengteng>. It has a bitter and slightly sweet taste with a "warm" property. It is blood-stimulant, stasis-discutient, analgesic, hemostatic, and tissue-generative. Hence, it is used to treat wounds, injuries and traumatic hemorrhage. It is a folk remedy for asthma and heart diseases.

CHEMICAL COMPOSITION

<Xishengteng> contains many alkaloids; the major ones are hayatine, about 0.1%, hayatinine and hayatidine. It also contains cyclanoline (cissamine) and cissampareine.

Two alkaloids were separately isolated from the herb produced in China. After being methiodized, they were called hayatine A and hayatine II. These two alkaloids were said to be identical to hayatine (1).

PHARMACOLOGY

1. Striated Muscle Relaxant Effect

The iodomethane salt of hayatine had a muscle relaxant effect; its efficacy in inducing head drop in rabbits was found to be 2.13 times stronger than that of curarine; its efficacy in paralyzing striated muscles in cats and dogs was 1.14 times that of curarine (2). About one minute after injection of hayatine A 0.1–0.15 mg/kg IV or hayatine II 0.1379 mg/kg IV to rabbits, headdrop, relaxation of the extremities, prostration, shallow and slow breathing occurred. After 4–5 minutes the muscle tone of the animals gradually recovered and they became active again as usual. The efficacy of the drugs was similar to that of curarine (3). As determined in the net-climbing test of albino mice, the ED_{50} of hayatine A was determined to be 0.161±0.0124 mg/kg IP, an efficacy 1.5 times that of curarine (4). the contractile response of tibialis anticus to stimulation of the sciatic nerve became weakened in rats given hayatine A 0.1 mg/kg IP. The degree of blockade was dose related. Hayatine A at 0.25 mg/kg produced a neuromuscular blockade of 96.80±3.19%, and hayatine II 5 mg/kg IV caused neuromuscular blockade of 81.6±8.76% which lasted about 15–19 minutes. This effect was abolished by injection of 0.1 mg/kg of neostigmine and antagonized by succinylcholine. The relaxant effect of hayatine could also be antagonized by neostigmine and potentiated by curarine. On the other hand, the muscle relaxant effect of hayatine A could be potentiated by repeated medication, suggesting that hayatine A is a nondepolarizing muslce relaxant. The action potential on the electromyogram began to decrease 3–5 minutes after injection of hayatine II 0.3 mg/kg IV. The lowest level was reached in 12 minutes and thereafter it started to rise. During the effective period of hayatine II, rapid stimulation (25 times/second) for tens of seconds succeeded by slow stimulation (1 or 5 times/minute) caused post-tetanic facilitation which is a characteristics of nondepolarizing blockade. After administration of hayatine II, neostigmine can still increase the amplitude of muscle action potential and virtually eliminate the waning phenomenon, suggesting a complete antagonism (5,6).

2. Histamine-Releasing Effect

Hayatine is capable of releasing histamine. The intravenously injected drug caused marked and sustained hypotension in cats (7). An average of 3.8 µg of histamine per gram of rat diaphragm could be released by hayatine A 1:1000. In histamine-release studies on cats, hayatine II caused milder hypotension than an equal dose of d-tubocurarine. Subcutaneous injection of hayatine A 0.1 mg also caused histamine release (3).

3. Miscellaneous Actions

Hayatine A at 0.4 mg/kg IV had no significant effect on the blood pressure of rabbits and dogs but lowered that of cats to 40.7–63% of the original readings. It did not significantly affect the heart rhythm and rate but increased the cardiac contractility of rabbits (3). Hayatine II at the concentration of 5×10^{-4} increased the contractility of the isolated frog heart and stimulated the isolated guinea pig ileum (5). Cissampareine was shown to inhibit cultured human nasopharyngeal cancer cells (8).

4. Toxicity

The LD_{50} of hayatine A in albino mice was 0.4457±0.0255 mg/kg IP. Its therapeutic index for muscle relaxation was 2.77 and that of d-tubocurarine was 1.7, indicating a wider safety range of the former than the latter (3,4). Both hayatines A and II caused diaphragm paralysis. They produced respiratory paralysis in rabbits and monkeys at 0.317 and 0.325 mg/kg, respectively. This effect was found to be reversible. Voluntary breathing can be restored within 3 minutes by means of artificial respiration in case of respiratory arrest (5).

CLINICAL STUDIES

1. Muscle Relaxation in Surgery

Hayatines A and II may be combined with various general anesthetics and herbal anesthetics in operations to produce muscle relaxation and to fascilitate control of respiration. Either drug may be repeatedly injected at doses of 0.2–0.3 mg/kg IV. The drug effects appeared in 3–5 minutes and lasted for 20–30 minutes. It is useful in abdominal and thoracic operations, and in other short operations demanding muscle relaxation. Hundreds of clinical cases showed that the drug has a short latent period, reasonable effective time, easy control and no ill effects on circulation (9).

2. Wounds, Injuries and Bleeding

Sufficient amounts of the crushed frest root or stem, or the dry powder, may be dressed over the wound once daily.

ADVERSE EFFECTS

Hayatines A and II at 0.2 mg/kg markedly inhibited respiration and at 0.3 mg/kg caused respiratory arrest. The use of this agent usually requires assisted respiration (10). Insufficient recovery of respiration after surgery can promptly be corrected by intravenous injection of neostigmine 1.0 mg (11). Overdosage may cause the release of histamine. One patient reportedly developed erythema over the upper chest immediately after receiving hayatine II 0.83 mg/kg, which was attributed to histamine release. A child developed bronchial spasm following hayatine II 0.6 mg/kg. The use of hayatine II also caused mydriasis, and in individual patients unequal pupil sizes but they gradually recovered with drug elimination. Hayatine II was discovered to accumulate. Thus, repeated medication with small doses caused significant respiratory depression (9).

REFERENCE

1. Editorial Group. Applications of and Discussions on Chinese Traditional Anesthetics. Shanghai People's Publishing House. 1973. p. 63.

2. Pradhan SN. British Journal of Pharmacology 1953 (8):399.

3. Muscle Relaxant Research Unit, Beijing Medical College. Proceedings of the National Seminar on Chinese Traditional Anesthetics. 1971. p. 217.

4. Zhang BH et al. Abstracts of the Symposium of the Chinese Society of Physiology. 1964. p. 29.

5. General Hospital of Kunming Military Region. Chinese Traditional and Herbal Drugs Communications 1974 (1):27.

6. Chinese Traditional Anesthesia Research Group, Jiangsu Hospital. Zhongma Tongxun (Communications on Chinese Traditional Anesthesia) 1975 (2):9.

7. Kupchan SM et al. Journal of the American Pharmacology Association 1960 (49):727.

8. Kupchan SM et al. Journal of Pharmacological Science 1965 (54):580.

9. Anesthesia Unit, Second Teaching Hospital of Kunming Medical College. Selected Information (Kunming Medical College) 1975 (1):23.

10. General Hospital of Kunming Units of the Chinese PLA. Chinese Medical Journal 1974 51(10):633.

11. General Hospital of Kunming Military Region. Chinese Traditional and Herbal Drugs Communications 1974 (2):24.

(Fang Zhiping)

JINJIER 錦鷄兒

<Jinjier>, also known as <Yangquehuagen> and <Jinquehuagen>, is the root of *Caragana sinica* (Buchoz.) Rehd. (Leguminosae). The root of other species such as *C. microphylla* Lam., *C. intermedia* Kuang, and *C. franchetiana* Kom. are also used as <Jinjier>.

<Jinjier> has a sweet taste and a "mild" property. It is vital-energy- and "kidney"-tonifying, blood-stimulant, menstruation-corrective, and antirheumatic. It is principally employed in the treatment of shortness of breath, palpitation, edema, tuberculosis, and leukorrhea. It is also a popular folk tonic. Thus, in some places it is called <Tuhuangqi> or used as the drug, <Huangqi> (1). The flower which is known as <Jinquehua> or <Yangquehua> is a common folk remedy for dizziness and vertigo.

CHEMICAL COMPOSITION

Preliminary chemical assay showed that <Jinjier> contains alkaloids, flavonoid glycosides, coumarin lactones and phytosterols. The chemical composition and the amount of the constituents vary widely with the varieties of the plant (2).

PHARMACOLOGY

1. Hypotensive Effect

The ethanol or ether extract of <Jinjier> had a relatively strong hypotensive effect. The ethanol extract at 1 g/kg IP (equivalent to 30 g/kg of the crude drug) decreased the blood pressure of anesthetized cats by 30–60% within 30–120 minutes, whereas the ether extract 0.15–0.3 g/kg lowered the blood pressure by 35–60% within 30–60 minutes. The hypotensive effect lasted longer than 4 hours. No significant alteration of the respiration and heart rate was seen during hypotension. Repeated medication produced no tachyphylaxis. Hypotension was also produced in some experimental rabbits and rats. <Jinjier> did not potentiate the hypotensive effect of acetylcholine; its hypotensive effect was unaltered by bilateral vagotomy or small doses of atropine. This herb has no ganglionic blocking action; therefore, its hypotensive mechanism is unrelated to the peripheral cholinergic system. It is also unrelated to histamine release because its hypotensive effect was not modified by diphenhydramine. <Jinjier> produced no hypotension in spinal cats, but low doses of it administered into the 4th cerebral ventricle not only produced significant hypotension but also suppressed and reversed the pressor reflex due to blockade of the carotid artery. <Jinjier>, moreover, intensified the hypotensive reflex elicited by stimulation of the carotid sinus. The action site is therefore believed to be located centrally. Pretreatment with atropine in large doses antagonized the hypotensive action of <Jinjier>, but no such effect was produced if atropine was administered during the effective hypotensive period. Thus, it appears that the herb competes with atropine for the same receptor in the reticular formation of the brain stem.

In addition, <Jinjier> potentiated the pressor effects of epinephrine or stimulation of major splanchnic nerves (3,4).

2. Anti-inflammatory Effect

A marked inhibitory action against formaldehyde-induced paw swelling was achieved by oral administration of the <Jinjier> decoction 50 g/kg daily in rats. It reduced the edema during the exudation period but did not significantly affect tissue degeneration and necrosis during late inflammatory stage, nor did it inhibit granulation of implanted cotton balls in rats. <Jinjier> was shown to have no glucocorticoid effect or any enhancing effect on the adrenocortical function, because it failed to decrease the thymic weight of young mice and the vitamin C content in the rat adrenal gland (5).

3. Miscellaneous Actions

In experiments on guinea pigs with asthma induced by histamine aerosol, oral administration of the <Jinjier> decoction at the dose of 12.5 g/kg markedly prolonged the latent period of asthma symptoms such as dyspnea, convulsion and prostration, suggesting the presence of an antiasthmatic effect. No antitussive or expectorant effect was exhibited by this agent in experiments on mice with cough induced by ammonia aerosol and in the phenol red method (6). In addition, *in vitro* studies showed that the <Jinjier> decoction was inhibitory to *Staphylococcus aureus* (7), alpha and beta *Streptococcus hemolyticus*, *Diplococcus pneumoniae*, and *Neisseria catarrhalis* (8).

4. Toxicity

<Jinjier> has a very low toxicity. The LD_{50} of its ethanol extract was determined to be 10.4 g/kg IP in mice which was equivalent to 309.7 g/kg of the crude drug (3).

CLINICAL STUDIES

1. Hypertension

A marked antihypertensive effect was obtained from the clinical treatment of various types of hypertension with the herb decoction (9), syrup (10), ethanol extract (11), or the compound prescriptions containing this herb as the principal ingredient (12,13). For instance, out of 81 cases of second- and third-stage essential hypertension treated with the tablet of the ethanol extract of

<Jinjier>, 66 cases benefitted, including 42 cases of marked improvement. The blood pressure in 19 cases started to descend after the first week of medication and 53 cases in 4 weeks (10). In another group of 100 cases of hypertension, the syrup given by mouth at 21–30 g/day was effective in the second and third stages, in renal and postpartum hypertension. The aggregate effective rate was 73% for blood pressure lowering and 79% for symptomatic improvement. It was particularly effective for the second-stage hypertension. Either increasing the dosage or prolonging the treatment period potentiated the antihypertensive effect. In cases of hypertension with myocardial damage, <Jinjier> not only lowered the blood pressure but also improved or corrected ECG aberration. The therapeutic effect of <Jinjier> was markedly potentiated when combined with other drugs, such as dihydrochlorothiazide and potassium chloride (14), leaf of Ginkgo biloba, reserpine (11), or the ripe seed of Cassia tora, and the root of Aristolochia debilis, (13).

2. Lupus Erythematosus

All 36 cases of lupus erythematosus including 10 discoid type and 26 systemic type obtained satisfactory therapeutic results following treatment with <Jinjier> as the chief remedy. The decoction of 120 g of <Jinjier> was given in three doses. Fourteen cases achieved complete remission, 16 amelioration and 1 case ineffective; 5 cases died (15).

3. Chronic Bronchitis

Oral administration of the decoction of <Jinjier> 100 g/day in 420 cases of chronic bronchitis was effective in relieving cough, expectoration, and dyspnea; an aggregate effective rate of 86.7% and marked effective rate of 40.2% were obtained. During the treatment period some patients experienced improvement in sleep and appetite, increase in urine output, subsidence of edema, decrease in the heart rate, and lowering of the blood pressure (mainly diastolic) (16).

ADVERSE EFFECTS

Allergic manifestations may occur in a minority of patients such as pruritus, urticaria, and allergic dermatitis; other symptoms are xerostomia, drowsiness, dizziness, vomiting, etc. These disappeared after discontinuing the drug (10,11,16).

REFERENCE

1. Editorial Group. National Collection of Chinese Materia Medica. Vol. 1. People's Medical Publishing House. 1976. p. 763.

2. Phytochemistry Section, Baotou Medical School. Baotou Yiyao (Baotou Medical Journal) 1977 (1):65.

3. Cardiovascular Research Group, Hubei College of Traditional Chinese Medicine et al. Hubei Pharmaceutical Industry 1973 (1):15.

4. Hubei College of Traditional Chinese Medicine et al. Selected Research Information on Traditional Chinese Medicine (Hubei Health Bureau) 1975 (6):23.

5. Pharmacology Section, Baotou Medical College et al. Baotou Yiyao (Baotou Medical Journal) 1977 (1):79.

6. Chronic Bronchitis Coordinating Research Group of Baotou Medical College. Baotou Yiyao (Baotou Medical Journal) 1977 (1):52.

7. Zhejiang People's Academy of Health. In vitro antibacterial tests of more than 200 kinds of Chinese traditional drugs. 1971.

8. Microbiology Section, Baotou Medical College. Baotou Yiyao (Baotou Medical Journal) 1977 (1):63.

9. Qichun County (Hubei). National Exhibition of Chinese Traditional Drugs and New Therapeutic Methods (Technical Data). Committee of the National Exhibition of Chinese Traditional Drugs and New Therapeutic Methods. 1971. p. 151.

10. Internal Medicine Department, Staff Hospital of Wuhan Steel Works. New Medical Communications (Hubei College of Traditional Chinese Medicine) 1974 (1):25.

11. Teaching Hospital of Hubei College of Traditional Chinese Medicine. Health Journal of Hubei 1972 (1):55; Hubei Pharmaceutical Industry 1973 (1):18.

12. Wuhan Ninth Hospital. Wuhan Journal of New Chinese Medicine 1972 (3):19.

13. Qizhuo Branch of Qichun County People's Hospital. Health Journal of Hubei 1974 (6):74.

14. Cardiovascular Group, Hubei College of Traditional Chinese Medicine. Compiled Information on Combined Western and Traditional Chinese Medicine (Teaching Hospital of Hubei College of Traditional Chinese Medicine) 1979 (2):23.

15. Internal Medicine Department, 291st Hospital of the Chinese PLA. Baotou Science and Technology — Health Edition 1975 (3–4):35.

16. Baotou Coordinating Research Group on Jinjier Therapy of Chronic Bronchitis. Baotou Yiyao (Baotou Medical Journal) 1977 (1):68.

(Deng Wenlong)

MANSHANXIANG 滿山香

<Manshanxiang>, also known as <Paicaoxiang>, is the rhizome or the whole plant of *Lysimachia capillipes* Hemsl. (Primulaceae). It is sweet and has a "mild" property. It is antirheumatic, antitussive, and menstruation-corrective. Hence, it is mainly used for common cold, cough, rheumatism, and irregular menstruation.

CHEMICAL COMPOSITION

<Manshanxiang> contains volatile oil and non-volatile components.

PHARMACOLOGY

1. Inhibitory Effect on Influenza Virus

The decoction of the rhizome was reported to have a marked inhibitory and inactivating effects on influenza viruses (1–4). The decoction inhibited Jingke 68–1 strain and many other strains of influenza virus in chicken embryos. The herb was active irrespective of whether it was given before or after viral inoculation. But the effect was most conspicuous when the drug was allowed to act on the virus *in vitro* for a period of time before they were inoculated into the embryos.

The potency of its effect closely correlated with both the titre of the inoculated viruses and the drug concentration (1). A dose of 70 mg per embryo infected with 160 EID_{50} of type A Asian influenza virus Jingke 68–1 strain inactivated the virus but a lower dose only suppressed its multiplication, the ED_{50} being 33 ± 9.9 mg per embryo (2). When viruses were introduced into the chicken egg allantois, injection of the drug into the yolk sac still produced a very striking antiviral action, suggesting other mechanisms besides direct inactivation. The inhibitory effect was still very marked even if treatment was started 60 minutes after the viral infection, implying that the herb does not prevent viral adsorption onto the cells but that it probably acts on certain early stages of the viral replication process (1,3).

A pronounced antiviral effect was also exhibited by some extracts of <Manshanxiang> (3,5). For example, addition of the 0.3% aqueous extract of <Manshanxiang> 60 minutes after the viral inoculation still suppressed the multiplication of influenza virus in the monolayer culture of human embryonic kidney epithelial cells. Very pronounced inhibitory effect was exhibited by this extract against 7, 30 and 40 median tissue culture infective doses ($TCID_{50}$) of "Yuefang" 72–243, England 72–42, and "Ganke" 74–4 viral strains (3). The <Manshanxiang> decoction repeatedly delayed the death and lowered the mortality rate of mice infected with 1.3–3.0 LD_{50} of virus. The crude extract of this herb also protected mice against infection of influenza virus; the protective rates in two out of five experiments were 45.4 and 56.1%, respectively, which were significantly different from the results in the control group (3,6).

It was discovered during clinical therapies using <Manshanxiang> that in patients diagnosed by the clotting inhibition and serum antibody tests to be infected with type A Asian influenza virus, the positive viral isolation rate after <Manshanxiang> administration was significantly lowered from 98 to 36.8% (7). However, this result was not reproduced in another study. <Manshanxiang> administration was unable to decrease the viral isolation rate in subjects inoculated with the active influenza vaccine. It was also reported that influenza patients treated with <Manshanxiang> had significantly lower antibody level than those receiving conventional drugs (6). In summary, these results of experimental and clinical studies indicate that the antiviral action of <Manshanxiang> still awaits confirmation through in-depth studies.

2. Antipyretic Effect

One report claimed that the orally or intramuscularly administered ethanol extract of the stem and leaf produced antipyretic effect on rabbits with fever induced by bacterial vaccine. The alkaloids and volatile oil of this extract were found to be inactive but the residual fluid was still active. On the other hand, the decoction of the stem and leaf was devoid of antipyretic activity (8). However, later studies demonstrated that the root decoction at 24 g/kg had a marked antipyretic effect in rabbits with fever induced by typhoid and paratyphoid vaccines. The body temperature was significantly lowered one hour after medication, and the temperature was below normal at the second hour and continued to descend on the fifth hour. In contrast, the body temperature of the control animals started to drop 3 hours after medication and normal temperature was not yet attained on the fifth hour. The root at 25 g/kg was equipotent to 200 mg/kg of aminopyrine. The stem, leaf and root also had antipyretic activity at 19.2 g/kg but were inactive below 10 g/kg (6).

3. Miscellaneous Actions

The ethanol extract of the stem and leaf (minus the tannins) was found to have no inhibitory action against 11 kinds of bacteria including *Staphylococcus aureus*. No analgesic effect was exhibited by <Manshanxiang> in mice with peritoneum irritated by chemicals (8).

4. Toxicity

The LD_{50} of the ethanol extract of the root (minus the tannins) was 1.12 g/kg IV in mice, and the lethal dose was 10 g/kg IV. The LD_{50} of the decoction of the stem and leaf was 72.0±4.1 g/kg PO, that of the ethanol extract 58.3±7.6 g/kg PO, and that of the extract devoid of tannins 2.24±0.17 g/kg IV or 20 g/kg IP (8).

CLINICAL STUDIES

1. Influenza and Common Cold

<Manshanxiang> was reported to have good prophylactic and curative effects for influenza and common cold (6,9–15). For example, in 114 cases of type A Asian influenza treated with the decoction of <Manshanxiang> at 30–60 g/day in 2–4 doses, and effective rate of 81.6% was achieved in which 58.1% were relieved of fever within 24 hours and 41.9% within 48 hours. In contrast, out of 50 control cases treated with antibiotics and antipyretics, only half of them responded (10). In a group of 109 cases of common cold treated with the 1:1 decoction 50 ml twice daily, an effective rate of 67.9% was achieved compared with 31% in 100 cases treated with compound aminopyrine 0.9 g per day (11). Optimal results were also achieved in 522 cases of influenza and common cold treated with <Manshanxiang> in combination with the root and rhizome of *Cynanchum stauntoni* and the rhizome of *Helminthostachys zeylanica*. Fever subsided within 1 day in 61.1% and within 2 days in 23.4% of the cases (12). Moreover, <Manshanxiang> was reported to have a good prophylactic effect against influenza and common cold, e.g., in 604 subjects given the compound formula of <Manshanxiang>, the 30-day incidence rate was 6.95% in contrast to 13.95% in the control group (13).

2. Epidemic Encephalitis B

Out of 93 cases of encephalitis B treated with the granule preparation of <Manshanxiang>, 81.3% were cured within 5 days. With respect to the average number of days required for the subsidence of fever and the relief of spasm, the average course of illness, cure rate and the mortality rate, this granule is superior to a heat-clearing and detoxifying compound formula used in 89 control cases (16).

3. Edema

The treatment of various kinds of edema with the decoction of the toot has been reported (17).

ADVERSE EFFECTS

<Manshanxiang> produces certain gastrointestinal side effects; the main symptoms were dry pharynx, dizziness, oral numbness, nausea, vomiting, abdominal pain, and diarrhea. The incidence of adverse reactions after oral administration for 2 days was reported to be 11.1–23.7% but all reactions were rather mild, requiring no special management and would not interfere with the treatment (18).

REFERENCE

1. Zheng YK et al. Acta Microbiologica Sinica 1973 13(2):162.

2. Microbiology-Etiology Section, Jiangxi Medical University. New Medical Practice (Jiangxi Medical University) 1973 (2):48.

3. Virus Group, Jiangxi Office for Prevention and Treatment of Chronic Bronchitis. Chinese Traditional and Herbal Drugs Communications 1976 (11):29.

4. Zhejiang Sanitation and Anti-epidemic Station. Information on the Prevention and Treatment of Influenza. Zhejiang Coordinating Research Group on Common Cold. 1975. p. 50.

5. Materia Medica Research Unit, Jiangxi Second People's Hospital. Jiangxi Medical Information 1975 (7):101.

6. Jiang ZS et al. Jiangxi Yiyao (Jiangxi Medical Journal) 1980 (5):6.

7. Virus Group, Jiangxi Office for Prevention and Treatment of Chronic Bronchitis. Jiangxi Medical Information 1973 (2):41.

8. Pharmaceutical Factory, Jiangxi Second People's Hospital. Jiangxi Information on Chronic Bronchitis (Jiangxi Office for Prevention and Treatment of Chronic Bronchitis) 1973 (4):73.

9. Common Cold Prevention and Treatment Group of Fuzhou District. Fuzhou Yiyao (Fuzhou Medical Journal) 1974 (2–3):32.

10. Staff Hospital of Jiangxi Cotton Textile and Dyeing Factory. Xinyiyaoxue Zazhi (Journal of Traditional Chinese Medicine) 1974 (1):29.

11. Common Cold Prevention and Treatment Group of Fuzhou District et al. Jiangxi Medical Information 1975 (7):69.

12. Lean County Health Bureau. Jiangxi Medical Information 1972 (2):9.

13. Beiliu County Supervisory Group on Prevention and Treatment of Chronic Bronchitis. Revolution in Health (Yulin District health Bureau, Guangxi) 1975 (4):11.

14. Zhejiang Sanitation and Anti-epidemic Station et al. Science and Technology — Medicine and Health (Information Institute of Zhejiang Bureau of Science and Technology) 1976 (1):19.

15. Nanchang District Coordinating Research Group on Prevention and Treatment of Common Cold. Jiangxi Medical Information 1975 (7):71.

16. Jiangxi Coordinating Research Group on Lysimachia capillipes Therapy of Epidemic Encephalitis B. Chinese Traditional and Herbal drugs Communications 1979 (7):22.

17. Jiang SQ et al. Guangdong Zhongyi (Guangdong Journal of Traditional Chinese Medicine) 1960 5(11):512.

18. Lean Pilot Area for Prevention and Treatment of Chronic Bronchitis. Jiangxi Information on Chronic Bronchitis (Jiangxi Office for Prevention and Treatment of Chronic Bronchitis) 1973 (5):33.

(Deng Wenlong)

BINGLANG 檳榔

<Binglang>, the seed of *Areca catechu* L. (Palmae), is bitter and puckery to the taste and has a "warm" property. It has digestant, anthelmintic, "jiangqi" (antiflatulent) and diuretic actions. The herb is mainly used as a remedy for abdominal distention due to dyspepsia; taeniasis, fasciolopsiasis, and edema.

CHEMICAL COMPOSITION

<Binglang> contains 0.3–0.6% of alkaloids, mainly arecoline, guvacoline, arecolidine and isoguvacine. It also contains condensed tannin 15%, fat 14%, aread red, starch and resin.

The raw <Binglang> contains much more alkaloids than processed seeds. The difference may reach 50%.

PHARMACOLOGY

1. Anthelmintic Effect

In vitro, the 30% <Binglang> decoction caused rigidity and even death of dog dwarf tapeworms in 40 minutes (1). The 1–2% extract of <Binglang> devoid of tannic acid caused flaccid paralysis of pork tapeworm (*Taenia solium*), beef tapeworm (*Taenia saginata*) and dwarf tapeworm (*Hymenolepis nana*). The head and immature proglottides of the worms were more sensitive to the drug than the mature proglottides (3). The site of action is believed not the muscles but the nervous system (4). The relatively poor result seen on beef tapeworms may be due to the large size of the gravid proglottides (3). The <Binglang> decoction also paralyzed rat pinworms. At 25% it rendered them immobile in 45 minutes, and after being transferred to Ringer's solution for 30 minutes 60% of the worms recovered (5). Another report stated that arecoline at concentrations of 2×10^{-7} M and 5×10^{-6} M paralyzed the suckers and somatic muscles of *Schistosoma mansoni* (6). Likewise, *in vivo* studies showed that arecoline hydrobromide 0.44 mg/kg PO expelled 95% of helminths (7). An anthelmintic activity against *Diphyllobothrium latum* and *Diplogonoporus grandis* was also exhibited in laboratory cats by arecoline bismuth iodide 48.5 mg PO in mice (4). The <Binglang> decoction expelled dwarf tapeworms and, concurrently, pinworms (5,8). Both <Binglang> and the seed of *Cucurbita moschata* paralyzed tapeworms and were found to be synergistic (2). In mice with experimental schistosomiasis 98% of the schistosomes shifted to the liver 1.5 hours after oral administration of the <Binglang> decoction. Synergism was observed between the <Binglang> decoction and furapromide in the treatment of schistosome cercariae in rabbits (6).

2. Effect on Cholinergic Receptors

Arecoline is a muscarinic receptor agonist. Consumption of <Binglang> increased the gastrointestinal smooth muscle tone, intestinal peristalsis, digestive juice secretion, and the appetite (9). Oral administration of <Binglang> decoction 9.9 g/kg in dogs caused purgation in a mean of 65 minutes for a mean of 5.4 bowel movements. Thus, the herb may enhance worm expulsion (10). The <Binglang> injection induced marked contraction of the isolated as well as the *in situ* gallbladders of dogs and cats. The combined use of this agent and an injection of the rhizome of *Rheum palmatum* would further enhance the contraction of the common bile duct and bile flow, implying a beneficial effect on the passing of choledocholiths (11).

Moreover, arecoline decreased the heart rate, and caused constriction of the coronary artery as well as contraction of the uterine smooth muscle in rabbits (12). It potentiated the vasoconstricting effect of atropine on the mouse hind limbs (13), and stimulated the nicotinic receptors manifested as excitation of skeletal muscles, nerve ganglions and carotid bodies. The agent also produced central cholinergic effects (14). Injection of the arecoline hydrobromide 10 mg/kg SC caused salivation and tremor in mice (15). Intravenous injection of small doses of arecoline in cats elicited cortical arousal reaction which could be reduced or blocked by atropine (14). Subcutaneous injection of arecoline minimized pentetrazole-induced convulsion, or impaired memory due to brain injury in mice (16). It was reported that cholinergic receptors were present in the muscles of *Schistosoma mansoni* and that stimulation of them by <Binglang> paralyzed the schistosomes; this effect was blocked by atropine (6).

3. Antimicrobial Effect

The 1:1 aqueous extract of <Binglang> inhibited skin fungi such as *Schlemn's Dermatomyces favosa, Trichophyton violaceum* to different extents (17). In experiments with chicken embryos, <Binglang> was shown to be active against influenza virus with an *in vitro* MIC of 0.08 mg/ml and *in vivo* MIC of 25 mg/embryo (18). The active antiviral substance might be tannins. The <Binglang> extract instilled into the nose and mixed with the drinking water for mouse was effective against influenza virus PR_8 infection (19–21).

4. Miscellaneous Actions

The ethyl acetate extract of <Binglang> caused uterine spasm in pregnant rats (22). It was reported that arecoline hydrolysate might be carcinogenic (23,24).

5. Toxicity

The LD_{50} of the <Binglang> decoction in mice was 120 ± 24 g/kg PO (6). The MLD of arecoline in mice, dogs and horses were 100, 5 and 1.4 mg/kg PO, respectively (25). The MLD of the bismuth iodide of this herb in rats was 1 g/kg PO; salivation, diarrhea, tachypnea, and restlessness appeared 15 minutes after medication, followed by death in 1.5–2 hours (4). Oral administration of arecoline hydrobromide to dogs might cause vomiting and convulsion (7).

CLINICAL STUDIES

1. Taeniasis

1.1 *Taenia solium infection.* The usual dosage of <Binglang> decoction is 75–100 g PO. It was reported to be 94.1% effective in 50 cases (26). Therapeutic effects were also achieved in 22 cases treated with the aqueous extract, in 10 cases with the extract, in 6 cases with a decoction and in 6 cases with the bismuth iodide of this herb (2).

1.2 *Hymenolepis nana infection.* The usual dosage of <Binglang> decoction is 80–100 g PO. Divergent therapeutic results have been reported. One paper claimed that all 16 cases were cured by this medication (27). In 32 other cases, the stool examination of 82.8% became negative for the ova (28). But, another report stated that only 3 out of 6 (26), and again 3 out of 14 cases were cured. Studies revealed that the therapeutic effect was influenced by the time of storage, quality, and method of preparation of the drug as well as to vomiting elicited by it (26).

1.3 *Taenia saginata infection.* Usually the dosage of <Binglang> decoction is 120–200 g PO taken on an empty stomach; the cure rate was only 30–50%(2,25,26,29). However, a cure rate as high as 95.19% was achieved in 96 cases treated with the seed of *Cucurbita moschata* in combination with <Binglang> (2). Satisfactory results were also reported on the use of this herb with the seed of *Cucurbita moschata*, the peel of *Punica granatum*, (2,26) or of this herb with the sclerotium of *Mylitta lapidescens* (30), as well as with quinacrine hydrochloride (31).

A single intraduodenal infusion of a decoction of 200 g of <Binglang> produced good therapeutic effect with minimal side effects in adult patients with *Taenia solium*, *Hymenolepis nana*, and *Taenia saginata* (32,33). Another report claimed that the decoction of 200 g of <Binglang> could expel *Diphyllobothrium latum* (34).

2. Fasciolopsiasis

Oral administration of <Binglang> decoction at adult doses of 40–50 g to 64 cases cured 33 by a single treatment, and 95.4% were cured after 3 treatments (35). A cure rate of 47.2% was achieved in 72 adult patients treated with a decoction of 31–93 g of <Binglang> (devoid of tannins) (36). <Binglang> with chilli and bephenium produced a cure rate of 60.71–95.9% (37–40).

3. Other Parasitic Diseases

Different degrees of therapeutic effect were achieved with <Binglang> and its compound prescriptions in treating ancylostomiasis (41–43), schistosomiasis (6,44), trichuriasis (45), and ascariasis (43,46).

4. Glaucoma

A 100-ml eye drops prepared from 200 g of <Binglang> was used to treat 4 cases, achieving an effect similar to the pilocarpine eye drops (47).

ADVERSE EFFECTS

The common adverse reactions are nausea and vomiting (20–30%), abdominal pain, dizziness, and nervousness. Vomiting may be minimized if the <Binglang> decoction is taken cold (26). A very rare side effect is peptic ulcer with hematemesis (10,26). Overdosage causes salivation, vomiting, drowsiness, and seizure. The treatments for oral dosage-induced side effects include gastric lavage with potassium permanganate solution and injection of atropine.

REFERENCE

1. Han WC et al. Research on Chinese Materia Medica. Northeastern Medical Publishers. 1953. p. 292.

2. Feng LZ. Chinese Medical Journal 1956 42(2):138.

3. Pharmacology Department, Jiangsu Medical College. Acta Academiae Medicinae Jiangsu 1957 (4):242.

4. Feng LZ et al. Peking Natural History Bulletin 1949 17:233.

5. Feng YS et al. Journal of Shandong University 1956 2(3):102.

6. Pharmacology Department, Faculty of Pharmacy of Zhejiang Medical College. Acta Academiae Medicinae Zhejiang 1980 9(1):1.

7. Batham EJ. Parasitology 1946 37:185.

8. Wang YZ et al. Chinese Journal of Health 1954 (5):390.

9. Qiu XT. Journal of the Formosan Medical Association 1933 36(6):857.

10. Shanghai Institute of Natural Sciences. Information on Areca catechu and Quisqualis indica. 1955.

11. Qingdao Institute of Medical Sciences. Xinyiyaoxue Zazhi (Journal of Traditional Chinese Medicine) 1979 (6):26.

12. Sirsi M et al. Chemical Abstracts 1969 70:113690p.

13. Sirsi M et al. Chemical Abstracts 1964 60:4658d.

14. Goodman LS et al. The Pharmacological Basis of Therapeutics. 3rd edition. The Macmillan Company. 1965. p. 471.

15. Nieschulz O et al. Chemical Abstracts 1968 68:113138y.

16. Nieschulz O. Chemical Abstracts 1968 68:28302c.

17. Cao RL et al. Chinese Journal of Dermatology 1957 (4):286.

18. Liu GS et al. Acta Microbiologica Sinica 1960 (2):164.

19. Wang SY. Kexue Tongbao (Science Bulletin) 1958 (3):90.

20. Wang SY. Kexue Tongbao (Science Bulletin) 1958 (5):155.

21. Wang SY. Kexue Tongbao (Science Bulletin) 1958 (11):343.

22. Kumari HL et al. The Indian Journal of Pharmacy 1964 26(10):248.

23. Boyland E. Chemical Abstracts 1969 70:18207c.

24. Jiang TL. Chinese Traditional and Herbal Drugs 1980 (9):425.

25. Zhu Y. Beijing Zhongyi (Beijing Journal of Traditional Chinese Medicine) 1953 2(6):23.

26. Xu YM. Zhongji Yikan (Intermediate Medical Journal) 1958 (3):15.

27. Feng LC. Peking Natural History Bulletin 1949 18(1):63.

28. Zhang L et al. Chinese Medical Journal 1963 49(2):92.

29. Wang HX. Chinese Medical Journal 1954 40(9):719.

30. Li FX. Modern Research of Traditional Chinese Medicine (Hebei Medical College) 1976 (1):21.

31. Xu XD et al. Chinese Medical Journal 1953 39(9):715.

32. Wang SM et al. Chinese Medical Journal 1953 39(12):954.

33. Wang SM et al. Chinese Medical Journal 1956 42(2):148.

34. Sha RH et al. Chinese Medical Journal 1953 39(12):957

35. Wu PN et al. Peking Natural History Bulletin 1950 18(3):151.

36. Teng B et al. People's Health Care 1959 (9):807.

37. Clinical Microbiology Section, Medical Department of Jiangsu College of New Medicine. Selected Information on Scientific Research (Jiangsu College of New Medicine) 1976 (1):86.

38. Shen RS. Zhejiang Journal of Traditional Chinese Medicine 1960 39(2):67.

39. Mobile Medical Team, Jinshan County (Shanghai) People's Hospital. Xinyiyaoxue Zazhi (Journal of Traditional Chinese Medicine) 1975 (5):30.

40. Liao YQ. Journal of Traditional Chinese Medicine 1959 (4):52.

41. Wang SM et al. Chinese Medical Journal 1956 42(12):1151.

42. Cai HE. Chinese Medical Journal 1957 43(5):371.

43. Nanjiang County Center of Schistosomiasis Control. Jiangsu Zhongyi (Jiangsu Journal of Traditional Chinese Medicine) 1962 (10):39.

44. Research Committee of Shanghai institute of Schistosomiasis Control. Shanghai Zhongyiyao Zazhi (Shanghai Journal of Traditional Chinese Medicine) 1959 (4):11.

45. Yong NS. Chinese Medical Journal 1958 44(6):626.

46. Qiu CB. New Compilation of Chinese Materia Medica (Summary of Researches). Shanghai: Qianqingtang Bookstore. 1955. p. 349.

47. Beijing Mobile Medical Team. Gansu Health Communications 1972 (4):51.

(Zhou Shufang)

SUANZAOREN 酸棗仁

<Suanzaoren> is the seed of *Ziziphus jujuba* Mill. (Rhamnaceae). It is sweet and "mild". Its actions are considered to be sedative, tranquilizing, "yin"-tonifying and anhidrotic. It is indicated for insomnia due to asthenia and anxiety, palpitation, hyperhidrosis, and thirst.

CHEMICAL COMPOSITION

<Suanzaoren> contains 0.1% of saponins, which is composed of jujubosides A and B. Hydrolysis of jujuboside B yields jujubogenin, and further hydrolysis yields ebelin lactone. <Suanzaoren> also contains triterpenoids betulin and betulic acid, and a large amount of fixed oil (31.8%).

PHARMACOLOGY

1. Sedative and Hypnotic Effects

<Suanzaoren> has been reported to have excellent sedative and hypnotic effects on various animal species including mouse, rat, guinea pig, rabbit, cat, and dog, as well as man (1–14). By means of the tremble cage recording method and photocell recording method as well as through direct observation of the activity of the test animals, it was showed that <Suanzaoren> strongly inhibited the spontaneous activity of the animals. For instance, in the tremble cage experiment, the sedation index of the <Suanzaoren> decoction at 5 g/kg PO was determined to be 1.65 and at 20 g/kg PO was 1.95, whereas that of the ethanol extract solution at 5 g/kg PO was 1.58 (1). In caffeine-induced hyperactivity of mice, intragastric administration of <Suanzaoren> 1 g/kg gave a sedation index of 2.43 in contrast to 6.54 by intraperitoneal injection (2). Likewise, sedative and hypnotic effects in rats were achieved by intragastric or intraperitoneal administration of the <Suanzaoren> decoction given to normal or caffeine-stimulated animals irrespective of the time of the day (3). <Suanzaoren> also markedly inhibited, in a dose-dependent manner, the passive motility of the test animals, i.e. fall from the rolling cylinder (4).

<Suanzaoren> synergized with many sedatives and hypnotics. For instance, the <Suanzaoren> decoction given intragastrically to mice greatly prolonged pentobarbital sodium-induced sleep (1), and increased the number of mice responsive to the subthreshold dose of pentobarbital sodium for abolishing the righting reflex (4). The decoction given subcutaneously synergized with thiopental sodium in that subthreshold dosage of the latter was sufficient to induce anesthesia (5). Injection of the decoction 3 g/kg IP also offset the manic response of cats to morphine (5).

A report pointed out that <Suanzaoren> influenced higher nervous activities; it markedly decreased the frequency of conditioned avoidance reflex in mice (5), caused spreading of internal inhibition, eliminated the conditioned reflexes, and prolonged the latent period of nonconditioned avoidance reflex. In the climbing test, hole test, and sleep potentiation method, it was discovered that the different constituents of <Suanzaoren> exhibited different degrees of sedative effect (7), and that the active components were the jujubosides (8).

Although <Suanzaoren> has marked sedative and hypnotic effects, it was never reported to induce anesthesia in animals even in very large doses (2). According to a report, administration of <Suanzaoren> to mice for 6 days caused a progressively shallower and shorter sleep, and on the sixth day it no longer induced sleep, indicating the development of tolerance from prolonged administration. However, there was no cross tolerance between this herb and amobarbital, and the developed tolerance readily disappeared one week after discontinuation of the medication (9). There is an old saying that the raw herb be prescribed for somnolence and the stir-fried herb for insomnia. Experiments on the active and passive activities of mice, however, showed that the crude herb had no stimulant effect at all (3), while both the raw and stir-fried herb had a sedative effect (10,11). Another author reported that the sedative effect of <Suanzaoren> is lost when its oil is destroyed by prolonged stir-frying (3). However, γ-ray irradiation did not affect the sedative action of this herb (12).

2. Anticonvulsant, Analgesic, and Hypothermic Effects

The soluble extract of <Suanzaoren> greatly reduced the convulsion rate and mortality rate of animals given the ED_{50} of pentylenetetrazole for inducing convulsion. In case of strychnine-induced convulsion, the same agent only prolonged the latent period of convulsion and delayed the death of the test animals; it did not significantly after the mortality rate (4). However, it was reported that <Suanzaoren> decoction at 5 g/kg IP significantly reduced the strychnine-induced mortality rate in mice (5). <Suanzaoren> did not protect rabbits from caffeine- or electric shock-induced convulsion (10). It was proved in the hot plate experiment that <Suanzaoren> decoction 5 g/kg had a significant analgesic effect in mice (5). In addition, a hypothermic effect was produced by intraperitoneal injection of 2.5 or 5 g/kg of the decoction in rats or by oral administration of 40 g/kg in cats (5).

3. Effect on the Cardiovascular System and Smooth Muscles

Intravenous injection of <Suanzaoren> decoction promptly caused a drastic and prolonged hypotension in anesthetized dogs (6,15). In rats with experimental renal hypertension, the stir-fried herb 20–30 g/kg given *ad lib* before or on the next day of operation also produced marked reduction in the blood pressure (16). Moreover, <Suanzaoren> caused heart block and marked uterine excitation (6,17). The leaf of *Ziziphus jujuba* could improve myocardial ischemia and increase the tolerance of myocardium to hypoxia (18).

4. Effect on Burns

The ethanol extract of <Suanzaoren> used alone or with the fruit of *Schisandra chinensis* increased the survival rate and prolonged the survival of scalded mice. Best effect was achieved when <Suanzaoren> 5 g/kg was used with the fruit of *Schisandra chinensis* 1 g/kg. <Suanzaoren> also markedly checked the deterioration of edema in mice due to scald. It also delayed the onset of shock in rats due to napalm burns and prolonged the life of these animals (19).

5. Toxicity

<Suanzaoren> and its extract are of very low toxicity if given orally (3–5,7). At 50 g/kg PO in mice, the decoction did not produce any toxic symptoms (5). No death occurred after intragastric administration of the 15 g/ml soluble extract at 1 ml/20 g (4). Chronic administration of <Suanzaoren> in rats produced marginal toxicity (5). However, its toxicity was greatly increased when the herb was given parenterally; the LD_{50} of the decoction was determined to be 14.3±2.0 g/kg IP (5). Mice died within 30–60 minutes after injection of the 50% ethanol extract at 20 g/kg SC (13). All guinea pigs given 10–15 g/kg of the decoction were killed. Intravenous injection of 0.1–0.2 ml of the 50% decoction to mice resulted in immediate death (10).

CLINICAL STUDIES

1. Neurasthenia and Insomnia

<Suanzaoren> is an important drug in traditional Chinese medicine for fidget and insomnia, and mainly for palpitation and insomnia due to lack of nourishment in the heart caused by anemia and flaring up of the asthenic fire. It ca be used by itself (20) but is usually used with the sclerotium of *Poria cocos*, the kernel of *Biota orientalis*, the root of *Salvia miltiorrhiza*, the processed root of *Rehmannia glutinosa*, etc., e.g., Ziziphus jujuba Decoction. There are many reports available regarding the use of <Suanzaoren> as the chief therapeutic agent in the management of insomnia due to neurasthenia (21–24). For example, insomnia was improved in 209 cases of neurasthenia treated with Ziziphus Kernel Powder, Ziziphus Kernel-Licorice Mixture, and Compound Ziziphus Kernel Decoction (21).

2. Climacteric Syndrome

Climacteric syndrome was effectively treated with Lilium-Ziziphus Decoction and acupuncture (25).

REFERENCE

1. Hu CJ. Acta Academiae Medicinae Wuhan 1957 (1):125.

2. Tang S et al. Acta Academiae Medicinae Jilin 1959 (4):99.

3. Huang WX. Shandong Medical Journal 1957 (1):4.

4. Pharmacology Section, Shandong Institute of Traditional Chinese Medicine and Materia Medica. Studies on Traditional Chinese Medicine (Shandong Institute of Traditional Chinese Medicine and Materia Medica) 1975 (8):35.

5. Huang HP et al. Abstracts of the Symposium of the Chinese Society of Physiology (Pharmacology). 1964. p. 103.

6. Sun SX. Abstracts of the Second National Congress of the Chinese Pharmaceutical Association. Vol. 2. 1956. p. 43.

7. Shibata M et al. Journal of the Pharmaceutical Society of Japan (Tokyo) 1975 (4):465.

8. Shibata S. The Journal of the Society for Oriental Medicine in Japan 1974 25(1):1.

9. Wang JH et al. Compiled Medical Information. Xuzhou Medical College. 1961.

10. Sun K. Chinese Medical Journal 1958 44(12):1168.

11. Pharmacology and Chinese Traditional Drugs Processing Sections, Shandong Institute of Traditional Chinese Medicine and Materia Medica. Studies on Traditional Chinese Medicine (Shandong Institute of Traditional Chinese Medicine and Materia Medica) 1975 (8):47.

12. Pharmacology and Medicinal Chemistry Sections, Faculty of Chinese Materia Medica of Chengdu College of Traditional Chinese Medicine. Chengdu Zhongyi Xueyuan Xuebao (Journal of Chengdu College of Traditional Chinese Medicine) 1978 (1):61.

13. Zheng CG. Acta Academiae Medicinae Dalian 1960 (1):53.

14. Shibata M. Japan Centra Revuo Medicina 1972 285:569.

15. Internal information of Sichuan Institute of Chinese Materia Medica. 1965.

16. Liu JF et al. Acta Pharmaceutica Sinica 1962 9(11):657.

17. Feng PC et al. Journal of Pharmacy and Pharmacology 1964 16(2):115.

18. Scientific Research Group, 153rd Hospital of the Chinese PLA. People's Military Medicine 1976 (1):58.

19. Tao JY. Acta Pharmaceutica Sinica 1963 10(9):531.

20. Zhao XD et al. Chinese Pharmaceutical Bulletin 1953 (4):162.

21. Yu CZ et al. Shandong Medical Journal 1965 (9):27.

22. Sun K. Shanghai Zhongyiyao Zazhi (Shanghai Journal of Traditional Chinese Medicine) 1966 (4):156.

23. Liu HM. Shandong Medical Journal 1957 (1):1.

24. Gao DY. Barefoot Doctor (Changwei District Health Bureau, Shandong) 1976 (2):21.

25. Shan JM. New Chinese Medicine 1973 (12):626.

(Deng Wenlong)

HANCAI 蔊菜

<Hancai> is the whole plant of *Rorippa montana* (Wall.) Small or *R. indica* (L.) Hiern. (Cruciferae). The former is also known as <Ganyoucai> and the latter <Jiangjiandaocao>. The herb is pungent, "warm" and nontoxic. It is noted for its "cold"-discutient and mucolytic actions and is thought to relieve thoracic distress. It is used to treat cough with expectoration and dyspnea, fever of common cold, and pharyngolaryngitis. It is used topically for dermatitis thus and snake bites.

CHEMICAL COMPOSITION

<Hancai> mainly contains rorifone and rorifamide. It also contains 6 crystalline substances (2 neutral substances and 4 organic acids). Rorifone and rorifamide have been synthesized, and so were a few decyanated derivatives.

PHARMACOLOGY

1. Antitussive, Expectorant, and Antiasthmatic Effects

The phenol red excretion test indicated that one-fifth of the LD_{50} of rorifone given to rabbits intragastrically caused expectoration (1); the amount of phenol red excreted by mice orally given 100 mg/kg of the natural or synthetic rorifone was at least triple that in the control. However, this effect was lost when a cyanide antidote sodium thiosulfate was given concurrently (2). The intragastrically administered rorifone (natural or synthetic) 80 mg/kg produced an insignificant antitussive effect in mice with sulfur dioxide-induced cough (2). Asthma induced in guinea pigs with the aerosol of a mixture of histamine and acetylcholine was markedly suppressed by the natural or synthetic rorifone 160 mg/kg PO as evidenced by prolongation of the mean latent period of convulsion from 2 minutes to 5 minutes and 33 seconds. Nevertheless, at this point, the test animals already showed toxic reactions (2–6).

2. Antibacterial Effect

In the plate dilution experiment, rorifone at a concentration of 5 mg/ml inhibited *Diplococcus pneumoniae*, *Staphylococcus aureus*, *Hemophilus influenzae*, *Pseudomonas aeruginosa*, and *Escherichia coli* (1,5).

3. Pharmacokinetics

In mice administered with an oral dose of 72 mg/kg of ^{14}C-rorifone, the blood radioactivity peaked in 6–8 hours; the highest radioactivity between 2–24 hours was found in the gastric tissue, the lowest in the brain; radioactivity equivalent to 87% of the administered dose was excreted in urine in 24 hours, indicating rapid elimination. Paper and thin layer chromatograms of the urine of rats and rabbits orally given rorifone revealed large amounts of thiocyanates. The radioactive substance in blood and urine of mice and rats 6 hours after intragastric administration of ^{14}C-rorifore, as detected by paper chromatography, consisted of the original drug and thiocyanates. The 24-hour urine of rats after oral administration of rorifone 400 mg/kg was analyzed by silica gel thin layer chromatography, gas chromatography and infrared spectrometry. It was discovered to contain a decyanated metabolite of rorifone which resembled the synthetic rorifone degradation product 3-mesylpropanoic acid. Incubation of rat liver slices with rorifone at 37°C for 4 hours produced the detoxified product thiocyanate; this product, however, was not produced by liver homogenate, indicating that the catalyzing enzyme strictly requires an intact cellular condition (2,6).

4. Toxicity

The LD_{50} of natural rorifone in mice was 423–302 mg/kg PO and those of three batches of synthetic rorifone were 379–335, 377–271, and 427–258 mg/kg, respectively. The toxic symptoms were respiratory depression followed by stimulation and then depression again, ataxia, convulsion, and death within 24 hours. Rabbits appeared normal after an oral dose of 100 mg/kg of natural rorifone. The dose 200 mg/kg PO killed 2 of 4 rabbits and the 300 mg/kg dose killed all in 4 hours. The same pre-death symptoms as in mice were seen. With the appearance of toxic symptoms about half an hour after the LD (400 mg/kg PO) in rabbit the cyanide antidote sodium thiosulfate was promptly given intravenously; this completely restored the normal state of animals. A single oral dose of 100 mg/kg of rorifone in dogs caused mild reactions such as sedation, weakness and anorexia, which usually disappeared on the next day; a single oral dose of 200 mg/kg caused vomiting in 30 minutes and stronger reactions which also disappeared on the next day; a dose of 300 mg/kg resulted in repeated vomiting with large amounts of the administered drug vomited (2,6).

The decyanated derivative of rorifone was at least 10 times less toxic than rorifone (7). *Subacute toxicity.* Intragastric administration of 60 mg/kg of rorifone to rabbit for 10 days did not cause abnormalities on the ECG and of the gross appearance. Intragastric administration of 20 and 50 mg/kg of rorifone to separate groups of dogs for 30 days resulted in no abnormality in liver and kidney functions, blood count, ECG, and histological examinations (2,5,6,8).

CLINICAL STUDIES

Rorifone is chiefly used for treating chromic bronchitis. The daily dosage of 200–300 mg of natural or synthetic rorifone is to be given in 4 doses, for a course of 10 days. Usually, three therapeutic courses are required. In treatment of more than 300 cases, the expectorant effect was good but the antiasthmatic and anti-inflammatory effects were insignificant. Following the treatment, sputum was greatly decreased. Microscopic examination of sputum showed marked changes in acid mucopolysaccharides and DNA. The former then consisted of scattered short threads in contrast to the pretreatment thread bundles; the latter did not show increase in the percentage of fibers. There were no significant alterations in the neutrophilic, eosinophilic and collagen cells in the sputum, in the blood and urine routine examinations, liver function, and pulmonary function. Furthermore, the severity of illness had no bearing on the therapeutic effect (7–13).

ADVERSE EFFECTS

Rorifone has few side effects and no specific reactions. Only transient xerostomia and mild gastric discomfort, which did not interfere with the medication, were experienced by individual patients (2,11,12).

REFERENCE

1. Chinese Academy of Medical Sciences. Medical Research Communications 1972 (3):19.
2. Shanghai Institute of Materia Medica. Proceedings of the Symposium on the Identification of Rorifone. December 1974.
3. Shanghai Institute of Materia Medica. Chinese Traditional and Herbal Drugs Communications 1972 (4):27.
4. Shanghai Institute of Materia Medica. Chinese Medical Journal 1973 (2):73.
5. Shanghai Group for the Pharmacology of Chronic Bronchitis. Studies on the Prevention and Treatment of Chronic Bronchitis. 2nd edition. Shanghai People' s Publishing House. 1972. p. 153.
6. Shanghai Institute of Materia Medica. The Pharmacology of Rorifone (internal information). 1975.
7. Dai PX. New Medical Information (Jiangxi College of Traditional Chinese Medicine) 1973 (6):29.
8. Information Department of the Chinese Academy of Medical Sciences. Medical Research Information 1972 (3):19.
9. National Institute of Scientific and Technological Information of the People' s Republic of China. Keji Xiaoxi (Scientific and Technological News) 1974 (1):54.
10. Tang ZJ et al. Scientia Sinica 1974 (1):15.
11. Shanghai Group for the Clinical Study of Senile Chronic Bronchitis. Research Information. Shanghai Sixth People' s Hospital. 1972.
12. Shanghai Sixth People' s Hospital. Shanghai Exhibition on Achievements in Combined Western and Traditional Chinese Medicine. Shanghai Exhibition Group. 1974. p. 10.
13. Beijing Institute of Pharmaceutical Industry. Beijing Pharmaceutical Industry 1975 (2):29.

(Song Yongtian)

XIXIANCAO 豨薟草

<Xixiancao> is the whole plant of *Siegesbeckia pubescens* Makino, or *S. orientalis* L. (Compositae). The plant, *S. glabrescens* Makino, is also used medicinally. <Xixiancao> tastes bitter and has a "cold" property. It is reputed to be antirheumatic and to relieve myalgia and ostalgia.

It is a remedy for functional impairment of the liver and "kidney", limb paralysis, ostalgia, weakness of the knee, and various sores due to "damp-wind". Externally, it is used to treat pyogenic infections of the skin, and furuncle.

CHEMICAL COMPOSITION

<Xixiancao> contains 5 diterpenes including darutoside and its aglycone darutigenol, pimar-8(14)-ene-6β,15,16,18-tetraol and 16,17-dihydroxy-16β-(-)-kauranoic acid (1). It also contains alkaloids (2).

PHARMACOLOGY

1. Anti-inflammatory Effect

A 5 or 10 g/kg dose of the decoction or ethanol extract of <Xixiancao> administered to rats orally produced no significant inhibitory effect on formaldehyde- or egg white-induced paw swelling. But a pronounced effect was obtained when the young leaf and branch of *Clerodendron trichotomum* were used in combination (3) (refer to the monograph on <Chouwutong>). 16,17-Dihydroxy-16-β-(-)-kauranoic acid, recently isolated from *Siegesbeckia pubescens*, administered to rats by mouth was proved by egg white heat coagulation and rat paw swelling methods to have anti-inflammatory activity. Two analogues of this compound also had anti-inflammatory effect (1).

2. Hypotensive and Vasodilatory Effects

Intraperitoneal injection of the <Xixiancao> decoction in cats caused hypotension which started 10 minutes after medication and lasted for about 1.5 hours (4). The aqueous extract and ethanol-water extract were also active (5). Hypotension was also induced by oral administration of dihydroxykauranoic acid in renal hypertensive rats; the other diterpenes of this herb were devoid of this effect (1).

The <Xixiancao> extract dilated the blood vessels in rabbit ears with intact nerves and also blocked the vasoconstriction due to nerve stimulation. No vasodilatory response was elicited in isolated rabbit ears. Therefore, the effect is postulated to be caused by inhibition of the sympathetic vasoconstrictor nerves. The extract antagonized vasoconstriction induced by norepinephrine; hence, it did not act on the adrenergic receptors of the vascular smooth muscle (6).

CLINICAL STUDIES

1. Rheumatic Arthritis

Siegesbeckia-Clerodendron Pill (Herba Siegesbeckiae and Folium Clerodendri Trichotomi) is a famous Chinese prescription used to treat rheumatism. In 15 cases treated with an initial dose of 6–8 g, and gradually adjusted to 12–15 g, twice daily for 18 days on average, 9 cases become asymptomatic and 5 cases achieved marked improvement (7). The herb was also effective when used in combination with the stem of *Piper futokadsura*, etc. (8).

2. Hypertension

Sixty-seven cases of hypertension were treated with the concentrated decoction of <Xixiancao> 3 g and the root bark of *Lycium chinenses* 10 g divided into 2–3 doses, or with its tablet preparation 1.5 g 2–3 times a day; 35 of them (52.5%) had their diastolic blood pressure lowered by more than 20 mmHg and 22 of them (32.8%) by more than 10 mmHg. The neurotic symptoms were also improved to different extents (4).

3. Malaria

<Xixiancao> had therapeutic value in 63 cases of malaria (9). However, this may not be reliable.

ADVERSE EFFECTS

There were no known adverse effects after prolonged oral administration of this herb (4,7).

REFERENCE

1. Han KD et al. Chemical Abstracts 1976 84:130259m.
2. Fu FY et al. Abstracts of the 1956 Academic Conference of the Chinese Academy of Medical Sciences. Vol. 2. 1956. p. 70.
3. Liu GT et al. Acta Pharmaceutica Sinica 1964 11(10):708.
4. Xu W. Chinese Journal of Internal Medicine 1960 (2):115.
5. Li GC et al. Abstracts of the 1956 Academic Conference of the Chinese Academy of Medical Sciences. Vol. 2. 1956. p. 70.
6. Huang HX et al. Journal of the Bethune University of Medical Sciences 1979 (3):17.
7. Tao WG. Journal of Traditional Chinese Medicine 1957 (11):608.
8. Hu TX. Jiangxi Zhongyiyao (Jiangxi Journal of Traditional Chinese Medicine) 1955 (4):29.
9. Shuanggang Commune (Boyang County) Health Centre. New Medical Information (Jiangxi School of Pharmacy) 1972 (2):40.

(Xue Chunsheng)

CHANTUI 蟬蛻

<Chantui> is the slough of cicada or *Cryptotympana atrata* Fabricius (Cicadidae). Also known as <Chanyi>, the drug is sweetish and salty with a "cool" property. It has diaphoretic, antipruritic (by inducing the eruption of measles at the early stage of the disease) and nebula-resolving effects. Thus, it is recommended for the treatment of common cold due to pathogenic "wind-heat", aphonia due to cough, non-eruptive measles, convulsion, epilepsy, pruritus in measles, cataract and nebula.

CHEMICAL COMPOSITION

The cicada slough mainly contains keratin and amino acids. Its aqueous extract showed reactions characteristic to acids and phenolic compounds (1).

PHARMACOLOGY

1. Anticonvulsive and Sedative Effects

In rabbits with tetanin induced tetanus, oral administration of <Chantui> decoction or Wuhu Zhuifeng Powder in which this herb is the chief ingredient, whether given concurrently with the intramuscular tetanin injection or 2 days after the appearance of tetanus, delayed the death of the test animals, prolonged their mean survival period, but did not alter the mortality rate. No synergism was displayed by Wuhu Zhuifeng Powder and tetanus antitoxin used in combination. In tetanin induced seizures, intramuscular injection of the <Chantui> decoction or Wuhu Zhuifeng Powder produced a marked anticonvulsive effect which became apparent 30 minutes after medication and more prominent after 1.5 hours; the effect gradually tailed off after 5 hours. It was therefore postulated that the therapeutic effect of these two drugs for tetanus seen in clinical practice was due to their anticonvulsive action (2).

Other experiments also proved that the <Chantui> fluidextract and the <Chantui> decoction slightly delayed the death of mice injected with tetanin (3). Further studies indicated that intraperitoneal injection of Wuhu Zhuifeng Powder markedly lowered the mortality rate in mice suffering from convulsions induced by strychnine, pentylenetetrazole, cocaine, and nicotine, and also markedly antagonized the muscular tremor induced by nicotine in rabbits. It was also shown that only <Chantui>, among the ingredients of this recipe, reduced strychnine-induced mortality of mice (4). The body of the cicada slough was more potent than the head and limbs (5). Intraperitoneal injection of <Chantui> partially relieved nicotine-induced muscular tremor in rabbits. None of the ingredients of Wuhu Zhuifeng Powder could combat lethality of pentylenetetrazole (4).

These two agents also had marked sedative action; they significantly inhibited the spontaneous activity of mice, considerably prolonged anesthesia induced in mice by cyclobarbital sodium, and induced sleep in mice given subthreshold doses of pentobarbital sodium. The intraperitoneally injected dose diminished the animals' activity, produced a tranquilizing effect, reduced the tension of abdominal and extremity muscles, and dulled the righting reflex. These effects were more pronounced if the <Chantui> decoction was injected intravenously. In addition, <Chantui> was believed to have analgesic activity as it increased the reaction time of mice to heat (4,5).

2. Antipyretic Effect

At 1 g/kg PO, <Chantui> decoction produced an antipyretic effect in rabbits with fever induced by expired typhoid vaccine. In terms of potency, the head and limbs ranked first, followed by the whole slough, and then the body.

3. Miscellaneous Actions

The <Chantui> decoction injected intraarterially into anesthetized cats blocked the superior carotid sympathetic nerve ganglions as proved by the nictitating membrane contraction test, but failed to alter the pressor effect of epinephrine and the hypotensive effect of acetylcholine (4). In addition, <Chantui> selectively inhibited the growth of cancer cells without affecting normal cells *in vitro* (6).

CLINICAL STUDIES

1. Tetanus

Wuhu Zhuifeng Powder (Periostracum Cicadae 30 g, Rhizoma Arisaematis 6 g, Rhizoma Gastrodiae 6 g, Scorpio (with tails) 7 pieces, Bombyx Batryticatus 7 pieces) is Shi Chuan'en's secret recipe for tetanus. It is given orally as a decoction with 1.5 g of Cinnabar and some yellow wine (7). It was confirmed effective in many clinical trials (8–11). Convulsion was mitigated or arrested in 65 cases after 0.5–3 days of treatment with <Chantui> used as the chief agent in a regimen of combined Chinese and Western medicines. Further treatment with <Chantui> alone also yielded satisfactory results (9,12–13). Six cases were cured with the fine powder of the baked body of <Chantui> 9–15 g/dose PO together with yellow wine thrice daily (12). Some authors reported the salutary effect of <Chantui> in combination with other Chinese medicines in treating tetanus (13–15).

2. Corneal Opacity

The injection is effective for nebula either as eye drops or injected subconjunctivally (1,16). It was effective in 110 cases (125 eyes); marked effects were achieved in 60 eyes and moderated effects in

35 others; the aggregate effective rate was 76%. It is useful for visual disturbances due to corneal opacity of various causes; it is particularly effective for nebula and less so for keratoleukoma. The injection was injected under the bulbar conjunctiva once daily or on alternate days, 10 injections as one therapeutic course. The proper injection site should be beneath the bulbar conjunctiva adjacent to the corneal opacity (16). The eye drops is also effective (1). Good results were achieved from the use of Double Slough Injection, prepared from cicada and snake sloughs, in the treatment of 50 eyes; marked effects were achieved in 15 and improvement in 30 eyes (17).

3. *Allergic Skin Diseases*

<Chantui> or its compound formula were relatively effective in many kinds of allergic skin diseases such as urticaria, eczema, drug rashes, and paint allergy (18–22). For instance, more than 10 cases of urticaria were cured with <Chantui> 3 g and glutinous rice wine 50 g without any relapse (18). In 30 cases of chronic urticaria treated with honeyed pills of <Chantui> or with <Chantui> plus the fruit of *Tribulus terrestris*, 7 cases were cured, 15 had marked effect, and 5 were improved (19). In 39 cases of urticaria, eczema and drug rashes treated with the decoction of the stem of *Ephedra sinica* and cicada slough or its modification, 37 cases were cured, 1 improved, and 1 ineffective (20,21).

4. *Bell's Palsy*

Ten cases were treated with "Fengchan Powder" (<Xiongfengchan> 3 pieces and gypsum 3 g ground separately into fine powders) by mouth with hot yellow wine at bad time; 9 of them were cured (23). The modified "Qianzheng Powder" which contains <Chantui> was also effective (24).

5. *Others*

The combined use of <Chantui> and batryticated silkworm had antipyretic effect on hyperpyrexia of influenza (25). Fifty-four out of 68 cases of acute nephritis were cured by the modified Cicada-Spirodela Decoction (26). Daily oral administration of 9 g of <Chantui> was said to be effective for the treatment of cataract (27).

REFERENCE

1. Li YW. Studies on Chinese Proprietary Medicine 1980 (2):14.

2. Pharmacology Section. Acta Academiae Medicine Zhejiang 1960 3(2):89.

3. Jiangsu College of New Medicine. Encyclopedia of Chinese Materia Medica. Vol. 2. Shanghai People's Publishing House. 1977. p. 2558.

4. Pharmacology Section. Acta Academiae Medicinae Zhejiang 1960 3(2):93.

5. Pharmaceutical Department, Jintan County People's Health Centre et al. Selected Information (Jiangsu College of New Medicine) 1975 (2):104.

6. Sato A. Kampo Kenkyu 1979 (2):51.

7. Wu SZ. Journal of Traditional Chinese Medicine 1955 (10):21.

8. Qu K. Chinese Medical Journal 1956 42(10):937.

9. Yongji County (Shanxi) Health Centre. Chinese Journal of Surgery 1959 (1):15.

10. Feng LX et al. Journal of Traditional Chinese Medicine 1963 (5):15.

11. Huang BF. Mindong Yiyao (Eastern Fujian Medical Journal) 1977 (3–4):1.

12. Wanrong County (Shanxi) Health Centre. Chinese Journal of Surgery 1959 7(4):367.

13. Zheng YZ et al. Fujian Zhongyiyao (Fujian Journal of Traditional Chinese Medicine) 1963 (1):46.

14. Wang LB et al. Journal of Traditional Chinese Medicine 1964 (4):23.

15. Guan S. Xinzhongyi (Journal of New Chinese Medicine) 1981 (2):45.

16. Zhang DS. Shanxi Medical and Pharmaceutical Journal 1979 (4):60.

17. Li YZ et al. Journal of Traditional Chinese Medicine 1980 (6):36.

18. Liu JZ. Xinzhongyi (Journal of New Chinese Medicine) 1980 (4):43.

19. Jiangsu Institure of Dermatology. Dermatological Research Communications 1972 (3):215.

20. Xia ZF. Chinese Medical Journal 1956 42(10):939.

21. Wang JY. Journal of Traditional Chinese Medicine 1964 (7):7.

22. Qin LF. Shanghai Zhongyiyao Zazhi (Shanghai Journal of Traditional Chinese Medicine) 1979 (6):43.

23. Yao ZC et al. Barefoot Doctor (Changwei District Institure of Medical Sciences, Shandong) 1977 (4):27.

24. Weng WJ et al. Zhenjiang Journal of Traditional Chinese Medicine 1964 (6):17.

25. Wei KB. Zhenjiang Zhongyi Xueyuan Tongxun (Communications of Zhejiang College of Traditional Chinese Medicine) 1977 (4):30.

26. Xu YC. Liaoning Zhongji Yikan (Liaoning Journal of Paramedics) 1980 (8):7.

27. Ophthalmology Department, Luda First People's Hospital. Yiyao Yisheng (Medical Doctor) (Luda Health Bureau) 1976 (6):48.

(Deng Wenlong)

XIONGDAN 熊膽

<Xiongdan> is the dried gallbladder with bile of bear *Selenarctos thibetanus* Curvier or *Ursus arctos* L. (Ursidae). It tastes bitter and has a "cold" property. It is latent-heat-clearing, antipyretic, hepatic-depressant and vision-improving. The drug is used for convulsion, and externally, for acute conjunctivitis and pharyngolaryngitis.

CHEMICAL COMPOSITION

The bile contains mainly of ursodeoxycholic acid and less of chenodeoxycholic acid, deoxycholic acid and cholic acid. They are mostly conjugated form), and the amount of free bile acids is minute. The bile also contains cholesterol, bilirubin and inorganic salts (1).

PHARMACOLOGY

1. Cholagogic and Choleretic Effects

The chief pharmacological action of the bile salts is promotion of bile secretion. In experiment with anesthetized rabbits, intravenous injection of the aqueous solution of the bear bile significantly increased the amount of bile secreted (2). Oral administration of chenodeoxycholic acid in monkeys greatly increased the secretion of bile and bile salts (3). Secretion of bile and bile salts was also increased in anesthetized dogs and dogs with biliary fistula by intravenous injection of ursodeoxycholic acid and chenodeoxycholic acid (4). In addition, the bile acid perfused into the pig liver markedly increased bile secretion (5).

Studies on the common bile duct with intact Oddi's sphincter showed that various bile salts at concentration of 10^{-4} relaxed the common bile duct and sphincter muscle. The potencies in decreasing ·· were sodium deoxycholate > sodium chenodeoxycholate > sodium ursodeoxycholate > sodium ·odium taurocholate > sodium glycinocholate. The passage of bile into duodenum in · was probably facilitated by this relaxant effect (6).

ng Effect

l that the 5% sodium deoxycholate solution dissolved the human gallstones '7). Experiments in monkeys indicated that chenodeoxycholic acid increased l lecithin to cholesterol in bile, increased the dissolving power of bile for e biosynthesis of cholesterol, and increased the bile secretion. Through leoxycholic acid dissolved gallstones and reduced their formation (3).

Cholecystography of cholelithic patients orally treated with chenodeoxycholic acid confirmed that the drug has stone-dissolving activity (3,8). It was also reported that ursodeoxycholic acid has stone-dissolving activity in patients with cholelithiasis (9).

3. Effect on Gastrointestinal Motility

The 5×10^{-5} solution of the bear bile powder had spasmolytic action on acetylcholine-induced spasm of the isolated mouse small intestine. In studies using the same method to evaluate the spasmolytic potency of the various bile salts in terms of ID_{50} (half inhibitory dose), it was found that sodium deoxycholate > sodium ursodeoxycholate > sodium taurodeoxycholate > sodium chenodeoxycholate > sodium cholate. Experimental analysis revealed that their spasmolytic mechanisms resembled that of papaverine (10). The bile salts of <Xiongdan> relaxed the isolated common bile duct and Oddi's sphincter but not gallbladder strips of pigs (6). In these experiments on isolated smooth muscles, it was also found that the spasmolytic effect of the bile salts was weakened to different degrees when they were conjugated with taurine or glycine (6,10). Application of cholic acid, deoxycholic acid, or other bile acids to the mucosa of isolated guinea pig ileum and colon caused intestinal peristalsis at low dosages and spasm at higher dosages (11). The bile salts applied to the mucosal surface of isolated and *in situ* stomach, small and large intestines of rabbits increased their motility, but when applied to the serosa caused inhibition (12). Refer to the monograph on <Zhudan> for the action of the bile salts on digestion.

4. Effect on the Heart

The 0.1% aqueous solution of <Xiongdan> increased the myocardial tone and slightly increased the contraction amplitude of the isolated frog or toad heart; concentrations of 2.5% and above caused cardiac inhibition or initial transient stimulation followed by inhibition and, lastly, cardiac arrest at the diastolic phase (13). The cholic acid and calcium cholate at 10^{-3} stimulated the isolated toad heart, whereas the same concentration of deoxycholic acid and its sodium and calcium salts, chenodeoxycholic acid, sodium taurocholate, sodium taurodeoxycholate, and bilirubin caused marked cardiac inhibition (14). Low concentration (3.33×10^{-5}) of calcium cholate stimulated the isolated guinea pig heart and slightly decreased the coronary flow (15).

5. Hypotensive Effect

Calcium cholate at 3.2×10^{-4} and calcium deoxycholate at 3.1×10^{-4} dilated the blood vessels in isolated rabbit ear; the effect of the former was more prominent. When injected to anesthetized rabbits at 5 mg/kg IV, both cholic acid and sodium taurocholate caused mild hypertension, whereas taurodeoxycholic acid produced no significant effect. On the other hand, calcium cholate, deoxycholic acid and its sodium and calcium salts, chenodeoxycholic acid, and bilirubin caused different degrees of hypotension; this effect generally lasted a few minutes. Calcium cholate and calcium deoxycholate definitely antagonized epinephrine-induced hypertension (14). In case of unanesthetized rats having idiopathic hypertension, oral administration of calcium cholate 100 mg/kg lowered the caudal arterial blood pressure by 50 mmHg for 3–4 days (15). Calcium cholate and calcium deoxycholate also caused hypotension in unanesthetized normal rats (14).

6. Antidotic Effect

Sodium ursodeoxycholate 200 mg/kg injected subcutaneously to mice caused elevation of the LD_{50} of strychnine nitrate by 2.7-fold, indicating a marked detoxifying effect. The effect was potentiated by sodium ursodeoxycholate, sodium chenodeoxycholate and sodium cholate (16).

7. Miscellaneous Actions

The chenodeoxycholic acid, cholic acid and deoxycholic acid possessed bacteriostatic, anti-inflammatory, antiallergic, antitussive, expectorant, antiasthmatic, and digestant actions, all described under the monograph of <Zhudan>. For the sedative, anticonvulsant and antipyretic actions of <Xiongdan>, refer to <Niuhuang>.

8. Toxicity

The bile salts of the bear bile are low in toxicity. The LD_{50} of sodium ursodeoxycholate and sodium chenodeoxycholate in mice were determined to be 1250 and 961 mg/kg SC, respectively (16). No death occurred in monkeys given chenodeoxycholic acid 10–100 mg/kg PO daily for one month, though the animals in high-dose group had diarrhea and slight decrease in body weight. The following laboratory findings in all cases were within the normal range: blood count, blood urea nitrogen, plasma albumin, SGOT, and lactic dehydrogenase. Liver biopsy showed no significant abnormality. The long-term toxicity experiment with chenodeoxycholic acid indicated liver damage due to 6 months' continuous medication (3,17). A report claimed that administration of chenodeoxycholic acid to pregnant monkeys caused hepatic, renal, and adrenocortical damages in the animals' fetuses (3). The toxicities of cholic acid and deoxycholic acid may be found in the monograph on <Niuhuang>.

CLINICAL STUDIES

1. Biliary Tract Diseases

A decoction of bear bile decocted with the root tuber and rhizome of *Curcuma longa* and the young shoot of *Artemisia capillaris* was effective for cholelithiasis, biliary tract infection and jaundice

(18). Chenodeoxycholic acid has been successfully synthesized and can be used for cholesterol cholelithiasis. According to foreign reports, stones were passed or diminished in 93 out of 234 cases treated with 0.75–1 g of chenodeoxycholic acid daily divided in 3–4 doses for a course of 3–18 months, as revealed by cholecystography; the effective rate being 39.7% (3,19). Chenodeoxycholic acid was tried in 36 cases in China at daily doses of 0.25 g on an empty stomach in early morning for a course of 6–12 months; for some cases livonal was given additionally. Repeated cholecystography of 22 of these cases showed stone dissolution in 10 cases (45.4%) (8). Another paper reported that 17 cases (47.2%) out of 36 cases were effectively treated with 0.1–2.0 g of ursodeoxycholic acid daily for a course of 4–24 months (9).

2. Acute Renal Hypertension

The dry powder of bile 0.5 g was given twice daily to 5 children of schooling age with acute renal hypertension; 4 of them obtained excellent results, with their blood pressure restored to normal level in a mean of 4–5 days (20).

3. Eye Diseases

Comparatively good therapeutic effects were achieved by subconjunctival injection of the 20% bear bile injection 0.2 ml/dose in treating lens opacity, fundal hemorrhage, and optic neuritis. Better effects were reportedly attained in treating corneal nebula with Bear Bile-Musk Injection, prepared from bear bile and a small amount of musk (21).

4. Miscellaneous

Bear bile had been traditionally used by Chinese herbalists to treat acute infantile convulsion, coma due to trauma, and neurotic stomachache. Bear bile mixed well with borneol and pig bile can be applied locally to treat toothache due to dental caries, and hemorrhoid (18). Bear Bile-Musk Pill can be used to treat infantile malnutrition.

ADVERSE EFFECTS

Bear bile had a low toxicity. Due to its fishy and bitter taste that may induce vomiting, the bear bile should be given as capsules (20). The bear bile injection is irritating and so may cause pain when injected subconjunctivally; it should be injected after anesthesia with 2% tetracaine (21). No significant toxic effects occurred with the therapeutic doses of chenodeoxycholic acid. A common side effect is diarrhea. A few patients may develop gastric upset. Based on toxicity studies on animals, chenodeoxycholic acid should be contraindicated in pregnant women and in patients with acute and chronic liver diseases. It is also contraindicated in those with functional disturbances of intestines (3,8).

REFERENCE

1. Scientific and Technological Information Room, Shenyang College of Pharmacy. Basic Studies and Uses of Bile — A Chinese Traditional Drug. Shenyang College of Pharmacy. 1973.

2. Sato K. Journal of Kyoto Prefectural University of Medicine 1935 13:676.

3. Hu KJ. References on Medicine Abroad — Pharmacy (Hunan Institure of Medical and Pharmaceutical Industry) 1977 (3):173.

4. Yanagiura S. Folia Pharmacologica Japonica 1976 72:689.

5. Lu SZ. Information of Foreign Research on Chinese Materia Medica (Hunan Institute of Medical and Pharmaceutical Industry) 1975 (6):18.

6. Kimura M. Journal of the Pharmaceutical Society of Japan (Tokyo) 1967 87(5):550.

7. Acute Abdomen Research Unit, Zunyi Medical College. Communications on Combined Western and Traditional Chinese Therapy of Acute Abdomen 1977 (2):49.

8. Acute Abdomen Research Unit, Anhui Medical College. Communications on Combined Western and Traditional Chinese Therapy of Acute Abdomen 1977 (2):29.

9. Chen C. References on Medicien Abroad — Surgery 1977 (2):93.

10. Kimura M et al. Journal of the Pharmaceutical Society of Japan (Tokyo) 1967 87(7):801.

11. Meyer AE et al. Chemical Abstracts 1948 42:8311d.

12. Sasaki K. Chemical Abstracts 1955 49:11142.

13. Wu TK. Collections of Research Information. 2nd edition. Sichuan Institure of Chinese Materia Medica. 1959. p. 78.

14. Iwaki R et al. Folia Pharmacologica Japonica 1964 60(6):529.

15. Iwaki R et al. Journal of the Pharmaceutical Society of Japan (Tokyo) 1965 85(10):899.

16. Kuboki N et al. Yakugaku Kenkyu 1959 31(6):65.

17. Dyrszka H et al. Gastroenterology 1975 69:333.

18. Lin LH. Medicinal Animals of Guangxi. Guangxi People' s Publishing House. 1976. p. 255.

19. Editorial Department. Communications on Combined Western and Traditional Chinese Therapy of Acute Abdomen 1977 (2):38.

20. Ren BJ. Harbin Zhongyi (Harbin Journal of Traditional Chinese Medicine) 1959 2(16):4.

21. Pharmacy of Xi' an Fourth Hospital. Chinese Pharmaceutical Bulletin 1959 7(3):122.

(Duan Meifen and Liu Wenqing)

HUJISHENG 槲寄生

<Hujisheng> refers to the whole plant of *Viscum coloratum* (Kom.) Nakai., *V. coloratum* (Kom.) Nakai f. *lutescens* Kitag., *V. coloratum* (Kom.) Nakai f. *rubroaurantiacum* Kitag., or *V. album* L. (Loranthaceae). Bitter and "mild", the herb is antirheumatic, liver- and "kidney"-tonifying, and muscle- and bone-fortifying. It is a remedy for rheumatism, soreness and weakness of the lumbar and knee, and for abnormal fetal movements. It is also used as a substitute for the herb <Sangjisheng>, yet the drug differ chemically.

CHEMICAL COMPOSITION

<Hujisheng> contains oleanolic acid, β-amyrin, mesoinositol, flavonoids, lupeol and β-sitosterol. *V. album* contains proteins, lipids, polysaccharides, visotoxin, vescerin, α-viscol, β-viscol, oleanolic acid, ursolic acid, alkaloids, choline, acetylcholine, propanylcholine, butyric acid, and pinitol.

PHARMACOLOGY

1. Effect on the Cardiovascular System

The 10% solution of the ethanol extract of the fresh leaf of *Viscum coloratum* f. *lutescens* in normal saline (equivalent to 0.83 g of the crude drug per ml) injected to dogs or rabbits at 1 ml/kg IV decreased the blood pressure by a mean of 32% for 3 minutes. The hypotensive effect of the solution at 5 ml/kg lasted more than 1 hour (1). *V. album* also has hypotensive action (2). The hypotensive effect of *V. coloratum* and *V. album* was thought due to a multiple of substances contained in these herbs; the mechanism of action, however, is still unknown. It may be due to inhibition of the medullary vasomotor center or of the interoceptors of the circulatory system which causes feedback inhibition of the vasomotor center. Some workers believed that the aqueous extract of *V. album* had cholinergic hypotensive feature (1–3). The hypotensive action of <Hujisheng> was greatly enhanced when used with the fruit of *Crataegus pinnatifida*, garlic, and the leaf of *Clerodendron trichotomum* (4).

2. Antineoplastic Effect

The chief constituents of *V. album* proteins, polysaccharides, and lipids can directly inhibit tumor cells. Both *in vivo* and *in vitro* studies indicated that the <Hujisheng> protein has a special antineoplastic action not possessed by other cell inhibitors. The solution of *V. album* extract also promoted specific and nonspecific immunologic functions (5).

CLINICAL STUDIES

1. Hypertension

No significant hypotensive effect was observed in 100 cases of hypertension treated with the 20% <Hujisheng> tincture, 20–40 drops 2–3 times a day, although subjective symptoms were improved in most patients with no attendant side effects (3). Other authors believed that *V. album* can regulate the blood pressure and therefore had therapeutic value for both hypertension and hypotension (2).

2. Cancer

Satisfactory results have been obtained in recent years with <Hujisheng> preparations used to treat cancer. Marked therapeutic effects were obtained with a preparation of the whole plant of *V. album*, Iscador, in preventing postoperative relapse as well as in treating advanced cancer (5). The regimens were described as follows.

Cancer patients were injected with Iscador before operation for a few weeks, and preventive treatment with the same agent started soon after operation for several years. The interval between therapeutic courses was gradually increased. Iscador increased the 5-year postoperative survival rate of patients with gastric cancer, even of advanced cases with metastasis to the lymph nodes. The 5-year postoperative survival rate of patients with colon cancer was also greatly increased. Comparing 37 cases treated with Iscador postoperatively with 41 control cases, it was found that 15 treatment patients were still alive 6–8 years after the operation, whereas only 6 control patients were alive for the same period. The average survival period of the dead Iscador-treated patients was 22.8 months in contrast to 6.1 months of the control. In malignant pleural effusion, several treatments with the 5% Iscador injection 1.0 ml following each thoracentesis caused rapid resorption of the effusion and disappearance of cancer cells. Comparison of 319 Iscador-treated and 253 control cases of breast cancer showed the 5-year therapeutic effect of Iscador was comparable to the best results reported in literature, and a 10-year therapeutic effect better than the average results in the past. In inoperable advanced cancer cases, Iscador at least prolonged the patients' survival, improved the symptoms, caused remission, and greatly relieved pain. In patients with good general condition and not too large tumor mass this drug often arrested or slowed down tumor growth, allowing the patients to survive despite bearing cancer. In 32 cases of III stage ovarian cancer with extensive metastasis to the abdominal organs treated with Iscador and 17 cases treated with Cytoval, 7 cases of the former group survived for 3 years with an average survival period of 23 months, whereas only 3 cases of the latter group survived for one year with an average survival period of 8 months. Iscador also greatly prolonged the live of patients with inoperable advanced rectal cancer. In 20% percent of patients with cancer of the urinary bladder, the drug reduced the tumor diameter by 25–100% and in some cases changed the cancer cells benign. A similar phenomenon was seen in treating colon cancer.

REFERENCE

1. Zhu Y. Pharmacology and Applications of Chinese Medicinal Materials. People's Medical Publishing House. 1954. p. 160.

2. Petkov V. The American Journal of Chinese Medicine 1979 7(3):197.

3. Zhang CS. Modern Research on Chinese Materia Medica. Chinese Scientific Books and Instruments Company. 1954. p. 63.

4. Zou TF. Acta Academiae Medicine Shandong 1957 (1):14.

5. Lerol R. British Homeopathic Journal 1978 (3):167; Guowai Yixue (Medicine Abroad — Traditional Chinese Medicine and Materia Medica 1979 (2):35.

(Huang Heng)

HECAOYA 鹤草芽

<Hecaoya> refers to the winter bud of *Agrimonia pilosa* Ledeb. var. *japonica* (Miq.) Nakai. (Rosaceae). It is an anthelmintic used for taeniasis.

CHEMICAL COMPOSITION

The drug contains the phenolic substance agrimophol.

PHARMACOLOGY

1. Parasiticidal Effect

1.1 *Taeniacidal effect.* The underground winter bud and the root of *A. pilosa* are lethal to tapeworms and bladder worms. Agrimophol, the active component, acted chiefly on the head but also on neck proglottides (1–2). Agrimophol was shown to be lethal to isolated *Cysticercus cellulosae*, young *Taenia solium, Moniezia expansa, Diphyllobothrium latum*, and *Taenia serrata* of dogs. A taeniacidal effect was also achieved by agrimophol used in rats with experimental infection of *Hymenolepis nana*. It was more potent against adult worms than against larvae and cysticerci. Compared to bithionol, this drug has a lower toxicity, quicker action, and is more potent. Its effect is characterized by rapid paralysis of the suckers of the tapeworm, rapid contraction and spastic paralysis of the worm body, causing expulsion of the worm out of the host. Experiments showed that agrimophol inhibited glycogenolysis of the worm, markedly inhibited the aerobic and anaerobic respiration and markedly inhibited the formation of the cellular metabolic product, succinic acid. Since succinic acid is closely related to the formation of ATP, the energy source for worm motility, the taeniacidal mechanism of agrimophol may therefore be attributed to the marked and sustained inhibition of the metabolism of worm body cells, thus cutting off the energy supply required for the maintenance of life (2,3).

1.2 *Schistosomicidal Effect.* Agrimophol not only promoted the migration of schistosomes towards the liver of the host, but also killed adult worms. However, the therapeutic effect of agrimophol was reported to be unsatisfactory; but it could be greatly potentiated if small doses of niridazole were used concurrently. Thus, in infected dogs treated with this combination, the female worms were reduced by 98–100% (4).

Agrimophol significantly decreased the glycogen content of the worm body, but the level was rapidly restored after discontinuation of medication. It increased the RNA content of the worm body initially but rapidly decreased it afterwards. It also decreased DNA and protein contents to a certain extent (5).

1.3 *Antimalarial effect*. The crude agrimophol given to rats intragastrically was active against *Plasmodium berghei*, the ED_{50} being 34 g (crude drug)/kg; it also markedly inhibited *Plasmodium inui* (6).

1.4 *Ascaricidal effect*. Agrimophol had a prolonged stimulant effect on the isolated ascarides of pigs (2).

2. Pharmacokinetics

The intragastrically administered suspension of agrimophol was very slowly absorbed in rats; 58.2% still remained in the gastrointestinal tract 12 hours after ingestion. The alkaline solution of agrimophol was twice as easily absorbed as the suspension. After absorption it was distributed in various tissues, predominantly in the liver and least in the brain. The drug was mainly excreted into bile and more slowly into urine. Peak excretion occurred 4–12 hours after medication. Incubation of rat liver slices revealed that the hepatic metabolism of this drug was greatly enhanced in the presence of oxygen. Agrimophol was also rapidly transformed in mice with a half-life of 54 minutes (7).

3. Toxicity

The LD_{50} of agrimophol was 435±88 mg/kg PO in mice. Repeated oral administration of this drug 120–150 mg/kg in rabbits resulted in reduction of food intake, watery stool, prostration and death. Administration of agrimophol 10–15 mg/kg/day PO to dogs with schistosomiasis resulted in anorexia, vomiting and watery diarrhea. One dog of the 15 mg/kg group developed mydriasis and lost the light reflex 4–5 days after treatment, and another dog died after one dose. Similar toxic reactions were seen in three rhesus monkeys treated with agrimophol preparation starting from 25 mg/kg/day with daily increment for 20, 22, and 25 days, respectively. No vision abnormality or alteration of light reflex occurred (4).

Agrimophol caused elevation of GPT in some dogs, which returned to normal levels one month after discontinuation of the treatment. There was no effect on the renal function. Some of these dogs and monkeys developed bradycardia and T wave inversion (4).

CLINICAL STUDIES

Taeniasis

In 275 cases of taeniasis (236 cases infected with *Taenia solium*, 37 with *Taenia saginata*, and 2 with *Hymenolepis nana*) treated with the powdered winter bud, its extract or agrimophol, an aggregate cure rate of 94.5% was achieved; 5.5% relapsed (1,8).

ADVERSE EFFECTS

Some patients developed nausea and vomiting (8).

REFERENCE

1. Shenyang College of Traditional Chinese Medicine et al. Chinese Traditional and Herbal Drugs Communications 1972 (1):34.

2. Shenyang Institute of Materia Medica et al. Journal of Shenyang College of Pharmacy 1975 (1):19.

3. Feng YS et al. Chinese Traditional and Herbal Drugs Communications 1978 (1):32.

4. Wang GF et al. Acta Pharmaceutica Sinica 1979 14(6):379.

5. Pan XQ et al. Chinese Traditional and Herbal Drugs Communications 1979 (5):29.

6. Shanghai Institute of Materia Medica et al. Brief summary of the antimalarial study of Agrimonia pilosa var. japonica. 1972.

7. Pharmacology Department, Shenyang College of Pharmacy. Journal of Shenyang College of Pharmacy 1975 (1):58.

8. Fushun Fourth Hospital. Chinese Medical Journal 1974 50(6):344.

(Chen Quansheng)

JIANGCAN AND JIANGYONG 殭蠶與殭蛹

<Jiangcan> refers to the dried larva of silkworm *Bombyx mori* L. (Bombycidae) infected with *Beauveria bassiana* (Bals.) Vuill. Also known as <Baijiangcan>, it is pungent, salty and has a "mild" property. It is anticonvulsant, mucolytic, and discutient. It is reported to be useful in laryngitis, tuberculosis, lymph node tuberculosis, infantile convulsion and night crying, various sores and scars, wind rash and erysipelas. <Jiangyong> is the silkworm pupa artificially infected with *B. bassiana* (1), which in recent years had been used clinically as a substitute for <Jiangcan>.

CHEMICAL COMPOSITION

The white powder of the dried larva contains ammonium oxalate, proteins and fat.
The cultured *B. bassiana* can produce pyridine-2,6-dicarboxylic acid and large quantities of oxalic acid and fat.

PHARMACOLOGY

1. Hypnotic and Anticonvulsant Effects

Hypnotic effect was achieved with the ethanol-water extract of <Jiangcan> either injected subcutaneously, intraperitoneally or administered orally to albino mice, or injected intravenously to rabbits. At 2.5 g/kg PO or 0.25 g/kg SC in mice, the extract produced a hypnotic effect similar to that of phenobarbital 50 mg/kg SC (2). Intragastric administration of the <Jiangcan> decoction (1:1) 30 g/kg, or <Jiangyong> decoction 20 g/kg, or Wuhu Zhuifeng Powder (Bombyx Batryticatus, Periostracum Cicadae, etc.) increased the mortality of mice with strychnine-induced convulsion (3–5). <Jiangyong> was even more potent than <Jiancan> (3). However, they did not significantly antagonize convulsion induced by electric shock, pentylenetetrazole and caffeine (4). The antagonistic effect of the <Jiangcan> or <Jiangyong> decoction against convulsion induced by strychnine was lost if ammonium oxalate was removed. The reason why <Jiangyong> was more potent than <Jiangcan> is because the former contains more ammonium oxalate than the latter. Ammonium oxalate is therefore believed to be the active principle for antagonizing strychnine-induced convulsion (4).

2. Miscellaneous Actions

In vitro studies showed that <Jiangcan> and <Jiangyong> have weak activity against *Staphylococcus aureus*, *Escherichia coli*, and *Pseudomonas aeruginosa*. In antineoplastic experiments, daily intragastric administration of 20% and 50% <Jiangyong> decoction 0.2 ml/mouse/day starting 24 hours after inoculation of sarcoma 180 inhibited the tumor growth, but the animals had lost weight (3).

3. Toxicity

No toxic reactions were observed after injection of the ethanol extract of <Jiangcan> 0.5–5 g/kg IP to mice and rats (6). The LD_{50} of the <Jiangyong> decoction was 44.5±1.4 g/kg PO mice. The 35 g/kg-dose produced toxic symptoms in animals manifested as gradual reduction of activity, lying down and remain quiet, and in some animals cyanosis (7). After oral administration of <Jiangyong> 2 g/kg (equivalent to 10 times the adult dose) daily for 22 days in mice, autopsy revealed no abnormalities of the liver, kidneys, and spleen (3).

CLINICAL STUDIES

1. Epilepsy

One hundred cases of epilepsy, in which 46 were primary and 54 symptomatic, were treated with the defatted-<Jiangyong> tablet (Type 718-II); 26 of them no longer had seizure after treatment and 51 cases had fever or milder attacks; the effective rate was 77%. *Dosage and administration*: The 718-II Tablet 0.9–1.5 g thrice daily, adequately reduced in children (8). Another report stated that 64 (73.5%) out of 87 cases of epilepsy were effectively treated with ammonium oxalate tablet (Type 718-III) alone (9). Thus, the defatted <Jiangyong> tablet and ammonium oxalate tablet had similar therapeutic effect.

2. Relieve Infantile Convulsion

The herb(s) had been used with scorpion, centipede, etc. to treat tetanus, and acute and chronic infantile convulsion. It was also used with hook-bearing twigs of *Uncaria rhynchophylla*, pearl powder, etc. as in "Wuhu Zhuifeng Powder" and Silkworm-Pearl Sedative Decoction, which are well-known prescriptions for children (10).

3. Upper Respiratory Tract Infections

In 37 cases treated with the <Jiangyong> tablet, the body temperature mostly descended in 1–2 days and the longest in 4 days. In 8 of them with rather severe pharyngitis, throat swelling and pain disappeared after 2 days of medication. Seventy of 94 cases of chronic bronchitis experienced alleviation of cough and thinning of sputum, yet the long-term therapeutic effect was not as good (3).

4. Diabetes Mellitus

In 27 cases of diabetes millitus of 1 week to 30 years' course treated with <Jiangcan>, 24 cases had remission of symptoms, 9 cases became negative for glucosuria and 1 case had glucosuria improved. More satisfactory results were achieved in mild and moderately severe patients who responded poorly to diet therapy than in severe patients (11).

5. Hypercholesterolemia

The herb(s) was tried in 25 cases of arteriosclerotic heart disease, hypertension, and fatty liver with elevated serum cholesterol levels; 14 of them had reduction in cholesterol level after 20–30 days of medication; β-lipoprotein was shown by turbidimetry to be decreased and α and β-lipoproteins were also decreased as shown by electrophoresis (3).

6. Miscellaneous

In 51 cases of mumps treated with a 7-day course of <Jiangyong> tablet, 43 cases responded. Generally, fever subsided in 1–2 days and swelling disappeared in 2–3 days (3). It had also been used in epidemic encephalitis B, sequelae of encephalitis, enuresis, urticaria, nephritis and hematuria, cervical lymphadenitis (3), and chronic liver diseases (12). <Jiangcan> was often used in combination with drugs having "heat-clearing and detoxicant" actions such as the fruit of *Forsythia suspensa*, the root of *Isatis tinctoria* and the root of *Scutellaria baicalensis* to treat furuncles and carbuncles (10).

ADVERSE EFFECTS

A minority of patients may experience xerostomia, nausea, impairment of appetite, and lassitude after administration of <Jiangyong>.

REFERENCE

1. Bombyx mori Section, Institute of Zoology of the Chinese Academy of Sciences. Dongwu Liyong Yu Fangzhi (Uses and Health Care of Animals) 1972 (5):15.

2. Neurology and Psychiatry Section, Dalian Medical College. Acta Academiae Medicinae Dalian 1961 2(2):26.

3. Institute of Zoology, Chinese Academy of Science et al. Chinese Traditional and Herbal Drugs Communications 1972 (6):5.

4. Neurology Section of the Pharmacology and Phytochemistry Department, Institute of Materia Medica of the Chinese Academy of Medical Sciences. Chinese Traditional and Herbal Drugs Communications 1978 (12):24.

5. Shan PN et al. Acta Academiae Medicinae Zhejiang 1959 3(2):93.

6. Siddiqui HH. The Indian Journal of Pharmacy 1962 24(8):183.

7. Institute of Materia Medica, Chinese Academy of Medical Sciences. Preliminary Studies of the Pharmacological Actions and Active Components of Jiangcan and Jiangyong (Bombyx mori). Chinese Academy of Medical Sciences. October 1974.

8. Chen JJ. Jiangsu Yiyao (Jiangsu Medical Journal) 1976 (2):3.

9. Internal Medicine Department, Friendship Hospital of Beijing et al. Internal information.

10. Zhongshan Medical College. Clinical Applications of Chinese Traditional Drugs. 1975. p. 477.

11. Ward of Combined Western and Traditional Chinese Medicine, Internal Medicine Department of Wuxi First People' s Hospital. Wuxi Yiyao(Wuxi Medical Journal) — Special Issue on Combined Western and Traditional Chinese Medicine 1976 (12):29.

12. Shanghai Coordinating Research Group on Hepatitis. Chinese Traditional and Herbal Drugs Communications 1976 (2):32.

(Yuan Wei)

YIYIREN AND YIYIGEN 薏苡仁與薏苡根

The kernel of *Coix lachryma-jobi* L. var. *ma-yuen* Stapf (C. *lachryma-jobi* L. var. *frumentacea* Makino) (Gramineae) is the Chinese herb <Yiyiren>, also known as <Yiyimi>. The root of the plant is also used as medicine. <Yiyiren> has a sweet and bland taste and a slightly "cold" property. It is spleen-invigorative, diuretic, and pus-discharging. It is used for diarrhea due to "splenic" asthenia, myalgia, ostalgia, arthralgia, edema, leukorrhea, pulmonary abscess, and intestinal abscess (*such as acute appendicitis).

CHEMICAL COMPOSITION

<Yiyiren> contains 4.65% of fixed oil which contains coixenolide and coixol. The root contains fixed oil, coixol, stigmasterol, β-sitosterol, and γ-sitosterol.

PHARMACOLOGY

1.Antineoplastic Effect

Intraperitoneal injection of the ethanol extract of <Yiyiren> to mice inhibited Ehrlich ascites carcinoma and prolonged the survival period of the test animals (1). Two components which inhibited Ehrlich ascites carcinoma cells of mice were isolated from the ethanol extract; one of them caused degenerative changes of plasma and the other stopped the nuclear division at metaphase (1,2). A small dose of this extract was tried in the case of cancerous peritonitis; the ascitic fluid aspirated 24 hours later showed marked degenerative changes in the protoplasm of cancer cells (1). Ehrlich ascites carcinoma in mice was also inhibited by the acetone extract of this herb. The test animals survived after daily intraperitoneal injection of 10.3 mg/day/animal. The ethyl acetate and chloroform extracts were less potent, and the petroleum ether, ether, and methanol extracts were inactive (3). Other reports stated that the acetone extract of the herb markedly inhibited cervical cancer U_{14} and HCA solid tumor of mice (4,5). The antineoplastic constituent isolated from the acetone extract was proved to be coixenolide (3,5).

2. Effect on Skeletal Muscle

The contraction amplitude of neuromuscular specimens of the frog hind limb continuously stimulated by electricity was found to be smaller after treatment with the <Yiyiren> oil, in comparison to the control. Moreover, the muscles were easily tired; hence, <Yiyiren> inhibits muscular contraction.

Further studies proved that it acts on the muscle fiber and not the neuromuscular junction (6). In order to elucidate the active constituents of this oil, emulsions of the acetate of various fatty acids were prepared and studied by the same methods for their blocking effect on muscle contraction. The results showed that all saturated fatty acids containing 10–18 carbon atoms inhibited muscular contraction and those with less carbon atoms were more potent, whereas the unsaturated fatty acids were inactive. These results suggest that the inhibitory effect of <Yiyiren> oil on muscular contraction was related to the saturated fatty acids (8).

Coixol also markedly inhibited contraction of the frog muscles (7). In experiments with rat diaphragms, coixol lowered the oxygen uptake of the diaphragm muscle and inhibited glycolysis. ATP-induced contraction of myosin isolated from the homogenate of rabbit psoas muscle in capillary glass tubes was inhibited by coixol (7).

3. Effect on the CNS

Coixol has the following central effects:

3.1 *Sedation*. Injection of coixol 100 mg/kg IV to mice reduced the animals' spontaneous activity. When injected at 20 mg/kg IV to rabbits, it caused high-amplitude slow waves on the EEG, denoting cortical depression.

3.2 *Inhibition of polysynaptic reflex*: Injection of coixol 5 mg/kg IV to anesthetized cats inhibited the contraction of gastrocnemius muscle induced by electrical stimulation of the contralateral afferent sciatic nerve.

3.3 *Hypothermia and antipyretic action*: Injection of coixol 50–100 mg/kg IP in rats decreased the normal body temperature; it also had antipyretic effect against experimental fever in rats.

3.4 *Analgesia*. A pronounced analgesic effect was exhibited in mice (electrical stimulation method) and rats (radiation heat method) by coixol at 100 mg/kg IP (7). The aqueous extract of the kernel, stem and leaf, or root of *Coix lachryma-jobi* also exhibited analgesic activity in mice (hot plate method) (8).

4. Cardiovascular Effect

<Yiyiren> oil at low concentrations stimulated the hearts of isolated frogs and guinea pigs, while at high concentrations it inhibited them (9). Coixol inhibited the isolated toad heart, decreasing its contraction amplitute and rate (7). <Yiyiren> oil at low concentrations caused contraction and at high concentrations caused dilation of the blood vessels of isolated rabbit ear (9), but coixol had no significant effect (7). Anesthetized rabbits intravenously injected with <Yiyiren> oil or coixol developed transient hypotension accompanied by respiratory stimulation (7,9).

5. Miscellaneous Actions

Low doses of the <Yiyiren> oil stimulated the isolated rabbit small intestine while high doses had an early-phase stimulant effect followed by a late-phase inhibitory effect (9). Coixol inhibited both the *in situ* and isolated small intestines of rabbits (7). The <Yiyiren> oil increased the tonicity and contraction amplitude of isolated uteri of rabbits and guinea pig uteri (9). The <Yiyiren> oil and coixol were also shown to have a weak hypoglycemic action in rabbits (6,7). The oil also decreased, though weakly, the blood calcium of rabbits (6). *In vitro* tests indicated that the juice of the fresh whole herb or the decoction of the dried root were active against *Staphylococcus aureus*, beta *Streptococcus hemolyticus, Bacillus anthracis* and *Corynebacterium diphtheriae* (10).

6. Toxicity

The tolerance dose of the oily acetone-extract of <Yiyiren> was 10 ml/kg PO in mice (5). A single injection of coixol 500 mg/kg IP in mice resulted in transient sedation but no death. A single dose of coixol 100 mg/kg IV caused no death or any abnormal manifestations. There was no toxic reaction after administration of 20, 100, or 500 mg/kg PO for 30 days (7).

CLINICAL STUDIES

1. Lung Abscess

A paper reported that 3 cases of lung abscess were radically cured with <Yiyigen> (11). "Qianjin Weijing Decoction" which contains <Yiyiren> was also found effective in this disease (12).

2. Verruca Plana

<Yiyiren> was tried in 27 cases of verruca plana; 9 cases were cured, 11 improved, and 7 unresponsive. *Dosage and administration*: Decoction of 10–30 g of <Yiyiren> daily as a single dose for 2–4 weeks (13). In another series of 23 cases, <Yiyiren> 60 g cooked together with adequate amounts of husked rice was given as one meal once every day; 11 of these cases were completely cured after 7–16 days, 6 cases not assessed and the remaining 6 cases unchanged after a trial course of 3 weeks. Prior to their disappearance, the skin lesions of most patients became enlarged and red, and the inflammation exacerbated, but these reactions usually disappeared after a few days without discontinuation of therapy (14).

3. Treatment of Cancer

A compound formula composed of <Yiyiren>, <Tengliu>, the fruit of *Terminalia billerica*, and the pulp of *Trapa bispinosa* was used to treat 168 of digestive tract cancer including postoperative and advanced inoperable cases. The decoction of these drugs was taken in 3 doses daily. Patients experienced increase of appetite and temporary improvement in general condition. The decoction was also effective in 30 of 36 cases who took the drug for more than 3 months. No significant side effects were known during the treatment course (15).

4. Miscellaneous

Coix-Aconitum-Patrinia Decoction (Semen Coicis, Radix Aconiti, Herba Patriniae) is one of the effective formulae commonly used by Chinese herbalists in the treatment of appendicitis. The 1:1 fluidextract of the decoction of <Yiyigen> at the total dose of 50 ml to be taken once or in 3 doses before meals was effective for ascariasis (16). Another report stated that chewing and eating the root induced labor at mid-term pregnancy (17).

ADVERSE EFFECTS

This herb has a very slight toxicity (7). In general, no adverse reactions has resulted after ingesting this herb (5,13,15), except when used in verruca plana (14).

REFERENCE

1. Nakayama M. Journal of Japanese Surgical Society 1960 61(2):234.

2. Nakayama T. The Journal of the Japan Medical Association 1959 41(2):945.

3. Ukita T et al. Chemical and Pharmaceutical Bulletin 1961 9(1):43.

4. Zhang RL. The References of Traditional Chinese Medicine 1974 (4):43.

5. Pharmacy, Zhongshan Hospital of Shanghai First Medical College. Proceedings of the Pan-China Regional Symposium on Pharmacy (Botany). Chinese Pharmaceutical Association (Shanghai Branch). 1978. p. 56.

6. Hano K et al. Journal of the Pharmaceutical Society of Japan (Tokyo) 1959 79(11):1412.

7. Hano K et al. Journal of the Pharmaceutical Society of Japan (Tokyo) 1960 80(8):1118.

8. Miura K/T et al. Yakugaku Kenkyu 1968 39(1):17.

9. Terasaka M. Japan Centra Revuo Medicina 1928 26:197.

10. Lingling District Sanitation and Anti-epidemic Station. Hunan Yiyao Zazhi (Hunan Medical Journal) 1974 (5):49.

11. Zhang GX. Fujian Zhongyiyao (Fujian Journal of Traditional Chinese Medicine) 1959 (6):20.

12. Paediatrics Department, Tengxian People' s Central Hospital. Shandong Yiyao (Shandong Medical Journal) 1978 (1):13.

13. Li CX. Chinese Journal of Dermatology 1958 4(6):492.

14. Qu KZ et al. Chinese Journal of Dermatology 1959 7(1):34.

15. Ye JQ. Jiangsu Zhongyi (Jiangsu Journal of Traditional Chinese Medicine) 1962 (1):29.

16. Ding SJ. Zhejiang Journal of Traditional Chinese Medicine 1960 (2):66.

17. Shuitianba District Health Centre (Zigui County, Hubei). New Chinese Medicine 1975 (4):218.

(Liu Wenqing)

BOHE 薄荷

<Bohe> is the herb obtained from *Mentha haplocalyx* Briq. (*M. aroensis* L. var. *haplocalyx* Briq.), or M. *haplocalyx* Briq. var. *piperascens* (Malinvaud) C. Y. Wu et H. W. Li (*M. arvensis* L. var. *piperascens* Malinvaud.) (Labiatae). Pungent and "cool", the herb has "wind-heat"-discutient and vital-energy-stimulant (or carminative) actions; it is noted for its ability to induce eruption of measles at the early stage of the disease. It is used for the treatment of common cold due to pathogenic "wind-heat", headache and conjunctivitis, pharyngolaryngitis, dyspepsia, flatulence, and measles.

CHEMICAL COMPOSITION

<Bohe> contains volatile oil which mainly contains 8 isomers of menthol (mentha camphor), followed by menthone and isomenthone. The herb also contains menthenone, camphene, pinene, limonene, rosmarinic acid, and azulen.

PHARMACOLOGY

1. Local Effect

Both menthol and menthone are irritating to the skin (1,2). Menthol applied to the skin initially produced a cold sensation and then mild prickly burning sensation due to its stimulant effect on the nerve ending receptors. During this time, the skin temperature did not drop but even slightly elevated. The drug gradually penetrated the skin, produced sustained congestion which, in turn, initiated deep vascular changes, and regulated the vascular function, thus attaining therapeutic effects (1,3,4). Anti-inflammatory and analgesic effects were produced by local application of compound prescription of menthol (5).

2. Diaphoretic and Antipyretic Effects

The orally administered <Bohe> in small amounts dilated the cutaneous capillary vessels through stimulation of the CNS. This effect promotes perspiration and heat dissipation, thus producing diaphoretic and antipyretic effects (4).

3. Antibacterial and Antiviral Effects

3.1 *Effect on virus.* In a primary culture of renal epithelial cells of suckling rabbits, <Bohe> decoction inhibited infection by 10–100 times the $TCID_{50}$ (median tissue culture infection dose) of herpes simplex virus, but failed to do if infection dose was increased. At 100 mg/ml, <Bohe> exhibited cytotoxicity (6). Experiments with the aqueous extract of *Mentha piperita* on chicken embryos showed that the herb inhibited herpes simplex, variola, Semliki forest and mumps viruses, but not influenza viruses A and B (7).

3.2 *Antibacterial effect.* The <Bohe> decoction was proved *in vitro* to be active against *Staphylococcus aureus, Staphylococcus albus*, alpha streptococcus, beta streptococcus, *Neisseria catarrhalis, Neisseria enteritidis, Shigella flexneri, Bacillus anthracis, Corynebacterium diphtheriae, Salmonella typhi, Pseudomonas aeruginosa, Escherichia coli, Proteus vulgaris*, and *Candida albicans* (8–11).

3.3 *Anthelmintic Effect.* The <Bohe> oil was reportedly an effective anthelmintic for ascariasis of dogs and cats (12).

4. Effect on the Respiratory System

In urethane-anesthetized rabbits, inhalation of menthol vapour 81 mg/kg increased mucous secretion from the respiratory tract and decreased its specific gravity. Inhalation of a dose of 243 mg/kg, conversely, decreased the mucous secretion. This effect was probably due to a direct action on mucous cells of the respiratory tract (13). Menthol can decrease foaming of blood and saponins and when used in bronchitis also decreased the foamy sputum in the respiratory tract so that it enlarges the effective lumen. In rhinitis and laryngitis, menthol diluted the thick and sticky mucus by promoting secretion, causing marked remission of symptoms (14).

5. Effect on the Digestive System

<Bohe> oil had a spasmolytic effect on the isolated intestinal muscle of mice. But in intact animals it failed to enhance propulsive intestinal peristalsis and at times even produced inhibition. <Bohe> oil has a stomachic effect which may be secondary to its stimulant effect on the olfactory and gustatory senses (15). Both menthol and menthone inhibited the isolated intestinal muscle of rabbits, but the latter agent was twice as potent as the former (16). At 260 mM/kg PO in rats, either menthol or menthone produced a strong choleretic effect; 3–4 hours after administration of menthol, the bile excretion was increased by about 4 times, but thereafter the effect weakened. Menthone exhibited an identical but more prolonged effect, increasing bile excretion by 50–100% 5 hours after medication (17,18).

In rats with CCl_4-induced liver damage, subcutaneous injection of the <Bohe> injection significantly decreased the SGPT activity, though the achieved level was far from normal. Though the treatment group had milder cloudy swelling and vacuolization of hepatocytes compared with the control group, it had worse necrotic pathological changes (19). Azulen, an agent obtained by distilling <Bohe> oil, had a therapeutic value on butadione-induced gastric ulcer of rats (20).

6. Miscellaneous Actions

Early-pregnancy of mice may be terminated by <Bohe> (21). Azulen exhibited an anti-inflammatory effect on burns of rabbit ears (20). *In vitro*, the infusion of this herb inhibited human cervical cancer JTC-26 strain (22).

7. Toxicity

The LD of natural menthol were 5–6 g/kg SC in mice and 1 g/kg SC in rats and that of the suspension was 800–1000 mg/kg PO or IP. The LD of synthetic menthol were 1.4–1.6 g/kg SC in mice and 1.5–1.6 g/kg PO or IP in cats (23). dl-Menthol 7500 or 4000 ppm added to feed of rats or mice for 103 weeks did not produce a carcinogenic effect (24).

CLINICAL STUDIES

1. Topical Use

Menthol may be used topically in headache, neuralgia, and pruritus.

2. Common Cold

Compound formulae which contain this herb such as Lonicera-Forsythia Powder, Lonicera-Forsythia Detoxicant Pill, Schizonepeta-Ledebouriella Detoxicant Powder and Morus-Chrysanthemum Decoction are widely used drugs for common cold (25–30). Fumigation of house and rooms with a solution of rice vinegar and <Bohe> in water was effective for the prevention of common cold (31).

3. Sore Throat

More than 100 cases of sore throat were cured with the modified Solidago decurrens Decoction (Herba Solidago, Herba Menthae, Rhozoma Belamcandae, Herba Rhodeae, Herba Peristrophis, Radix Ardisiae, Radix Glycyrrhizae). One to three doses usually cured the disease. All the crude drugs listed above may also be used alone to treat sore throat (32).

4. Acute Mastitis

Filtrate of the decoction of <Bohe> and the leaf of *Platycodon grandiflorum* each 60 g may be applied with a towel as a hot compress over the disease site in the morning and evening. Over 40 non-ulcerated cases so treated achieved good therapeutic results (33).

5. Miscellaneous

Satisfactory results were obtained with modified formulae of this herb such as Schizonepeta-Ledebouriella Detoxicant Decoction in treating allergic dermatitis, pruritus, urticaria, psoriasis, and eczema (34). Three Fresh Herb Decoction (fresh Folium Isatidis, fresh Herba Artemisiae Annuae, fresh Herba Menthae) was effective to a certain extent for epidemic encephalitis B (35).

ADVERSE EFFECTS

The toxic and side effects of this herb were very rare. One case of injudicious ingestion of 20 ml of <Bohe> oil to relieve abdominal distention developed 15 minutes later dizziness, blurred vision, nausea, vomiting, and numbness of the extremities and eventually became unconscious with slight drop of blood pressure (70/60 mmHg). The patient recovered on the next day after intravenous infusion of fluid and administration of central stimulants (36).

REFERENCE

1. Masaki T et al. Nihon Yakubutsugaku Zasshi 1943 38(2):2.
2. Masaki T et al. Nihon Yakubutsugaku Zasshi 1948 43(3):80.
3. Sollmann T. A Manual of Pharmacology. 7th edition. 1948. p. 211.
4. Editorial Group. National Collection of Chinese Materia Medica. People's Medical Publishing House. 1975. p. 924.
5. Carosin S. Chemical Abstracts 1979 90:29027h.
6. Chen ZJ et al. Journal of Traditional Chinese Medicine 1980 21(2):73.
7. Herrmann EC et al. Proceedings of the Society for Experimental Biology and Medicine 1967 124:874.
8. Lingling District Sanitation and Anti-epidemic Station et al. Hunan Yiyao Zazhi (Hunan Medical Journal) 1974 (5):49.
9. Leptospirosis Research Unit, Chengdu College of Traditional Chinese Medicine. Scientific Research Compilation. 3rd edition. Chengdu College of Traditional Chinese Medicine. 1972. p. 71.
10. Microbiology Department. Journal of Nanjing College of Pharmacy 1960 (5):10.
11. Microbiology Section. Acta Academiae Medicinae Shandong 1959 (8):24.
12. Tanabe T. Japan Centra Revuo Medicina 1942 79:14.
13. Boyd EM et al. Archives Internationales de Pharmacodynamie et de Therapie 1969 182(1):206.
14. Sollmann T. A Manual of Pharmacology. 8th edition. 1957. p. 202.
15. Haginiwa et al. Journal of the Pharmaceutical Society of Japan (Tokyo) 1963 83(6):624.
16. Zhao YR. Japan Centra Revuo Medicina 1956 121:652.
17. Moersdorf K. Chemical Abstracts 1967 66:74701p.
18. Pasetsnik Ikh. Farmakologiia I Toksikologiia 1966 29(6):735.

19. Liver Diseases Research Group. Medical and Health Communications (Shanxi Medical College) 1977 (2):8.

20. Maksimenko GN. Farmakologiia I Toksikologiia 1964 27(5):571.

21. Academy of Traditional Chinese Medicine. Selected Information on Science and Technology. 1972. p. 145.

22. Sato A. Kampo Kenkyu 1979 (2):51.

23. Spector WS. Handbook of Toxicology 1956 1:184.

24. National Cancer Institute. Chemical Abstracts 1979 91:50817w.

25. Guo ZQ. Zhejiang Journal of Traditional Chinese Medicine 1959 (36):28.

26. Ye JH. Shanghai Zhongyiyao Zazhi (Shanghai Journal of Traditional Chinese Medicine) 1958 (5):14.

27. Ye RG et al. Guangdong Zhongyi (Guangdong Journal of Traditional Chinese Medicine) 1959 (2):56.

28. Wang ZC. Fujian Zhongyiyao (Fujian Journal of Traditional Chinese Medicine) 1959 (10):6.

29. Han DW. Journal of Traditional Chinese Medicine 1957 (12):653.

30. Wang GL. Medicine and Health (Shaoxing District Centre of Medical and Health Information, Zhejiang) 1979 (2):17.

31. Sun M. Journal of Barefoot Doctor 1977 (12):14.

32. Shi ZL. Medicine and Health (Shaoxing District Centre of Medical and Health Information, Zhejiang) 1978 (1):44.

33. Liang ZS. Guangxi's Barefoot Doctor 1977 (1):43.

34. Wu SM. Xinyiyaoxue Zazhi (Journal of Traditional Chinese Medicine) 1978 (6):26.

35. Mao ZQ. Zhejiang Zhongyiyao (Zhejiang Journal of Traditional Chinese Medicine) 1977 (3):18.

36. Wang SY. Chinese Journal of Internal Medicine 1960 8(4):386.

(Gong Xuling)

ZANGQIE 藏茄

<Zangqie> is derived from the root and seed of *Anisodus tanguticus* (Maxim.) Pascher (*Scopolia tanguticus* Maxim.) (Solanaceae). The whole plant may also be used as medicine<Zangqie> has a bitter taste and "warm" property. Its actions are considered to be analgesic, spasmolytic, blood-stimulant, stasis-eliminative, sedative, tranquilizing, antiasthmatic and antitussive. It is used for anesthesia, septic shock, visceral colic, ulcer, and vasospasm.

CHEMICAL COMPOSITION

Hyoscyamine, anisodamine (654), anisodine (AT-3), scopolamine and cuscohygrine were isolated from the root and aerial part of *A. tanguticus* (1,2). Hyoscyamine is levorotatory, and its biological activity is thrice that of atropine. Since hyoscyamine readily racemizes during preparation and storage, it is often racemized as atropine for clinical use.

Synthetic anisodamine is called 654–2; it was reported to produce mydriasis and xerostomia more pronounced than that caused by the natural compound (3). Anisodine, a new anticholinergic, is first isolated in China. Cuscohygrine was isolated abroad for more than a century, but its pharmacological activity is extremely low. In China, cuscohygrine was hydrogenated to form cuscohygrinol and esterified to form cuscohygrinyl acetylamygdalate (abbreviated as cuscohygrinol ester); they have significant pharmacological activity (4–6). Anhydroatropine and a few new alkaloids with unknown chemical structure were recently isolated in China (7).

PHARMACOLOGY

1. Effect on the CNS

Anisodine, anisodamine, scopolamine, and atropine, all caused synchronization of the electroencephalic activity in unanesthetized cats with the electroencephalogram showing irregular high amplitude slow waves. These agents blocked the arousal EEG and, in addition, caused dissociation of the electroencephalic pattern and behaviour; they also have antitremor effect (8–10) and antagonized the analgesic action of tremorine (8,9). These agents also inhibited the conditioned avoidance reflex of rats (8–10). The order of potency is: scopolamine > atropine > anisodine > anisodamine (9). It is postulated that their potency is affected by their ability to cross the blood-brain barrier (11). Scopolamine and anisodine were chiefly central depressive. Used with hibernation-inducing agents, either of them induces clinical anesthesia, which may be attributed to blockade of the cholinergic receptor of the neurons in the sensory and motor areas (12). It was discovered in recent years that anisodine markedly increased the efflux of acetylcholine from the cortex of cats;

this probably played an important role in compound intravenous anesthesia (13). However, some workers believed that scopolamine does not act on the cortex but on the subcortical area, particularly around the mildline between the midbrain and diencephalon (14), and that the anesthetic action was probably related to the blockade of cholinergic activating system of the brain stem reticular formation and to the ascending adrenergic dorsal tract (15,16). Anisodamine was shown to have a rather weak central depressant action while atropine was strong. Cuscohygrine had no central activity; but cuscohygrinol and cuscohygrinol ester had sedative effect. In large doses, they greatly decreased the spontaneous activity of animals and synergized with sodium pentobarbital (5,6).

2. Effect on the Digestive System

Scopolamine had the strongest antagonistic action against the contractile effect of acetylcholine on isolated intestinal strips of rats and rabbits; the potencies of anisodine and anisodamine were similar to that of atropine (8,10). Large doses of cuscohygrinol, cuscohygrinol ester, and cuscohygrine also produced an antispasmodic effect; cuscohygrinol was about five times more potent the other two agents (6). The half inhibitory doses of atropine, cuscohygrinol, cuscohygrinol ester and cuscohygrine against the motility of mouse intestines *in situ* were determined to be 4.9, 23, 44, and 62 mg/kg IP, respectively (5,6). Cuscohygrinol ester also inhibited gastric secretion in rats (5). In inhibiting salivary secretion, atropine showed the strongest action, followed by anisodine and weakest by anisodamine and cuscohygrinol ester (5,8,10).

3. Effect on the Respiratory System

Anisodine and atropine have no antitussive effect on mice with cough induced by ammonia water but showed an antiasthmatic action. They effectively prevented histamine-induced asthma in guinea pigs; the effect of anisodine 10 mg/kg was equivalant to that of atropine 5 mg/kg (17). The antiasthmatic activity of cuscohygrinol ester was slightly weaker (5).

4. Effect on the Circulatory System

Injection of anisodine or anisodamine 2 mg/kg IV to anesthetized dogs did not alter the heart rate and blood pressure (10,17), but intravenous (5) or intramuscular (18) injection of cuscohygrinol ester significantly lowered the blood pressure. Anisodine and anisodamine completely antagonized the hypotensive effect of acetylcholine (10,17). Cuscohygrinol ester in large doses only decreased but not entirely abolished the action of acetylcholine (5). Anisodine (17), and to a lesser extent cuscohygrinol ester (5), increased the contractility of the isolated rabbit heart. The latter compound also increased the coronary flow but not the myocardial nutritional blood flow. It exerted no significant antagonistic action against pituitrin-induced myocardial ischemia of rats (5). Anisodine exerted biphasic action on the blood vessels of isolated rabbit ears; low concentrations caused vasodilation and high concentrations caused vasoconstriction (17). In contrast, high concentrations of cuscohygrinol ester caused vasodilation (5). Scopolamine, atropine, anisodine, and anisodamine caused vasodilation of the rat hind sole in descending order (19). Anisodine dilated the cerebral cortical blood vessels of rabbits (20); it increased the cerebral blood flow and improved cerebrovascular resistance as shown in cerebral hemodromogram (21). Atropine and anisodamine improved the microcirculation of the nailfold (22), and anisodine improved the microcirculatory disorders due to traumatic hemorrhage in anesthetized hamster (20).

5. Mydriatic Effect

The mydriatic activity of anisodine in mice was 5 times that of anisodamine, but weaker than that of atropine (8,17). Cuscohygrinol ester had the weakest mydriatic effect, about 1/100 that of atropine (5).

6. Antagonism to Organic Phosphates

Anisodine, anisodamine and atropine increased the LD_{50} of DFP, dipterex, parathion and acephate, antagonized or mitigated their toxic effects, and precluded the death of intoxicated mice; anisodine was found to be most potent (8,10,17).

7. Pharmacokinetics

The tropane alkaloids are readily absorbed from the gastrointestinal and other mucosal surfaces (23). The "half absorption time" of the orally administered dose of 100 mg/kg was 3.5 hours (24). Anisodine was more rapidly absorbed from the gastrointestinal tract than anisodamine (25) but more slowly than scopolamine (26). Injection of anisodamine at the same dose resulted in a plasma level lower than that of atropine; this might be due to the more rapid excretion of the former (24). The serum half-life of scopolamine, anisodine, anisodamine, and cuscohygrinol ester were 95 (26), 70 (26), 40 (24), and 40 (27) minutes, respectively. After intravenous injection of scopolamine and anisodine, the concentration in the brain was found to be higher than that in plasma. Higher concentrations appeared in the corpora striata, cerebral cortex and hippocampi, next in the septal area and diencephalon, and low levels in the lower brain stem and cerebellum. The level of scopolamine in the brain was significantly higher than that of anisodine, whereas atropine distributed evenly in the brain; such difference in distribution may be a reflection of their differences in central effect (26). Twenty-four hours after intravenous injection of anisodamine, 38.8% of the parent drug was excreted in the urine; this percentage was more than twice higher than that of atropine (17.4%) (24). Five hours after intramuscular injection of cuscohygrinol ester, 56.6% of the drug was excreted in the urine (27); the 48-hour urinary excretion of anisodine by intravenous injection and oral administration were 23 and 26%, respectively; those of scopolamine and atropine were 1.2 and 18%

and 0.55 and 33%, respectively (25). The tropane alkaloids were eliminated primarily by biotransformation; biotransformation of about 50% of hyoscyamine and 70% of anisodine occurred in the body (24,25). Scopolamine was transformed faster than anisodine (26).

8. Toxicity

Refer to the table below for the acute LD_{50} (mg/kg) of the following drugs by intravenous injection in mice (5,8,10,17,18,28).

Atropine	Scopolamine	Anisodamine	Anisodine	Cuscohy-grine	Cuscohy-grinol	Cuscohy-grinol ester
135.9		149.7	595.4	123.3	42.5	87.1
97.7	80*	123.3	363.1			
61.3						

*MLD in dogs.

The oral doses were less toxic. The LD_{50} of cuscohygrinol ester in mice was about 3000 mg/kg PO (18); in mice the MLD of anisodamine and atropine was 1600 and 700 mg/kg, respectively (10). Subacute toxicity studies indicated that anisodine, anisodamine, and cuscohygrinol ester had no significant effect on the blood picture, liver and kidney functions (5,8,10,17), nervous system, and internal organs (17) of laboratory animals.

CLINICAL STUDIES

1. Chinese Traditional Anesthesia

Scopolamine is the chief active constituent of a Chinese herbal anesthetic, the flower of *Datura metel*. It can therefore be used as a substitute for the herb in Chinese traditional anesthesia (refer to the monograph on <Yangjinhua>. In concert with hibernation drugs and muscle relaxants, anisodine can be employed in surgical anesthesia. According to a report of 200–odd cases, intravenous compound anesthesia of anisodine had the advantages of fast induction, stable anesthesia, wide safety range, fast and reliable arousal, and anti-shock, although the anesthesia so induced was not deep enough despite the increased dosage (29–31).

2. Septic Shock

Atropine and anisodamine have been widely used for the treatment of septic shock. They are effective in improving the microcirculation and increasing the tissue blood flow (23).

3. Visceral Colic

Atropine had marked spasmolytic and analgesic effects (23); intramuscular injection of 50–100 mg of cuscohygrinol ester relieved gastrointestinal, biliary, and urinary colics in 178 clinical cases; the aggregate effective rate was as high as 70–90% (32).

4. Peptic Ulcer

In 21 in-patients of gastric ulcer treated by intramuscular injection of 50 mg of cuscohygrinol ester thrice daily, a 6-week cure rate of 52.4% and an aggregate effective rate of 85.7% confirmed by optic gastroscopy were achieved; the effective rate could be further increased if gastropine (an antacid) was concurrently used (33). Four other cases were also cured with rectal suppositories of cuscohygrinol ester (33). However, ineffective treatment of out-patients was also reported (34). The therapeutic effect in in-patients with duodenal ulcer was also better than that in out-patients (32).

5. Migraine-Type Vascular Headache

In 50 cases treated with anisodine intravenously, intramuscularly or orally, 1–6 mg each time, the marked effective rate was 70% and the aggregate effective rate was 96% (35).

6. Organic Phosphate Poisoning

Atropine is an important antidote for organic phosphate poisoning; it promptly and effectively relieves serious symptoms and is life-saving (23). Anisodine was also quite effective; it markedly improved the nervous sequelae of organic phosphate poisoning (36).

7. Miscellaneous

Atropine is useful as an antiarrhythmic agent (23), and anisodine in vasospasm of retinal and optic nerves (37), cerebrovascular ischemia (38,39), poliomyelitis (40), parkinsonism (41), motion sickness (42), and chronic bronchitis (43). Anisodamine is also employed in vertigo (23); cuscohygrinol ester can be used for sedation and hypnosis (44).

ADVERSE EFFECTS

The common manifestations are xerostomia, dizziness, headache, blurred vision, lassitude, drowsiness, and palpitation, and occasionally dysuria. Anisodine, anisodamine and cuscohygrinol ester have fewer side effects than atropine. Acute poisoning produces hyperthermia, quick and thready pulse, mydriasis, dry and flushed skin, mania, delirium, hallucination, convulsion, and coma. Treatment includes, apart from general symptomatic measures, administration of cholinomimetic agents such as physostigmine which is able to cross the blood-brain barrier to antagonize the central anticholinergic toxicity of tropane alkaloids.

REFERENCE

1. Tianjin Institute for Drug Control and Tianjin Institute of Materia Medica. Resources of medicinal plants containing anisodine. In: Information of the Conference on the Identification of Anisodine. 1975.

2. Chengdu No. 1 Pharmaceutical Factory. Production techniques of anisodine hydrobromide. In: Information of the Conference on the Identification of Anisodine. 1975.

3. Pediatrics Department, Friendship Hospital of Beijing et al. Chinese Medical Journal 1973 53(5):259.

4. Liu RH. Studies on a new anticholinergic drug — cuscohygrinol ester. In: Proceedings of the 1979 Symposium of the Chinese Pharmaceutial Association (Chengdu Branch).

5. Wang YS et al. Abstracts of the First National Symposium of the Society of Pharmacology. 1979. p. 3.

6. Wang YS et al. Abstracts of the First National Symposium of the Society of Pharmacology. 1979. p. 3.

7. Yang JS et al. Chinese Pharmaceutial Bulletin 1980 15(7):44.

8. Neurology Section of the Pharmacology Department, Institute of Materia Medica of the Chinese Academy of Medical Sciences. Zhonghua Yixue Zazhi (National Medical Journal of China) 1975 55(11):795.

9. Neurology Section of the Pharmacology Department, Institute of Materia Medica of the Chinese Academy of Medical Sciences. Zhongma Tongxun (Communications on Chinese Traditional Anesthesia) 1975 (4):10.

10. Pharmacology Department, Institute of Materia Medica of the Chinese Academy of Medical Sciences. Chinese Medical Journal 1973 53(5):269.

11. Peng JZ. Abstracts of the First National Symposium of the Society of Pharmacology. 1979. p. 2.

12. Jin GZ. Zhongma Tongxun (Communications on Chinese Traditional Anesthesia) 1975 (2):41.

13. Huang JH et al. Abstracts of the First National Symposium of the Society of Pharmacology. 1979. p. 1.

14. Chinese Traditional Anesthesia Research Unit, Nanjing College of Pharmacy. Abstracts of the First National Symposium of the Society of Pharmacology. 1979. p. 10.

15. Pharmacology Section, Xuzhou Medical College. Zhongma Tongxun (Communications on Chinese Traditional Anesthesia) 1975 (4):17.

16. Bian CF et al. Abstracts of the First National Symposium of the Society of Pharmacology. 1979. p. 4.

17. Pharmacology Section, Sichuan Medical College et al. Chinese Traditional and Herbal Drugs Communications 1975 (6):27.

18. Chengdu No. 1 Pharmaceutical Factory. Chinese Traditional and Herbal Drugs Communications 1971 (3):26.

19. Qinghai Institute of Medical Sciences. The vasodilatory action and mechanism of anticholinergic drugs anisodine and tropane alkaloids on rat paws. In: Information of the Conference on the Identification of Anisodine. 1975.

20. Neurology and Psychiatry Department, Sichuan Medical College et al. Information on Medical Sciences and Technology (Sichuna Medical College) 1975 (3):40.

21. Neurology Department, Teaching Hospital of Sichuan Medical College et al. Information on Medical Sciences and Technology (Sichuan Medical College) 1975 (3):36.

22. First Research Unit, Teaching Hospital of the Chinese Academy of Medical Sciences. Chinese Medical Journal 1973 53(5):264.

23. Shanghai First Medical College et al. Medical Pharmacology. 1st edition. People' s Medical Publishing House. 1977. pp. 379–385.

24. Pharmacology Department, Institute of Materia Medica of the Chinese Academy of Medical Sciences et al. Chinese Medical Journal 1973 53(5):274.

25. Pharmacology Department, Institute of Materia Medica of the Chinese Academy of Medical Sciences et al. Chinese Medical Journal 1977 57(7):422.

26. Yue TL et al. Acta Pharmaceutica Sinica 1979 14(4):208.

27. Central Laboratory, Chengdu First Pharmaceutical Factory et al. In vivo animal studies of the absorption, distribution and excretion of the cuscohygrinol ester injeciion. In: Information of the Conference on the Identification of Cuscohygrinol Ester. 1979.

28. Tianjin Institute for Drug Control and Tianjin Institute of Materia Medica. Zhongma Tongxun (Communications on Chinese Traditional Anesthesia) 1975 (4):33.

29. Ningbo District (Zhejiang) Coordinating Research Group on Chinese Traditional Anesthesia. Anisodine in compound anesthesia by IV injection. In: Information of the Conference on the Identification of Anisodine. 1975.

30. Central Hospital of the Shanghai Bureau of Railways. Clinical uses of anisodine in compound anesthesia by IV injection. In: Information of the Conference on the Identification of Anisodine. 1975.

31. Chinese Traditional Anesthesia Group, Shanghai Second Hospital of Tuberculosis. Anesthesia by anisodine and Datura by IV injection in fifty cases of thoracic surgery. In: Information of the Conference on the Identification of Anisodine. 1975.

32. Clinical uses of ' 701' — a brief summary. In: Information of the Conference on the Identification of Cuscohygrinol Ester. 1979.

33. Zhang JF et al. Clinical Study on the treatment of gastric ulcer with ' 701' . In: Information of the Conference on the Identification of Cuscohygrinol Ester. 1979.

34. Digestion Research Unit of the Internal Medicine Department, First Teaching Hospital of Chongqing Medical College. Clinical and endoscopic studies of cuscohygrinol ester in therapy of gastric ulcer. In: Information of the Conference on the Identification of Cuscohygrinol Ester. 1979.

35. Neurology Department, Teaching Hospital of the Sichuan Medical College et al. Information on Medical Sciences and Technology (Sichuan Medical College) 1975 (3):15.

36. Zhu HM et al. Report on anisodine therapy of three cases of nervous system sequelae of organic phosphate poisoning. In: Information of the Conference on the Identification of Anisodine. 1975.

37. Ophthalmology Department, General Hospital of the Chinese PLA. The clinical use of anisodine hydrobromide in ophthalmology. In: Information of the Conference on the Identification of Anisodine. 1975.

38. Neurology and Psychiatry Section, Sichuan Medical College. Information on Medical Sciences and Technology (Sichuan Medical College) 1975 (3):1.

39. First, Second and Third Teaching Hospitals of Chengdu Medical College. Anisodine hydrobromide therapy of twenty-one cases of cerebrovascular ischemia. In: Information of the Conference on the Identification of Anisodine. 1975.

40. Chengdu Hospital of Infectious Diseases. Clinical efficacy of anisodine in the treatment of poliomyelitis. In: Information of the Conference on the Identification of Anisodine. 1975.

41. Neurology Department, First Teaching Hospital of Chengdu Medical College. Clinical efficacy of AT-3 in the treatment of Parkinson's disease. In: Information of the Conference on the Identification of Anisodine. 1975.

42. 173 Beijing Unit of the Chinese PLA. Preliminary studies on the efficacy of anisodine hydrobromide and other drugs for seasickness. In: Information of the Conference on the Identification of Anisodine. 1975.

43. 38th Army Hospital of the Chinese PLA. Brief summary of one hundred and eighty-four cases of chronic bronchitis treated with anisodine hydrobromide. In: Information of the Conference on the Identification of Anisodine. 1975.

44. Mu SH. Clinical efficacy of cuscohygrinol ester in insomnia. In: Information of the Conference on the Identification of Cuscohygrinol Ester. 1979.

(Ye Songbai)

QUMAI 瞿麥

<Qumai> is derived from the root or plant of *Dianthus superbus* L. or *D. chinensis* L. (Caryophyllaceae). The herb is bitter, "cold", and nontoxic. It is latent-heat-clearing, antipyretic, diuretic, anticoagulant, and channel-deobstruent. It is mainly used to treat strangury, urinary retention, edema, and eczema.

CHEMICAL COMPOSITION

The whole plant contains saponins and a small amount of alkaloids. The flower contains benzyl salicylate, methyl salicylate and volatile oil which is mainly composed of eugenol, phenylethanol, and benzyl benzoate.

PHARMACOLOGY

1. Diuretic Effect

The <Qumai> decoction had a diuretic effect in rats, rabbits, anesthetized and unanesthetized dogs (1–3). A 2 g/kg-dose of the spike decoction given orally to rabbits markedly increased the urinary output and urinary chloride excretion; the spike was found to be more potent than the stem (3–6). The <Qumai> decoction increased the urinary output by 1–2.5 times in anesthetized dogs and by 5–8 times in unanesthetized dogs (2). It is controversial as to what component caused diuresis; one worker believed that the ash and glucose content caused diuresis (1). Others discovered that <Qumai> had a more potent kaliuretic than natriuretic effect in unanesthetized dogs (2) and in rats (3). <Qumai> was found to contain 500 mg% of potassium (2); its diuretic and natriuretic activities in laboratory rats were not much different from those of the ash (4). Consequently, the diuretic effect was presumed to be due to the potassium salts.

2. Effect on Smooth Muscles

Studies on isolated rabbit intestine, *in situ* intestinal tract of anesthetized dogs, and chronic intestinal fistula of dogs indicated that <Qumai> decoction had marked stimulant effect on intestines which could be antagonized by diphenhydramine and papaverine. The stimulant effect of <Qumai> on the isolated intestines was primarily characterized by increased tone, whereas on *in situ* intestinal tract of anesthetized dogs and in chronic intestinal fistula of dogs this manifested as increased peristalsis without increasing the tone (5).

3. Effect on the Heart and Blood Vessels

The decoction of the spike had a pronounced inhibitory effect on isolated frog and rabbit hearts; it sometimes caused atrioventricular block irreversible by epinephrine. Injection of the decoction 0.5 g/kg IV to anesthetized dogs decreased the blood pressure probably due to depression of the heart, which was accompanied by brief renal vasoconstriction. However, transient renal vasodilation occurred during the peak hypotensive effect, and renal blood volume returned to normal along with the normalization of blood pressure (5).

4. Schistosomicidal Effect

In vitro studies showed that the 10% decoction directly killed the parasites in 8–12 minutes. Thirty-four percent of the schistosome-infected rabbits were found to have residual worms after treatment with the herb decoction 4 g/kg PO daily for 4 weeks, in contrast to 59.75% of the control. The liver pathological changes were also found to be milder in the treatment group (6). But a contrary report claimed that daily intragastric administration of the tolerance dose of the ethanol extract of this herb to schistosome-infected mice produced no therapeutic effect (7).

CLINICAL STUDIES

1. Acute Urinary Tract Infection and Cystitis

<Qumai> can be used with the plant *Polygonum aviculare* and the spores of *Lygodium japonicum*.

2. Blood Stasis and Amenorrhea

The root of *Salvia miltiorrhiza*, the root of wild *Paeonia lactiflora* and the plant of *Leonurus heterophyllus* may be used with this herb (8).

3. Cancer of Esophagus and Rectum

Decoction of the fresh root of *D. chinensis* 30–60 g (or 24–30 g of the dried root) alone, or with ginseng, the sclerotium of *Poria cocos*, rhizome of *Atractylodes macrocephala*, and licorice was reportedly effective against cancer of the esophagus and rectum (9).

REFERENCE

1. Rao MR. Chinese Medical Journal 1959 45(1):67.

2. Wang LW et al. Compiled Information on Medical Research. Luda Health Bureau. 1959. p. 364.

3. Wang LW et al. Chinese Traditional and Herbal Drugs 1980 (5):272.

4. Wang LW et al. Acta Academiae Medicinae Dalian 1965 5(1):19.

5. Rao MR. Acta Academiae Medicinae Primae Nanjing 1959 (1):27.

6. Schistosomicides Section, Zhejiang People' s Academy of Health. Zhejiang Health Communications 1955 (13):2.

7. Zang QZ et al. Shizhen Yuanxun (Communications of Li Shizhen Society) (Sichuan Institute of Chinese Materia Medica) 1958 (3):5.

8. Nanjing College of Pharmacy (editor). Chinese Traditional Pharmacy. Vol. 2. Jiangsu People' s Publishing House. 1976. p. 200.

9. Hefei Processing Factory of Chinese Medicinal Materials (Anhui). National Collection of Chinese Materia Medica. 1972. p. 419.

(Li Jizhen)

CHANSU 蟾酥

<Chansu> refers to the venom of the toad *Bufo bufo gargarizans* Cantor or *B. melanostictus* Schneider (Bufonidae). It has a sweet and pungent taste and a "warm" property. It is anti-inflammatory, detoxicant, detumescent, and analgesic. It is principally used to treat pernicious ulcers, carbuncle, furuncle, and pharyngolaryngitis. Externally, it is useful as a hemostatic.

CHEMICAL COMPOSITION

The chemical composition of the toad venom is complex. The major cardiotonic components are glycosides, that is, bufotoxins. Hydrolysis of bufotoxins yields the aglycones bufogenins and bufagins. Bufogenins and bufagins are sterols, the composition of which varies slightly with the species. There are more than 10 kinds of aglycones which are often distinguished by prefixing with their species name. Thus, aglycones obtained from Chinese toads are called cinobufagin, cinobufatalin, telocinobufagin, cinobufalin and cinobufotalin. Aglycones obtained from Japanese toads are called gamabufogenin and gamabufotalin, and others are called resibufogenin, bufotalin, bufotanine, bufalin, bufotalinin and bufotalidin.

The toad venom also contains epinephrine and indole derivatives bufotenine, bufotenidine and serotonin (1–3).

PHARMACOLOGY

1. Cardiotonic Effect

Small doses of toad venom enhanced the contractility of the isolated toad heart, and in anesthetized cats, dogs and frogs; large doses induced bradycardia followed by arrhythmia, atrioventricular block and lastly cardic arrest at the systolic phase. ECG revealed prolongation of the P-R interval, T wave inversion, ectopic beat, bundle branch block, and ventricular fibrillation. Among various cardiotonic components telocinobufagin was found to be the most potent and the next were bufalin and cinobufagin. The cardiotonic effect of <Chansu> resembled that of digitalis but it had no cumulative effect (4–11).

2. Effect on Blood Pressure and Respiration

Bufalin, cinobufagin, and resibufogenin elevated the blood pressure and stimulated the respiration in various anesthetized animals (8,12–15). Resibufogenin had a stronger respiratory stimulant action than lobeline and nikethamide; it also antagonized the respiratory depressant effect of morphine and barbiturates. The repiratory stimulant effect was unaltered by sectioning of the carotid sinus and vagus nerves. Therefore, the main site of action might be located at the respiratory center of the brain stem (7,8,16,17). Cinobufagin had a pressor effect similar to that of epinephrine, which was also blocked by α-receptor blockers (18,19). Bufotenine caused the release of epinephrine and increased the sensitivity of the animals to epinephrine (20).

3. Effect on the CNS

Injection of resibufogenin into the lateral ventrical or vein of conscious or anesthetized rabbits resulted in desynchronization of the EEG; this effect was prolonged with increased dosages, reflecting the pronounced stimulant effect of this drug on cerebral cortex (21). It also antagonized the central depressant action of pentobarbital sodium (7). Bufalin induced convulsion (22). Bufotenine, a derivative of serotonin, showed LSD-like hallucinating effect. The onset and disappearance of the hallucination of bufotenine given intravenously were even quicker than those of mescaline (23). Bufotenine also prolonged chloral hydrate-induced sleep (24). Moreover, <Chansu> also had an analgesic action because it elevated the pain threshold of mice in the hot plate experiment and central functional summation studies in rabbits (25).

4. Local Anesthetic Effect

The 80% ethanol extract of <Chansu> is a local anesthetic. As shown in rabbit cornea and human tongue tests, its effect was stronger and more persistent than cocaine. The most potent constituent of which was bufalin, approximately 90 times more potent than cocaine; the next were cinobufotalin and cinobufagin. In the skin wheal test, their infiltrative anesthetic effect was found to be several hundred times greater than that of procaine (4,26–30).

5. Antineoplastic Effect

Satisfactory inhibitory effect was achieved with the extract of toad skin against mouse sarcoma 180, as well as rabbit B and P tumors (31,32). The *in vitro* methylene blue test and breathing methods revealed that it had a relatively strong inhibitory action against leukemic cells (33). No inhibitory effect was, however, shown against spermatogonia, ascitic carcinoma cells, and hepatoma of mice. But the skin extract prolonged the survival, strengthened the reticuloendothelial function, resulting in the focal hypertrophy of the adrenocortical zona fasciculata of some mice, and it increased glycolysis (34). Nevertheless, data on the absence of significant inhibitory action by <Chansu> against sarcoma 180, Ehrlich ascites carcinoma, hepatoma, skin basal cell cancer, lung cancer, and cervical cancer are available, although it reportedly strengthened to different extents the tumor-inhibitory effect of antineoplastic drugs such as cyclophosphamide (35,36).

6. Anti-inflammatory Effect

The subcutaneous "granuloma" of rats induced by filter paper pledget impregnated with formaldehyde was strongly inhibited by <Chansu> (37). <Chansu> and its various constituents suppressed the increase of vascular permeability induced by acetic acid (38,39). The spreading of infection in rabbis caused by type A *Streptococcus hemolyticus* or *Staphylococcus aureus* may be stopped by intramuscular injection of the injection prepared from fresh postauricular secretion of toads or from the total water-soluble components of <Chansu>, thus causing the subsidence of the inflammation (40,41). In culture experiments (paper disc method) of sputum of patients with pulmonary heart disease complicated with infection, the injection of the total glycosides of <Chansu> was shown to inhibit *Proteus vulgaris, Pseudomonas aeruginosa*, tetrads, *Staphylococcus albus*, and *Neisseria catarrhalis* (42).

7. Effect on Striated and Smooth Muscles

Bufagins and bufogenins had a stimulant effect on striated muscles. Low concentration of bufalin (10^{-4}) enhanced the presynaptic release of acetylcholine from rat diaphragm, while high concentrations caused initial enhancement followed by suppression of the release. It also partially antagonized the neuromuscular blocking effect of Mg^{++} but did not inhibit cholinesterase (43). Both bufotenidine and resibufogenin caused contraction of the frog musculi rectus abdominis. The potency of bufotenidine ranked between those of nicotine and acetylcholine; its muscle contracting effect was blocked by curare and not strengthened by physostigmine. Meanwhile, the contraction induced by resibufogenin was accompanied by changes in membrane potential and was inversely related to the extracellular Ca^{++} concentration. Resibufogenin enhanced potassium ion-induced muscle contraction, but contraction did not occur without the presence of K^+ (44). <Chansu> caused contraction and then relaxation of the intestinal and bronchial smooth muscles. It antagonized histamine- and acetylcholine-induced contractions and excited the uterus and ureter, and even caused abortion of rabbits (4,45).

8. Leukocytotic and Antiradiation Effect

Injection of the aqueous preparation of <Chansu> 0.25 mg/kg IM in dogs, intraperitoneal injection of the 1:2 toad skin extract 0.4 ml or of the 2% <Chansu> oil solution in mice produced significant prophylactic and therapeutic effects against ^{60}Co-induced acute radiation sickness. These treatments markedly increased the survival rate and prolonged the survival time of the laboratory animals, particularly of the female animals, and also improved the decreased total peripheral WBC count (36,46,47). Normal dogs given the <Chansu> injection in various doses also showed increase in peripheral WBC (47).

9. Antitussive, Expectorant, and Antiasthmatic Effects

The aqueous extract of <Chansu> had an antitussive effect in mice with sulfur dioxide-induced cough; it was more effective than Toad Powder but less effective than morphine (45). The antitussive effect of <Chansu> decoction was stronger than its expectorant effect (48). Subcutaneous injection of bufotenine markedly protected guinea pigs from serotonin-induced bronchospasm but not from bronchospasm induced by histamine and acetylcholine (49).

10. Miscellaneous Actions

<Chansu> produced diuresis (45); it inhibited the secretion of sweat and salivary glands, and inhibited epinephrine-activated thyroid adenyl cyclase. Like insulin, it enhanced glycogenesis, inhibited lactic acid formation, and antagonized the lipolytic action of norepinephrine (4). *In vitro*, it inhibited the motility of schistosomes but did not affect their oxygen consumption (50). It had an antihypersensitivity effect on allergy of isolated guinea pig uterus or ileum to egg white (51). <Chansu> also increased the cellular and humoral immunity of mice (36).

11. Pharmacokinetics

The orally administered <Chansu> was easily absorbed, and the onset and disappearance of its action were rapid; it had no cumulative effect. The radioactivity in various tissues at different intervals following intravenous injection of tritiated resibufogenin into mouse caudal vain was high in the liver and intestine, lower in the stomach, heart, kidneys, brain, and muscles in descending order. The plasma half life was short, only 7.5 minutes. Autoradiography of intact animals showed the highest radioactivity in the contents of gallbladder and upper small intestine, suggesting substantial biliary excretion. Comparatively small amounts (4.4 and 1.93% of the injected dose) were excreted in the urine in 24 hours, while fecal excretion (43.3 and 28.8% of the injected dose) was considerable (52–53). Autoradiography of mice given the injection of 131I labelled <Chansu> total glycosides revealed the highest drug level in the heart, and lower in the spleen, brain, lungs, liver, and kidneys in descending order. The drug was also primarily excreted through the kidney; the highest renal content appeared in 8 hours after the injection. Excretion was almost complete in 24 hours (42). The metabolism of <Chansu> in the body is still not clear (53).

12. Toxicity

Mice given intravenous or intraperitoneal injection of <Chansu> developed tachypnea, muscular cramp, convulsion, arrhythmia, and finally death from paralysis (5,38). Atropine had detoxifying effect whereas epinephrine was ineffective. Boiling greatly decreased the toxicity of <Chansu> (5).

In animal studies, the toad skin preparation caused myocardial hemorrhage, and in pigeons and dogs vomiting (31). The LD_{50} (mg/kg) of <Chansu> and its various contituents in mouse are listed in the following table (7–11,14–16,27,32,40,54,55).

	IV	SC	IP	PO
<Chansu>	41.0	96.6	26.81, 13.74	
Resibufogenin	6.01	124.5	11.5, 16.3	64.0
Cinobufagin			4.38	
Bufotalin	0.36(dog)			0.98(dog, MLD)
Bufalin			2.2	
Bufotenidine	1.3			
Deacetylbufotalin		6.95		24.5

CLINICAL STUDIES

1. Respiratory and Circulatory Failure

<Chansu> was proven effective in poisoning of hypnotics and anesthetics, hypotension due to surgical bleeding, pulmonary heart disease, toxic pneumonia, carbon monoxide poisoning, respiratory and circulatory failures in neonatal asphyxia. It has the following advantages: strong respiratory stimulation; reliable, rapid, stable and sustained pressor effect; can increase the renal, cerebral, and coronary blood flows; and superior to epinedrine and related vasoconstricting drugs (7,14,15,18,53,56). <Chansu> 4–8 mg 2–3 times daily was used to treat 13 cases of heart failure; with the exception of one, 12 cases had improvement in symptoms and signs after 2–48 hours, evidenced by decrease of the pulse rate, increase of urine output, subsidence or amelioration of edema, and reduction of hepatomegaly. In another report, Cardiotonic Powder (Venenum Bufonis:Poria, 1:9) was used in 30 cases of heart failure of various etiologies; 12 cases had marked effects, 14 moderate effects, and 4 ineffective; the aggregate effective rate was 86.7% (45). Five hundred cases of various kinds of shock were treated with resibufogenin in Tianjin city; up to 90% of the cases had their blood pressure elevated. Marked effects (normalization of blood pressure or elevation of systolic pressure of over 30 mmHg) was achieved in 40%; the blood pressure rise was both quick and sustained and there was no excessive increase. This agent markedly stimulated the respiration and increased pulmonary ventilation; hence, it was believed to be superior to lobeline or nikethamide (53). When used with Chinese anesthetics, this agent stimulated the respiration, reduced tachycardia during anesthesia, and minimized the side effects (57–59).

2. Cancer

<Chansu> prepartions have short-term therapeutic effect in the treatment of cancer. Skin cancer and basal cell carcinoma were more sensitive than squamous epithelioma to the drug. The therapeutic effect was enhanced when the drug was used with radiotherapy and chemotherapy, and the attendant

side effects were reduced (45). Twenty-seven cases of cancer (cancer of lungs, liver, and breast and lymphosarcoma, etc.) responded to treatment with the 2% <Chansu> in sesame oil given intramuscularly at 2 ml 1–2 times daily for a therapeutic course of 8–26 days; 17 of them showed improvement or stabilization of the original blood picture, and abatement or improvement of symptoms; 10 or them were either unresponsive or had deteriorated (60). Good results were also achieved with <Chansu> in sesame oil used with other antineoplastic drugs against nasopharyngeal cancer, undifferentiated lung cancer, and other poorly differentiated squamous epithelioma. It delayed or reversed the chemotherapy-induced leucopenia (61). Eight out of 35 cases of skin cancer had a short-term cure after topical application with the 20% ointment of <Chansu> (35).

3. Anesthesia in Tooth Extraction and Oral Inflammatory Diseases

Anesthesia can be attained in approximately 3 minutes after application of <Chansu> tincture on the gingiva and periodontal sac of the diseased tooth. This medication was found to be satisfactory in the elderly, weak, or phobic patients and in those allergic to procaine (62). It may also be used in necrotic stomatitis, gingivitis, acute periodontitis, gum bleeding, and sore throat (45).

4. Miscellaneous

Fifty-nine cases of pulmonary tuberculosis were treated with the injection of the aqueous extract of <Chansu>; most of the patients become asymptomatic or improved with increase in appetite. However, the closing of cavities were unsatisfactory. More satisfactory therapeutic effects were attained when it was used with isoniacid in those unresponsive to long-term treatment with various antitubercular agents (63). Unsatisfactory results, however, were also reported (64). Two cases of advanced schistosomiasis complicated with colon cancer were markedly improved with reduced abdominal mass after treatment with <Chansu> (Chansu Pill and bufotalin) (65). <Chansu> can also be used in acute suppurative infections (41).

ADVERSE EFFECTS

Toxicity is relatively low when the therapeutic dose and the speed of injection are appropriate. Very rapid injection and excessive dosage caused dizziness, malaise, chest discomfort, restlessness, numbness of the mouth, lips and extremities, or upper abdominal distress, nausea, and vomiting. Serious reactions include palpitation, extreme nervousness, and arrhythmia. The ECG may show atrioventricular block, ST segment depression, and distorted T wave —changes typically seen in digitalis poisoning. In some cases shortness of breath, mental dullness, tearing, salivation, convulsion, coma, and death occurred. Atropine has a detoxifying action in these cases. The emergency treatment is basically the same as in digitalis poisoning (5,7,45,53). In addition, exfoliative dermatitis was reported to develop after oral administration of <Chansu> (66). Since <Chansu> has uterus-contracting effect, it is contraindicated in pregnancy (18,53).

REFERENCE

1. Kamano N. The Journal of Japanese Chemistry 1970 24(4):57.

2. Kamano N. The Journal of Japanese Chemistry 1970 24(5):27.

3. Hunan Institute of Medical and Pharmaceutical Industry. Chinese Traditional and Herbal Drugs Communications 1975 (5):60.

4. Suga T. Metabolism and Disease (May Supplement); The References of Traditional Chinese Medicine 1976 (4):39.

5. Wu GD et al. Proceedings of the Symposium on Medical Sciences. Health Division of the Logistics Department of Nanjing Military Region. 1959. p. 69.

6. Chen KK et al. Chemical Abstracts 1951 45:5812g.

7. Xue KX. Zhongma Tongxun (Communications on Chinese Traditional Anesthesia) 1976 (4):47.

8. Okada M et al. Folia Pharmacologica Japonica 1959 55(6):172.

8. Okada M et al. Folia Pharmacologica Japonica 1959 55(6):172.

9. Ueda M et al. Chemical Abstracts 1957 51:15789i.

10. Takamura S et al. Folia Pharmacologica Japonica 1971 67(2):18p.

11. Ueda G et al. Folia Pharmacologica Japonica 1957 53(2):70p.

12. Raymond-Hamet. Chemical Abstracts 1944 38:1796(5).

13. Powell CE et al. Chemical Abstracts 1955 49:13527d.

14. Tianjin Conference on the Identification of ' Laisujing' . Medical Trends (Chinese Academy of Medical Sciences) 1976 (4):5.

15. Tianjin Institute of Chinese Materia Medica. Developments in Chinese Traditional Drugs 1976 (8):4.

16. Scientific Research Unit, Rugao County (Jiangsu) People' s Hospital. Chinese Traditional and Herbal Drugs Communications 1977 (8):35.

17. Okada M et al. Japan Centra Revuo Medicina 1962 176:555.

18. Science and Technology Unit, Ningbo District Health Bureau. Medical Literature 1976 (9):64.

19. Raymond-Hamet. Chemical Abstracts 1943 37:2465(5).

20. Raymond-Hamet. Chemical Abstracts 1943 37:4470(6).

21. Xue KX. National Medical Journal of China 1978 58(11):678.

22. Yoshida et al. Folia Pharmacologica Japonica 1972 68(1):2p.

23. Howard DF et al. Science 1956 123:886.

24. Fastier FN. Experientia 1956 12(12):351.

25. Zhao Y et al. Journal of Military Medicine 1958 (1):25.

26. Okada M et al. Folia Pharmacologica Japonica 1961 57(1):13.

27. Liu ZY. Jiangxi Yiyao (Jiangxi Medical Journal) 1965 5(3):665.

28. Okada M. Chemical Abstracts 1969 70:36154n.

29. Okada M et al. Chemical Abstracts 1961 55:16798d.

30. Okada M et al. Chemical Abstracts 1960 54:2582b.

31. Shanghai No. 3 Pharmaceutical Factory. Proceedings of the National Symposium on Antineoplastic Drug Research. Henan Office of Antineoplastic Drug Research. Mar 1971. p. 60.

32. Guangzhou No. 5 Pharmaceutical Factory. Proceedings of the National Symposium on Antineoplastic Drug Research. Henan Office of Antineoplastic Drug Research. March 1971. p. 52.

33. First Teaching Hospital of Xuzhou Medical College. Zhongliu Fangzhi Cankao Zhiliao (References on the Prevention and Treatment of Cancer) 1972 (5):21.

34. Pathology Section, Hebei University of New Medicine. Research on New Chinese Medicine 1972 (1):41.

35. Qingdao Coordinating Research Group on Cancer. Qingdao Yiyao Keji Jianbao (Qingdao Bulletin of Medical Sciences and Technology) 1972 (8):1.

36. Wang DC et al. Chinese Pharmaceutical Bulletin 1980 (9):42.

37. Kimura M et al. Journal of the Pharmaceutical Society of Japan (Tokyo) 1968 88(2):135.

38. Kimura M. Metabolism 1973 (May Supplement) 10:37; The References of Traditional Chinese Medicine 1976 (1):36.

39. Kimura M et al. Journal of the Pharmaceutical Society of Japan (Tokyo) 1968 88(11):1367.

40. Bing CZ et al. Papers of Nantong Medical College. 1963. p. 45.

41. Ni JQ et al. Chinese Traditional and Herbal Drugs Communications 1976 (5):15.

42. Tian JT. Acta Academiae Medicinae Jiamusi 1977 (3):49.

43. Yoshida et al. Folia Pharmacologica Japonica 1971 67(5):133p.

44. Okada M et al. Folia Pharmacologica Japonica 1966 62(2):99.

45. Xue KX. Xinyiyaoxue Zazhi (Journal of Traditional Chinese Medicine) 1974 (1):39.

46. 709 Scientific Research Group. Selected Information (Jiangsu College of New Medicine) 1973 (1):77.

47. Shanghai Institute of Industrial Health. Radiomedicine and Radiation Protection 1974 (2):19.

48. Huimin District Institute for Drug Control. Huimin Yiyao (Huimin Medical Journal) 1973 (2):15.

49. Courvoisier S et al. Chemical Abstracts 1960 54:17725n.

50. Zhang CS. Chinese Medical Journal 1956 42(5):409.

51. Fink MA et al. Proceedings of the Society for Experimental Biology and Medicine 1958 97:554.

52. Faculties of Chemistry and Biology, Beijing Normal University. Proceedings of the National Symposium on the Techniques of the Use of Radioisotopes. July 1977.

53. Tianjin Bureaux of Science and Technology, and Health et al. The References of Traditional Chinese Medicine 1976 (3):52.

54. Okada M et al. Chemical Abstracts 1960 54:2582d.

55. Raymond-Hamet. Chemical Abstracts 1959 53:3477g.

56. Fan GH. Health Journal of Hubei 1980 (5):51.

57. Chinese Traditional Anesthesia Unit, Rugao County (Jiangsu) Hospital. Zhongma Tongxun (Communications on Chinese Traditional Anesthesia) 1977 (1):15.

58. Chinese Traditional Anesthesia Unit, Rugao County (Jiangsu) Hospital. Zhongma Tongxun (Communications on Chinese Traditional Anesthesia) 1976 (4):29.

59. Scientific Research Group, Rugao County (Jiangsu) Hospital. Zhongma Tongxu (Communications on Chinese Traditional Anesthesia) 1977 (11):36.

60. Hangzhou Chinese Medicine Factory et al. Notes on Science and Technology — Medicine and Health (Information Institute of Zhejiang Bureau of Science and Technology) 1971 (12):13.

61. Tumor Prevention and Treatment Group of 1042 Liaoning Unit of the Chinese PLA. Medical Research 1972 (2):26.

62. Sanduo Commune Health Centre (Gaoyou County, Jiangsu). Chinese Traditional and Herbal Drugs Communications 1978 (9):30.

63. Jiangsu Hospital et al. Chinese Traditional and Herbal Drugs Communications 1978 (3):29.

64. 161st Hospital of the Chinese PLA. Tuberculosis 1973 (2):42.

65. Changde District Center of Schistosomiasis Control. Hunan Information on Science and Technology — Medical Series 1972 (15):50.

66. Xu XS et al. Dermatology Research Communications 1974 3(1):32.

(Wang Jingsi)

SHEXIANG 麝香

<Shexiang> is the dried musk from the male musk deer, *Moschus berezovskii* Flerov, *M. sifanicus* Przewalski, or *M. moschiferus* L. (Cervidae). It is pungent and "warm" with a very strong aroma. It is analeptic, blood stimulant, channel-deobstruent, discutient and analgesic. It is used in convulsion of febrile diseases, coma in apoplexy, sharp pain of the epigastrium and abdomen, abdominal mass, numbness and pains of limbs, injuries and wounds, carbuncle, furuncle, pyogenic infections and ulcers of skin.

CHEMICAL COMPOSITION

Musk contains about 0.5–2% of muscone which can be synthesized. Musk also contains normuscone, muscopyridine and the recently isolated compounds 3β-hydroxyandrost-5-en-17-one, 5α-androstane-3,17-dione, 3β-hydroxy-17-keto-5α-androstane and 3β-hydroxy17-keto-Δ^5-androstene and its 3-acetate (1). Eleven androstane derivatives were isolated from the ether extract (2). Musk-anti-inflammatory I (musk-65), which is composed of 15 kinds of amino acids and has a molecular weight of 5000–6000, was isolated from the aqueous extract (3). It also contains cholesterol, calcium carbonate, calcium phosphate and proteins.

PHARMACOLOGY

1. Effect on the Circulatory System

The synthetic and natural muscone as well as the ether extract of musk injected intravenously to toads increased the contractility of the heart *in situ* (4). A dose of the 1% normal saline solution of musk 1–30 mg increased the contractility of the isolated frog heart, but did not alter the heart rate. In case of the isolated rabbit heart, doses of 0.3–0.5 mg increased the contraction amplitude by 50% but did not markedly modify the heart rate and perfusion volume (5). A recent paper reported that perfusion of natural musk 0.5–2 mg/ml to the isolated frog heart increased the contraction amplitude, contractility, and cardiac output, but perfusion of muscone at a concentration of 0.4 mg/ml weakened the cardiac contractility dose-dependently. These results indicated that muscone, unlike the natural musk, has no cardiotonic activity (6). Intravenous injection of the 1% musk tincture at 0.02 ml/kg to rabbits, or to dogs at 0.03 ml/kg, increased the blood pressure and respiration rate (7). Intravenous injection of either the synthetic or natural muscone 0.006–0.6 μg/kg produced no significant effect on the blood pressure and respiration of dogs, but elevated the blood pressure and increased the respiratory rate and tidal volume of cats. In this respect the synthetic muscone was weaker than the natural agent (4). Intravenous injection of musk at 1 mg/kg decreased the blood pressure, increased the heart rate, and increased the frequency and depth of respiration in cats (8).

2. Effect on the CNS

Low dosage (0.002 mg/kg) of natural or synthetic muscone did not significantly affect the conditioned feeding reflex in rats; moderate dosage (0.01–0.05 mg/kg) prolonged the latent period of the positive conditioned reflex or even abolished it altogether, improved the differentiation phase in most animals but inhibited it in individual animals; high dosage (1 mg/kg) caused poisoning in most animals, irregularity or disappearance of the positive conditioned reflex, and inhibition of the differentiation phase (4). Intraperitoneal injection of the aqueous solution or intragastric administration of the suspension of musk to mouse increased the mortality rate of the animals poisoned by central stimulants amphetamine (5), strychnine (9) and the leaf of *Illicium lanceolatum* (10).

Intraperitoneal injection of musk at doses 25, 50 or 100 mg/kg (5), of synthetic or natural muscone at doses of 0.02–0.5 mg/kg, or of natural musk 2 mg (4) into mice shortened the cyclobarbital sodium (5) or pentobarbital sodium induced sleep (4). Conversely, sleep of mice induced by pentobarbital sodium was prolonged by synthetic and natural muscone at doses of 100–500 mg/kg or by natural musk at 1 g/kg. The effect of synthetic muscone in either shortening or prolonging sleep was the weakest. Consequently, it is considered that musk exerts a biphasic action on the CNS, stimulation at low dosage and depression at high dosage (4). This fact apparently rationalized the use of this drug by Chinese herbalist in the treatment of stroke, as well as in epilepsy and convulsion.

Injection of musk 50 or 100 mg/kg IP into rats prolonged the latent period of heat and pain reaction by 57–63% but had no significant effect on the body temperature (5). It was also reported that musk and its ether extract had antipyretic activity in normal rats and rabbits, and also in rabbits with peptone-induced fever (11,12).

3. Effect on b-Adrenergic Receptors

3.1 *Effect on palillary muscle of cats and bronchial smooth muscle.* The papillary muscle of cats and bronchial smooth muscle of guinea pigs have β-adrenergic receptors primarily. In experiments, the aqueous extract of musk 0.1 mg/ml did not affect the papillary muscle and bronchial smooth muscle, but pretreatment of these tissues with this agent for 10 minutes enhanced the contraction of papillary muscle and the relaxation of the bronchial muscle induced by isoproterenol, epinephrine and norepinephrine. Its potentiation of catecholamines was strongest for isoproterenol, weaker for epinephrine, and least for norepinephrine (8,13,14). Another study showed that intraperitoneal injection of the aqueous extract of musk 0.5 g/kg to mice slightly reduced the myocardial uptake of ^{86}Rb but, subcutaneously, the same agent slightly increased the ^{86}Rb uptake. However, these changes had no statistical significance. When musk and isoproterenol were used in combination, the myocardial uptake of ^{86}Rb was greatly increased, indicating that musk enhanced the sensitivity of the cardiac β-receptors to isoproterenol (12).

3.2 *Effect on vascular and spermatic duct smooth muscles.* The smooth muscles of blood vessels and vas deferens have α-adrenergic receptors. Musk 0.1 mg/ml had no direct action on the thoracic aortic smooth muscle of rabbits. Pretreatment of the specimen with this agent for 10 minutes failed to antagonize vasoconstriction due to α-agonistic activity of epinephrine and norepinephrine. Therefore, it was considered that the β-agonistic activity of musk was not due to blockade of α-receptors. On the other hand, in experiment with the lower abdominal (genitofemoral) nerve-vas deferens specimen of guinea pigs, musk did not enhance the contraction of the spermatic duct smooth muscle evoked by electrical stimulation of the sympathetic nerves (8,13).

The crude aqueous extract of musk (MO) enhanced the action of isoproterenol but not that of the selective β$_2$-agonist, salbutamol, on the heart and trachea (salbutamol also antagonizes COMT). A refined extract of musk, W5-a, significantly enhanced the cardiac effect of isoproterenol but not the effect of isoproterenol and salbutamol on the bronchial smooth muscle, indicating that W5-a selectively acts on the cardiac β$_1$-receptor. Hence, musk probably also contains some other constituents agonistic to the bronchial β$_2$-receptors, and these constituents were at least partially inhibitory to COMT. Two kinds of constituents may be present in musk, one specific to β$_1$- and the other β$_2$-receptors (15).

3.3 Studies on the β-receptor agonistic mechanism.

3.3.1 *Effect on catecholamine storage.* The sympathomimetic amines such as tyramine can pass through nerve membranes into synaptic vesicles to displace norepinephrine and cause its release which in turn enhances the contraction of cat papillary muscles. Cocaine can antagonize the action of tyramine, whereas musk cannot. Therefore, unlike cocaine, musk is incapable of interfering with the storage of norepinephrine in the nerve endings (8,13). In reserpinized and then cocaine treated papillary muscles of cats, musk can still enhance the effect of isoproterenol (13). It was found that musk did not disrupt the uptake of ^{3}H-isoproterenol into the cells of the isolated rat heart but tended to increase it. Thus, the agonistic effect of musk on β-receptors is unrelated to the storage of catecholamines (8).

3.3.2 *Effect on catecholamine metabolism.* Experiments showed that there was no correlation between the COMT-inhibitory and β-receptor agonistic effects of musk. The II-W5 fraction of musk No. II had a weaker COMP-inhibitory effect than musk No. II itself, but it had a stronger potentiating effect to isoproterenol. These results indicate that the adrenergic agonistic effect of musk was not mainly due to inhibition of COMT (15).

3.3.3 *Effect on adrenergic receptors.* The agonistic effect of musk is not due to blockade of α-receptors. Further studies showed that pretreatment with a β-receptor blockader, pronethalol, did not attenuate the potentiating effect of musk on isoproterenol activity, whereas the potentiating effect of musk on pyrogallol was significantly weakened. Therefore, it cannot be said that the adrenergic receptors are involved in the actions of musk (8).

To sum up, being a substance of multiple constituents, musk exerts a complex action on adrenergic receptors. However, authors differ in this regard and further studies are essential.

4. Anti-inflammatory Effect

Experiments showed that musk affects three stages of the inflammatory process: increased vascular permeability, leukocytic migration, and granulation. The aqueous extract of musk markedly inhibited the increase of capillary permeability in mice; it was trice as potent as rutin and 40 times as strong as sodium salicylate (12). Liu Shen Pill which contains musk had a significant inhibitory effect on capillary permeability stronger than hydrocortisone and rutin. Marked synergism was displayed by musk, <Chansu>, and bovine bezoar used in combination (16). Administration of the aqueous extract of musk intraperitoneally and musk-65 or musk-51 intravenously to mice had an anti-inflammatory activity six times that of hydrocortisone on croton oil-induced ear inflammation. Chemical analysis showed that musk-65 may be a polypeptide with molecular weight >10,000, which upon hydrolysis by trypsin lost its anti-inflammatory activity (17). Similarly, a marked inhibitory effect on mouse ear inflammation induced by croton oil was also exhibited by musk suspension or suspension of the ether extract of musk given intraperitoneally (18).

In vitro, musk was 10 times as potent as sodium salicylate and 20 times as potent as hydrocortisone in inhibiting migration of guinea pig leukocytes (8). Another paper reported that a polypeptide with a molecular weight of about 1000 isolated from musk was 40 times as potent as hydrocortisone in inhibiting migration of guinea pig leukocytes (17,19).

Studies using the formaldehyde-filter paper method indicated that the musk suspension weakly inhibited granuloma formation during the late inflammatory stage in rats; its strength was only one-tenth that of cortisone acetate (20). Nevertheless, a subcutaneous dose of musk emulsion 1–2 mg/rat markedly inhibited croton oil-induced granulation, and 2 mg of musk was as potent as 1 mg of hydrocortisone acetate (21). The formaldehyde-filter paper method also showed that "Liu Shen Pill" which contains musk had a more powerful inhibitory effect on rat granulation than musk itself. The results indicated that the anti-inflammatory activity of "Liu Shen Pill" is attributable to the synergistic effect of the different components of the pill (20). Another experiment showed that musk had a higher anti-inflammatory activity than phenylbutazone for adjuvant-induced arthritis in rats (22).

In conclusion, musk and its crude extract are effective in inflammation at various stages especially at the early and middle stages. However, more studies are required to determine whether the components active on each inflammatory stages are identical. It can be preliminarily concluded that the inhibitor for leukocytic migration resides in the soluble polypeptide fraction. Muscone was shown to be inactive against granuloma formation.

5. Effect on Uterus

The 5% ethanol extract of musk markedly stimulated the isolated uteri of pregnant and nonpregnant rats, guinea pigs, and rabbits, and also of the *in situ* uterus of pregnant rabbits. The uteri of pregnant animals, particularly the *in situ* uteri at late pregnancy, showed greater sensitivity to the drug than those of nonpregnant animals. The stimulant effect on nonpregnant uteri was slow in onset but was prolonged (23). Muscone at 50 μg/ml also markedly stimulated the isolated uteri of nonpregnant rats and mice, and at 10 μg/ml it increased the excitability of uteri of pregnant rats and markedly enhanced and prolonged the duration of its spontaneous contraction. Musk was inactive at the same concentration (24).

6. Antibacterial Effect

A 1:400 dilution of the 2% musk tincture had been reported to inhibit *Vibrio cholerae-suis, Escherichia coli* and *Staphylococcus aureus in vitro* (7). Studies in recent years using the well and paper disk diffusion techniques, however, failed to find any bacteriostatic action from the 20% musk suspension against *Staphylococcus aureus*, sarcinae, and *Bacillus subtilis* (11).

7. Androgenic Effect

Early studies evaluating the androgenic action of various drugs by measuring the surface area of the cockscomb of castrated fouls discovered that the 10% olive oil solution of musk 0.2 ml painted on the cockscomb had an adrogenic effect equipotent to that of dehydroandrosterone 100 mg, whereas muscone was inactive (25,26). It was reported in recent years that subcutaneous injection of 1 mg of the ether extract of musk or 74 mg of synthetic muscone daily for 7 days, or of the compounds isolated from musk 3β-hydroxyandrost-5-en-17-one, 5α-androstane-3,17-dione, 3β-hydroxy-17-ketoΔ^5-androstene-3-acetate, and 3β-hydroxy-17-keto-5α-androstane increased the weight of prostate and seminal vesicle of castrated rats (11).

8. Antineoplastic Effect

Incubation of Ehrlich ascites carcinoma cells and sarcoma 180 cells of mice with concentrated musk suspension 17 mg/ml for 15 minutes killed the tumor cells. Electron microscopy also revealed marked wrinkling and cracking of the membrane of Ehrlich ascites carcinoma cells, uneven projection of protoplasm and fusion of cells. No such changes were observed in cancer cells from the same mouse that had not been treated with musk. Various preparations of natural and synthetic muscone also inhibited the cellular respiration of mouse Ehrlich ascites carcinoma, sarcoma 37 and sarcoma 180. However, *in vivo* studies on animals produced no therapeutic effect (27).

9. Miscellaneous Actions

Using the metabolism of pentobarbital sodium as a criterion, it was found that the liver homogenate of rats treated with natural or artificial musk contained much less pentobarbital sodium than the control. This effect of musk was abolished by destroying the hepatic drug transforming enzymes with thioacetamide. The result suggests that both natural and artificial musk have enzyme inducing activity (28). Intravenous injection of the aqueous preparation of musk 0.59 mg/kg to normal rats increased the plasma cAMP, which peaked in 15 minutes after medication, for 2 hours (29).

10. Toxicity

The LD_{50} of natural and artificial musk in mice by intravenous injection was 172 and 152 mg/kg, respectively, and by intraperitoneal injection 270 and 290 mg/kg, respectively (6). The LD_{50} of the aqueous preparation of musk in mice was 331,1 mg/kg IP (5). Intragastric administration of musk 60 mg/kg in rats or 62 mg/kg in rabbits daily for 15 days or of musk suspension 2 g/kg in rats for 16 days did not affect body weight, blood picture, and liver and kidney functions (9,11). Intramuscular injection of synthetic muscone 400 or 800 mg/kg/day (equivalent to 5–10 times the adult dosage) to dogs for 14 days increased the animals' appetite but no effect on their normal activity. No reddening, swelling or nodule formation occurred at the injection site. There were no significant changes in the liver and kidney functions, the blood picture, and histology of various organs. No toxic reactions developed in monkeys receiving injections of the same agent at 1.2 g/animal/day for days (30).

CLINICAL STUDIES

1. Angina Pectoris

Artificial musk sublingual tablets (4.5 mg of musk each) were tried in 119 cases of angina pectoris. The patients were instructed to take 1–2 tablets sublingually (or swallow in individual patients) during anginal attack or having signs of impending attack. Drug effect appeared in 5–10 minutes in most patients. It was effective in relieving feeling of suffocation, but its action in relieving anginal pain was weaker and slower than that of nitroglycerin (31). Oral ingestion of artificial musk was also effective in 410 cases of angina pectoris (32–36). Two hundred and forty cases were treated with artificial musk aerosol; better results were seen in those patients with shortness of breath and chest discomfort due to coronary insufficiency. The aerosol dosage form was superior to the tablets in preventing anginal attack (37–43).

2. Vascular Headache

Twenty-five cases of migraine and vascular headache were treated with muscone sublingual tablets (1.5 mg/tablet) 2–3 times a day taken sublingually during the first indication of attack with additional one or more tablets during the attack; individual patients were additionally injected with synthetic muscone 1 mg 1–2 times daily. Four cases had marked improvement and 16 cases improved (44).

3. *Neoplasm*

Ninety-six cases of cancer of the esophagus, stomach, liver, colon, and rectum were treated with implants of musk (retroperitoneal, anteperitoneal, and subcutaneous). The treatment was believed effective in improving appetite, clinical symptoms, and anasarca in patients with alimentary tract cancer (45). Implant and injection of musk in 40 cases of alimentary tract cancer were reported to have short-term therapeutic effect for early- and middle-stages of alimentary tract cancer (46). Another report claimed that 22 out of 46 cases of alimentary tract cancer treated similarly deteriorated and died. These medications had poor efficacy for the advanced cases but had better effect for the middle-stage cases. Since the duration of the follow-up of these cases did not exceed two years, it is therefore difficult to draw any conclusion on the effectiveness of the musk implantation therapy (27).

REFERENCE

1. Pharmacology Section of the Chinese Materia Medica Research Division, Shanghai Medicinal Materials Company. Internal information. 1979.

2. Do JC et al. Chemical and Pharmaceutical Bulletin 1975 23(3):629.

3. Yu DQ et al. Acta Pharmaceutica Sinica 1980 15(5):306.

4. Zhu Y et al. Abstracts of the 1962 Symposium of the Chinese Pharmaceutical Association. 1963. p. 299.

5. Mukhopadhyay A et al. The Indian Journal of Pharmacy 1973 35(6):169.

6. Guo GW et al. Chinese Pharmaceutical Bulletin 1980 (6):41.

7. Guo ZJ et al. Monographs and Literature on Veterinary Medicine in Traditional Chinese Medicine. Vol. 2. 1959.

8. Kimura M et al. Metabolism 1973 10(5) supplement:745.

9. Institute of Materia Medica, Zhejiang Academy of Health. Brief summary of the collaborative research on the substitution of musk with civet secretion (internal information). 1979.

10. Wu Ym et al. Abstracts of the 1962 Symposium of the Chinese Pharmaceutical Association. 1963. p. 300.

11. Beijing Institute of Materia Medica. Internal information. 1979.

12. Zhu XY et al. Internal information. Institute of Materia Medica of the Chinese Academy of Sciences. 1979.

13. Zhu XY et al. Journal of the Pharmaceutical Society of Japan (Tokyo) 1968 88(2):130.

14. Kimura M et al. The Japanese Journal of Pharmacology 1966 16(1):129.

15. Kimura M. Journal of the Pharmaceutical Society of Japan (Tokyo) 1978 98(4):466.

16. Kimura M. Journal of the Pharmaceutical Society of Japan (Tokyo) 1968 88(11):1367.

17. Zhu XY et al. Acta Pharmaceutica Sinica 1979 14(11):685.

18. Cao WR et al. Studies on Chinese Proprietary Medicine 1980 (3):38.

19. Kimura M et al. Journal of the Pharmaceutical Society of Japan (Tokyo) 1978 98(4):442

20. Kimura M. Journal of the Pharmaceutical Society of Japan (Tokyo) 1968 88(2):135.

21. Hishra RK et al. Journal of Pharmacy and Pharmacology 1962 14:830.

22. Siddiqui HH. The Indian Journal of Pharmacy 1965 27(3):80.

23. Zhang JQ et al. Acta Academiae Medicinae Wuhan 1965 (6):477.

24. Liu Y et al. Internal information. 1979.

25. Sano T. Journal of the Pharmaceutical Society of Japan (Tokyo) 1936 56(11):913.

26. Sano T. Journal of the Pharmaceutical Society of Japan (Tokyo) 1937 57(9):851.

27. Beijing Coordinating Research Group on the Antineoplastic Studies of Musk. People's Military Medicine 1917 (7):54.

28. Shanghai Institute for Drug Control. Proceedings of the Seminar on Artificial Musk. 1975. p. 1.

29. Cheng YS et al. Abstracts of the First National Symposium of the Society of Pharmacology. 1979. p. 85.

30. Shanghai Experimental Drug Factory. Brief Summary of the Toxic Effect of Muscone Injection. 1977.

31. Coordinating Research Unit on Systematization of Chinese Traditional Drug Information, Petrochemical Industry Department. Development in Chinese Traditional Drugs 1977 (2):7.

32. Internal Medicine Department, Shanghai Eighth and Fifth Hospitals. Clinical Studies of Artificial Muscone. 1977. p. 19.

33. 411th Naval Hospital of the Chinese PLA. Clinical Studies of Artificial Muscone. 1977. p. 13.

34. Zhongjin Pharmaceutical Factory. Guangdong Medical Information (Guangdong Institute of Medicine and Health) 1976 (3):60.

35. Beijing Hospital of Workers, Peasants and Soldiers. Selected Information on Coronary Disease. Beijing Coordinating Research Group on Coronary Disease. 1975. p. 7.

36. Beijing Institute of Chinese Materia Medica. Integrated Information. 1975.

37. Tianjin First Central Hospital. Clinical Studies of Artificial Muscone. 1976. p. 1.

38. Peace Hospital of Tianjin. Clinical Studies of Artificial Muscone. 1976. p. 12.

39. Hedong Hospital of Tianjin. Clinical Studies of Artificial Muscone. 1976. p. 13.

40. Second Teaching Hospital of Tianjin Medical College. Clinical Studies of Artificial Muscone. 1976. p. 9.

41. Internal Medicine Department, Shanghai Sailors' Hospital. Clinical Studies of Artificial Muscone. 1977. p. 16.

42. Cardiovascular Group of the Internal Medicine Department, Ruijin Hospital of Shanghai Second Medical College. Clinical Studies of Artificial Muscone. 1977. p. 7.

43. Internal Medicine Department, Changhai Hospital of Second Military College. Clinical Studies of Artificial Muscone. 1977. p. 9.

44. Neurology Department, First Teaching Hospital of Hunan Medical College. Clinical Studies of Artificial Muscone. 1977. p. 20.

45. Information Department, Chinese Academy of Medical Sciences. The References of Traditional Chinese Medicine 1975 (4):22.

46. Chen SS. People's Military Medicine 1976 (3):60.

(Yuan Wei)

INDEX OF SCIENTIFIC NAMES

INDEX OF PHARMACOLOGICAL ACTIONS

Anthelmintic

Antiadrenergic

Antiallergic agent

Antiamebic

Antiarrhythmic

Antiasthmatic

Antibacterial

Anticholinergic

Anticholinesterase

Anticoagulant

Anticonvulsant

Antiemetic

Antifertility agent

Antifluke agent

Antifungal

Anti-inflammatory agent

Antilipemic

Antimalarial

Antineoplastic

Antipneumosilicosis

Antipyretic

Antipyrotic and vulnerary

Antiradiation agent

Antischistosomal

Antishock agent

Antitoxin

Antitrichomonal

Antitussive

Anti-ulcer agent

Antivenin

Antiviral

Bitter stomachic and digestant

Cardiotonic

Cathartic

Central stimulant

Choleretic and cholagogue

Cholinergic

Coagulant and hemostatic

Coronary vasodilator

Detoxicant

Diuretic

Elevator of leucocyte count

Emetic

Enhancer of the tolerance to hypoxia

Expectorant of mucolytic

Fracture-healing promotor

Gastrointestinal smooth muscle stimulant

Hematinic

Histamine-releasing agent

Hyperglycemic

Hypoglycemic

Hypotensive

Hypothermic agent

Immunoadjuvant

Immunosuppressant

Insecticide

Litholytic and lithagogue

Liver-protective agent

Local anesthetic

Peripheral vasodilator

Photosensitizer

Pressor

Promotor of anabolism

Promotor of leukocytic phagocytosis

Promotor of reticuloendothelial phagocytosis

Sedative and hypotic

Sex-hormone-like agent

Smooth muscle inhibitor or spasmolytic

Striated muscle relaxant

Tranquilizer

Uterine inhibitor

Uterine stimulant

INDEX OF CHINESE DRUGS

* Plant name